IMMUNOLOGICAL TOLERANCE
TO SELF AND NON-SELF

ANNALS OF THE NEW YORK ACADEMY OF SCIENCES

Volume 392

IMMUNOLOGICAL TOLERANCE TO SELF AND NON-SELF

Edited by Jack R. Battisto, Henry N. Claman, and
David W. Scott

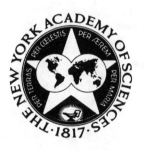

The New York Academy of Sciences
New York, New York
1982

Library of Congress Cataloging in Publication Data

Main entry under title:

Immunological tolerance to self and non-self.

(Annals of the New York Academy of Sciences; v. 392)

"The result of a conference entitled Immunological Tolerance to Self and Non-self, held by the New York Academy of Sciences from October 19 to October 21, 1981"—P.

1. Immunological tolerance—Congresses.
I. Battisto, Jack Richard, 1922–   . II. Claman, Henry N., 1930–   . III. Scott, David W., 1943–   . IV. New York Academy of Sciences. V. Series.
Q11.N5 vol. 392 [QR188.4] 500s [616.07'9]

82–12457

ISBN 0–89766–174–5
ISBN 0–89766–175–3 (pbk.)

PCP

Printed in the United States of America
ISBN 0-89766-174-5 (Cloth)
ISBN 0-89766-175-3 (Paper)

ANNALS OF THE NEW YORK ACADEMY OF SCIENCES

VOLUME 392

September 8, 1982

IMMUNOLOGICAL TOLERANCE TO SELF AND NON-SELF *

Editors and Conference Chairmen
JACK R. BATTISTO, HENRY N. CLAMAN, AND DAVID W. SCOTT

——————◆——————

CONTENTS

* This volume is the result of a conference entitled Immunological Tolerance to Self and Non-Self, held by the New York Academy of Sciences from October 19 to October 21, 1981.

Financial assistance was received from:

- BURROUGHS WELLCOME CO.

- E. I. DU PONT DE NEMOURS & COMPANY

- ICI AMERICAS, INC.

- OFFICE OF NAVAL RESEARCH

- ORTHO PHARMACEUTICAL CORPORATION

- SCHERING-PLOUGH CORPORATION

- SEARLE RESEARCH AND DEVELOPMENT

The New York Academy of Sciences believes that it has a responsibility to provide an open forum for discussion of scientific questions. The positions taken by
the scientists whose papers are presented here are their own and not necessarily
those of The Academy. The Academy has no intent to influence legislation by
providing such forums.

OPENING REMARKS AND APPRECIATION

Jack R. Battisto

Department of Immunology
Cleveland Clinic Foundation
Cleveland, Ohio 44106

As a member of the organizing committee, which includes Drs. Henry Claman and David Scott, it is my distinct pleasure to welcome all of you to this conference on tolerance. In addition, it gives me a great deal of pleasure to introduce to you Dr. Merrill W. Chase, my former mentor, whom we are honoring at this meeting. We honor him here because he is a pioneer in this area of immunological unresponsiveness.

While many present today may know Dr. Chase, some of the younger investigators may not. In order for you to be able to identify him, I shall display this photo. This picture of Dr. Chase was taken relatively recently. You can see from his healthy appearance that his habit of working long hours in the laboratory agrees with him. Now, I know that Dr. Chase is a very modest man, and he is undoubtedly squirming under the shower of attention that we will be giving him throughout this meeting. The fact that he is squirming is precisely what gives me great pleasure. Finally, the shoe is on the other foot! It's retribution for the manner in which he has caused those of us who were students in his laboratory to squirm under his scrutiny. He is, without doubt, a one-man surveillance mechanism, and, at the same time, a most productive investigator.

Born in Rhode Island in 1905, Dr. Chase was educated at Brown University, where he received his undergraduate and graduate degrees. His doctoral thesis was concerned with liberating toxins from enteric bacteria. Following a year as an Instructor of Biology at Brown, he entered Dr. Karl Landsteiner's laboratory at the Rockefeller Institute for Medical Research. He remained at the Institute (now the Rockefeller University) throughout his career—rising through the ranks to become a Professor of Immunology and Microbiology in 1965. As head of the Laboratory of Immunology and Hypersensitivity, Dr. Chase has trained and influenced several pre- and post-doctoral students who have become well-known productive investigators. Above all, Dr. Chase thrived in the laboratory setting.

His first paper on anaphylaxis to the simple chemicals picryl chloride and dinitrochlorobenzene was published with Dr. Karl Landsteiner some forty-four years ago. Many of his findings on hypersensitivity to simple chemicals since that time were summarized in his Harvey lecture of 1966. Today, as a result of his spade work with these haptens, they are commonly referred to, even by fledgling medical students, by abbreviations such as TNP and DNCB.

I shall not recount Dr. Chase's many contributions to our area of common interest, except to single out two observations crucial to this meeting. Most of us know that one of his findings is the transference of delayed type hypersensitivity using intact white blood cells. This adoptive transfer system is fundamental to a wide variety of experiments done daily in laboratories throughout the world. It is so essential to experimental protocol that I would guess that

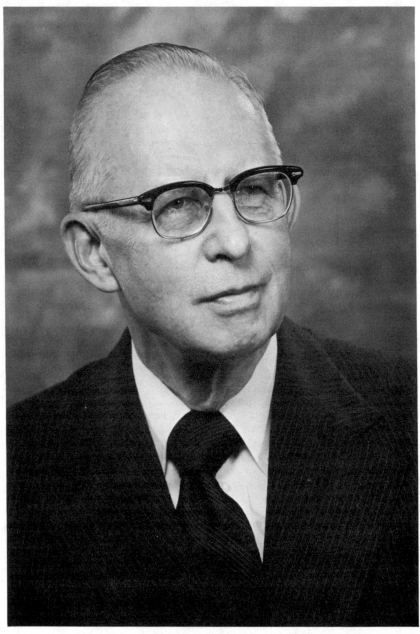

MERRILL W. CHASE

the majority of speakers on our program will refer to adoptive transfers in their presentations.

Dr. Chase's other major finding pertinent to this meeting is that haptens, introduced *via* the gastrointestinal route, induce a profound and long-lasting specific unresponsiveness. One segment of our program is devoted to this feeding method for inducing tolerance. Indeed, Dr. Chase himself will speak on that topic.

Now, it is said that "each of us has drunk from wells we haven't dug and been warmed by fires we haven't built." Dr. Chase is one of those who has helped to dig the wells and build the fires from which we have all benefited. Thus, we are indeed fortunate to have with us and to honor an individual such as Dr. Chase who is so thoroughly identified with the subject matter of our conference.

Our conference has been in the planning stage for slightly more than one year. The organizing committee has put together a team of speakers and fashioned a poster session that we feel are representative of a wide cross-section of thought on the subject of tolerance to self and non-self. Our decision-making process had to cope with limitations of program time, distances over which prospective speakers must travel, and availability of funds. These three items severely restricted our capability to have additional investigators on the program. So, unfortunately, some individuals who have contributed to our concepts and who should be represented here are not.

At the outset, we planners thought that the conference should fulfill several functions. We have charged the speakers, as well as the poster presenters, with the responsibilities of reviewing the existing body of knowledge, while, at the same time, adding new information to it. From them we anticipate learning what changes have occurred in our understanding of the mechanisms of tolerance. We will want to know whether clonal elimination and receptor blockade are achievable under natural conditions *in vivo*. Have the suppressor cell circuits diverted all the energy away from the other mechanistic possibilities? Is the balance between responsiveness and tolerance simply reducible to a titration of helper *versus* suppressor factors? How close are the methods for tolerance induction to clinical applicability?

We, in the audience, must prod the speakers and poster presenters with questions and suggestions so as to discharge our duty of contributing to the proceedings.

Overseeing this process of verbal give and take are the session chairmen. They are responsible for seeing that each of the presentations is properly introduced, timed, and discussed so as to meet our tight schedule. To tell us how successful we have been at exchanging information, Dr. David Scott has accepted the unenviable task of delivering a summary statement on our last meeting day. He will capsulize the proceedings and help us assess the level at which we have arrived as a consequence of our having met.

This conference would not have been possible without review and approval by a subcommittee of the New York Academy of Sciences that consisted of Drs. Gregory Siskind, Herbert Kayden, and Carmia Borek. Furthermore, highly competent advice came from the Academy's conference director, Ellen A. Marks, and her staff, Renée Wilkerson and Erna Levine. The executive editor, Bill Boland, and the administrative editor, India Trinley, helped with many of the details of publication. Finally, the skill of associate editor Frederick H. Bartlett has been invaluable to the appearance of the Annal. The help of all these individuals is gratefully acknowledged.

RECOGNITION AND REGULATION
BY MODIFIED SELF

David W. Scott, Timothy L. Darrow, and Brigitte Grouix

Division of Immunology
Department of Microbiology and Immunology
Duke University Medical Center
Durham, North Carolina 27710

Lawrence A. Wilson

Department of Microbiology and Immunology
Louisiana State University Medical Center
New Orleans, Louisiana 70112

The starting point for much of the work to be discussed in this meeting, and especially for our work, is the fact that the immune system does not overtly respond to its own self antigens. It will become quite clear that this process of "self tolerance" is an active one. It has been our hypothesis during the course of our work over the last decade that foreign antigens associated with self antigens would therefore be nonimmunogenic; indeed, that they would be tolerogenic. A corollary to this hypothesis is that the major guideposts for this process are self histocompatibility antigens. While the data to be presented at this meeting will generally support this notion, it is clear that this hypothesis is an oversimplification. Nevertheless, we believe that the underlying concepts of this hypothesis are still valid and, as we shall see during the course of this meeting, hold enormous promise for future clinical applications.

These concepts emanate from the original observations by Merrill Chase that the administration of a reactive hapten by an appropriate systemic route would induce unresponsiveness to subsequent sensitization to that same hapten.[1] Following his lead, Battisto and Bloom showed that haptens and complete antigens could each be coupled directly to self cellular components *in vitro;* such complexes led to the production of an unresponsive state in regard to both the humoral and the cellular effector phases of the immune response.[2] The combination of direct coupling to self cell surfaces and systemic administration led us to reproduce these findings in rat and murine systems with similar results in terms of both plaque-forming cells and delayed hypersensitivity.[3, 4] Moreover, these modified-self conjugates were able to abrogate an ongoing immune response.[3]

We subsequently determined that the induction of a hyporesponsive state by modified self *in vivo* required the presence of T cells, since nude mice and cyclophosphamide-treated mice both failed to generate any suppression of the immune response.[5] In addition, we established that the unresponsiveness induced in intact animals was relatively stable *in vitro,* but could be reversed by the simple removal of Thy 1 positive cells.[6] These studies also implicated the role of T cells bearing the Lyt 1 and Lyt 2 alloantigens in this process.[6]

Observations using *in vitro* systems led to interesting parallels and initially pointed out the importance of self histocompatibility antigens as restricting elements in the immune system. In 1970, Naor *et al.*[7] showed that hapten-

1

0077–8923/82/0392–0001 $1.75/0 © 1982, NYAS

modified spleen cells effectively blocked the *in vitro* antibody response to hapten.[7] Shearer's observation that hapten-modified self lymphoid cells stimulated the generation of cytotoxic T cells, which are restricted in their effector function to the class I histocompatibility antigens,[8, 9] led us to determine whether these modified-self conjugates would simultaneously inhibit the B cell response and stimulate the generation of cytotoxic T cells.[4] This was indeed the case, and led to our suggestion that recognition of H-2 antigens by T cells may be important in the suppression of the B cell response.[10]

The role histocompatibility antigens played as guideposts in this suppression process was emphasized in the work of several groups, including our own.[10-13] It was subsequently shown that H-2 negative cell lines were inefficient in inducing suppressor cells.[14, 15] Moreover, Jandinski *et al.*, using an *in vitro* system, demonstrated that the blockage and/or modulation of H-2 K/D antigens on the stimulator cells would abrogate the suppression induced *in vitro*;[16] indeed, in some experiments, help for a trinitrophenyl (TNP)-specific antibody response was induced in the absence of extrinsically added TNP immunogen. Formal evidence that histocompatibility antigens were important during the induction phase of this suppressor process came from work performed in our lab by James Li. In these experiments, TNP-modified spleen cells were cultured overnight and the material shed from these cells was harvested and passed through affinity columns to remove H-2, Ia, immunoglobulin, and complexes containing TNP. The material that passed through the column was examined for the generation of suppressor cells *in vitro*. These studies showed that only the removal of TNP or H-2 (presumably coupled with TNP) led to the abrogation of suppressor cell induction.[17]

How then do these T suppressor cells (Ts) act? What is their specificity and are they restricted in any way? Our earlier studies had indicated that suppression was entirely specific both *in vivo* and *in vitro*.[10] Using doubly haptenated antigens (*i.e.*, both TNP and fluorescein (FL) coupled to the same immunogenic carrier, such as lipopolysaccharide (LPS) or ficoll), we established that the suppression of the anti-TNP response still remained highly specific. This suggests, but does not prove, that the suppressor cells, once induced, do not interfere with antigen-presenting cells in carrying out their function, since antigen that displays both TNP and FL would be presented by the same accessory cell. However, if suppressor cells act on a B cell that has bound TNP to its surface Ig receptors, one might also expect Ts activity to occur with a B cell that has bound the same TNP-FL-antigen complex to its surface by means of an anti-FL receptor. Since we still see specific suppression, we tentatively conclude that the interference by suppressor cells that occurs in the immune response could simply be mediated at one level by factors that compete for the hapten. This is supported by observations that we and many other groups have made that modified-self-induced suppressor cells can be purified by panning on hapten-coated petri dishes and that suppressor factors (or at least some suppressor factors) only recognize hapten.

While *in vitro* studies showed that the conditions for the induction of suppression were very similar to those required for the generation of H-2 restricted cytotoxic T cells,[4, 8, 18] several lines of evidence indicated that suppressor cells were not merely reflecting a function of cytotoxic T cells.[5, 19] Nevertheless, to examine this point further, we investigated whether conditions could be found under which cytotoxic T cells are not generated but which still lead to significant suppression *in vitro*. For these studies, we elected to use thymocytes as a source of responder cells, since this population contains few alloreactive cytotoxic precursors and since, in our laboratory, very little nonspecific suppression is generated when thymocytes are cultured *in vitro* (FIGURE 1). The data presented in TABLE 1, using heat-killed stimulator cells, demonstrate that thymocytes are still able to recognize hapten-modified self on these cells in such a way as to generate significant suppression of the subsequent B cell response. However, under these conditions, no significant cytotoxicity is observed. Thus, cytotoxic cells do not seem to be involved in this *in vitro* suppression model.

Since thymocytes do not yield significant alloreactive responses *in vitro*, we chose this system for the investigation of the putative restriction of modified self suppressor cells. It should be noted that allogeneic carriers have been used by a number of workers investigating the restriction of suppressor cells affecting delayed-type hypersensitivity (DTH) responses.[12, 20, 21] Such experiments are difficult to do when measuring the B cell response because of the potent allogeneic effects that can be elicited *in vivo* and that can lead to either nonspecific

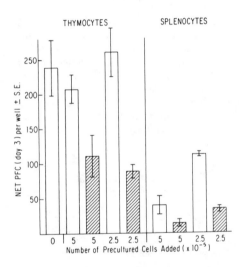

FIGURE 1. Absence of nonspecific suppression in precultured thymocytes. Thymocytes or spleen cells (SC) were cultured at a 10:1 ratio with irradiated normal (open bars) or TNP-modified spleen cells (cross-hatched bars). Two days later, they were harvested and washed three times before being added to 5×10^6 fresh normally responding spleen cells, which were challenged with 100 ng ml^{-1} TNP-LPS. The net PFC response was determined on day 3.

suppression or a polyclonal activation of B cells.[22-24] However, when thymocytes are cultured *in vitro* with TNP-modified syngeneic stimulator cells, suppressor cells are induced that are able to specifically suppress the anti-TNP response of both syngeneic and totally allogeneic responder cells (TABLE 2). Interestingly, as in the DTH models, when thymocytes are cultured with allogeneic TNP-modified cells, suppressor cells are induced, but they appear to be restricted to target cells that are identical to the original stimulating cell. At the present time, we do not know whether the restricting elements in this allogeneic suppressor system are H-2K or H-2D molecules or both, or whether immunoglobulin allotypes play a role in this restriction process. These studies are in progress but have been hampered by antigen carryover in some *in vitro* experiments (Darrow and Scott, unpublished). Hopefully, the restriction of Ts can be confirmed with cloned suppressor cell hybridoma lines.

Work in a number of different laboratories has indicated that suppressor cells that recognize idiotypic determinants can be generated by the administra-

TABLE 1

SUPPRESSION IS NOT DUE TO CYTOTOXIC T CELLS

CBA Suppressor Donor	CBA Stimulator (Irradiated)	Percentage Control Response *	Percentage Cytotoxicity †
THY	TNP-SC	41	37
THY	ΔTNP-THY ‡	44	<5

* Precultured cells (48 h) were added to fresh responding spleen cells at 1:2 (suppressor:responder), and stimulated with TNP-LPS; their PFC was measured 3 d later. The control PFC response was 166 PFC per well.

† Precultured cells (5 d) were tested in a ^{51}Cr release assay at 20:1 (E:T). The background ^{51}Cr release on RDM-4 cells was 1%.

‡ Stimulators heat treated 56° 45'.

tion of highly purified idiotype-bearing molecules coupled to self carrier cells.[25-27] This has been established primarily in the DTH system but also for humoral responses with both the azobenzene arsonate and 4-hydroxy-3-nitrophenylacetyl haptens.[27, 28] One of the best-characterized systems involving a major group of idiotypes is the response of Balb/c mice to α 1 → 3 dextran, as exemplified by the MOPC-104E predominant response to dextran B1355.[29, 30] We have chosen this system to investigate idiotypic control in our model instead of the anti-TNP response because the latter is extremely heterogeneous. In these studies, MOPC-104E myeloma proteins (μ:λ) are coupled to syngeneic spleen

TABLE 2

H-2 RESTRICTION OF SUPPRESSOR CELL-TARGET INTERACTION

Stimulator Spleen Cells *	Target Spleen Cells	Target H-2	Net PFC	Percentage of Control
A. Syngeneically induced CBA (H-2^k) suppressors				
CBA	CBA	k	208	100
TNP-CBA	CBA	k	70	34
CBA	B6D2	bd	193	100
TNP-CBA	B6D2	bd	90	41
B. Allo-induced CBA (H-2^k) suppressors				
B6D2	CBA	k	170	100
TNP-B6D2	CBA	k	152	89
B6D2	B6D2	bd	243	100
TNP-B6D2	B6D2	bd	101	42

* Control CBA thymocytes were incubated with unhaptenated syngeneic CBA or allogeneic B6D2 spleen cells. Suppressor cells were induced by incubating CBA thymocytes with TNP-modified syngeneic CBA or allogeneic B6D2 spleen cells. After 2 d, control and suppressor cells were washed separately three times and then added to fresh normal CBA or B6D2 responding spleen cells. Cultures were either unstimulated or challenged with 100 ng ml^1 TNP-LPS and the PFC response was determined on day 3.

cells and injected intravenously, as in the TNP model. Mice so treated are subsequently challenged with both B1355 and FL-ficoll as a specificity control. The plaque-forming cell (PFC) responses of these mice, as well as those of mice pretreated with a monoclonal IgM antifluorescein (F9–4)–coupled syngeneic spleen cells, were then determined with respect to both fluorescein- and dextran-specific plaque-forming cells. In addition, we determined the percentage of MOPC-104E idiotype-positive cells by plaque inhibition using a monoclonal anti-idiotype generously provided by Dr. John Kearney (University of Alabama).

The data presented in TABLE 3 indicate that this idiotype-modified self treatment leads to a suppression of the predominant idiotypic response to dextran B1355, with no detectable inhibition of the total anti-dextran response. It should be noted that the anti-fluorescein response is normal in these mice and is also normal in the control group treated with monoclonal anti-fluorescein coupled to syngeneic spleen cells. Presumably, however, that portion of the anti-fluorescein response which bears the F9–4 idiotype is inhibited, but is

TABLE 3

SUPPRESSION OF THE MOPC-104E IDIOTYPE BY PRETREATMENT WITH MOPC-104E COUPLED SPLEEN CELLS *

Exp.	Pretreatment	Anti-FL	Anti-Dextran	Percentage MOPC-104E Idi^{+ve}
1	MOPC–104E–SC	1108	576	19
	F9–4–SC	1409	329	$63^{p<0.01}$
2	MOPC–104E–SC	1441	3175	32
	F9–4–SC	1429	2376	$76^{p<0.01}$

* CAF$_1$ (exp. 1) and Balb/c (exp. 2) mice were injected on day 7 and day 6 with 2.5×10^7 syngeneic spleen cells coupled with MOPC-104E or F9-4 (a monoclonal IgM anti-fluorescein). On day 0, these groups of mice were immunized with 100 μg dextran B1355 and 10 μg FL-ficoll. Five days later, PFC were determined in the presence or absence of monoclonal anti-MOPC-104E idiotype (SJL18-1, from Dr. John Kearney). This anti-Id inhibited dextran-specific PFC but not FL-specific PFC. Data presented as PFC per 10^6 spleen cells.

undetectable under our assay conditions. We also have found that none of the antifluorescein PFC are inhibited by monoclonal anti-MOPC-104E idiotype (data not shown), which is an indication of the specificity of this reagent. These are the first studies demonstrating that regulation of a predominant idiotypic response can be induced by application of the modified self approach in the polysaccharide system. Further evidence for this idiotypic regulation in other antigenic models will be presented by others later on in this volume.

The ability to manipulate the immune response to haptens or complete antigens by the association of these antigens (or idiotypes) with syngeneic membranes has great potential application to the manipulation of clinically undesirable responses.[10, 31, 32] Since the cytotoxic response to haptens such as TNP is not dramatically altered by procedures that lead to B cell unresponsiveness,[4, 10] we asked whether the humoral immune response in a more complicated antigenic system, that of herpes simplex virus, could be manipulated in the same way as we have demonstrated for rat histocompatibility antigens.[31] In these experiments, detergent-solubilized glycoproteins from purified herpes virions were coupled by means of the chromic chloride method to syngeneic spleen cells. After the administration of these conjugates or mock-coupled cellular conjugates intravenously, animals were challenged either with herpes glycoproteins in complete Freund's adjuvant or with live virus. The data in FIGURE 2 indicate that such pretreatment causes a greater than twofold diminution in the subsequent humoral response to herpes virus with either challenge. Interestingly, no significant effect on the subsequent cytotoxic response to infectious virus has been noted in these experiments (data not shown; Wilson and Scott, in preparation, 1982). It remains to be determined whether

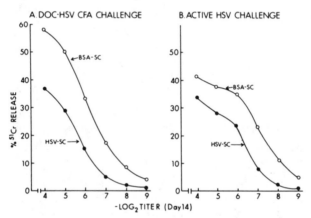

FIGURE 2. Suppression of the anti-herpes humoral response by pretreatment with soluble HSV glycoprotein-coupled syngeneic spleen cells (●). Control C3H/HeJ mice were treated with BSA-coupled spleen cells (○). Seven days after treatment, the groups were challenged either with deoxycholate (DOC)-solubilized HSV in adjuvant (A) or with active viral infection (B). Complement-mediated cytotoxicity was measured on day 14 by means of serum samples.

such modified-self pretreatment using viral antigens will have a potential therapeutic effect in terms of clinical infection and survival. At the least, this approach will allow us to modulate the humoral response to herpes virus.

In summary, we have shown that the modified self model is a potent system for the modulation of the humoral immune response to simple antigens as well as complex viral glycoproteins. This system involves the generation of suppressor cells that initially recognize hapten in the context of self histocompatibility antigens and that are antigen-specific and non-H-2 restricted in their eventual effector function. Production of antigen-specific and idiotype-specific cell lines with suppressor function should prove most useful in understanding the mechanism of modified self regulation and in the eventual therapeutic modulation of clinically undesirable immune responses.

REFERENCES

1. CHASE, M. W. 1946. Proc. Soc. Exp. Biol. Med. **61:** 257.
2. BATTISTO, J. & B. BLOOM. 1966. Fed. Proc. Fed. Am. Soc. Exp. Biol. **25:** 152.
3. LONG, C. A. R. & D. W. SCOTT. 1977. Eur. J. Immunol. **7:** 1.
4. SCOTT, D. W. & C. A. LONG. 1976. J. Exp. Med. **144:** 1369.
5. SCOTT, D. W. 1978. Cell. Immunol. **37:** 327.
6. JANDINSKI, J. J. & D. W. SCOTT. 1979. J. Immunol. **123:** 2447.
7. NAOR, D., R. I. MISHELL & L. WOFSY. 1970. J. Immunol. **105:** 1322.
8. SHEARER, G. M. 1974. Eur. J. Immunol. **4:** 527.
9. SHEARER, G. M., T. G. REHN & C. GARBARINO. 1975. J. Exp. Med. **141:** 1348.
10. SCOTT, D. W., C. LONG, J. J. JANDNISKI & J. T. C. LI. 1960. Immunol. Rev. **50:** 275.
11. GREENE, M. I. & B. BENACERRAF. 1980. Immunol. Rev. **50:** 163.
12. MOORHEAD, J. W. 1979. J. Exp. Med. **150:** 1432.
13. CLAMAN, H. N., S. D. MILLER & M-S. SY. 1977. J. Exp. Med. **146:** 49.
14. PIERRES, A., J. S. BROMBERG, M-S. SY. 1980. J. Immunol. **124:** 343.
15. LI, J. T. C. & D. W. SCOTT. 1980. J. Immunol. **125:** 2385.
16. JANDINSKI, J. J., J. LI, P. J. WETTSTEIN, J. A. FRELINGER & D. W. SCOTT. J. Exp. Med. **151:** 133.
17. SCOTT, D. W. & J. T. C. LI. 1981. Cellular and Molecular Mechanisms of Immunologic Tolerance. T. Hraba Ed. Marcel Dekker. New York. In press.
18. FORMAN, J., E. S. VITETTA & D. A. HART. 1977. J. Immunol. **118:** 803.
19. SCOTT, D. W. & T. L. DARROW. 1982. Compendium in Immunology, Vol. 3. Lazar M. Schwartz, Ed. Van Nostrand Reinhold. Princeton, N. J. In press.
20. BROMBERG, J. S., B. BENACERRAF & M. I. GREENE. 1981. J. Exp. Med. **153:** 437.
21. MILLER, S. D., M-S. SY & H. N. CLAMAN. 1978. J. Exp. Med. **147:** 788.
22. KATZ, D. H. & D. P. OSBORNE. 1972. J. Exp. Med. **136:** 455.
23. ORNELLAS, E. P. & D. W. SCOTT. 1974. Cell. Immunol. **11:** 108.
24. BYFIELD, P., G. CHRISTIE & J. G. HOWARD. 1973. J. Immunol. **111:** 72.
25. SY, M-S., J. W. MOORHEAD & H. N. CLAMAN. 1979. J. Immunol. **123:** 2593.
26. GREENE, M. & M-S. SY. 1980. Fed. Proc. Fed. Am. Soc. Exp. Bilo. **39:** 2458.
27. NISONOFF, A. & M. GREENE. 1980. Prog. Immunol. **4:** 58.
28. SHERR, D. H., S-T. JU, J. Z. WEINBERGER, B. BENACERRAF & M. E. DORF. 1981. J. Exp. Med. **153:** 640.
29. CARSON, D. & M. WEIGERT. 1973. Proc. Nat. Acad. Sci. USA **70:** 235.
30. HANSBURG, D., D. E. BRILES & J. M. DAVIE. 1976. J. Immunol. **117:** 569.
31. BOLLINGER, R. R. & D. W. SCOTT. 1980. Transplantation **29:** 449.
32. SANTORO, T., D. W. SCOTT & D. PISETSKY. 1981. J. Immunol. **127:** 690.

DISCUSSION OF THE PAPER

J. A. BERZOFSKY (*National Institutes of Health, Bethesda, Md.*): In the studies in which you used membrane preparation from TNP-modified cells to induce suppressor cells, you indicated that, if you passed the membrane fragments over an anti-H-2K column or over an anti-TNP column, you removed the activity. I wonder if you were able to mix the effluents from the two columns to see whether you could regenerate the activity or whether, in fact, both the TNP and H-2K had to be on the same complex?

SCOTT: That's a very good question. We have independently shown and

Jim Forman very elegantly demonstrated that, under the conditions of our experiments, the H-2 molecules are quite heavily trinitrophenylated. The experiment you describe has not been done. Nor have we tried to elute the activity from the anti-H-2K column. This can, however, be attempted, since we used the 11–4.1 monoclonal, which is easy to work with; we could then show exactly what that molecule looks like and show that it has the suppressor activity that you want it to have.

A. SCHWARTZ (*Tufts University, Boston, Mass.*): David, in your studies with heated stimulator-induced suppressors I think it's important to be concerned about what is actually induced in such cultures. We have studied, to a very limited degree, the TNP-modified self system. In our reactive suppressor-inducing system, we have found that heated stimulators will not induce killer effectors, but will cause clonal expansion and the induction of suppressor-resistant cytotoxic T cell precursors. It's essentially an arrest of the Tc precursor at a later stage. From other studies that we've done, I can agree with your conclusion that the killer isn't doing the suppressing. But there will be killer cells that will differentiate upon exposure to TNP in the second culture.

SCOTT: That's a good point.

QUESTION: David, are you able to suppress transplantation immunity by your system?

SCOTT: Randy Bollinger worked with that in my laboratory. Using a rat model with solubilized histocompatibility antigens, he showed that we could "suppress" an alloantibody response. By using deoxycholated AgB, which was lectin purified and then coupled to syngeneic spleen cells, we could modulate the alloantibody response to injected allogeneic cells. It was very effective. I cannot tell you what happens in terms of the cellular aspects in that system. Presumably we would be able to modulate delayed hypersensitivity. From everything I've said we probably won't modulate cytotoxic cells. We can then get into a basic argument over whether you believe that cytotoxic cells are involved in transplantation rejection. Those studies are being pursued by Randy right now.

J. CHILLER (*Scripps Clinic and Research Foundation, La Jolla, Calif.*): With respect to mechanisms of this suppression, is the suppressor effect that you're seeing directed toward B cells *per se* or toward a helper population that is necessary for the induction of these cells? You really didn't address yourself to that point at all.

SCOTT: The model in which we examined suppression of a B cell response has primarily been thymus-independent responses. We don't have any direct evidence that helper cells are being affected by the suppressor cells because we haven't examined it.

CHILLER: But if you compare, for example, the response of T cell–dependent and T-independent antigens, as you said you did in certain cases, do both responses reflect similar sorts of restrictions? Are both responses identical in this way?

SCOTT: The only thing I can tell you is that we can suppress both T cell–dependent and T cell–independent responses. We, ourselves, have not examined the restriction for the T cell–dependent response. I think we may hear more on that later.

THE EFFECT OF AUTOLOGOUS SERUM PROTEINS ON THE IMMUNE RESPONSE AND THE INDUCTION OF TOLERANCE IN MICE TO THE 2,4-DINITROPHENYL DETERMINANT

H. Francis Havas

Department of Microbiology and Immunology
Temple University School of Medicine
Philadelphia, Pennsylvania 19140

INTRODUCTION

In early studies of tolerance, living cells,[1] bacteria,[2] proteins,[3, 4] and pneumococcal polysaccharides [5] were used. However, because of their complexity, it became preferable to employ simpler, well-defined molecular models, namely, antigens in which antibody response to an individual determinant could be analyzed, *e.g.*, conjugates of chemically defined haptens coupled to protein carriers.[6-8]

In our initial studies, we investigated the role of the carrier in enhancing or suppressing the immune response to the 2,4-dinitrophenyl ligand (DNP),[6] and found that the magnitude of the anti-DNP response was dependent upon the immunogenicity of the carrier protein.[6] Mouse gamma globulin (MGG), mouse serum albumin (MSA), and even bovine serum albumin (BSA) were effective carriers for inducing tolerance,[6-8] while little if any tolerance was achieved with the highly immunogenic hemocyanin (Hcy).[6] Conversely, the most effective carrier for immunizing against DNP was Hcy.[6] The ligand DNP was chosen because it is a small molecular probe, its epitope density can be easily monitored, and its immunological properties have been well characterized.[9]

The earlier studies were performed in collaboration with A. Pickard, a former graduate student, and Dr. T. Hraba, a guest investigator.[7, 8, 10] In these studies we found that, after the first and even after the second challenge with DNP-Hcy, tolerized mice had significantly lower numbers of indirect plaque-forming cells (PFC) and hemagglutination titers than did controls.[6, 7] When serum antibody levels were quantitated by radioimmunoassay and the affinity was determined by equilibrium dialysis, neonate and adult tolerized mice showed significantly lower levels of antibody of lower affinity than did controls.[10, 11] However, regardless of the regime used to induce tolerance, only partial tolerance was achieved.

Although many of the studies reported here have been published previously,[6-8, 11] they are incorporated with later findings and interpreted in an integrated framework.

MATERIALS AND METHODS

Mice. Neonate or eight- to twelve-week-old Balb/c AnIcr (Balb/c) mice of both sexes from our stock colony were used.

Antigens. All DNP-derivatized proteins were maximally substituted by coupling for 24 h as described by Eisen,[9] except that the protein concentration was

9

0077–8923/82/0392–0009 $1.75/0 © 1982, NYAS

determined by the dry weight and by the optical density at 360 nm for calculating the degree of substitution. The number of DNP groups per protein molecule varied somewhat with each antigen preparation; subscripts denote the number of DNP groups per protein molecule. In the initial studies, MGG was used as the carrier (DNP_{35}-MGG).[6, 7] In later experiments, DNP was coupled to MSA (DNP_{31}-MSA), because MSA polymerized less readily, was more easily available, and proved to be a more effective tolerogen in our experiments.[8]

Immunization. Mice were immunized i.m. or i.p. with 0.1 mg DNP_{31}-Hcy (per 100 000 M.W. of Hcy) in incomplete Freund's adjuvant.[6-8]

Tolerance Induction. Mice were tolerized by different concentrations of DNP_{35}-MGG,[6, 7] DNP_{31}-MSA,[8] and DNP_{27}-BSA,[10, 11] as reported in the tables. Adult mice were tolerized by either one or multiple injections of the appropriate antigen concentration in saline. Neonates were tolerized by two i.p. injections given within 72 h of birth. Littermates were divided into tolerant and control groups and their immune responses were monitored following a challenge with DNP-Hcy.[8, 10, 11]

Plaque-Forming Cell Assay Against DNP. The Jerne PFC assay was used to detect anti-DNP antibody-secreting cells. Initially, 1-fluoro-2,4-dinitrobenzene was coupled to sheep red blood cells (SRBC)[7, 8] by a modification of the method of Merchant and Hraba.[12] Later, the Rittenberg procedure was used,[13, 14] coupling 2,4,6-trinitrobenzene sulfonate to SRBC. Both direct and indirect PFC of individual spleens were enumerated and the geometric mean $\overset{x}{\div}$ antilog standard deviation (S.D.) of logs or arithmetic mean $\pm$ S.D. was calculated, and the data are presented in TABLES 1–7.[7, 8]

Inhibition. The inhibition tests of the PFC assay were performed by adding equal concentrations of serial dilutions of 10^{-5} to 10^{-10} M DNP-lysine to both the top and bottom agar layers.[8]

In Vitro TESTS FOR SERUM ANTIBODY

Hemagglutination. Mice were bled on the day of the PFC assay or on the days indicated. Sera were heat inactivated and tested by Stavitsky's passive tanned SRBC hemagglutination test using DNP coupled to heterologous proteins, as described in Reference 6.

Radioimmunoassay. Serum anti-DNP antibody concentrations were determined by radioimmunoassay, as described in Reference 11, on duplicate samples of individual mouse sera. DNP-lysyl-bromacetyl cellulose was used as the immunoadsorbent and ^{125}I-rabbit anti–mouse immunoglobulin Fab fragment (kindly donated by Dr. Klinman, Scripps Clinic and Research Foundation, La Jolla, Calif.) was used to detect bound anti-DNP antibody.

Antibody Affinity. After determining the concentration of anti-DNP antibody by radioimmunoassay, antibody-hapten association constants were measured by equilibrium dialysis on an ammonium sulfate precipitated immunoglobulin fraction with ϵ-N-(2,4-dinitro-3,5,6-T-phenyl)-L-lysine (New England Nuclear). Average intrinsic association constants (K_o) were calculated by a least squares linear regression analysis of equilibrium dialysis data according to the Sips equation,

$$\log[r/(n-r)] = \alpha \ \log \ c + \alpha \ \log \ K_o,$$

where r is the number of moles of bound hapten per mole of antibody at free hapten concentration c and α is the Sips heterogeneity index $(0 < \alpha \leq 1)$. The standard free energy, ΔF°, was calculated from the expression $\Delta F^\circ = -RT\ln K_0$, in which R is the gas constant and T is the absolute temperature (283.15 K).[10, 11]

RESULTS AND DISCUSSION

In earlier studies, we found that the level of anti-DNP response was related to the immunogenicity of the carrier molecule.[6] MGG [6, 7] and MSA [8] were the most effective carriers for inducing tolerance to the DNP ligand, regardless of the route of administration. Even when DNP-MGG was administered i.m. in adjuvant, no antibody against DNP only could be detected following challenge with DNP-Hcy, as measured by passive hemagglutination with DNP-heterologous carrier-sensitized erythrocytes.[6] However, all mice were found to have antibody against the hapten carrier DNP-MGG when rechallenged with DNP-MGG. The data confirmed that even haptens on nonimmunogenic carriers are not inert, since they can induce tolerance to the hapten and, in adjuvant, induce an immune response to the hapten-homologous carrier.[6, 15]

Studying the kinetics of DNP-specific PFC four, six, eight, and ten days following the two challenges, we found that the numbers of both direct and indirect PFC in the DNP-MGG pretreated mice were significantly lower than in the immune control on all days tested, but lower than in the untreated controls only on days four and six. However, the number of DNP-specific PFC detected was low in both groups due to the DNP-coupling procedure used in the initial PFC assays.

Partial Tolerance to DNP in Adult and Neonatal Mice

Because the immune response following the two challenges of mice pretreated with a single injection of DNP-MGG sometimes paralleled that of the controls,[7] multiple injections of DNP-MSA were used at both low (10 μg) and high (1 mg) doses in order to increase the level of tolerance. It can be seen (TABLE 1) that, while individual values vary in both the low- and high-dose pretreated groups, the mean number of indirect PFC of both pretreated groups is significantly different from that of the controls. The ratio of direct to indirect PFC was consistently higher in the pretreated mice than in the controls, largely because the number of indirect PFC was three to five times lower in the pretreated mice than in the controls (TABLE 1).[8]

In order to achieve a more profound degree of tolerance, neonatal mice were tolerized within three days of birth by two injections of 1.25 mg DNP_{31}-MSA, and their immune response following a second challenge ten weeks later was compared to that of the untreated littermate controls (TABLE 2). Although the number of direct PFC did not differ significantly from that of the controls,[8] the number of indirect PFC was significantly reduced in all mice in the neonatally tolerized group, and, again, because of the lower number of indirect PFC the ratio of direct to indirect PFC was significantly higher in the tolerized mice than in the controls (TABLE 2).[8]

When splenocytes from mice pretreated with multiple injections of low

TABLE 1

DNP-Specific PFC/Spleen Four Days after Second Challenge Following Pretreatment with High and Low Doses of DNP-MSA

	Low dose *		High dose †		Controls	
	Indirect PFC	Direct/Indirect	Indirect PFC	Direct/Indirect	Indirect PFC	Direct/Indirect
	10 120	0.07	17 270	0.14	209 350	0.015
	48 110	0.12	27 560	0.20	97 670	0.20
	21 790	0.16	22 150	0.11	176 920	0.003
	44 140	0.02	38 680	0.17	160 240	0.001
	39 050	0.02	40 570	0.04	111 000	0.020
	14 810	0.23	43 060	0.21	142 240	0.004
	25 436 ×÷ 1.8 ‡	0.103 ± 0.083 §	29 885 ×÷ 1.4	0.145 ± 0.06	144 629 ×÷ 1.3	0.04 ± 0.078

* Mice were injected i.p. with 3×10 μg DNP-MSA per week for four weeks before being challenged with 0.1 mg DNP-Hcy in incomplete Freund's adjuvant.

† Mice were injected i.p. with 3×1.0 mg DNP-MSA per week for four weeks.

‡ Geometric mean of PFC ×÷ antilog of standard deviation (s.d.) of logs.

§ Arithmetic mean ± s.d. of ratios (from Reference 8).

(10 μg) or high (1 mg) doses of DNP-MSA were transferred into lethally irradiated recipients, their response following each antigenic challenge was variable, but generally paralleled that of the immunized controls. However, splenocytes of neonatally tolerized mice remained unresponsive following transfer, showing differences between the tolerant state induced in neonate mice and that induced in adult mice (unpublished data).

Inhibition of DNP-Specific PFC in Tolerant and Immune Mice

The specificity of the PFC assay was ascertained by the ability of DNP-lysine to inhibit both direct and indirect PFC with concentrations varying

TABLE 2

NEONATAL TOLERANCE

	Tolerant †		Controls	
Litter	Indirect * PFC/Spleen	Direct / Indirect	Indirect PFC/Spleen	Direct / Indirect
A	7 498	0.24	78 350	0.15
	12 150	0.12	68 237	0.05
B	10 230	0.36	46 200	0.12
	10 005	0.38	58 500	0.30
C	39 300	0.46	108 500	0.08
	21 900	0.19	62 300	0.03
	13 560	0.26		
D	6 275	0.22	68 466	0.07
	3 583	0.78	52 500	0.02
	11 045 $\overset{\times}{\div}$ 2.01 ‡	0.33 ± 2.01 §	65 792 $\overset{\times}{\div}$ 1.30	0.10 ± 0.09

* Indirect PFC four days after the second challenge with DNP-Hcy.
† Littermates in the tolerant group were injected twice with 1.25 mg DNP-MSA within the first three days of birth. Both groups were challenged six and ten weeks later with DNP-Hcy.
‡ Geometric mean $\overset{\times}{\div}$ S.D. of indirect PFC four days after the second challenge.
§ Arithmetic mean ± S.D. of the ratio of direct to indirect PFC (from Reference 8).

from 10^{-5} to 10^{-6} M (FIGURE 1). It can be seen that the concentration required to achieve 50% inhibition in four inbred Balb/c mice varied by almost one log (10^{-7} to 10^{-8} M).

When the ability of 10^{-6} M DNP lysine to inhibit direct PFC was compared in mice tolerized by low doses of DNP_{31}-MSA and control mice following a second challenge, no significant differences were observed.[8] However, significantly more hapten was required for inhibition of indirect PFC in tolerant than in control mice, as can be seen from the greater number of uninhibited indirect PFC in the tolerant mice (TABLE 3).

The degree of inhibition is affected by the quantity and affinity of antibody released per cell.[8] Direct PFC and PFC of low affinity require more hapten

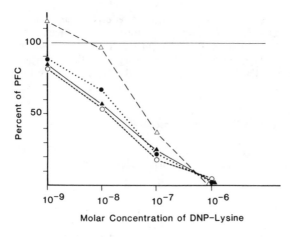

FIGURE 1. The inhibition of indirect DNP-specific PFC by DNP-lysine. (From Hraba *et al.*,[8] by permission.)

Molar Concentration of DNP–Lysine

for inhibition than indirect PFC and those of high affinity. Thus, more DNP-lysine was required for the inhibition of indirect PFC in neonatal and adult tolerant mice than in controls.[8] Since tolerance is preferentially induced in cells with high affinity receptors, the nontolerized cells remaining have low affinity.

In a recent study comparing the affinity of IgM and IgG it was found that the highest affinity of IgG receptors exceeded that of IgM receptors by a factor of at least 50.[16] This provides a valid explanation of the finding that, in general, the number of indirect (high-affinity) PFC was affected by tolerance induction, while the number of direct PFC paralleled that of the controls.

TABLE 3

INHIBITION OF DNP-SPECIFIC PFC IN LOW-DOSE TOLERANCE *

Uninhibited PFC					
Tolerant			Controls		
Uninhibited PFC (%)		Direct †	Uninhibited PFC (%)		Direct †
Direct	Indirect	Indirect	Direct	Indirect	Indirect
101	14	0.05	44	6	0.02
83	11	0.17	62	4	0.06
90	39	0.41	65	2	0.08
33	5	0.13	–	2	0.06
31	13	0.14	36	2	0.10
108	23	0.20	74	6	0.04
74 ± 34 ‡	17 ± 12	0.18 ± 0.12	56 ± 16	3.7 ± 2.0	0.06 ± 0.03

* Inhibition with 10^{-6} M DNP-lysine of four-day PFC after the second challenge.
† The ratio of the numbers of direct to indirect PFC in the *absence* of inhibitor (from Reference 8).
‡ Arithmetic mean ± S.D. of uninhibited PFC of six individual mice per group.

Affinity of Antibody in Partially Tolerant Adult Mice

Because inhibition studies revealed differences in affinity between tolerant and control mice, we investigated the thermodynamic aspects of partial tolerance further by measuring antibody affinity by equilibrium dialysis and by calculating the standard free energy change ($\Delta F°$) as described above. Both the antibody concentration of the individual mouse sera and the maturation of affinity were compared in neonate and adult tolerant mice.

It was found that adult tolerant mice showed significantly lower ($0.05 > p > 0.01$) antibody levels than controls 28 days after the first challenge and lower levels 8 and 28 days after the second challenge (TABLE 4). In both groups, maximum responses were found on the eighth day after the second challenge with DNP-Hcy.

TABLE 4

KINETICS OF THE RESPONSES OF ADULT TOLERIZED AND CONTROL MICE

Days after First Injection	Group *	Antibody Concentration † ($\mu g/ml$)	$K_o \times 10^{-5}$ ‡ (M^{-1})
8	AT	13 $\overset{\times}{\div}$ 8.42	ND §
	Control	6 $\overset{\times}{\div}$ 3.51	ND
28	AT	76 $\overset{\times}{\div}$ 2.80	0.74 $\overset{\times}{\div}$ 1.31
	Control	259 $\overset{\times}{\div}$ 1.78	3.00 $\overset{\times}{\div}$ 1.61
50 ‖	AT	25 $\overset{\times}{\div}$ 5.79	ND
	Control	18 $\overset{\times}{\div}$ 3.10	ND
58	AT	263 $\overset{\times}{\div}$ 1.60	3.52 $\overset{\times}{\div}$ 2.22
	Control	590 $\overset{\times}{\div}$ 1.90	13.80 $\overset{\times}{\div}$ 1.44
78	AT	146 $\overset{\times}{\div}$ 2.12	20.70 $\overset{\times}{\div}$ 1.94
	Control	372 $\overset{\times}{\div}$ 1.68	39.30 $\overset{\times}{\div}$ 1.72

* Both groups were immunized with 0.1 mg DNP-Hcy in incomplete Freund's adjuvant on day 0 at 12 weeks of age. There are eleven and twelve mice in the adult tolerized (AT) and control groups, respectively.
† Geometric mean of serum anti-DNP antibody concentration $\overset{\times}{\div}$ antilog S.D. logs.
‡ Geometric mean of average intrinsic association constant $\overset{\times}{\div}$ antilog S.D. logs.
§ Not determined.
‖ The secondary injection with 0.1 mg DNP-Hcy in incomplete Freund's adjuvant followed bleeding on day 50.

While the mean association constant K_o increased 28-fold for tolerized mice and only 13-fold for controls (TABLE 4), K_o was still only half of the controls even after second challenge.[11]

When the affinity ($\Delta F°$) to the DNP-hapten of adult immunized mice was compared with that of tolerant mice following each challenge with DNP-Hcy, it was observed that, while the average affinity increased with time in both groups, antibody of the partially tolerant mice remained at a significantly lower affinity ($p < 0.01$) at all times tested. However, there was considerable variation in the range of affinity of antibody produced by individual partially tolerized mice after primary immunization compared to the range of affinities expressed by nontolerized controls (TABLE 4 and FIGURE 2). The data thus show that induction of tolerance and recovery do not occur at the same rate in individual mice even in an inbred strain (Balb/c).

Affinity of Antibody of Neonate Tolerized Mice

When individual sera of neonate tolerized mice were tested seven weeks before the first challenge, they had no detectable antibody.[10, 11] After the first challenge with antigen, 8 of 13 mice responded with antibody levels comparable to those of the controls, while 5 of 13 were totally unresponsive (FIGURE 3). After the second challenge, both groups of tolerized mice responded, but at lower levels than their littermate controls throughout the period of observation until day 78.[11] It can be seen that, while affinities increased with time for all groups of mice until they overlapped at day 78, the $\Delta F°$ of the nonresponders increased much more slowly.

These studies demonstrated that both neonate and adult tolerized mice produce antibody with significantly lower affinity for the DNP-determinant than do immunized controls following antigenic challenge. At the cellular level, this indicates that tolerance is preferentially induced in cells producing high-affinity antibody. The data confirmed the observations of Siskind and Benacerraff in rabbits [17, 18] and extended them to neonate and adult mice. The affinity dependence of tolerization has also been confirmed by Venkataraman and Scott.[19] They demonstrated that tolerization inactivated only the high-affinity cells, leaving only low-affinity PFC precursor cells, which are susceptible to polyclonal activation by LPS. Only a reduced number of precursors that are susceptible to stimulation by a specific antigen remain.

Although affinities of antibody are initially low in tolerized mice, affinity maturation occurs in all animals, so neonate tolerized mice eventually produce

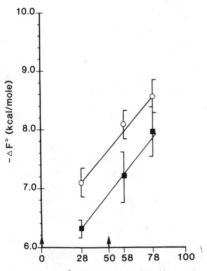

FIGURE 2. The change of antibody affinity (mean $\Delta F° \pm$ s.d.) in adult tolerized (■) and control (□) mice with time after primary immunization. Arrows represent DNP-Hcy injections. The number of individual sera tested ranged from 6 to 11 per group. (From Pickard and Havas,[11] by permission.)

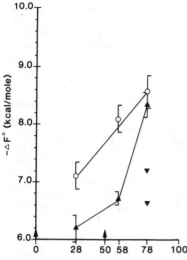

FIGURE 3. The change of antibody affinity (mean $\Delta F° \pm$ s.d.) in neonate tolerized responder (▲), neonate tolerized nonresponder (▼) and littermate control mice (△) with time after primary DNP-Hcy immunization. The number of individual sera tested ranged from 6 to 8 per group; arrows represent DNP-Hcy injections. (From Pickard and Havas,[11] by permission.)

Days after 1° immunization with DNP–HCY

antibody with affinities comparable to those of neonate littermate controls (FIGURE 3). Another interesting observation is that the Sips indices of heterogeneity (α) showed antibody made by neonate tolerized mice to be less heterogeneous than that of controls, suggesting that a more restrictive cell population is being stimulated.[11]

The differences seen in the kinetics of affinity maturation (K_0) between adult and neonate tolerized animals suggest that the slower recovery in adult tolerized mice may be caused primarily by the functional release of "tolerant" cells from an unresponsive state, possibly by deblocking receptors. The more rapid recovery in neonate tolerized animals may involve both release of unresponsive cells and the concomitant generation of new cells capable of responding to the DNP determinant.[11]

These results are consistent with predictions made by the antigen selection hypothesis presented by Siskind and Benacerraf [18] and Venkataraman and Scott [19] that antigens react preferentially with cells possessing high-affinity receptors regardless of whether an immunogenic or tolerogenic stimulus is provided.

Effect of Antithymocyte Serum (ATS) Treatment

In order to increase the level of tolerance induction and to delineate the role of the T cell, ATS was used both *in vivo* and *in vitro*. It was prepared in rabbits by the method of Levey and Medawar [20] by the repeated immunization of rabbits with 1×10^9 thymocytes prepared from thymuses of weanling mice.[21]

When tolerant and immune splenocytes were treated *in vitro* with ATS before adoptive transfer into irradiated recipients and then challenged with DNP-Hcy, PFC were not significantly decreased in the tolerant mice compared to the immune controls, which were decreased to less than one-third.[21] When tolerized mice and normal or immune controls were treated *in vivo* with ATS injections three times a week for one week, reduction of the indirect PFC occurred in all groups of mice and not preferentially in the tolerant group (TABLE 5). Because of these ambiguous results, the use of ATS was not pursued further.

Effect of Cyclophosphamide on Immune Response

In order to achieve higher levels of tolerance, different dosages ranging from 1 to 10 mg of DNP-MSA were administered in multiple injection schedules. It was found that the most suppressive regime was 1 mg DNP-MSA given three times weekly, which substantially lowered both the direct and the indirect PFC response, while single injections even of 10 mg DNP-MSA were less effective. In order to modulate the induction of tolerance, a series of experiments were undertaken using cyclophosphamide (Cy). Cy was either administered three

TABLE 5

EFFECT OF *In Vivo* ATS TREATMENT ON THE SIX-DAY PFC RESPONSE TO DNP *

	PFC/Spleen †	
	Direct	Indirect
Adult tolerant	2330 $\overset{\times}{\div}$ 1.35	3194 $\overset{\times}{\div}$ 1.33
Adult tolerant + ATS	1194 $\overset{\times}{\div}$ 1.84	402 $\overset{\times}{\div}$ 3.8
Normal control	5093 $\overset{\times}{\div}$ 1.47	10713 $\overset{\times}{\div}$ 1.22
Normal control + ATS	1203 $\overset{\times}{\div}$ 1.28	670 $\overset{\times}{\div}$ 1.74
Immune control	10657 $\overset{\times}{\div}$ 1.76	161868 $\overset{\times}{\div}$ 1.35
Immune control + ATS	8788 $\overset{\times}{\div}$ 3.9	3686 $\overset{\times}{\div}$ 3.7

* Mice were treated with 0.25 ml ATS three times per week for eight weeks following the first tolerizing or immunizing injection. All mice were injected with DNP-Hcy two days after the ATS treatment and assayed six days later.

† Geometric mean of PFC $\overset{\times}{\div}$ antilog of s.d. of logs.

times a week simultaneously with DNP-MSA or on day 28, the time of DNP-Hcy injection, after the three-week tolerizing regime. It can be seen that the strongest effect on reducing the number of direct PFC and hemagglutination titers was obtained when Cy was administered on day 28 (TABLE 6), presumably at a time of re-emergence of antigen-reactive cells.

In a previous study, we found that Cy either enhances or suppresses the immune response, depending on the dosage and on the timing of the administration with respect to the antigen.[22] When Cy was administered simultaneously with, or within two days of, antigen injection, it was totally suppressive, whereas the immune response was enhanced when Cy was given four days before antigen injection. Only small effects were observed at other times.[22]

Similar results were obtained when Cy was administered four days before or after a tolerizing injection of DNP-MSA. There was little effect on tolerance induction; on the contrary, the immune response was enhanced to the level of normal controls (TABLE 7). However, when Cy was injected on the same days as the tolerogen it profoundly reduced the number of indirect PFC to 20%

TABLE 6

EFFECT OF CY ON TOLERANCE INDUCTION BY DNP-MSA

Group	PFC/Spleen †		Percentage of Control Response		HA titer †
	Direct	Indirect	Direct	Indirect	
1. DNP-MSA *	3608 $\overset{\times}{\div}$ 1.6	2358 $\overset{\times}{\div}$ 1.9	32	22	1857 $\overset{\times}{\div}$ 1.7
2. DNP-MSA + Cy 1 mg 3 × per wk	2757 $\overset{\times}{\div}$ 2.7	2138 $\overset{\times}{\div}$ 2.8	24	23	1118 $\overset{\times}{\div}$ 1.4
3. DNP-MSA + Cy 3 mg day 28	2569 $\overset{\times}{\div}$ 1.2	692 $\overset{\times}{\div}$ 1.5	23	6	470 $\overset{\times}{\div}$ 1.9
4. Control	11046 $\overset{\times}{\div}$ 1.5	10365 $\overset{\times}{\div}$ 1.7	100	100	5815 $\overset{\times}{\div}$ 2.5

* All groups except controls were treated with 1 mg DNP-MSA three times per week for three weeks. All mice were injected with DNP-Hcy on day 28 and the PFC assay was performed on day 34.

† Geometric mean $\overset{\times}{\div}$ antilog of S.D. of logs.

of that of the controls. This effect parallels that seen on the immune response in normal mice, where the same dosage of Cy either enhanced or suppressed the immune response, depending solely on the time of its administration in relation to antigenic challenge.[22] These findings imply that, in addition to Cy's cytotoxicity, which depleted B and T cells equally,[23] its effect may be due to similar processes such as activation of suppressor cells or inactivation of antigen-responsive helper cells in both tolerant and immune mice.

TABLE 7

EFFECT OF CY ON INDUCTION OF TOLERANCE

	Six-Day Indirect Response	
	PFC/Spleen ‡	Percentage of Control Response
	Adult Tolerant * †	
Cy day − 4	5076 $\overset{\times}{\div}$ 2.54	138
Cy day − 2	3854 $\overset{\times}{\div}$ 1.76	105
Cy day − 0	959 $\overset{\times}{\div}$ 1.50	26
Cy day + 2	1208 $\overset{\times}{\div}$ 2.11	32
Cy day + 4	3222 $\overset{\times}{\div}$ 1.22	87
Tolerant control	3628 $\overset{\times}{\div}$ 2.40	98
	Controls	
Cy day 0, control	1747 $\overset{\times}{\div}$ 1.79	47
Control	3671 $\overset{\times}{\div}$ 1.59	100

* All tolerized mice were given one injection of 4 mg DNP-MSA on day 0 and 3 mg Cy on the days indicated.

† Mice in both groups were challenged with 0.1 mg DNP-Hcy six days before the PFC assay on day 21.

‡ Geometric mean $\overset{\times}{\div}$ antilog of S.D. of logs.

Because the intact host is a complex milieu, with many cell types and interacting factors, splenocytes were removed from tolerant hosts and placed in a defined environment in Marbrook chambers (as described in Reference 24). They were cultured for five days *in vitro* prior to the PFC assay (TABLE 8).

It can be seen that, even in the absence of antigen, the number of PFC of the tolerized mice was reduced compared to controls regardless of whether the mice had been tolerized with DNP-MSA alone or in combination with Cy (TABLE 8). Thus, Cy did not affect the subsequent *in vitro* response. These findings are in agreement with those of Howard and Shand, who found that Cy did not influence B cell tolerance induction.[25] Further *in vivo* and *in vitro* experiments are needed to clarify the role of Cy in tolerance induction.

SUMMARY AND CONCLUSIONS

The carrier plays a crucial role in determining whether immunity or tolerance ensues. MGG, MSA, and even BSA or weakly immunogenic proteins are

TABLE 8

EFFECT OF DNP-MSA AND Cy ON THE FIVE-DAY *In Vitro* IMMUNE RESPONSE

	Direct PFC *		Percentage of Control Response
	Per Culture	Per 10^6	
DNP-MSA †	505	131	48
DNP-MSA + Cy ‡	480	149	45
Control	1068	264	100

* Pooled spleen cells from each were placed in tissue culture two days after the last injection and assayed five days later.

† Donor mice were injected three times per week with 1 mg DNP-MSA in saline.

‡ Donor mice were injected three times per week with 1 mg DNP-MSA in saline and simultaneously three times per week with 1 mg Cy—geometric mean of six separate cultures.

the best carriers for inducing tolerance to DNP, while Hcy, the most immunogenic carrier, results in immunity. Tolerance was routinely induced with DNP coupled to isologous carriers such as MGG and MSA and, in one study, BSA.

Because single doses of DNP-MSA or DNP-MGG produced only a partial degree of tolerance, multiple injections of high and low doses were employed, which increased the tolerance level so that, even after the second challenge, low- and high-dose tolerized mice had only 17 to 20% of the indirect PFC of the controls. Direct PFC were less affected than indirect PFC, presumably because of their lower affinity.

Tolerance was preferentially induced in high-affinity antibody-producing cells, resulting in low levels of low-affinity antibody in the serum. However, in adult tolerant mice, antibody affinity matured in parallel with that of immune mice, but its recovery was more rapid in neonate tolerized mice.

ATS treatment *in vivo* lowered the responses of both immune and tolerant mice, whereas *in vitro* treatment had little effect.

Cy administered simultaneously with or two days after the tolerizing injection of DNP-MSA significantly lowered the numbers of both direct and indirect PFC, while prior injection resulted in enhanced responses.

The kinetics of the effect of Cy on tolerized mice parallel the effects on nontolerized controls, which suggests that similar mechanisms may be involved. Because only partial tolerance can be achieved, regardless of the regime of tolerance induction, Cy may be a valuable tool in modulating and enhancing the tolerant state.

REFERENCES

1. BILLINGHAM, R. W., L. BRENT & P. B. MEDAWAR. 1956. Nature (London) 178: 514–19.
2. NOSSAL, G. J. V. & G. L. A. ADA. 1964. Nature (London) 201: 580–81.
3. HAVAS, H. F. & K. SENFF. 1967. J. Immunol. 99: 1002–11.
4. GOLUB, E. S. & W. O. WEIGLE. 1971. J. Immunol. 102: 389–96.
5. FELTON, L. D., G. KAUFFMAN, B. PRESCOTT & B. OTTINGER. 1955. J. Immunol. 74: 17–26.
6. HAVAS, H. F. 1969. Immunology 17: 819–29.
7. HAVAS, H. F. & T. HRABA. 1969. J. Immunol. 103: 349–56.
8. HRABA, T., H. F. HAVAS & A. R. PICKARD. 1970. Int. Arch. Allergy Appl. Immunol. 38: 635–47.
9. EISEN, H. N. 1969. In Methods in Medical Research, vol. 10: 94–102. Year Book. Chicago.
10. PICKARD, A. 1972. Ph.D. Thesis. Temple University. Philadelphia.
11. PICKARD, A. & H. F. HAVAS. 1972. J. Immunol. 109: 1360–70.
12. MERCHANT, B. & T. HRABA. 1966. Science 152: 1378–79.
13. RITTENBERG, M. B. & K. L. PRATT. 1969. Proc. Soc. Exp. Biol. Med. 132: 576–81.
14. HAVAS, H. F. & G. D. SCHIFFMAN. 1978. Immunology 34: 1–8.
15. WALTERS, C. S., J. W. MOORHEAD & H. N. CLAMAN. 1972. J. Exp. Med. 136: 546–55.
16. MANDAL, C. & F. KARUSH. 1981. J. Immunol. 127: 1240–44.
17. SISKIND, G. W. 1969. In Immunological Tolerance. M. Landy and W. Braun, Eds.: 12. Academic Press. New York.
18. SISKIND, G. W. & B. BENACERRAFF. 1969. Adv. Immunol. 10: 1–50.
19. VENKATARAMAN, M. & D. W. SCOTT. 1979. Cell. Immunol. 47: 323–31.
20. LEVEY, R. H. & P. B. MEDAWAR. 1966. Proc. Nat. Acad. Sci. USA 56: 1130–37.
21. FLEISCHMANN, J. 1976. M. S. Thesis. Temple University. Philadelphia.
22. HAVAS, H. F. & G. SCHIFFMAN. 1981. Cancer Res. 41: 801–7.
23. HAVAS, H. F. & G. SCHIFFMAN. In Cellular and Molecular Mechanisms of Immunologic Tolerance, 19th Int. Symp. Biological Models, Brno, 1981. Marcel Dekker. New York.
24. PATEL, M. & H. F. HAVAS. 1982. Immunology. In press.
25. HOWARD, J. G. & F. L. SHAND. 1979. Immunol. Rev. 43: 43–69.

DISCUSSION OF THE PAPER

J. A. BERZOFSKY (*National Institutes of Health, Bethesda, Md.*): Did you look at all at the level of the density of hapten on MSA for inducing tolerance? What was the molar coupling ratio of hapten to protein carrier?

HAVAS: The molar coupling ratio was generally high. I believe it was 35 for mouse gamma globulin and 31 for mouse serum albumin. Generally, we did not use low coupling ratios.

Y. BOREL (*Harvard University, Cambridge, Mass.*): I wonder why you use mouse serum albumin as carrier, since you originally said that isologous gamma globulin was most effective as carrier. I think that you obtained partial tolerance because you used the wrong carrier. You need a very high dose of DNP-MSA to suppress indirect plaques. You need a very small dose of DNP-isologous gamma globulin to suppress both the direct and the indirect plaque response for a very long time. So I think that autologous gamma globulin is the most effective carrier to induce tolerance. I wonder why you have not pursued your original observation.

HAVAS: We only obtained partial tolerance when we used mouse gamma globulin. Presumably this is because we did not purify the mouse gamma globulin as you have done. We used mouse gamma globulin fractionated by ammonium sulfate precipitation. There is more mouse serum albumin per ml of serum and it has less of a tendency to polymerize than mouse gamma globulin. Really, our reasons are more practical than profoundly theoretical.

A. H. SEHON (*University of Manitoba, Winnipeg, Man.*): In relation to your answer to Dr. Borel's question, I'd like to say that we followed in your and his footsteps in the early 70's, and what we found was that the epitope density of the hapten on mouse gamma globulin was all-important. Now, if you do not control your epitope density, you will find that haptenated mouse gamma globulin is not always effective because we found that, below an epitope density of 4 and above one of 11, our hapten conjugates were not very effective.

HAVAS: It's not that we didn't control for epitope density, we just opted for using maximal substitution, which we obtained after coupling for 24 h. Whether or not that was a wise decision, we can't say. Perhaps we should have tried different epitope densities, but we did not.

SEHON: Well, the epitope density would control whether or not you also affect the PFC response. I think that it was clear from Dr. Borel's work that the Fc portion should not have been modified drastically in order to exert its best tolerogenic activity.

HAVAS: That may very well be why we did not get the degree of tolerance that Dr. Borel induced.

THE DEGREE OF CLONAL ELIMINATION IN VARIOUS TYPES OF SPECIFIC IMMUNOLOGICAL UNRESPONSIVENESS

Göran Möller, Susanne Bergstedt, Shouzi Dai,
Carmen Fernandez, Erna Möller, and Teresa Ramos

Department of Immunobiology
Karolinska Institute
Wallenberglaboratory
104 05 Stockholm, Sweden

INTRODUCTION

Since the first discovery of immunological tolerance in newborn mice injected with allogeneic cells [1] and the description of immunological paralysis against polysaccharide antigens in adult mice,[2] a variety of conditions leading to immunological unresponsiveness have been described. Immunological tolerance was initially thought to represent a "central," or—in modern nomenclature —to be caused by elimination of the antigen-specific T and B cells, as opposed to "afferent" or "efferent" inhibition of the immune response. There is no reason to believe that all the experimental conditions characterized by specific immunological unresponsiveness known today would all be caused by one mechanism only.

We will focus on experimental conditions leading to B cell unresponsiveness and concentrate on one parameter only: whether or not the particular B cell unresponsiveness leads to elimination or irreversible inhibition of the entire clone of B cells of a certain specificity. This is an important question if one is to analyze the mechanism of immunological unresponsiveness, since the only property common to all members of a B cell clone is the variable region of their antigen-specific immunoglobulin (Ig) receptor. If it can be shown that a particular phenomenon of immunological unresponsiveness eliminates or irreversibly inhibits the entire B cell clone it is highly probable that the mechanism of unresponsiveness is mediated by the Ig receptors. Contrariwise, if the entire clone is not eliminated, it is very likely that the mechanism does not directly involve the Ig receptors, but other receptors or properties of the B cells.

METHODS TO STUDY THE DEGREE OF CLONAL ELIMINATION

The most convenient way to establish whether a particular phenomenon of specific immunological unresponsiveness is due to clonal elimination or not is to use polyclonal B cell activators (PBA). These substances have the capacity to directly activate a large proportion of dormant B cells to antibody synthesis without interacting with the Ig receptors.[3] Different PBA act on different B cell subpopulations and the application of several PBA can, therefore, reveal the immunocompetence of most B cells belonging to a particular clone.[4] However, lipopolysaccharide (LPS) alone is usually sufficient, since this PBA can activate about 30% of the B cells. In certain cases it may be necessary to

23

0077-8923/82/0392-0023 $1.75/0 © 1982, NYAS

dissociate or remove the antigen from the Ig receptors before activating them with LPS, as will be described below. Thus, if a particular PBA can induce antibody synthesis against the relevant antigen, unresponsiveness cannot be due to a complete elimination of the clone.

A different approach uses thymus-independent and thymus-dependent forms of the same antigen. It is well known that these two types of antigens activate different B cell populations. If unresponsiveness to a thymus-independent form of an antigen can be broken by thymus-dependent forms of the same antigen, unresponsiveness does not affect the entire clone of B cells.

ANTIBODY-MEDIATED FEEDBACK SUPPRESSION OF IMMUNE RESPONSES

This is probably the oldest known specific mechanism for completely abolishing an immune response.[5] IgG antibodies, administered before or after the antigen, specifically suppress the immune response. The specificity of the phenomenon by itself suggested a role for the variable region of the IgG antibodies in suppression. Antibody feedback suppression has been found to be determinant specific. Thus, when antibodies were administered against only one determinant on a carrier molecule or cell, T cell–mediated reactions such as delayed hypersensitivity and allograft rejection were suppressed only with regard to that epitope, not other antigenic determinants on the same carrier.[6, 7] Whether this is also the case in humoral antibody synthesis has not yet been studied. However, since different Ig classes vary in their capacity to suppress and IgM antibodies actually enhanced rather than suppressed the response,[8] it seems likely that the constant regions of the antibodies play a role. In addition, there have been several studies indicating the importance of the Fc region of the suppressive antibodies (for reviews, see Reference 9).

An important finding for the understanding of the mechanism of antibody feedback suppression was the demonstration that B cells exposed to antigen-antibody complexes could not be activated by LPS into synthesis of antibodies against the antigen in the complex, whereas antibodies of all other specificities studied were induced.[10] Subsequent studies revealed that other PBA also failed to break unresponsiveness.[11] This clearly indicates that antibody feedback suppression of B cell responses represents a state of complete clonal elimination or irreversible suppression, thus focusing attention on the role of Ig membrane receptors on the B cells in this type of suppression. It was suggested that the Ig receptors of the B cells bound the antigen in the immune complex and by doing so were exposed to the Fc parts of the antibodies in the complex.[10] The Fc regions would interact with the Fc receptors on the B cells, which would result in negative signals. Since the affinity between the Fc region and the Fc receptors is low, it would be necessary to present the antibodies in the form of an immune complex in order to achieve sufficient stability of interaction between Fc regions and the corresponding receptors. This concept is in agreement with the observed role of the Fc region in suppression.

In an attempt to confirm the role of the Fc parts in suppression, IgG antibodies were treated with pepsin, and $F(ab)_2$ antibodies were mixed with the antigen (horse red blood cells), and the complex was added to B cells *in vitro*. In this case, LPS failed to activate antibody synthesis against horse red blood cells (FIGURE 1), whereas other specificities were induced (data not shown). We also tried to prevent the antigen-specific inhibition induced by immune complexes by treating them with protein A, which specifically interacts with the Fc part of several IgG subclasses (FIGURE 1). However, protein A–treated complexes also specifically suppressed polyclonally induced antibody synthesis against horse red blood cells. These findings argue against a role of the Fc fragment in suppression. However, in certain cases, as will be shown below for tolerance induction to dextran preparations, it is necessary to remove the antigen from the Ig receptors before activating the cells with LPS. Therefore, it is possible that unresponsiveness caused by $F(ab)_2$ antibodies is due to blocking of the B cell surface by immune complexes in such a way that they prevent LPS from activating the cells. Actually, it remains to be determined whether intact antibodies in the immune complex operate by the same mechanism.

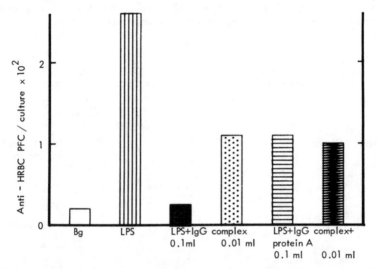

FIGURE 1. Immune complex suppression of polyclonal B cell activation. Spleen cells were cultured either alone (Bg) or together with 100 μg ml^{-1} LPS. Other groups received 0.1 or 0.01 ml of an immune complex between mouse IgG anti-horse erythrocytes and horse red blood cells in addition to LPS. In the last two groups (to the right) the immune complex was pretreated with 1 mg ml^{-1} of protein A. The PFC response against horse red blood cells was tested after two days.

Although the mechanism of suppression is not completely understood and it cannot yet be determined whether or not the clone is eliminated, it seems likely that suppression affects the whole clone and, thus, that the Ig receptors on the B cells must be involved in suppression. The originally proposed mechanism for suppression (blocking of the antigenic determinants by the IgG antibody without participation of their Fc regions) cannot account for suppression, since, in that case, polyclonal B cell activators would trigger the dormant noncomplex coated B cells to antibody synthesis. Most likely, an active suppressive mechanism that initially involves the Ig receptor on the B cells is operating. The steps subsequent to the initial binding of the immune complex to the antigen-specific B cells are not known in detail and several mechanisms may operate, including an Fc receptor–mediated negative signal.

SUPPRESSION INDUCED BY IMMUNIZATION WITH ALTERED SELF STRUCTURES

B cell immune responses against haptenated syngeneic lymphocytes in mice exhibit some unusual properties (for reviews, see Reference 12). When the hapten (fluoroscein isothiocyanate; FITC) was conjugated to spleen cells using three different concentrations of hapten (5, 0.5, and 0.05 mg ml^{-1}) only one concentration (0.5) induced a specific B cell response that was thymus-independent.[13] However, both immunogenic (5) and nonimmunogenic (0.05) conjugates induced a long-lasting state of unresponsiveness specific for the FITC epitope on the same carrier or on a thymus-dependent carrier (sheep—SRBC— or horse—HRBC—red blood cells). In contrast (TABLE 1), the same hapten conjugated with a thymus-independent carrier (native dextran) induced a FITC-specific response in suppressed animals that was either higher than or not significantly different from normal (nonsuppressed) controls.[13]

TABLE 1

EFFECT OF PREIMMUNIZATION WITH SC-FITC 0.05
ON THE RESPONSE TO THE SAME HAPTEN ON DIFFERENT CARRIERS

	PFC per 10⁶ Cells Mice Immunized Day 0 with	
Boosted Day 7 with	—	Syngeneic-FITC 0.05
Exp. 1 —	170 ± 9	143 ± 18
HRBC-FITC 0.5	1315 ± 172	685 ± 172
FITC-Dx 100 μg	6125 ± 175	7847 ± 508
Exp. 2 —	16 ± 3	13 ± 3
Syngeneic-FITC 0.5	124 ± 2	16 ± 2
FITC-Dx 100 μg	1582 ± 61	5159 ± 99
Exp. 3 —	32 ± 1	40 ± 10
Syngeneic-FITC 0.5	170 ± 28	54 ± 6
FITC-Dx 100 μg	2364 ± 1138	6506 ± 744
Exp. 4 —	22 ± 6	56 ± 18
SRBC-FITC 0.5	443 ± 133	212 ± 49
FITC-Dx	1195 ± 321	3225 ± 827

NOTE: In experiment 1, anti-SRBC-FITC 5 PFC were detected and, in experiments 2–4, anti-HRBC-FITC 5 PFC. Strain A/Sn was used in experiment 1 and (A × 5M)F₁ hybrids in experiments 2–4.

Since T cells were not responsible for the unresponsiveness against haptenated self structures (although major histocompatability complex–restricted T cells developed in normal immunized mice [15]), the finding that suppression did not completely abrogate the response to FITC when T cells were bound to dextran as a carrier suggests that suppression had not affected all anti-FITC-specific B cells; therefore, a complete clonal elimination is unlikely to be the mechanism of suppression. This in turn suggests that the Ig receptors alone cannot be responsible for suppression, although they are involved, since the phenomenon shows immunological specificity. However, it is possible that the anti-FITC antibodies induced by FITC-dextran and FITC-self do not belong to the same clone, even though they are detected on the same target cells. Only studies of the idiotypes would resolve this issue.

IMMUNOLOGICAL TOLERANCE

Specific immunological tolerance can be induced by antigen doses that are considerably larger than those needed for an immune response. Tolerance to thymus-dependent antigens can affect helper T cells and B cells differently, while tolerance to most thymus-independent antigens does not involve T cells. Although several different mechanisms can lead to a state of specific unresponsiveness after antigen contact, we will limit our discussion to the classical tolerance phenomenon generally considered to represent a crucial defect of immunocompetence. We will define immunological tolerance to thymus-independent antigens as an inability of B cells to respond to the antigen because they have received an active signal leading to irreversible inactivation or elimination of the reactive B cells.

The Immune Response to Dextran

Dextran B512 is a linear polymer of glucose in alpha 1–6 linkages. It is a thymus-independent antigen that gives rise to a mono- or pauciclonal immune response. The ability to respond is determined by one or several closely linked Igh-V genes; mice that lack or do not express the gene cannot respond.[15] An important point in this connection is that nonresponsive mice cannot make use of other V genes to produce antibodies against the alpha 1–6 epitope, since nonresponsive mice remain unresponsive during their life. In addition, young mice of highly responsive strains that possess the Igh-V gene do not express this gene or any gene coding for antibodies against dextran for a long time period after birth.[16] Unresponsiveness in these two situations is not due to suppressor T cells or other suppressive cells or influences, as shown by various types of mixing and transfer experiments described elsewhere.[17]

Induction of Tolerance to Dextran

The immunogenicity of dextran B512 varies with its molecular weight.[17] Dextran preparations above 70 000 daltons are immunogenic and immunogenicity increases with the M.W. up to native dextran (M.W. $10–100 \times 10^6$). The ability of dextran to act as a polyclonal B cell activator also increases with molecular weight in parallel with immunogenicity.[18]

Tolerance is regularly induced by injecting 5–10 mg of native dextran per mouse, *e.g.*, 1000 times the optimal immunogenic dose; tolerance is complete and long lasting.[19]

Tolerance is Caused by an Active Signal

We have shown before that tolerance is not induced immediately after injecting dextran into mice or after adding dextran to lymphocytes *in vitro*.

More than 2 and less than 24 h was required for tolerance induction.[20] In an attempt to determine whether tolerance is caused by an active signal or passive events, such as blocking of immunoglobulin receptors, we compared the tolerogenicity of native dextran with that of dextran M.W. 40 000, which is neither an immunogen nor a polyclonal B cell activator. Mice were given 10 mg native dextran or 100–150 mg dextran 40 000 and both groups were subsequently immunized with an immunogenic dose of native dextran. There was no response to the alpha 1–6 epitope in any group. However, when the tolerized mice were given dextranase and afterwards immunized with native dextran, the animals given high doses of dextran M.W. 40 000 responded, indicating that they had not been tolerized, whereas those given 10 mg of native dextran remained unresponsive even after dextranase treatment (Bergstedt et al., unpublished data).

These findings indicate that nonimmunogenic dextran preparations are nontolerogenic,[19] suggesting that tolerance requires a signal and cannot be explained by passive events such as immunoglobulin receptor blockade. However, if dextran was not removed by treating the animals with dextranase, the mice could not be immunized by native dextran, presumably because the immunoglobulin receptors on the specific B cells were blocked by the nonimmunogenic dextran. Thus, the intact mice were phenotypically tolerant after treatment with high doses of dextran 40 000, although all their dextran-specific B cells remained in a dormant state and could be activated by an immunogenic dextran preparation, provided that their immunoglobulin receptors had been cleared from the dextran by treatment with dextranase.

Breaking of Tolerance to Dextran

It is well known that immunological tolerance to thymus-dependent antigens can be broken by the injection of cross-reactive antigens.[21] A common explanation for this phenomenon is that tolerance primarily affects T cells and not B cells and, therefore, the cross-reactive antigen can interact with T cells directed against the new antigenic determinants.[22] Although this model is a sufficient explanation for the breaking of tolerance to thymus-dependent antigens, it cannot be applied to thymus-independent antigens. Therefore, we performed a study to determine whether or not tolerance to dextran could be broken by cross-reactive antigens.

Mice were tolerized with 10 mg native dextran and given dextranase at various times thereafter. They were subsequently immunized, either with native dextran or with dextran conjugated to different protein antigens. The molecular weight of the dextran molecules conjugated to proteins varied from 7000 (conjugated to edestin) to 70 000 (conjugated to BSA, protein A, staphylococcus bacteria, and others). It was shown that all the dextran-protein conjugates used were thymus-dependent.

It was consistently found that mice made tolerant to native dextran (and treated with dextranase) remained unresponsive when immunized with native dextran, but always gave an immune response to the thymus-dependent dextran-protein conjugates (FIGURE 2).[23] This immune response was indistinguishable from that obtained with native dextran in nontolerized mice. Since there appears to be only one or very few linked Igh-V genes coding for antibodies to dextran and since other genes are not used (see above), it seems highly unlikely that the response to dextran-protein conjugates in tolerized mice could be ascribed to antibodies of other affinities or specificities. It was actually shown that the anti-dextran antibodies possessed the same idiotype whether immunized with BSA-dextran or dextran. The only tenable conclusion is that tolerance to a thymus-independent antigen does not affect all B cells with immunoglobulin receptors reactive with dextran. However, tolerance affected some B cells in this clone, since native dextran did not induce an immune response. It seems likely, therefore, that tolerance induction to native dextran affected the B cells that could be activated by native dextran given in immuno-

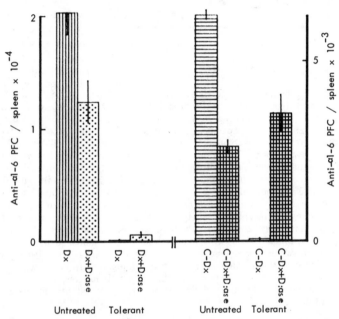

FIGURE 2. An immune response to the tolerogen can be obtained with dextran conjugates after dextranase treatment. C57BL mice were tolerized to native dextran by one injection of 10 mg. Five and seven days later, half of these mice, as well as untreated controls, were given injections of 20 units dextranase. Three days later, these mice and previously untreated controls were immunized with 2 μg native dextran or 0.2 ml of 10% suspension of Cowan dextran. The direct PFC response was determined five days later. Three mice were used per group. (From Möller and Fernandez,[23] with permission.)

genic concentrations, but not the B cells that are activated by T cell help. Thus, tolerance only affects some of the B cells specific for the alpha 1–6 epitope of dextran—namely, those having both activating and immunoglobulin receptors for dextran, whereas B cells with different activating receptors remain dormant (FIGURE 3). The latter B cells must be cleared of the dextran that has bound to their immunoglobulin receptors before they can be activated, as shown by the fact that no response occurred in thymus-dependent antigens if the tolerant mice had not been pretreated with dextranase, again indicating that blocking of im-

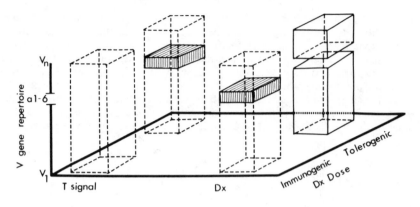

PBA receptor   repertoire

FIGURE 3. A schematic outline of the two levels of heterogeneity that determine the ability of B lymphocytes to become activated or tolerized to dextran. The heterogeneity of the V-gene repertoire is indicated on the y-axis and the V gene for alpha 1–6 antibodies is specifically indicated. The heterogeneity of the B cell subpopulation to become activated by different polyclonal B cell activators is depicted on the x-axis, where two subpopulations are illustrated, one responding to thymus-dependent antigens (T cell signals) and the other to native dextran. The dose of dextran is indicated on the z-axis, one being immunogenic and the other tolerogenic. The subpopulation of B cells responding to the PBA property of dextran is shown to the right. At immunogenic concentrations of dextran, only B cells in this subset having Ig receptors for alpha 1–6 are activated, the rest of the cells remaining dormant (broken lines), whereas, at tolerogenic doses, B cells with Ig receptors against alpha 1–6 are irreversibly tolerized, as indicated by the gap in the cube. However, when tolerogenic concentrations of dextran have been given, immunogenic doses of thymus-dependent dextran conjugates are competent to activate a specific alpha 1–6 immune response in the subpopulation responding to T signals (to the left). No cells in this subpopulation are activated at immunogenic concentrations of dextran.

munoglobulin receptors can make mice phenotypically unresponsive, in spite of the fact that they possess immunocompetent B cells to the antigen.

We have also shown that lymphocytes from dextran-tolerant mice can be activated into synthesis of antibodies against the tolerogen by polyclonal B cell activators such as LPS.[24] Again, it was necessary to clear the cells of the tolerogen by giving dextranase to them or by adding them to serum-free cultures for 24 h *in vitro* before contact with the polyclonal B cell activator.

AUTOANTI-IDIOTYPIC ANTIBODIES INDUCE CLONAL ELIMINATION

Attempts to induce a secondary response against dextran have consistently failed (FIGURE 4). Actually, no animal has an immune response to dextran after the primary response. This suppression is specific for the alpha 1–6 epitope of dextran.[25] Suppression can be passively transferred with serum from dextran-immunized mice, even when the anti-dextran antibodies have been removed.[25]

It was shown that suppression was caused by the spontaneous appearance of autoanti-idiotypic antibodies specifically reacting with anti-dextran antibodies.[26]

The dextran-specific prolonged immunosuppression after a primary immune response was found to be mediated by the autoanti-idiotypic antibodies. Immunosuppression affected the immune response to both thymus-independent and thymus-dependent dextran preparations, suggesting that the entire clone of anti-dextran-specific B cells had been affected, as would be expected from the fact that the autoanti-idiotypic antibodies were directed against the Ig receptors of the specific B cells.

However, the dextran-specific B cells had not been depleted or irreversibly inactivated, since the transfer of dextranase-treated spleen cells from dextran-immunized mice into untreated, lethally irradiated mice immunized with dextran resulted in an immune response.[25] Thus, at least for some time after immunization, the dextran-specific B cells remained in the mice and could be rescued by dextranase treatment and adoptive transfer. It remains to be determined whether the unresponsiveness induced by autoanti-idiotypic antibodies is mediated by the Fc parts of the antibodies or represents a passive blockade of the variable regions of the Ig receptors.

Summary

Several different types of antigen-specific immunosuppressive phenomena have been analyzed with regard to the degree of elimination of the entire B cell clone specific for the antigen. A complete clonal elimination would be a strong

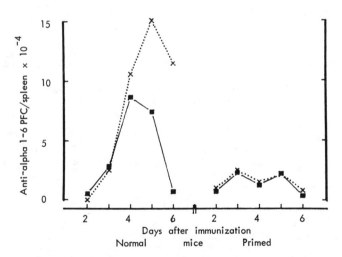

FIGURE 4. Primary and secondary IgM (solid lines) and IgG (dotted lines) responses to the alpha 1–6 epitope of dextran in C57B1 mice. Six days after primary immunization with dextran and horse erythrocytes, the mice and previously untreated controls were given 10 units of dextranase and, at day 14, they were immunized with the same antigen mixture. The primary response is shown to the left and the secondary response to the right.

argument for a direct role of the Ig receptors in causing suppression. In contrast, a partial elimination of the clone shows that the Ig receptors are not responsible for suppression and suggests that other B cell structures were responsible for suppression. The degree of clonal elimination was analyzed by the use of polyclonal B cell activators and thymus-independent and thymus-dependent forms of the same antigen.

Antibody-induced feedback suppression of the immune response affected the entire clone, although it cannot be determined if the clone was eliminated. Suppression of the immune response against the alpha 1–6 epitope of dextran that is mediated by autoanti-idiotypic antibodies affected the whole clone, but the B cells could respond to the antigen after dextranase treatment and adoptive transfer into irradiated recipients.

Induction of immunological tolerance in adult mice using dextran as the antigen did not result in a complete elimination of the antigen-specific B cell clone, indicating that the Ig receptors do not mediate tolerance. Suppression that occurs after immunization with altered self structures (using the hapten FITC conjugated to syngeneic cells) was broken after injection of cross-reactive antigens, but the possibility that different B cell clones responded to the cross-reactive antigen cannot be ruled out.

A third type of antigen-specific immunosuppression occurred after injecting large doses of nonimmunogenic dextran preparations into mice. Such animals exhibited complete tolerance to thymus-dependent and -independent dextran preparations, but responded normally to all dextran preparations when they had been injected with the enzyme dextranase. In this case, the Ig receptors were blocked by antigen molecules, but, after removal of the antigen by dextranase, the B cells responded normally to all dextran preparations, indicating that clonal elimination had not occurred at all.

REFERENCES

1. BILLINGHAM, R. E., L. BRENT & P. B. MEDAWAR. 1953. Nature (London) **172:** 603.
2. FELTON, L. D. & B. J. OTTINGER. 1949. J. Bacteriol. **43:** 99.
3. ANDERSSON, J., O. SJÖBERG & G. MÖLLER. 1972. Transplant. Rev. **11:** 31.
4. GRONOWICZ, E. & A. COUTINHO. 1975. Transplant. Rev. **24:** 3.
5. SMITH, T. J. 1909. J. Exp. Med. **11:** 241.
6. BENACERRAF, B. & P. G. H. GELL. 1959. Immunology **2:** 53.
7. MÖLLER, G. 1963. J. Nat. Cancer Inst. **4:** 65.
8. HENRY, C. & N. K. JERNE. 1968. J. Exp. Med. **128:** 133.
9. Immunol. Rev. 1980. **49:** 3–197.
10. OBERBARNSCHEIDT, J. & E. KÖLSCH. 1978. Immunology **35:** 151.
11. HOLMGREN, M. & G. MÖLLER. 1980. Scand. J. Immunol. **11:** 85.
12. Immunol. Rev. 1980. **50:** 3–309.
13. RAMOS, T. & G. MÖLLER. 1978. Scand. J. Immunol. **8:** 1.
14. RAMOS, T., E. MÖLLER & G. MÖLLER. 1979. Eur. J. Immunol. **10:** 100.
15. RAMOS, T. & E. MÖLLER. 1981. Scand. J. Immunol. **13:** 119.
16. FERNANDEZ, C., R. LIEBERMAN & G. MÖLLER. 1979. Scand. J. Immunol. **10:** 77.
17. FERNANDEZ, C. & G. MÖLLER. 1978. J. Exp. Med. **147:** 645.
18. HOWARD, J. G., G. VICARI & B. M. COURTENAY. 1975. Immunology **29:** 585.
19. HOWARD, J. G., G. VICARI & B. M. COURTENAY. 1975. Immunology **14:** 253.
20. FERNANDEZ, C. & G. MÖLLER. 1978. Scand. J. Immunol. **7:** 137.

21. WEIGLE, W. O. 1962. J. Exp. Med. **116:** 913.
22. WEIGLE, W. O., J. M. CHILLER & G. S. HABICHT. 1972. Transplant. Rev. **8:** 3.
23. MÖLLER, G. & C. FERNANDEZ. 1978. Scand. J. Immunol. **8:** 29.
24. FERNANDEZ, C. & G. MÖLLER. 1977. J. Exp. Med. **146:** 308.
25. FERNANDEZ, C. & G. MÖLLER. 1980. Scand. J. Immunol. **11:** 53.
26. FERNANDEZ, C. & G. MÖLLER. 1979. Proc. Nat. Acad. Sci. USA **76:** 5944.

DISCUSSION OF THE PAPER

E. DIENER (*University of Alberta, Edmonton, Alta.*): By clonal deletion, do you mean the physical disappearance of the clone or the functional elimination of the clone? Using a pulse system, we have been able to show that, when you induce tolerance, you do, in fact, get capping and the antigen is gone from the surface of these cells. New receptors are then generated, but they still cannot be triggered. Because your clone is still there with receptors, perhaps with antigen on the surface, I wonder whether you can, in fact, say that the Ig receptor is not involved. It could be involved metabolically, making the cell refractory to further challenge. But that doesn't mean that the receptor is not involved in causing the suppression.

G. MÖLLER: It is not possible to distinguish between the physical disappearance of a clone and the functional elimination of the clone. The Ig receptors are involved, since only B cells have both Ig and activation receptors for the antigen. Whether the Ig receptors do more than bind the antigen in the tolerance situation is not known.

J. S. COWDERY, JR. (*National Institutes of Health, Bethesda, Md.*): Although autoanti-idiotypic antibodies are produced in concert with a primary response to the TI-2 antigens, do you have any direct evidence that the inability of mice to respond to a second injection is, in fact, due to these autoanti-idiotypes, rather than anti-antigen?

G. MÖLLER: Yes. We can passively transfer suppression with serum taken from dextran-immunized mice even when the serum is absorbed with antigen. That also goes for the suppression of plaque-forming cells, which is done with antigen-absorbed antiserum.

QUESTION: Some people have suggested that, in immature B cells, a true clonal abortion, as opposed to deletion, exists. Your models have all been with more or less mature animals; perhaps there are differences there. Do you have any feeling about that?

G. MÖLLER: We have only studied adult animals. But I have definite feelings about it. With immature B cells, which are very easily tolerized, you should not be able to induce autoantibodies later in adult mice because all these cells will be gone. We all know that polyclonal B cell activators can induce autoantibodies to whatever antigen you look at. So then you say that it's only during the neonatal period that these immature B cells are tolerized and that they are not tolerized in adult organisms. If you don't take that way out, I think you have some difficulty in explaining autoantibody formation with B cell activators.

D. W. SCOTT (*Duke University Medical Center, Durham, N.C.*): I think that one could make a quantitative argument as to why one would be able to make autoantibodies. But we could probably talk for hours about that.

A. H. SEHON (*University of Winnipeg, Man.*): My question is in relation to your last observation that anti-idiotypic antibodies lead to suppression. On transfer of the cells into irradiated animals, the cells seem to be rescued. Have you studied the concentration effect of the antibodies? I can see that you do not have enough antibodies to silence the whole clone. On transfer into irradiated animals, some of the cells that were not silenced in the first place are now capable of generating a new clone. It's not an all or none phenomenon, anyway. You always have a little bit of background noise.

G. MÖLLER: Yes. That's possible. What we have seen before is how easy it is to clear B cell from its antigen. It requires an overnight incubation *in vitro* or transfer to an animal; that is enough. That was done with the dextran. That's why I think that the same mechanism operates with autoanti-idiotypic antibody. It's the same as an antigen. When it's cleared, the cell is normally responsive. It could also be quantitative, as you say.

CAN EXPERIMENTAL B CELL TOLERANCE SERVE AS A MODEL FOR SELF TOLERANCE?

E. Diener, U. E. Diner, R. C. von Borstel, and C. A. Waters

Department of Immunology
MRC Group on Immunoregulation
University of Alberta
Edmonton, Alberta, Canada T6G 2H7

INTRODUCTION

In recent years, the concept of self tolerance, envisioned as the clonal elimination of potentially anti-self reactive lymphocytes,[1] has gained new impetus through the revival of Lederberg's clonal abortion hypothesis.[2] In particular, the work from Klinman's and Nossal's laboratories supports the notion that certain multivalent antigens preferentially induce unresponsiveness in B cells in their development towards immunocompetence.[3, 4] Whether or not this predisposition towards tolerance induction in immature B cells is at all related to the absence of help, *i.e.*, Bretscher and Cohn's signal 2,[5] remains unanswered. Whatever conceptual differences exist between these two theories of self tolerance, neither theory puts any constraints upon the nature of the antigen or its mode of presentation to the B cell, as long as the latter is intrinsically "predisposed" towards being rendered unresponsive upon contact with antigen—this predisposition being defined by relative immaturity. Therefore, all antigens with multivalent epitopes, regardless of their carrier, should preferentially induce tolerance in immature receptor-bearing B cells. Experiments in support of clonal abortion have used the antigen concentration as the critical parameter when comparing degrees of tolerance susceptibility between mature B cells of the adult and immature B cells of the neonatal mouse.[3, 6] In contrast, the work described in this paper is based on what appears to us the most critical prediction of the clonal abortion theory: immature B cells, unlike adult B cells, should not be able to distinguish between epitopes whose tolerogenic or immunogenic potential is determined by the carrier.

Hapten-specific tolerance was induced in adult B cells *in vivo* and *in vitro* by nonimmunogenic dinitrophenylated carboxymethyl cellulose (DNP-CMC) or methyl cellulose (DNP-MC). Oxidation and the subsequent reduction of the vicinal hydroxyl groups of both these carriers abrogated the conjugate's tolerogenic potential, although they remained nonimmunogenic as well as multivalent. Both the native and the chemically modified antigens were shown to be linear polymers with the same molecular weight and to have the same avidity for free hapten-specific antibody and hapten-binding B cells. Contrary to the prediction of the clonal abortion theory, identical results were obtained in studies using both neonatal and adult mice that had been lethally irradiated and treated with either the native or the modified antigens during repopulation with 13-day-old fetal liver cells. Like adult mice, these immunologically immature animals were capable of distinguishing between carrier-controlled, tolerogenic, and nontolerogenic forms of each antigen. In agreement with these observations are other experiments from this laboratory (Waters *et al.*, in preparation),

0077-8923/82/0392-0035 $1.75/0 © 1982, NYAS

which show that the trinitrophenylated polyclonal B cell activator, lipopoly-saccharide (LPS), abrogates hapten-specific tolerance when induced in newborn mice with TNP-BSA but not with TNP-HGG. We argue that all the above results are incompatible with the clonal abortion hypothesis, since they demonstrate carrier-dependent susceptibility to tolerance induction not only in the adult but also in the immunologically immature mouse.

MATERIALS AND METHODS

Mice

Male CBA/CaJ mice bred at the Ellerslie Animal Farm, University of Alberta, newborn and 60 to 90 days of age, were used. They were killed by cervical dislocation and their spleens placed in Mishell-Dutton balanced salt solution (MDBSS).[7] Antigen and fetal liver cells were injected intravenously. Newborn mice were injected with antigen intraperitoneally. For repopulation of irradiated mice, 2×10^6 fetal liver cells (FLC) from 13-day-old syngeneic donors were injected. The mice were subjected to whole body irradiation of 950 rad (^{137}Cs source, Gamma cell 40 Irradiator, Atomic Energy of Canada Ltd., Ottawa, Ontario, Canada).

Tissue Culture

Spleen cell suspensions were obtained by gently squeezing the tissue through nylon gauze into the culture medium under sterile conditions. After removing debris by sedimentation at 1 g for 10 min, the cells were centrifuged at 400 g for 7.5 min and resuspended in Click's medium[8] prepared in our laboratory containing 10% v/v fetal calf serum (FCS) ("Rehatuin," Reheis Chemical Co., Phoenix, Arizona) and 5×10^{-5} M 2-mercaptoethanol. 5×10^6 cells were placed in each well of 24-well Linbro culture dishes (Flow Laboratories, Hamden, Connecticut) and cultured in Click's medium with 10% FCS and 5×10^{-5} M 2-mercaptoethanol. Cultures were kept for three days at 37° C in a 10% CO_2/air atmosphere. Viable cells were counted by eosin dye exclusion.

Assay for Antibody-Forming Cells

The number of antibody-forming cells (AFC) was determined by the Jerne plaque assay as modified by Cunningham and Szenberg.[9] Trinitrophenylated sheep red blood cells (TNP-SRBC) were used as targets for IgM-producing AFC.[10]

Antigens

Ficoll (F) (M.W. 400 000) was obtained from Pharmacia Fine Chemicals, Uppsala, Sweden. Trinitrobenzene sulfonic acid (TNBS), 2,4-dinitrofluoroben-zene, cyanogen bromide, carboxymethyl cellulose (CMC) (medium viscosity), methyl cellulose (MC) of 4000 centipoises, and N-2,4-dinitrophenyl-L-lysine were purchased from Sigma Chemicals, St. Louis, Missouri. The succinimide derivative of 4-hydroxy-3-iodi-5 nitrophenylacetic acid (NIPOSu) was purchased from Biosearch Laboratories, San Rafael, California. Burro red blood cells (BRBC) and sheep red blood cells were kept at 4° C in Alsever's solution. Preparation of the various conjugates is described in detail in a previous publication.[11] The vicinal hydroxyl groups of CMC and MC were oxidized with sodium periodate at pH 5 [12] at equal carbohydrate/periodate concentrations (2 mg ml^{-1}). The resulting aldehyde groups were reduced with 0.04 M sodium cyanoborohydride in 0.05 M carbonate buffer at pH 9.5. The number of aldehyde groups was estimated by determining the reducing number of the carbohydrate preparations.[13] The chemically treated materials were purified by Sephacryl (S-300; 0.9 × 70 cm) column chromatography and eluted with either water or saline at a flow rate of 10 ml h^{-1}. A spectrophotometric evaluation of the material was made by measuring the absorption of the effluent at 206 nm. Analytical ultracentrifugation was performed in a Beckman model E ultracentrifuge at 6000 rpm. LPS from *Salmonella typhosa* 0901 was purchased from Difco Laboratories, Detroit, Michigan. TNP-LPS was prepared as follows: 25 mg LPS was dissolved in 5 ml of 0.1 M carbonate buffer at pH 9, after which 30 mg trinitrobenzene sulfonic acid (TNBS) was added and the reaction mixture was allowed to stand at room temperature for 4 h. The solution was then dialyzed extensively against water and the conjugation ratio was calculated by dry weight determination and the absorption at 354 nm. For preparation of DNP-LPS, 20 mg LPS were dissolved in 5 ml of 0.11 M carbonate buffer at pH 9.5. 100 μl of a 2% (w/v) suspension of 2,4-dinitrofluorobenzene (DNFB) in absolute ethanol were added and the reaction mixture allowed to stand at room temperature for 15 min, whereupon it was dialyzed exhaustively against water. The conjugation ratio was calculated by dry weight determination and absorption at 360 nm.

SRBC were trinitrophenylated as follows: 30 mg TNBS was dissolved in 10 ml cacodylate buffer (0.28 M, pH 7) and 1.5 ml of packed SRBC added. The reaction mixture was left at room temperature for 10 min and poured into 20 ml phosphate-buffered saline (PBS) (0.01% CaCl$_2$, 0.01% MgCl$_2$ containing 30 mg glycyl-glycine). After 5 min, the cells were washed twice with PBS Ca Mg and resuspended in 10 ml MDBSS. Bovine serum albumin (BSA) and human γ-globulin (HGG) were purchased from Sigma Chemical Company, St. Louis, Missouri, and were trinitrophenylated as described previously.[14] TNP$_{10}$-BSA and TNP$_{10}$-HGG were precipitated on alum [14] and 0.5 mg of each was given intraperitoneally to animals along with 10^9 heat-killed *Bordetella pertussis* organisms (Connaught Laboratories, Willowdale, Ontario), the final injection volume being 0.2 ml. Nine days later, the above procedure was repeated and, five days after the second challenge, spleens were assayed as above for both IgM and IgG antibody-forming cells. Rabbit anti-mouse IgG, purchased from Cappel Laboratories, Cochranville, Pennsylvania, was used in the latter determination at a concentration found to be optimal. The hapten:carrier substitution ratio is given on a mole per mole basis, unless stated otherwise.

Binding Avidity between Multivalent Antigen and B Cells or Free Antibody

The binding avidity for B cells of DNP-MC, DNP-CMC, and their oxidized-reduced (OR) forms was measured by an antigen-binding competition assay with trinitrophenylated SRBC. Normal washed spleen cells at 20 × 10^6 cells ml^{-1} were incubated at 4° C for 30 min in MDBSS and different concentrations of either DNP-MC, DNP-MCOR, DNP-CMC, or DNP-CMCOR. The cells were subsequently washed three times by centrifugation at 400 g for 7.5 min, and resuspended in 1 ml MDBSS to which 10 μl of a 10% suspension of either normal SRBC or TNP-SRBC was added. The mixture was left for 60 min at 4° C and the rosettes were fixed with 0.05% glutaraldehyde. The binding avidity of antigen for antibody in solution was measured by fluorescence quenching, as per Eisen.[15]

RESULTS AND DISCUSSION

Hapten Derivatives of Carboxymethyl Cellulose and Methyl Cellulose Are Nonimmunogenic Tolerogens for Adult B Cells

As part of a systematic search of polymeric carbohydrates for tolerogenic carriers of hapten we found two compounds, CMC and MC, whose hapten derivatives are able to induce profound hapten-specific tolerance in mice (TABLE 1a). Like CMC, MC is composed of D-glucose pyranose molecules, lacking, however, carboxyl groups. Of particular significance for the interpretation of the data to be presented here is the absence of any immunogenic or mitogenic property associated with these tolerogenic carriers. Furthermore, their ability to induce tolerance in T cell–deficient nu/nu [11] or thymectomized, irradiated, FLC-repopulated mice (TABLE 1b) confirms their function as B cell tolerogens. In light of the one signal hypothesis on immune induction,[16] it is unexpected that neither MC nor CMC can act as polyclonal B cell activators (PBA) under conditions at which PBA activity by LPS could readily be shown (E. Diener et al., in preparation). T cell–independent antigens are said to induce tolerance in B cells by virtue of PBA activity and, hence, an ability to deliver an excess of inductive signals.[17]

The ability of an antigen to deliver a tolerogenic signal in the absence of immunogenicity suggests the existence of two distinct inductive pathways, one for immunity and another for tolerance, unless one postulates that tolerance induced by such an antigen is due to receptor blockade.[18] Experiments incompatible with receptor blockade in this system involve the abrogation of unresponsiveness by the hapten derivative of LPS at concentrations too low to trigger a polyclonal response (TABLE 2).[19] Such a result reflects the availability of "unblocked" hapten-specific receptors, the cells of which were either rendered reversibly unresponsive by the tolerogen or never rendered tolerant in the first place. Explanations supporting the latter possibility that are based on affinity differences between B cell subpopulations can be ruled out in light of the identical hapten affinity distribution profiles in normal and DNP-MC tolerant mice challenged with DNP-LPS. Whatever the reason for tolerance reversibility by DNP-LPS, receptor blockade, by definition, does not distinguish between tolerance-susceptible and -nonsusceptible B cell subpopulations and does not, therefore, account for our results.

Chemical Alteration of the Carriers CMC and MC Abolishes Their Ability to Induce Tolerance in Adult B Cells

We have fortuitously discovered that oxidation followed by subsequent reduction of the vicinal hydroxyl groups of CMC and MC abrogates the

TABLE 1

THE HAPTEN DERIVATIVE OF METHYL CELLULOSE INDUCES
HAPTEN-SPECIFIC TOLERANCE

	Pretreatment *	anti-NIP †	AFC per Spleen ± SEM (IgM)	
			anti-TNP	anti-BRBC
a.	MC	32 160 ± 3469	170 640 ± 18 419	n.d.
	DNP$_9$MC	25 200 ± 815	4950 ± 2000	n.d.
	MC	n.d.	54 000 ± 1774	162 400 ± 14 708
	DNP$_6$MC	n.d.	320 ± 89	190 400 ± 18 654
b.	MC	n.d.	82 333 ± 5735	3000 ± 288
	DNP$_9$MC	n.d.	5900 ± 2348	900 ± 431

NOTES: a. Normal mice. b. Thymectomized, irradiated, fetal liver–repopulated mice.
Normal adult CBA/CaJ mice were each injected with 250 μg of the tolerogen and
challenged with 20 μg DNP$_8$F * two days later.

For specificity control, NIP$_8$F * and burro red blood cells were used. Note that
thymectomized, irradiated, and fetal liver–repopulated mice are deficient in immunocompetence to BRBC.

* The subscripts indicate the number of haptens per 100 000 m.w. of carrier.

† Nitroiodophenyl.

tolerogenic potential of DNP-CMC and DNP-MC (TABLE 3). Interpretation
of these data critically depends on effects these chemical alterations may have
on the antigen's molecular weight and binding avidity for immunocompetent
cells as well as free antibody. Column chromatography of DNP-MC and DNP-
MCOR on Biogel B.6 revealed a single elution peak in the same position for
both antigens, indicating that chemical alteration of the native antigen did not

TABLE 2

LPS AND DNP-LPS ABOLISH HAPTEN-SPECIFIC TOLERANCE INDUCED BY
DNP-MC *In Vitro*

Pretreatment *	Challenge *	Anti-TNP AFC per Culture ± SEM (IgM)
DNP$_8$F	DNP$_8$F 100 ng ml^{-1}	3346 ± 395
DNP$_{12}$MC	DNP$_8$F 100 ng ml^{-1}	853 ± 200
DNP$_{12}$MC	LPS 10 μg ml^{-1}	3460 ± 200
DNP$_{12}$MC	LPS 1 ng ml^{-1}	294 ± 25
DNP$_{12}$MC	DNP$_3$LPS 1 ng ml^{-1}	4040 ± 232
—	LPS 10 μg ml^{-1}	2852 ± 740
—	LPS 1 ng ml^{-1}	106 ± 82
—	DNP$_3$ LPS 1 ng ml^{-1}	1240 ± 318

NOTES: LPS at a concentration of 1 ng ml^{-1} is inactive, whereas DNP$_3$LPS at 1
ng ml^{-1} is immunogenic.

Normal CBA/CaJ spleen cells were preincubated with 100 μg ml^{-1} antigen at
4° C, washed three times and cultured for four days in the presence of DNP$_8$F.*

* The subscript indicates the number of haptens per 100 000 m.w. of carrier.

TABLE 3

INDUCTION OF HAPTEN-SPECIFIC TOLERANCE BY DNP-MC AND DNP-CMC
BUT NOT DNP-MCOR AND DNP-CMCOR

		AFC per Spleen ± SEM (IgM)	
Pretreatment *	Challenge *	Anti-TNP	Anti-BRBC
a. *In vivo*			
Saline	DNP_8F	5400 ± 7174	162 640 ± 14 831
DNP_3MC	DNP_8F	6000 ± 538	60 640 ± 8722
$DNP_{10}CMC$	DNP_8F	400 ± 235	100 400 ± 14 373
DNP_3MCOR	DNP_8F	52 800 ± 9327	n.d.
$DNP_{10}CMCOR$	DNP_8F	23 600 ± 4000	n.d.

		AFC/culture ± SEM (IgM)	
		Anti-TNP	Anti-BRBC
b. *In vitro* (tested for haptenated MC and MCOR only)			
DNP_6F	DNP_8F	710 ± 150	200 ± 29
DNP_6MC	DNP_8F	< 1	320 ± 23
DNP_6MCOR	DNP_8F	1120 ± 158	310 ± 47

NOTES: a. Normal adult CBA/CaJ mice were each injected with 200 μg antigen or saline and challenged with 20 μg DNP_8F * two days later. For specificity control, BRBC were used.

b. Normal CBA/CaJ spleen cells were preincubated with 100 μg ml^{-1} antigen at 4° C, washed three times and cultured for four days in the presence of 100 ng ml^{-1} DNP_8F * and BRBC.

* The subscript indicates the number of haptens per 100 000 M.W. of carrier.

change its molecular weight. Identical results were obtained with DNP-CMC. Determination of sedimentation coefficients by ultracentrifugation at 6000 rpm indicated no change attributable to the chemical modification of CMC (DNP_6CMC, $S^0_{20w} = 1.60$; DNP_6 CMCOR, $S^0_{20w} = 1.61$)· Most important assessment of antibody binding avidity by the fluorescence quenching method [15] revealed a K_a for DNP_6MCOR ($K_a = 7.6 \times 10^8$ 1 mol^{-1}) that was 25 times higher than that for DNP_6MC ($K_a = 0.30 \times 10^8$ 1 mol^{-1}). Finally, competitive inhibition by DNP_9MC or DNP_9MCOR of TNP-rosette-forming B cells from normal mouse spleen yielded a binding avidity fifty times higher for DNP_9MCOR than for DNP_9MC. The same results were obtained with CMC and CMCOR as carrier. Taken together, these data lead one to the conclusion that the tolerance to DNP induced by the hapten derivatives of CMC or MC is entirely dependent on the nature of the carrier.

*Induction of Hapten-Specific Tolerance in Immature B Cells
is Carrier Dependent*

As explained in the introduction, the clonal abortion hypothesis predicts that immature B cells do not distinguish between antigens that are either intrinsically immunogenic or intinsically tolerogenic for mature B cells. It follows from the discussion of the previous section that induction of tolerance by one of our hapten-carrier conjugates in immunologically immature newborn or irradiated mice during hemopoietic repopulation with fetal liver stem cells is expected to occur independently of the carrier. This prediction, however, was not borne out in experiment. Tolerance induction during development of the immune system in either FLC-repopulated or newborn mice proved as carrier dependent as that in adult mice (TABLE 4). In support of these results, carrier dependency of tolerogenicity has also been demonstrated in newborn mice for hapten derivatives of T cell–dependent proteins (Waters *et al.*, in preparation). Hapten-specific tolerance was induced in newborn mice with TNP-HGG and TNP-BSA, as determined by challenge with the same antigens on alum with *B. pertussis*. However, upon challenge of these tolerant mice with an immuno-

TABLE 4

B CELLS, DURING THEIR DEVELOPMENT, CAN DISTINGUISH BETWEEN TOLEROGENIC NATIVE DNP-MC AND NONTOLEROGENIC DNP-MCOR

	Antigen Pretreatment *		Mean Anti-TNP AFC per Spleen $\pm$ SEM (IgM)
a.	MC	(100 μg)	88 000 $\pm$ 10 084
	DNP$_3$MC	(10 μg)	3440 $\pm$ 1502
	DNP$_3$MC	(100 μg)	200 $\pm$ 126
	MCOR	(100 μg)	63 216 $\pm$ 10 374
	DNP$_3$MCOR	(10 μg)	32 200 $\pm$ 3725
	DNP$_3$MCOR	(100 μg)	5440 $\pm$ 278
b.	MC		81 680 $\pm$ 5213
	MCOR		83 440 $\pm$ 11 239
	DNP$_{14}$MC		784 $\pm$ 385
	DNP$_{14}$MCOR		13 888 $\pm$ 3998
c.	MC		68 000 $\pm$ 6491
	DNP$_3$MC		1520 $\pm$ 751
	DNP$_3$MC		160 $\pm$ 167
	MCOR		148 800 $\pm$ 30 747
	DNP$_3$MCOR		19 920 $\pm$ 5454
	DNP$_3$MCOR		12 680 $\pm$ 3828

NOTES: a. Lethally irradiated fetal liver–repopulated CBA/CaJ mice were injected twice weekly from the time of repopulation with the tolerogen or its chemically modified form in amounts per injection as indicated. Challenge with 30 μg DNP$_8$F was in the fourth week following repopulation. Spleens were assayed for IgM AFC five days after the immunogenic challenge. Note that the loss of tolerogenicity of DNP$_3$MCOR, relative to DNP$_3$MC, is not complete. This is most likely due to the low reducing number of 100 for DNP$_3$MCOR. p values between: DNP$_3$MC (10 μg) and DNP$_3$MCOR (10 μg) < 0.001, DNP$_3$MC (100 μg) and DNP$_3$MCOR (100 μg) < 0.001.

b. Neonatal CBA/CaJ mice were injected twice weekly for four weeks with the tolerogen or its chemically modified form, challenged with 20 μg DNP$_8$F, and assayed for AFC as in a. Amounts of the putative tolerogen were adjusted to be equivalent to 100 μg per 30 g body weight. The reducing number of DNP$_{14}$MCOR is 140.

c. Normal adult CBA/CaJ mice were injected twice weekly with 100 μg of the tolerogen or its chemically modified form, challenged, and assayed for AFC as in a.

* The subscript indicates the number of haptens per 100 000 M.W. of carrier.

genic dose of TNP-LPS or TNP-*Brucella,* the state of tolerance remained stable only in mice that had been treated with TNP-HGG, but was significantly abrogated in those rendered unresponsive with TNP-BSA (TABLES 5 and 6). Since, in these experiments, both tolerogens bore the same hapten, the above difference in reversibility of tolerance must reflect carrier-dependent differences in mechanisms by which the two antigens induce unresponsiveness. Furthermore, these data also point out the possibility that the mammalian immunoglobulins, which have been the tolerogens of choice for most experimental work supporting clonal abortion, may induce unresponsiveness by unique mechanisms. These may involve an interaction between the Fc portion of the Ig molecule and its corresponding receptor on the B cell surface membrane.

CONCLUSION

Antigens are known to differ in their ability to induce tolerance in adults; such functional differences have frequently been attributed to the carrier portion of the molecule rather than to the nature of its epitopes. In contrast, for neonatal animals, the clonal abortion hypothesis predicts that differences in antigen structure are irrelevant with respect to the mechanisms presumed to induce tolerance. Contrary to these predictions, we must conclude from our data that the immature immune system is no different, in this case, from that of the adult; its susceptibility to hapten-specific tolerance induction is carrier-dependent. Furthermore, such dependence on the carrier was also evident from experiments in which tolerance, once induced, was reversed by LPS.

TABLE 5

NEONATAL TOLERANCE TO TNP-HGG IS NOT REVERSED BY TNP-CONJUGATED
T CELL–INDEPENDENT ANTIGENS

Neonatal Treatment	Challenge	Anti-TNP IgG PFC Per Spleen	p Value
a. None	TNP-HGG	96 117(117 761–78 451)	
1 mg TNP-HGG	TNP-HGG	840	< 0.001
b. None	TNP-LPS	110 561(140 727–86 861)	
1 mg TNP-HGG	TNP-LPS	1840(2503–1354)	< 0.001
c. None	TNP-BruA	156 495(185 117–132 298)	
1 mg TNP-HGG	TNP-BruA	2204(3303–1471)	< 0.001

NOTE: CBA/CaJ mice were injected within 24 h of birth and twice weekly thereafter with the indicated intraperitoneal doses of $TNP_{10}HGG$ (or $TNP_{10}BSA$) (TABLE 6). At 9–11 weeks of age, the groups were subdivided and challenged with one of the following three regimens: (a) 0.5 mg $TNP_{10}HGG$ (or $TNP_{10}BSA$) on alum with 1.5×10^9 killed *B. pertussis* organisms i.p. followed by a similar second challenge nine days later and assay of splenic response (PFC) five days later; (b) 50 μg TNP-LPS given i.v., assayed five days later for PFC, or (c) 4×10^9 TNP–*Brucella abortus* (strain 1119) given i.v., assayed seven days later for PFC.

TABLE 6 *

NEONATAL TOLERANCE TO TNP-BSA IS REVERSED BY TNP-CONJUGATED
T CELL–INDEPENDENT ANTIGENS

Neonatal Treatment	Challenge	Anti-TNP IgG PFC per Spleen	p Value
a. None	TNP-BSA	16 607(16 773–16 443)	
1 mg TNP-BSA	TNP-BSA	596(758–469)	< 0.001
b. None	TNP-HGG	153 674(170 784–138 278)	
1 mg TNP-BSA	TNP-HGG	37 299(43 278–32 146)	< 0.001
c. None	TNP-LPS	110 322(117 909–102 735)	
1 mg TNP-BSA	TNP-LPS	57 260(75 651–38 869)	< 0.005
d. None	TNP-BruA	205 116(217 492–193 445)	
1 mg TNP-BSA	TNP-BruA	170 098(180 926–159 919)	> 0.05
e.† None	NIP-BruA	93 400(102 261–84 539)	
1 mg TNP-BSA	NIP-BruA	79 417(83 454–75 380)	> 0.05

* For legend, see TABLE 5.
† Section e, 4 $\times$ 10^9 NIP–*Brucella abortus* used as immunogen.

SUMMARY

We have examined the abilities of the mature and immature immune systems to discriminate between tolerogenic and nontolerogenic forms of a hapten-carrier conjugate; both forms are multivalent nonimmunogenic polymers of the same molecular weight, and have the same avidity for free, hapten-specific antibody and hapten-binding B cells. Hapten-specific tolerance was induced in adult B cells by nonimmunogenic dinitrophenylated carboxymethyl cellulose or methyl cellulose. Oxidation and subsequent reduction of the vicinal hydroxyl groups of both carriers abrogated tolerogenicity, although they remained non-immunogenic. This chemical modification did not affect the carrier's molecular weight, and it did not reduce the binding avidity of their hapten derivatives to hapten-specific antibody or to antigen-binding B cells. The same experiments, when carried out in either neonatal mice or mice that had been lethally irradiated and given the above compounds during treatment with 13-day-old fetal liver cells, invariably yielded the same results. Like adult mice, these immunologically immature animals were capable of distinguishing between the tolerogenic and the nontolerogenic form of each antigen. It has also been shown (C. A. Waters *et al.*, in preparation) that neonatally induced tolerance to TNP-HGG is irreversible, whereas tolerance to TNP-BSA is reversible by challenge with TNP-LPS. These results are in conflict with the clonal abortion hypothesis.

REFERENCES

1. BURNET, F.M. 1959. The Clonal Selection Theory of Acquired Immunity. Cambridge University Press. New York.
2. LEDERBERG, J. 1959. Genes and antibodies: do antigens bear instruction for

antibody specificity or do they select cell lines that arise by mutation? Science **129:** 1649–53.

3. NOSSAL, G. J. V. & B. L. PIKE. 1975. Evidence for the clonal abortion theory of B lymphocyte tolerance. J. Exp. Med. **141:** 904–17.

4. METCALF, E. S. & N. R. KLINMAN. 1976. *In vitro* tolerance induction of neonatal murine B-cells. J. Exp. Med. **143:** 1327–40.

5. BRETSCHER, P. A. & M. COHN. 1970. A theory of self-nonself discrimination. Science **169:** 1042–49.

6. METCALF, E., A. F. SCHRATER & N. R. KLINMAN. 1979. Immunol. Rev. **43:** 143–83.

7. MISHELL, R. I. & R. W. DUTTON. 1967. Immunization of dissociated spleen cultures from normal mice. J. Exp. Med. **126:** 423–42.

8. CLICK, R. E., L. BENCK & B. J. ALTER. 1972. Immune response *in vitro.* 1. Culture conditions for antibody synthesis. Cell. Immunol. **3:** 264–76.

9. CUNNINGHAM, A. & A. SZENBERG. 1968. Further improvements in the plaque technique for detecting antibody forming cells. Immunology **14:** 599–600.

10. OKUYAMA, T. & K. SATAKE. 1960. On the preparation and properties of 2,4,6-trinitrophenyl-amino acids and peptides. J. Biochem. **47:** 454–66.

11. DINER, U. E., D. KUMIMOTO & E. DIENER. 1979. Carboxymethyl cellulose, a nonimmunogenic hapten carrier with tolerogenic properties. J. Immunol. **122:** 1886–91.

12. TE PIAO KING, L. KOCHOUMIAN, K. ISHIZAKA, L. M. LICHTERNSTEIN & P. S. NORMAN. 1975. Immunochemical studies of Dextran coupled ragweed pollen allergen, antigen E^1. Arch. Biochem. Biophys. **169:** 464–73.

13. SCHOCH, T. J. 1964. *In* Methods in Carbohydrate Chemistry. R. L. Whistler, Ed.: 64–68. Academic Press. New York.

14. WATERS, C. A., L. M. PILARSKI, T. G. WEGMANN & E. DIENER. 1979. Tolerance induction during ontogeny. I. Presence of active suppression in mice rendered tolerant to human γ-globulin *in utero* correlates with the breakdown of the tolerant state. J. Exp. Med. **149:** 1134–51.

15. EISEN, H. N. & J. E. MCGUIGAN. 1971. *In* Methods in Immunology and Immunochemistry. A. Williams and M. W. Chase, Eds.: 395–411. Academic Press. New York.

16. COUTINHO, A. & G. MÖLLER. 1974. Immune activation of B-cells: Evidence "for one nonspecific triggering signal" not delivered by the Ig receptor. Scand. J. Immunol. **1:** 133–46.

17. FERNANDEZ, C., L. HAMMERSTROM, G. MÖLLER, D. PRIMI & C. J. E. SMITH. 1979. Immunological tolerance affects only a subpopulation of the antigen-specific B lymphocytes. Evidence against clonal deletion as the mechanism of tolerance induction. Immunol. Rev. **43:** 3–41.

18. BOREL, Y. 1976. Isologous IgG-induced immunologic tolerance to haptens: A model of self versus nonself recognition. Transplant. Rev. **31:** 3–22.

19. COUTINHO, A. &. G. MÖLLER. 1975. Thymus-independent B-cell induction and paralysis. Adv. Immunol. **21:** 114–239.

———————◆———————

DISCUSSION OF THE PAPER

Y. BOREL (*Harvard University, Cambridge, Mass.*): We have exactly similar data with tolerance to DNP–mouse gamma globulin that cannot be reversed by DNP-LPS. It is not settled whether this is clonal abortion or something else. But I think the most critical question is the one you raised at the beginning of your talk. Do B cells become tolerant to natural antigens? As you know, there are very few systems that have addressed this question because it is so difficulty to study. In a model of genetically determined natural B cell tolerance, *i.e.*, the C5 model in the mouse, Dorothy Harris in our laboratory has found that B cells are completely responsive and not tolerant to C5. Only the T cells are tolerant. So, the question remains: Are B cells ever tolerant to an antigen? So far I don't think there is any definite answer.

DIENER: I like that model very much.

A. H. SEHON (*University of Manitoba, Winnipeg, Man.*): Erwin, what is the molecular weight of the methyl cellulose?

DIENER: 86 000.

SEHON: So in a molecule of 86 000 daltons you have 6 DNP groups. That is tolerogenic. Have you shown whether or not suppressor cells are involved?

DIENER: Yes, we have done transfer experiments and mixing experiments, the data of which are published. We could not show any evidence for active suppression. However, I'm not saying that there is no active suppression involved. It is very difficult to demonstrate with immature cells. You don't know what level of the biological model tolerance actually functions at. So, if you don't find suppressors, it may be because you need very, very few suppressors to affect your target cells.

SEHON: You show that the oxidized and reduced material is still pretty suppressive in relation to the control. If you had started with a material that would have been broken down, *e.g.*, cellulose or polyhydroxy material, you'd have been able to conclude that there is still suppression.

DIENER: Have you done these experiments?

SEHON: No.

DIENER: Because you refer to them.

SEHON: No. I think that you concluded that everything is relative. The reason I'm asking you this question is that we have used polyhydroxy materials, the polyvinyl alcohols. They are small molecules—3000 to 14 000 M.W.—and there we find both mechanisms: suppressor T cells, as well as silenced B cells. I'm just trying to see the similarities or dissimilarities between the two systems.

DIENER: I must say, with respect to suppression, that we can very effectively induce tolerance *in vitro*. This is done by incubating spleen cells with the putative tolerogen at 4° C and then washing it off. When we do that with anti-Thy 1 treated spleen cells, we still get exactly the same results. From all the evidence that we can come up with, it doesn't look like T cells are involved.

G. MÖLLER (*Karolinska Institute, Stockholm, Sweden*): I have two points. One is that I think that HGG may be a unique tolerogen and obey special rules. It may actually cause receptor-negative signals that work in the same way as antibody feedback suppression.

The second is this. Before one makes a statement about the state of B cells after immunization or after tolerance, I think it's necessary to clear the antigen from the B cell receptor. Only then can you really say that the B cell is tolerant, repressed, or just blocked. Otherwise, I don't think you can.

DIENER: I think I agree in principle with what you're saying. The methyl cellulose does cap off very readily, as easily as polymerized flagellin (POL). You can overload the system and prevent clearing of the antigen from the surface. But, as we showed with POL, that doesn't seem to have any effect at all with respect to the tolerogenic state. Whatever our compound is doing, the main message is that it's doing things that you would not predict according to the clonal abortion hypothesis.

W. O. WEIGLE (*Scripps Clinic and Research Foundation, La·Jolla, Calif.*): I'd like to point out that it takes a very small amount of antigen to make T cells tolerant and a very large amount to make B cells tolerant. The difference may be up to 2 logs.

DIENER: In the adult animal?

WEIGLE: In the adult animal and also in the neonatal animal. BSA has a half-life of around 12 hours, while HGG has a half-life of around 7–8 days; that may be why HGG is a unique tolerogen. It's very difficult to get enough BSA in the animal to get the B cells tolerant, even if you inject antigen daily or three or four times a day.

Also, if one looks at the tolerance to self antigens present in very small amounts, such as C5, one would not expect tolerance at the B cell level. However, you certainly would expect tolerance to your own serum albumin.

WATERS: I would only like to remind Bill Weigle that the half-life of MC and CMC is 34 hours *in vivo*, as we just showed. So if you're looking at a long-term tolerance state, you have very little CMC and MC in the serum. In fact, they could be said to be of the same order of magnitude as BSA. So you're left to explain the difference between them. We've done some autoradiography studies, which we presented at Brno in Czechoslovakia, in which we showed quite clearly that, even though the BSA does disappear from the serum relatively quickly, it is persistent in the spleen and thymus for quite some time. In fact, if given neonatally, the BSA persists quite demonstrably until about five weeks when you immunize, say at six weeks, and test for tolerance.

DIENER: In fact, Bill, I'll also remind you of Ada's studies. I'm sure you remember those, in which he very clearly showed that BSA stays in lymphatic organs just as long as HGG. Therefore, I don't think that serum levels have any bearing on the tolerant state of the animal. I think what really counts is where antigen localization occurs in the lymphatic system, and how long it persists there. With respect to the ease of T cell tolerance in the animals that are tolerized to HGG *in utero*, you don't find any difference at all between the breakdown of tolerance in T cells and in B cells. In fact, during the breakdown of tolerance, the antigen disappears at about eight weeks postnatally and you find that T cells become responsive at about the same time as B cells. I think that one would probably find a difference between the susceptibility of T cells and that of B cells to tolerance induction with different antigens. I also think that one would find a difference if one looked at completely immature animals, such as fetuses, which might be different from neonatal animals.

IMMUNOLOGICAL UNRESPONSIVENESS
TO HSA IN CHICKENS

Tomáš Hraba, Ivan Karakoz, and Jindřich Madar

Institute of Molecular Genetics
Czechoslovak Academy of Sciences
166 10 Prague 6, Czechoslovakia

In 1949, Burnet and Fenner anticipated the existence of immunological tolerance as a consequence of contact with antigen during the embryonic period.[1] However, when Burnet and his collaborators tested this hypothesis by introducing influenza virus, mammalian erythrocytes, and bacteriophage into chicken embryos, they failed to demonstrate it.[2] In 1957, when tolerance to allogeneic antigens had already been obtained by introducing them into chicken embryos,[3,4] Cohn was unsuccessful in similar experiments with different defined antigens, including haptenated bovine serum albumin (BSA). In the same year, Wolfe *et al.* induced tolerance in chickens by injecting large doses of BSA during the short interval after hatching. Even at six weeks, the earliest time of testing, this tolerance was partial, *i.e.*, tolerant fowls produced detectable anti-BSA antibodies, though in smaller quantities than did normal chickens. Similar results were obtained by injecting human serum albumin (HSA) into chick embryo yolk sacs [7] or by injections of this antigen after hatching.[8]

The availability of homogeneous inbred lines of chickens permitted us to study an active suppression of antibody formation in chickens unresponsive to HSA. Transfers of spleen cells from tolerant and normal donors to nonreactive syngeneic recipients, which had been irradiated [9,10] or treated with cyclophosphamide [11] after hatching, did not reveal that active suppression had any decisive role in this tolerant state.

Surgical bursectomy, the removal of the primary lymphoid organ responsible for B cell maturation in chickens, substantially increased the suppression of antibody formation and prolonged the duration of the tolerance induced by either BSA [12] or HSA.[9,13] On the other hand, surgical thymectomy carried out on the day of hatching influenced neither the degree nor the duration of tolerance to HSA in chickens.[14] We have concluded from these findings and from the relatively short duration of tolerance that T cells play no essential role in the tolerance to HSA induced in chickens after hatching and that the major mechanism responsible for the observed suppression of antibody formation is inactivation or elimination of B cells.

It was found earlier that the immunization of chickens tolerant to HSA with a crossreacting antigen, BSA, induced an earlier and more intensive anti-HSA antibody production than the challenge with HSA.[15,16] In this paper, we shall deal with the implications of this discovery for the understanding of the cellular mechanisms that are responsible for the inhibition of antibody formation in chickens unresponsive to HSA.

MATERIAL AND METHODS

Experimental Animals. Chickens used in the experiments were F_1 hybrids of two inbred chicken lines, CB and IC.[17,18]

47

0077–8923/82/0392–0047 $1.75/0 © 1982, NYAS

Antigens. Solutions were prepared from lyophilized HSA or BSA, or from a 20% HSA solution, all produced by the Institute of Sera and Vaccines, Prague, Czechoslovakia.

Tolerance Induction and Challenge. Tolerance was induced by one or four intraperitoneal injections of HSA (100 mg each). All tolerant chickens received one injection of HSA on the day of hatching. When tolerance was induced by four doses of HSA, the subsequent injections were given on days 4, 7, and 11 after hatching.

Challenge with HSA or BSA consisted of a single intraperitoneal injection of the antigen solution. The challenging dose of HSA or BSA was 20 mg per chicken (about 100 mg per kg body weight) at the age of 4 weeks, and 15 mg per chicken at 6 weeks of age (about 40 mg per kg body weight).

Antibody Assay. The hemagglutination technique was used to determine anti-HSA and anti-SRBC (sheep red blood cell) antibodies. The hemagglutination reactions were performed in a Takátsy microtitrator (Labor, Budapest, Hungary). For the detection of anti-HSA antibodies, syngeneic chicken erythrocytes were coupled with HSA by means of *bis*-diazotized benzidine.[11, 19]

RESULTS

We carried out most of the experiments in chickens rendered tolerant by four injections of HSA. The data obtained in experiments in which tolerant and normal chickens from the same hatchings were immunized in parallel with either HSA or BSA four or six weeks after hatching are summarized in TABLE 1. When HSA was used for challenge, the ability of tolerant chickens to form anti-HSA antibodies was low at both ages, reaching about 5% of the antibody production of normal chickens at six weeks. A much higher response to HSA was induced in tolerant chickens challenged with BSA. At four weeks, it was about one-fifth and, at six weeks, it was already two-thirds of the antibody production of normal chickens.

A simple mathematical model was proposed to describe the kinetics of tolerance to HSA in chickens.[20] It assumed that this tolerance is induced by irreversible inactivation of B cells and that the escape from tolerance was effected by differentiation of new B lymphocytes reactive to HSA from the stem cells. The observed recovery from tolerance in chickens challenged with HSA was much slower than that calculated according to this model. However, the calculated rate of escape from tolerance agreed well with the values obtained after challenge with BSA.[21] The computed kinetics of escape from tolerance to HSA induced by both one and four injections of antigen indicated maximum difference between the two tolerant groups at the age of four weeks. This prediction was verified in four experiments. In each of them, tolerance was induced in chickens from the same hatching group by either one or four injections of HSA. Tolerant and normal chickens were challenged with HSA or BSA at the age of four weeks. The results of these experiments are summarized in TABLE 2. After challenge with HSA, anti-HSA antibody formation was low in both groups of tolerant chickens and there was no significant difference between them. The production of anti-HSA antibodies induced by BSA challenge was higher when tolerance was induced by one dose than by four doses of antigen. However, the observed differences were statistically significant

TABLE 1

REACTIVITY OF TOLERANT CHICKENS TO HSA OR BSA CHALLENGE

Challenge with	Challenge at	
	Four Weeks	Six Weeks
HSA	< 2 *	4.8 ± 0.6
BSA	22.0 ± 5.3	69.8 ± 8.7
n †	7	2
	(8.4)	(9.5)

* Mean percentage of responsiveness ± s.e.
† Number of experiments (mean number of chickens per experimental group).

(p < 0.05) only in experiment 3, probably because of the high variations in titers of individual fowls. These variations were also responsible for the observed differences between individual experiments. The observed mean values did not differ substantially from the calculated ones.

We tested in parallel spleen cells from chickens rendered tolerant by both one and four doses of HSA in transfers to young irradiated recipients. In the three experiments of this kind, anti-HSA antibody production in the recipients of cells from both groups of tolerant donors was detectable only exceptionally. Differences between the reactions of the recipients of spleen cells from the two tolerant groups and those of the recipients of cells from normal fowls was statistically significant in all three experiments (p < 0.01). The results of one of them are shown in TABLE 3. These findings indicate that the tolerance induced by one dose of HSA is irreversible, as has already been seen when tolerance was induced by four doses of antigen.[22] However, we have not yet carried out other transfer experiments with cells from chickens rendered tolerant by one dose of HSA. Therefore, we cannot exclude the possibility that the mechanisms involved in the unresponsiveness differ in chickens rendered tolerant by one or four doses of HSA, although the agreement of experimental and calculated results suggests that the same mechanisms are operative in both groups of tolerant fowls.

TABLE 2

REACTIVITY OF CHICKENS RENDERED TOLERANT BY ONE OR FOUR INJECTIONS OF HSA AFTER CHALLENGE WITH BSA AT FOUR WEEKS OF AGE

Number of Tolerance-Inducing Doses of HSA	Experiment				Mean ± s.e.
	1	2	3	4	
4	44 *	25	8	10	21.5 ± 8.1
1	87	30	26	16	39.0 ± 15.5
n †	9.5	8.3	7.8	6.0	7.9

NOTE: After HSA challenge at four weeks of age, the mean percentage of reactivity of both tolerant groups was < 2.
* Mean percentage of responsiveness of the group.
† Mean number of chickens per experimental group.

TABLE 3

ANTIBODY FORMATION IN NEWLY HATCHED RECIPIENTS OF TRANSFERRED
SPLEEN CELLS

Antibody against	Donors of Transferred Cells		
	Tolerant		Normal
	4 × HSA *	1 × HSA	
HSA	0.17 ± 0.17 † (1/6)‡	0.17 ± 0.12 (2/18)	3.17 ± 0.72 (7/9)
SRBC	6.17 ± 0.17 (6/6)	5.36 ± 0.21 (18/18)	5.17 ± 0.66 (8/9)

NOTE: The recipients were irradiated with 500 r on the day of hatching. The next day they received 150 × 10⁶ pooled spleen cells from four-week-old donors intraperitoneally. HSA (2 mg per chicken) and SRBC (0.1 ml of a 20% suspension per chicken) were added to the injected cell suspension. Blood for antibody determination was collected from the recipients 10 d after the transfer.

* Number of tolerance-inducing HSA injections (100 mg each).

† Mean ± S.E. of —log₂ hemagglutinating antibody titer.

‡ Number of fowls with detectable antibodies per total number of fowls in group.

Our previous observations suggested that, in contrast to the findings obtained in rabbits, a simultaneous administration of the tolerated and cross-reacting antigen did not prevent the termination of tolerance. Further studies in chickens rendered tolerant by four injections of HSA showed that, although the presence of the tolerated antigen did not completely prevent the increase in anti-HSA antibody formation after challenge with BSA, it decreased the production of these antibodies compared to challenge with BSA only. The results of one of these experiments are shown in TABLE 4. The difference between the chicken and the rabbit tolerance model seems to be quantitative rather than qualitative, in this respect.

TABLE 4

EFFECT OF SIMULTANEOUS CHALLENGE WITH BSA AND HSA ON THE
TERMINATION OF TOLERANCE

Chickens	Challenge with		
	HSA	BSA	HSA + BSA
Tolerant	0 (0/9)‡	2.81 ± 0.78 † (6/8)	0.78 ± 0.66 (2/9)
Control	6.33 ± 0.71 (6/6)	5.00 ± 0.56 (8/8)	5.79 ± 0.84 (7/7)

NOTE: Tolerance was induced by four injections of HSA. The challenge was carried out at the age of four weeks.

†‡ See legend for TABLE 3.

DISCUSSION

In tolerance to heterologous serum proteins in mammals, challenge with a cross-reacting antigen often terminates the tolerance. This phenomenon was explained by the differential recovery of T and B cells from tolerance. It was supposed that activation of T helper cells specific for the cross-reacting antigen provides the necessary T cell help, which is absent due to the persisting tolerance in T cells specific for the tolerated antigen.[23] Therefore, the immune response to the tolerated antigen after challenge with a cross-reacting one was considered to be an indicator of the recovery of B cells from tolerance.[24]

The situation seems to be similar in chickens tolerant to HSA. They also recover the ability to form antibodies to the tolerated antigen after challenge with the cross-reacting antigen, the BSA. The values of B cell recovery from tolerance, which are calculated according to our mathematical model,[20] corresponded well to the observed anti-HSA antibody formation in tolerant chickens challenged with BSA. This finding suggests that this reactivity may be regarded as a measure of B cell recovery from tolerance in chickens, too. In contrast to the apparent thymus dependence of tolerance to heterologous serum proteins in mammals, T cells seem to play no significant role in tolerance to HSA in chickens. This conclusion is based on the following observations:

Thymectomy carried out on the day of hatching neither increased nor prolonged inhibition of anti-HSA antibody formation in tolerant chickens.[14]

Bacterial lipopolysaccharide was presumed to bypass the requirement for T cell help in tolerant mammals. The production of antibodies to the tolerated antigen induced by simultaneous injection of lipopolysaccharide was also regarded as a measure of B cell reactivity in tolerant animals.[25] The administration of different doses of bacterial lipopolysaccharide at the time of challenge with HSA did not increase the anti-HSA antibody production in tolerant chickens.[26]

There was no substantial recovery of anti-HSA antibody production when spleen cells from tolerant chickens were transferred into syngeneic recipients treated with cyclophosphamide after hatching.[11] It was observed that the bursa of Fabricius did not recover from this treatment with cyclophosphamide, but T cells regained their reactivity quickly.[27] The cyclophosphamide-treated recipients of cells from tolerant chickens were challenged with HSA four weeks after treatment with the drug. It could be assumed that their T cell reactivity had already recovered and that the recipients would be able to supply the required T cell help to the reactive B cells transferred from tolerant donors.

The findings of other authors suggest a T cell–independent character of the antibody response both to HSA[28] and BSA[29] in chickens.

Taken together, all these findings suggest that termination of tolerance to HSA in chickens by BSA challenge is not mediated by an interaction between T and B cells. It is improbable that a mechanism at the level of individual B cells could explain this termination of tolerance. It seems more promising to search for the mechanism responsible for this effect in other cellular interactions.

In the model of tolerance to a T cell–independent antigen, Diener *et al.* observed that adherent cells, probably macrophages, decided whether the B cell response to the antigenic stimulus was antibody formation or tolerance.[30] The "tolerant" adherent cells were able to initiate antibody production to other antigens.

Schott and Merchant described a carrier-specific immunological memory to a hapten in nude mice.[32] The carrier restriction of this memory seems to result from the interaction of B cells specific for the carrier determinants with hapten-specific B cells.

We wonder whether some similar interaction is not responsible for the differential reactivity of chickens tolerant to HSA. The cellular interaction could not cause an active inhibition of the immune response, because cells from tolerant chickens transferred into nonreactive recipients together with cells from normal donors did not inhibit their antibody production.[9–11]

SUMMARY

HSA injected into chickens after hatching induces suppression of anti-HSA antibody formation. Unresponsive chickens react by producing the anti-HSA antibodies earlier and more intensively after BSA challenge than after challenge with HSA. This effect cannot be ascribed to T cells, because they were found to play no substantial role in the unresponsiveness to HSA. Neither was active suppression, which could account for the depressed antibody production, detected. B cell inactivation seems to be the major mechanism involved in this unresponsiveness. However, some additional mechanism must prevent B cells of unresponsive chickens from producing anti-HSA antibodies after HSA challenge, although they are able to form them after immunization with BSA. We suggest that cellular interactions, either between B cells of different specificities or between B cells and macrophages, are responsible for this differential reactivity.

ACKNOWLEDGMENTS

The authors gratefully acknowledge the competent technical assistance of Ms. Mirka Madarová, Ms. Marie Miglová, and Ms. Jana Průšová.

REFERENCES

1. BURNET, F. M. & F. FENNER. 1949. The Production of Antibodies. Macmillan. Melbourne.
2. BURNET, F. M., J. D. STONE & M. EDNEY. 1950. The failure of antibody production in the chick embryo. Aust. J. Exp. Biol. Med. Sci. **28:** 291–97.
3. HAŠEK, M. 1953. Vegetative hybridization of animals by joining their blood circulations during embryonic development. (In Czech.) Čs. Biol. **2:** 265–77.
4. BILLINGHAM, R. E., L. BRENT & P. B. MEDAWAR. 1953. Actively acquired tolerance of foreign cells. Nature (London) **172:** 603–5.
5. COHN, M. 1957. The problem of specific inhibition of antibody synthesis in adult animals by immunization of embryos. Ann. N.Y. Acad. Sci. **64:** 859–76.
6. WOLFE, H. R., C. TEMPELIS, A. MUELLER & S. REIBEL. 1957. Precipitin production in chickens. XVII. The effect of massive injections of bovine serum albumin at hatching on subsequent antibody production. J. Immunol. **79:** 147–153.
7. STEVENS, K. M., H. C. PIETRYK & J. L. CININERA. 1958. Acquired immunological tolerance to a protein antigen in chickens. Brit. J. Exp. Pathol. **39:** 1–7.

8. HRABA, T. & J. IVÁNYI. 1963. A contribution to the study of immunological tolerance to protein antigen in the chickens. Folia Biol. (Prague) **9**: 354–63.
9. HRABA, T., I. KARAKOZ & J. MADAR. 1977. Attempts to characterize cellular mechanisms of immunologic tolerance to HSA in chickens. Folia Biol. (Prague) **23**: 336–46.
10. HRABA, T., I. KARAKOZ & J. MADAR. 1979. Cellular mechanisms of immunological tolerance to HSA in chickens. Folia Biol. (Prague) **25**: 347–48.
11. HRABA, T., I. KARAKOZ, Š. NĚMEČKOVÁ & J. MADAR. 1978. Persistence of immunological tolerance to HSA in chickens after cell transfer to immunosuppressed hosts. Folia Biol. (Prague) **24**: 173–84.
12. PETERSON, R. D. A., G. V. ALM & S. MICHALEK. 1971. The effect of bursectomy on the recovery from immunologic tolerance. J. Immunol. **106**: 1609–14.
13. IVÁNYI, J. & A. SALERNO. 1972. Cellular mechanisms of escape from immunological tolerance. Immunology **22**: 247–57.
14. BALCAROVÁ, J., I. KARAKOZ, T. HRABA & L. KOHOUTOVÁ. 1974. Avidity of antibodies formed in partially tolerant and neonatally thymectomized chickens. Folia Biol. (Prague) **20**: 392–97.
15. HRABA, T., I. KARAKOZ & J. MADAR. 1978. Termination of tolerance to HSA in chickens. Folia Biol. (Prague) **24**: 206–10.
16. KARAKOZ, I., J. MADAR & T. HRABA. 1979. Termination of tolerance to HSA in chickens by a cross-reacting antigen. Folia Biol. (Prague) **25**: 349–50.
17. HAŠEK, M., F. KNÍŽETOVÁ & H. MERVARTOVÁ. 1966. Syngeneic lines of chickens. I. Inbreeding and selection by means of skin grafts and tests for erythrocyte antigens in C line chickens. Folia Biol. (Prague) **12**: 335–42.
18. HÁLA, K., M. HAŠEK, I. HLOŽÁNEK, J. HORT, F. KNÍŽETOVÁ & H. MERVARTOVÁ. 1966. Syngeneic lines of chickens. II. Inbreeding and selection within the M, W and I lines and crosses between the C, M and W lines. Folia Biol. (Prague) **12**: 407–22.
19. IVÁNYI, J., T. HRABA & J. ČERNÝ. 1964. Immunological tolerance to human serum albumin (HSA) in chickens of adult and juvenile age. Folia Biol. (Prague) **10**: 198–205.
20. KLEIN, P., J. DOLEŽAL & T. HRABA. 1979. Compartmental model of immunological tolerance to HSA in chickens. Folia Biol. (Prague) **25**: 345–46.
21. KLEIN, P., J. DOLEŽAL & T. HRABA. 1981. A simple mathematical model of immunological tolerance to HSA in chickens. *In* Cellular and Molecular Mechanisms of Immunologic Tolerance. T. Hraba and M. Hašek, Eds.: 367–72. Marcel Dekker. New York.
22. HRABA, T., I. KARAKOZ & J. MADAR. 1981. Mechanisms of immunologic tolerance to a xenogeneic serum protein in chickens. *In* Cellular and Molecular Mechanisms of Immunologic Tolerance. T. Hraba and M. Hašek, Eds.: 361–66. Marcel Dekker. New York.
23. BENJAMIN, D. C. & W. O. WEIGLE. 1970. The termination of immunological unresponsiveness to bovine serum albumin in rabbits. I. Quantitative and qualitative response to cross-reacting albumin. J. Exp. Med. **132**: 66–76.
24. LEECH, S. H. & N. A. MITCHISON. 1976. Break-down of tolerance. Brit. Med. Bull. **32**: 130–34.
25. PARKS, D. E. & W. O. WEIGLE. 1980. Maintenance of immunologic unresponsiveness to human γ-globulin: Evidence for irreversible inactivation in B lymphocytes. J. Immunol. **124**: 1230–36.
26. MADAR, J., I. KARAKOZ, J. BALCAROVÁ, J. SEDLÁK & T. HRABA. 1975. Different effects of bacterial lipopolysaccharide on neonatal immunological tolerance to HSA in rabbits and chickens. Folia Biol. (Prague) **21**: 316–23.
27. LERMAN, S. P. & W. P. WEIDANZ. 1970. The effect of cyclophosphamide on the ontogeny of the humoral immune response in chickens. J. Immunol. **105**: 614–19.

28. IVÁNYI, J. & A. SALERNO. 1971. Impairment of humoral antibody response in neonatally thymectomized and irradiated chickens. Eur. J. Immunol. **1:** 227–30.
29. NAGASE, F., I. NAKASHIMA, N. KATO & K. YAGI. 1978. Studies on the immune response in chickens. I. Effect of various immunization procedures on the primary and secondary antibody responses to bovine serum albumin. Z. Immunitaetsforsch. **154:** 256–67.
30. DIENER, E., N. KRAFT, K.-C. LEE & C. SHIOZAWA. 1976. Antigen recognition. IV. Discrimination by antigen-binding immunocompetent B cells between immunity and tolerance is determined by adherent cells. J. Exp. Med. **143:** 805–21.
31. SCHOTT, C. F. & B. MERCHANT. 1979. Carrier-specific immune memory to a thymus-independent antigen in congenitally athymic mice. J. Immunol. **122:** 1710–18.

DISCUSSION OF THE PAPER

G. J. THORBECKE (*New York University School of Medicine, New York, N.Y.*): I think that your data are in very good agreement with the conclusion that we came to from studying T cell tolerance in the chicken. Injection of very small doses of protein antigen intravenously can induce tolerance at the level of delayed hypersensitivity. If you just immunize intravenously, even with the doses that induce tolerance for delayed type sensitivity, you get antibody production. And this antibody production is relatively normal in terms of primary response. If you then try to boost the chickens into good memory responses, you find that their 7S production is somewhat deficient, so the defect in helper activity is not nearly as noticeable in the chicken as in mammals. Although there is a carrier effect and there is certainly helper cell activity of the T cell, the B cell may be relatively less dependent on T cell help. So, with these antigens, chickens can make relatively good primary responses even if there is tolerance at the T cell level.

HRABA: Actually, we suspect that the T cell–independence of the anti-HSA antibody response in chickens could be effected by T cell tolerance induced by challenge with relatively high doses of HSA.

E. DIENER (*University of Alberta, Edmonton, Alta.*): I would recall the work carried out by Ramshaw in Australia, who showed the induction of suppression of the IgG response in cyclophosphamide-treated mice. This correlated with the increase in DTH after sensitization. Thus, I wonder to what extent, when we observe tolerance in the humoral immune response, we are in fact observing a switch from one immune class expression to another, such as humoral response to DTH. Have you tested your chickens to determine if they were, in fact, sensitive to DTH induction with this protein?

HRABA: We didn't work with agammaglobulinic chickens. In normal chickens, we observed strong immediate wattle reactions that overshadowed the DTH reactions, so we were unable to draw any conclusions from that work.

SUPPRESSION OF IgE ANTIBODIES WITH CONJUGATES OF HAPTENS OR ALLERGENS AND SYNTHETIC HYDROPHILIC POLYMERS *

A. H. Sehon

Department of Immunology
MRC Group for Allergy Research
Faculty of Medicine
University of Manitoba
Winnipeg, Manitoba, Canada R3E 0W3

INTRODUCTION

It is now generally accepted that common forms of hypersensitivity of the immediate type—such as extrinsic asthma, hay fever, rhinitis, urticaria, and some drug and occupational allergies [1-3]—are mediated primarily by IgE antibodies produced by allergic individuals in response to a wide spectrum of allergens. As documented by a number of investigators, crosslinking of IgE molecules [4] that are fixed tenaciously to mast cells or basophils by polyvalent antigens [5] leads to the degranulation of these cells and to the release of the mediators of anaphlaxis, *i.e.*, histamine,[6] slow reacting substance of anaphylaxis,[7] eosinophil chemotactic factor of anaphylaxis,[8] and the platelet activating factor.[9] It ought to be emphasized that, in addition to IgE, antibodies belonging to subclass(es) of IgG [10-12] and capable of sensitizing the above cells may also participate in the allergic response in experimental animals and man.

The symptoms of hypersensitivity conditions of the immediate type are a direct result of the interactions of the above-mentioned mediators of anaphylaxis with their target cells and may, in extreme cases, as in honeybee venom sensitivity, result in death due to anaphylactic shock. The two main forms of therapy currently practiced in relation to immediate allergies involve the administration of a variety of drugs (*e.g.*, cromoglycates, antihistaminics, bronchodilators, and corticosteroids), which may inhibit the release of these mediators from the patient's mast cells and basophils or antagonize the effects of the released vasoactive compounds, and long-term hyposensitization therapy, which consists of a series of injections of the extracts of the offending allergen in small doses, the currently used extracts being crude mixtures also containing constituents to which the patients may not be allergic before treatment. Obviously, the former form of therapy is at best palliative, since it treats the effects of the disease rather than the disease itself, and the latter is inconvenient to the patient, costly, and not consistently effective in bringing about a reduction of the level of IgE antibodies and the sensitivity of the patient's mast cells and basophils.

Clearly, suppression of the production of the appropriate sensitizing antibodies would represent the ultimate aim in developing effective therapeutic

* This research was supported by grants from the Medical Research Council of Canada and the National Institute of Allergy and Infectious Diseases of the National Institutes of Health of Bethesda, Maryland.

55

regimens for the cure, or at least alleviation, of immediate-type allergies. Some progress toward achieving this goal with modified allergens has been made in a number of laboratories in recent years; [13-20] regrettably, the appropriate papers cannot be reviewed here because of space limitations. This article, will, therefore, be limited to a survey of the results of two methods developed in recent years in the author's laboratory for the suppression of IgE responses in experimental animals by conjugates of antigens and haptens with nonimmunogenic, synthetic, hydrophilic polymers, *viz.*, conjugates of antigens with the monomethoxy derivatives of polyethylene glycols (PEG), referred to as mPEG, and conjugates of haptens with polyvinyl alcohols (PVA) or poly(*N*-vinylpyrrolidone) (PVP).

Rationale for Use of Conjugates of PEG and PVA with Allergenic Molecules

In the light of recent cellular and genetic studies of the mechanisms of immune responses, the immunological system may be visualized as a finely tuned homeostatic balance among different types of lymphoid and accessory cells that consists of a complex dynamic network of positive and negative circuits determined by the interaction of these cells *via* their appropriate Lyt and Qa-1 surface markers.[21-25] It is now generally accepted that collaboration between T helper (Th) cells and bursal equivalent lymphocytes (B cells) is a prerequisite for induction of IgM and IgG responses to most protein antigens, *i.e.*, T cell–dependent antigens, and, whereas B lymphocytes are the cells that eventually differentiate to become antibody-synthesizing and -secreting cells, the different subpopulations of T lymphocytes are the cells that are responsible for controlling the magnitude and duration of antibody responses.

Priming the immunological machinery with a carrier may generate, on balance, a population of Th cells that cooperates with B memory cells to produce a population of antibody-secreting cells, or a population of suppressor T (Ts) cells capable of specifically suppressing the antibody response; a third population of amplifier T cells (Ta cells) that enhances the effects of the Th and Ts cells has been also identified.[26a, 26b] Moreover, there is an increasing body of evidence favoring the hypothesis that potential Th cells possess two recognition units (receptors), one for the antigen and the other for the products of the MHC, and that activation of Th cells to most soluble antigens occurs only if the antigen is processed by the macrophages and presented to the T cell membrane in association with the appropriate gene product encoded in the I region of the MHC.[42-44] By contrast, the processing of antigens by macrophages does not seem to be necessary for the activation of Ts cells; in fact, the very opposite appears to be the case.[38, 44]

Accordingly, to test the hypothesis that an antigen in a nonimmunogenic form favors the selective activation of Ts cells, we explored, in our earlier studies, the possibility of converting immunogenic protein antigens to nonimmunogenic derivatives by covalent conjugation with PEG or, in more recent experiments, with mPEG. The choice of PEG was based on the report that catalase and bovine serum albumin (BSA) lost their immunogenicity after conjugation with PEG.[27a, 27b] This concept was further extended to experiments involving conjugates of haptens with the chemically polyfunctional polymers, PVA and PVP; the haptenic groups used for this purpose were the benzylpenicilloyl (BPO), the 2,4-dinitrophenyl (DNP), and the 4-hydroxy-3-iodo-5-nitrophenylacetyl (NIP) groups.

Antigen-PEG Systems

In the initial studies, ovalbumin (OA) and the nondialyzable constituents of ragweed pollen (RAG) were coupled, with the aid of cyanuric chloride, to two batches of PEG with average molecular weights of 6000 and 20 000 daltons, referred to as PEG_6 and PEG_{20}, respectively.[28, 29] These conjugates were shown to be, indeed, nonimmunogenic. Thus, the i.v. administration of OA-PEG and RAG-PEG conjugates into mice did not elicit antibodies to OA and RAG. In addition, these conjugates persisted in circulation for extended periods of at least one month and were capable of suppressing, in an immunologically specific manner, the capacity of the animals to mount primary, as well as secondary, IgE responses to sensitizing doses of DNP_3-OA and RAG. For example, the i.v. administration of a single injection of 1 mg of OA-PEG into mice 4 h before immunization with a sensitizing dose of DNP_3-OA completely suppressed the primary anti-DNP and anti-OA IgE responses and these mice responded very poorly to a further sensitizing dose of DNP_3-OA. By contrast, injection of free PEG_6, of PEG_{20}, or of OA that had been subjected to treatment with the coupling agent (cyanuric chloride) in the absence of PEG, had no effect on the ability of the animals to mount IgE responses to DNP_3-OA. Furthermore, this tolerizing regimen also abrogated the ongoing anti-DNP and anti-OA IgE responses in mice that had been sensitized with DNP_3-OA.[30] However, the anti-DNP response was not affected if these animals were immunized with a sensitizing antigen consisting of DNP coupled to a carrier other than OA. It is also worth noting that administratioin of PEG conjugates also dampened the IgM and IgG antibody responses, but to a much lesser extent than the IgE response. Moreover, it was shown that the transfer of 3×10^7 normal syngeneic spleen cells into mice that had been immunosuppressed even 21 d earlier with OA-PEG_6 did not break their tolerance, *i.e.*, these mice retained their state of immunological refractoriness with respect to the carrier OA in spite of receiving an additional sensitizing dose of DNP_3-OA.

Since PEG has two hydroxyl groups and cyanuric chloride also has two, if not three, reactive groups, the conjugation of allergens to PEG by this method inevitably produces a heterogeneous mixture of high molecular weight copolymers of ill-defined composition, which may contain both inter- and intramolecularly crosslinked allergens. Consequently, in order to produce PEG-allergen conjugates that would consist of PEG molecules grafted directly onto the allergen molecules, without the additional complication of crosslinking the latter, a new coupling procedure was designed using the monofunctional succinylated derivative of mPEG ($mPEG-OCOCH_2CH_2COOH$) and the mixed anhydride method described elsewhere.[31]

With a view to evaluating the general applicability of this method to the preparation of mPEG conjugates of common allergens of clinical relevance, mPEGs with average molecular weights of 2000, 5000, 10 000, and 20 000 were coupled to a series of diverse antigens, *i.e.* OA, RAG, dog albumin (DA), bovine pancreatic ribonuclease, the nondialyzable constituents of the aqueous extracts of Timothy grass pollen (Tim), *Ascaris suum*, and *Micropolyspora faeni*. All these mPEG conjugates markedly depressed the ongoing IgE antibody formation in sensitized animals in spite of additional injections of the sensitizing dose of the appropriate antigen.[31] It should also be pointed out that grafting mPEG molecules onto these antigens led to the abolition of, or a marked reduction in, their allergenicity,[32, 33] which is a highly desirable property of an immunosuppressive preparation if it is to be used for therapeutic purposes; this effect was probably due to the masking or chemical modification of some of the determinants of the original antigenic molecules. Almost coincidentally with the earlier studies conducted in the author's laboratory, King *et al.* reported that their mPEG conjugates of antigen E of RAG, designated as AgE, were significantly less allergenic than AgE [34] and subsequently they confirmed that these mPEG conjugates were capable of inducing a long-lasting depression of IgE antibodies in mice.[35] It is also worth noting that Smorodinsky and coworkers very recently reported that PVP conjugates of Tim suppressed the established IgE response to these allergens in mice.[36] Hence, it would appear that conjugation of different nonimmunogenic hydrophilic polymers with a wide variety of allergens may lead to the production of the corresponding immunosuppressive derivatives.

In an attempt to gain an insight into the molecular characteristics that determine the tolerogenicity of mPEG conjugates, some conjugates of DA and OA of varying degrees of substitution were prepared with mPEG of different molecular weights, and their immunological properties were assessed; the term "degree of substitution" refers to the average number of mPEG molecules grafted onto a protein antigen molecule. Although the effect of these two parameters on the ongoing IgE response was not investigated exhaustively, it appeared, as indicated in TABLE 1, that, for a series of tolerogenic conjugates of the same antigen (*e.g.,* OA) there existed some inverse relationship between the degree of substitution and the molecular weight of mPEG. In other words, a high level of tolerogenicity with a concomitant reduction in or total loss of allergenicity was achieved with a lower degree of substitution using mPEG of increasing molecular weights. On the other hand, subjecting the antigens alone—*i.e.,* in the absence of mPEG-OCOCH$_2$CH$_2$COOH—to the conditions of the coupling reaction did not result in their acquiring tolerogenic properties. Similarly, with the exception of DA, none of the other antigens exerted a detectable suppressive effect when they were administered in their free form in amounts equivalent to the antigen contents of the suppressive doses of the corresponding mPEG conjugates. In spite of the tolerogenic capacity of DA alone, it must be pointed out that the DA-mPEG conjugates had the advantage, over free DA, of having either a markedly reduced or no allergenicity.[31] This result is a further indication that, upon conjugation with mPEG, some of the determinants of the antigenic molecule are modified or rendered sterically inaccessible to antibodies preformed to the original antigen. Hence, in relation to the potential therapeutic use of these conjugates, they are to be preferred to the unmodified antigen that may lead to systemic reactions.

With the aim of establishing the cellular mechanisms underlying the suppression by conjugates of OA-mPEG, the spleen cells of tolerized mice as well as their splenic T and B cell subpopulations were transferred into normal syngeneic recipients that were subsequently immunized with a sensitizing dose of DNP$_3$-OA. As is evident from the results of the experiment illustrated in TABLE 2, whereas splenic B cells of tolerized donors did not possess any suppressive capacity, the unfractionated spleen cell population, as well as the T cells of immunosuppressed mice, undermined the capacity of normal recipients to mount

TABLE 1

THE DEPENDENCE OF TOLEROGENICITY AND ALLERGENICITY OF OA-mPEG$_w$ CONJUGATES ON THE DEGREE OF SUBSTITUTION AND MOLECULAR WEIGHT OF mPEG *

Day	−28	−1	0	PCA 7	PCA 28 — 35
Treatment †	DNP$_3$-OA + Al(OH)$_3$	OA or OA-mPEG$_w$	DNP$_3$-OA + Al(OH)$_3$		DNP$_3$-OA + Al(OH)$_3$

Compound Injected	Degree of Substitution	Anti-OA PCA Titers (Test/Control) ‡		Percentage of Neutralization of PCA §			
		Secondary Response	Tertiary Response	1 µg	10 µg	100 µg	200 µg
OA	0	5430/5880	5790/6460	60	100	100	100
OA-mPEG$_2$	20	980/5880	1430/6460	0	0	90	100
OA-mPEG$_5$	10	2100/11 950	3020/11 750	0	0	0	50
OA-mPEG$_5$	16	870/11 950	850/11 750	0	0	0	50
OA-mPEG$_{10}$	2.8	2820/14 630	3180/12 720	0	0	0	50
OA-mPEG$_{10}$	5.1	1830/14 630	1410/12 720	0	0	0	60
OA-mPEG$_{20}$	2.8	1410/5750	730/5120	0	0	0	50

* The subscript w denotes the average molecular weight of a given mPEG preparation in thousands of daltons.

† A single i.p. dose of the test compound (OA or conjugate; 1 mg per mouse) was injected into primed mice one day before administering the second sensitizing dose of DNP$_3$-OA; control mice received saline instead of the test compound. The sensitizing dose consisted of 1 mg DNP$_3$-OA in the presence of 1 mg Al(OH)$_3$.

‡ The PCA titers refer to the reaginic antibodies in sera at day 7 after secondary and tertiary immunizations.

§ Various amounts of the compounds listed were added to 0.1 ml volumes of the mouse reaginic serum of known anti-OA titer (PCA = 2560) and diluted to a volume of 1.0 ml, and the residual free anti-OA IgE antibodies were determined by PCA assay.[31,32]

TABLE 2

THE NATURE OF SUPPRESSOR CELLS INDUCED WITH OA-mPEG$_{10}$

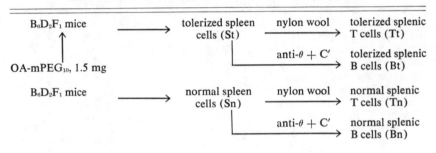

Cells Transferred Into Normal Recipients	PCA Titers	
	Anti-DNP	Anti-OA
No cells	1600	1600
Sn (2×10^7)	1280	1280
Bn (2×10^7)	1280	1260
Tn (2×10^7)	1280	900
St (2×10^7)	160	90
Bt (2×10^7)	1500	1620
Bt (4×10^7)	1590	1700
Tt (6×10^6)	310	290
Tt (2×10^7)	90	120

vigorous anti-DNP and anti-OA IgE responses. Hence, it may be concluded that the immunosuppression caused by injection of OA-mPEG in saline was due primarily, if not exclusively, to the activation of Ts cells. On the other hand, in another experiment, administration of tolerogenic OA-PEG conjugates with Al(OH)$_3$ into normal mice was shown to induce helper activity, as determined by the fact that further immunization of these animals with an injection of DNP$_3$-OA in the presence of Al(OH)$_3$ resulted in both anti-DNP and anti-IgE responses equivalent to those seen in animals that had received two sensitizing injections of DNP$_3$-OA.[37] These findings are reminiscent of the earlier results of Takatsu and Ishizaka who showed, in adoptive transfer experiments, that spleen cells of mice that had been injected with urea-denatured OA in the presence of Al(OH)$_3$ exerted a helper function for anti-DNP IgE and IgG responses when the mice were subsequently immunized with DNP$_3$-OA.[38]

The interpretation that the immunosuppressive effects of the cells transferred from tolerized mice may have been due to the carry-over of tolerogenic quantities of mPEG conjugates, rather than to OA-specific Ts cells, was dispelled by the results illustrated in TABLE 3, which demonstrate that treatment of the recipients of tolerized cells with cyclophosphamide two days before cell transfer obliterated the suppressive capacity of these cells after transfer.[37] This interpretation is based on a previous report by Chiorazzi and colleagues that Ts cells were sensitive to cyclophosphamide.[39] By contrast, pretreatment of the recipients of normal cells with an equivalent dose of cyclophosphamide did not impair the capacity of these animals to mount normal IgE responses and, hence, these results further support the conclusion that the suppression caused by tolerogenic mPEG conjugates was due to carrier-specific Ts cells. Moreover, in preliminary experiments, it has been recently shown that incubation of spleen cells of mice, which had been tolerized with OA-mPEG, with Sepharose-OA conjugates at 37° C for 5 h resulted in the release of soluble factor(s) into the cell-free supernatant, which was capable of suppressing the anti-DNP and anti-OA IgE responses of normal mice receiving this factor before immunization with a sensitizing dose of DNP_3-OA. Further experiments are underway to characterize the physicochemical and immunological nature of this suppressor factor.

Although the exact mechanism responsible for the induction of suppressor cells by OA-mPEG conjugates has yet to be elucidated, it may be concluded that tolerogenic mPEG conjugates led to the activation of carrier-specific Ts cells, which prevented—either directly or *via* soluble factor(s)—the cooperative effect of Th-B_ϵ cell interactions, which normally underly the production of the corresponding strongly T cell–dependent IgE antibody responses.[40, 41] In ac-

TABLE 3

ELIMINATION OF OA-SPECIFIC SUPPRESSOR CELLS BY TREATMENT WITH
CYCLOPHOSPHAMIDE

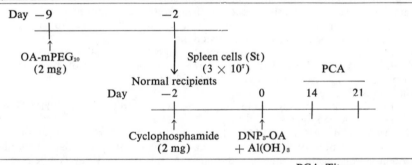

Treatment of Recipient Mice	Day	PCA Titers	
		Anti-DNP	Anti-OA
Day 0: DNP-OA + Al(OH)₃	14	1740	1470
	21	960	1700
Day −2: Cyclophosphamide (2 mg)			
Day 0: DNP-OA + Al(OH)₃	14	1740	1280
	21	1580	1620
Day −2: Normal spleen cells (3 × 10⁷)			
Day 0: DNP-OA + Al(OH)₃	14	1480	1590
	21	870	1590
Day −2: St (3 × 10⁷)			
Day 0: DNP-OA + Al(OH)₃	14	350	320
	21	360	700
Day −2: Cyclophosphamide (2 mg) and St (3 × 10⁷)			
Day 0: DNP-OA + Al(OH)₃	14	1970	1950
	21	1780	1820

cordance with the hypotheses reviewed above, it may be suggested that the immunosuppressive capacity of these conjugates is due to their not being processed readily by macrophages, as evidenced by their extended clearance time. This view is also supported by the experimental results, which indicate that treatment of mice with OA-PEG$_6$ in the presence of Al(OH)$_3$ preferentially stimulated Th cells, whereas injection of mice with OA-PEG$_6$ in the absence of adjuvant predominantly elicited Ts cells.[37] Clearly, the role of the antigen-presenting cells, i.e., of macrophages,[27, 45] in the induction of tolerance with allergen-mPEG conjugates should be investigated.

Hapten-PVA Systems

Whereas, as described above, PEG or mPEG conjugates of common antigens proved to be tolerogenic, DNP$_{1.5}$-PEG conjugates were shown in this laboratory to be devoid of the capacity to suppress the production of anti-hapten IgE antibody responses even in normal mice. Clearly, the epitope density of hapten-PEG conjugates cannot exceed two, since PEG contains only two terminal hydroxyl groups. Hence, a search for synthetic polymers capable of acting as tolerogenic carriers for haptens was initiated. It was thus discovered that the administration of conjugates of haptenic groups (viz., DNP and BPO residues) with the hydrophilic and nonimmunogenic polymer, PVA,[46-50] resulted in an immunologically specific suppression of the corresponding anti-hapten responses not only with respect to IgE antibodies, but also with respect to antibodies belonging to other classes of immunoglobulins. The choice of PVA was based on the fact that PEG and PVA consist, respectively, of the isomeric units (CH$_2$CH$_2$O) and (CH$_2$CHOH); the average molecular weights of the polyvinyl alcohols, PVA$_w$, used were 3000–14 000 daltons, the subscript w representing thousands of daltons.

For these studies, mice were immunized with appropriate sensitizing doses of hapten-OA conjugates, consisting of 1 μg DNP$_3$-OA or 10 μg BPO$_4$-OA in the presence of Al(OH)$_3$). In addition to the fact that the corresponding tolerogenic hapten-PVA conjugates did exclusively suppress hapten-specific responses, i.e., without affecting the anti-OA IgE antibody levels, their most remarkable feature was that they were immunosuppressive even at the low average epitope density of about one. The suppressive effectiveness of these tolerogenic conjugates was dose dependent. Thus, while a single dose of 0.1 mg DNP$_{1.4}$-PVA$_{14}$ significantly depressed an ongoing anti-DNP IgE response, complete suppression of this response was achieved with 1 mg of the conjugate; as would be expected, significantly lower amounts of the conjugate were needed to dampen the primary anti-DNP IgE response.[46, 47]

The unresponsive state of the spleen cells of mice that had been rendered tolerant to DNP was maintained even after cell transfer into x-irradiated (650 rad) syngeneic mice. Moreover, the results listed in TABLE 4 demonstrate that, whereas, in adoptive transfer experiments, the interaction of DNP-specific B cells with OA-specific T cells of primed mice resulted, on challenge of the cell recipients with a sensitizing dose of DNP$_3$-OA, in a marked anti-DNP IgE response, the B cells of mice that had been treated with DNP-PVA cooperated poorly with OA-specific T cells and produced only a low level of anti-DNP IgE antibody; and the B cells of tolerized mice did not affect the cooperation of B and T cells of immune mice in the production of IgE responses.[47] Furthermore, as illustrated in TABLE 5, in x-irradiated, syngeneic recipients (1) the capacity of immune spleen cells to mount a secondary anti-DNP IgE response was suppressed by spleen cells of mice tolerized with DNP-PVA seven days before transfer and (2) the suppressive activity of spleen cells of tolerized mice was due to T cells but not to B cells.

TABLE 4

DEMONSTRATION OF TOLERANCE INDUCTION IN B_ϵ CELLS WITH $DNP_{1.7}$-PVA_{14} IN ADOPTIVE CELL TRANSFER

Day: -120 0 $\rightarrow$ Spleen Cells $\xrightarrow{\text{Anti-}\theta + C'}$ $B_{DNP(p)}$

      $\uparrow$
     DNP-ASC
     $+$ Al(OH)$_3$

Day: -120 -7 0 $\rightarrow$ Spleen Cells $\xrightarrow{\text{Anti-}\theta + C'}$ $B_{DNP(t)}$

      $\uparrow$ $\uparrow$
     DNP-ASC $DNP_{1.7}$-PVA_{14}
     $+$ Al(OH)$_3$ (2 mg)

Day: -90 0 $\rightarrow$ Spleen Cells $\xrightarrow{\text{Nylon Wool}}$ $T_{OA(p)}$

   $\uparrow$
  OA
  $+$ Al(OH)$_3$

Cells (10^7 of Each Type) Transferred into X-Irradiated Recipients	Anti-DNP PCA Titers §
$B_{DNP(p)}$*	< 10
$T_{OA(p)}$†	< 10
$B_{DNP(t)}$‡	< 10
$B_{DNP(p)} + T_{OA(p)}$	380
$B_{DNP(t)} + T_{OA(p)}$	40
$B_{DNP(t)} + B_{DNP(p)} + T_{OA(p)}$	370

    * DNP-primed B cells, designated $B_{DNP(p)}$, were obtained by treatment with anti-θ serum and complement of spleen cells of mice that had been primed with DNP-ASC and Al(OH)$_3$ 120 d before being killed.
    † The OA-primed helper T cells, designated $T_{OA(p)}$, were prepared by passage over a nylon wool column of spleen cells of mice that had been primed with 1 μg OA and 1 mg Al(OH)$_3$ 90 d before being killed.
    ‡ The tolerized spleen cells were obtained from mice that had been primed as described above,* but which also received an i.p. injection of 2 mg $DNP_{1.7}$-PVA_{14} 7 d before being killed. For the preparation of the tolerized B cells, designated $B_{DNP(t)}$, the T cells were destroyed by treatment with anti-θ serum and complement.
    § The x-irradiated recipients were immunized with 10 μg DNP_8-OA immediately after cell transfer and their IgE responses were measured 14 d later.

It is important to stress that, in another experiment, the transfer of spleen cells from mice that had been treated with DNP-PVA seven days before being killed even into normal, nonirradiated, syngeneic mice was shown to result in the impairment of the recipients' capacities to mount an anti-DNP IgE re-

TABLE 5

DEMONSTRATION OF SUPPRESSOR T CELLS IN ADOPTIVE TRANSFER SYSTEM

```
                    7 d
  ────────────┼──────────────→ Tolerized Spleen
              ↑                  Cells (St)
  DNP₁.₄-PVA₁₄
```

$$DNP_{1.4}\text{-}PVA_{14} \xrightarrow{7\ d} \text{Tolerized Spleen Cells (St)} \begin{cases} \xrightarrow{\text{Anti-Ig} + C'} \text{Tolerized Splenic T Cells (Tt)} \\[2ex] \xrightarrow{\text{Anti-}\theta + C'} \text{Tolerized Splenic B Cells (Bt)} \end{cases}$$

$$DNP_{3}\text{-}OA + Al(OH)_{3} \xrightarrow{69\ d} \text{Primed Spleen Cells (Sp)}$$

Groups	Cells Transferred into X-Irradiated Recipients *	PCA Titers † Anti-DNP	PCA Titers † Anti-OA
I	Sp (10⁷)	6460	7250
II	Sp (10⁷) + Sn (4 × 10⁷)	5950	5750
III	St (4 + 10⁷)	< 10	< 10
IV	Sp (10⁷) + St (4 × 10⁷)	1580	7470
V	Sp (10⁷) + Tt (4 × 10⁷)	320	6760
VI	Sp (10ʳ) + Bt (4 × 10⁷)	2580	6840

* The primed spleen cells (Sp) were obtained from mice that had been immunized with a sensitizing dose of DNP₃OA 60 d before being killed. The tolerized spleen cells (St) were obtained from mice that had been treated with 2 mg DNP₁.₄-PVA₁₄ 7 d before being killed. The splenic T (Tt) and B (Bt) cells were prepared by treatment of St with anti-Ig and anti-θ sera, respectively, in the presence of complement. The spleen cells of normal mice are designated Sn.

† Immediately after cell transfer, all x-irradiated recipients were immunized i.p. with 1 μg DNP₃-OA in the presence of 1 mg Al(OH)₃ and their IgE responses were measured 14 d later.

sponse upon immunization with a sensitizing dose of DNP_{3}-OA (*i.e.*, in the presence of 1 mg $Al(OH)_{3}$) without affecting, however, their anti-OA IgE responses. Moreover, the unresponsive state of mice that had been treated 22 days earlier with DNP-PVA could not be broken by the transfer of either normal or immune spleen cells and an additional sensitizing dose of DNP_{3}-OA.[48]

In another experiment, it was shown that treatment of mice presensitized to BPO_{3}-OA with 1 mg $BPO_{1.6}$-PVA_{10} completely abrogated the ability of all these animals to mount a secondary anti-BPO IgE response without affecting the IgE response to OA.[49] Moreover, within nine days of the injection of the tolerogenic conjugate, these animals had become systemically and specifically desensitized, as demonstrated by their refractoriness to i.v. challenge with the polyvalent conjugate of BPO with mouse γ-globulins. By contrast, all the control animals that had received saline instead of BPO-PVA died of anaphylaxis upon injection of this polyvalent conjugate. Similarly, mice in both test and control groups underwent anaphylaxis upon challenge with OA. These findings thus provide further evidence for the specificity of the immunosuppressive effect of hapten-PVA conjugates for the appropriate haptenic determinant.

In more recent experiments, it was demonstrated that a soluble suppressor factor(s) could be isolated from the suppressor cells activated by DNP-PVA by disruption of the cells by sonication, or by freezing and thawing.[50] For this purpose, the suppressor cells were induced by i.p. injection of 1 mg DNP_2-PVA_{14} into mice 14 d before being killed and a suspension of the tolerized spleen cells (St) was prepared in minimum essential medium buffered with 20 mM HEPES (MEM-H) and separated by centrifugation on a Ficoll-Metrizoate density gradient.[51] After being washed twice with MEM-H, the St cells were resuspended in MEM-H at a concentration of 1×10^8 ml^{-1}. A soluble factor was then isolated from these cells by sonication or by six cycles of freezing and thawing of the cells at 78° C and 37° C, respectively. After centrifugation at 15 000 rpm for 15 min, each supernatant (1 ml) was injected i.p. into normal, nonirradiated recipients, which were immunized with a sensitizing dose of DNP_3-OA 4 h later. The IgE responses were measured 14 and 21 d after sensitization. From the results listed in TABLE 6, it is obvious that a soluble factor obtained from St cells by sonication, or by freezing and thawing, was capable of dramatically suppressing the anti-DNP IgE response of the recipients. Moreover, the specificity of the suppression was demonstrated by the fact that the anti-OA IgE response was not affected.

In recent exploratory experiments,[52] the hapten-specific suppressor factor(s) isolated from these St cells (by either sonication or freezing and thawing) have been shown to be nondialyzable, to be precipitable with ammonium sulfate at 50% saturation, and to have a molecular weight of 20 000–50 000, as estimated by gel filtration. Moreover the injection of the suppressor factor(s) from spleen cells of C3H (H-2^k) mice that had been tolerized with DNP-PVA into $B_6D_2F_1$ (H-2$^{b/d}$) mice markedly suppressed the formation of anti-DNP IgE antibodies of the latter. Hence, it may be inferred that the effect of the suppressor factor(s) induced by DNP-PVA is not strain-restricted, as was the case for the IgE class-specific suppressor factor released from Ts cells that had been

TABLE 6

ISOLATION OF SOLUBLE SUPPRESSIVE FACTOR FROM SPLEEN CELLS OF MICE
TOLERIZED WITH DNP_2-PVA_{14}

Treatment of Normal Recipients	Day	PCA Titers	
		Anti-DNP	Anti-OA
Control	14	2000	1900
	21	900	950
Soluble factor *	14	90	1400
	21	40	880
Soluble factor †	14	100	1660
	21	70	1280

* Supernatant (1 ml) from spleen cells (1×10^8 ml^{-1}) of tolerized mice after freezing and thawing six times.

† Supernatant (1 ml) from sonicated spleen cells (1×10^8 ml^{-1}) of tolerized mice; the Biosonik Sonicator (Bronwill Scientific, Rochester, N.Y.) was used at the setting of 50% for 3 min to disintegrate the cells.

generated by injection of conjugates of DNP with *Mycobacterium tuberculosis*.[53] Suppressor factors have also recently been generated by incubation with hapten–Sepharose 4B conjugates of Ts cells from spleens of animals immunosuppressed with hapten-PVA conjugates.

Taking an overall view of the findings reported in this section, these results may be interpreted as indicating that treatment of mice with hapten-PVA conjugates resulted in (1) hapten-specific tolerance of B cells and (2) induction of hapten-specific Ts cells that were capable of strikingly depressing the potential of normal mice, or of immune spleen cells in adoptive transfer experiments, to mount an IgE response to the hapten in question. The latter interpretation, rather than the alternate possible suggestion that the observed dampening of the immunological capacity of the cell recipients was due to the carry-over of the tolerogen along with the transferred cells, was further supported by the finding that the suppressive effect of these cells was eliminated by treatment of the normal recipients with cyclophosphamide two days before cell transfer.[48]

It is also worth noting that conjugates of haptens with three other water-soluble polymers, *viz.*, PVP, polyacrylic acid, and the copolymer of ethylene and maleic anhydride, were shown to behave immunologically in a manner analogous to PVA-hapten conjugates.[54, 55] Thus, all these conjugates induced hapten-specific suppression and the mechanism underlying the down regulation of the corresponding anti-hapten IgE responses was shown to be mediated by suppressor cells.

As stated above, suppressor factor(s) were released from splenic T cells of tolerized mice by disruption of the cells or by exposure of the cells to hapten–Sepharose 4B conjugates. Hence, it may be inferred that these Ts cells and their factor(s) express idiotypic determinants and that the corresponding IgE responses are regulated *via* an idiotype network. Accordingly, it may be visualized that the idiotype positive (id+) Ts cells, and/or their factors, may interfere with the function of id-specific Th cells or, alternatively, may stimulate the activation of second-order idiotype-specific (id-specific) Ts cells.[56] The first suggestion is supported by the recent demonstration that id+ Ts cells regulate the anti-ABA (azobenzene arsonate)[56] and anti-NP (4-hydroxy-3-nitrophenyl-acetyl)[57, 58] delayed-type hypersensitivity responses in A/J and C57BL/6 mice, respectively, and that this type of cell may also underly the mechanism of a number of humoral antibody responses.[59-64]

SUMMARY

A variety of allergens and allergenic haptens can be converted to non-immunogenic and tolerogenic derivatives by conjugation to nonimmunogenic, hydrophilic, synthetic polymers, such as mPEG, PVA, and PVP. The resulting conjugates of common allergens and of small molecules, such as those responsible for drug allergies, can potentially be used therapeutically for the specific suppression of the IgE antibodies that mediate the corresponding allergic manifestations of the immediate type. All these conjugates exert their immunosuppressive effect in mice by activating suppressor T cells; hapten-PVA and hapten-PVP conjugates—as distinct from antigen-mPEG conjugates—also appear to inactive the hapten-specific B cell population.

ACKNOWLEDGMENTS

The studies in the author's laboratory described in this article were conducted in collaboration with his former associate. Dr. W. Y. Lee. The excellent technical assistance of Ms. V. J. Cripps and the expert secretarial assistance of Ms. B. A. Krochak are gratefully acknowledged.

REFERENCES

1. BUTCHER, B. T., J. E. SALVAGGIO, H. WEILL & M. ZIZKIND. 1976. J. Allergy Clin. Immunol. 58: 89–100.
2. CHANG-YEUNG, M., J. J. ASHLEY, P. COREY, G. WILLSON, G. DORKEN & S. GRYZBOWSKI. 1978. J. Occup. Med. 20: 323–27.
3. MACCIA, C. A., I. L. BERNSTEIN & E. A. EMMET. 1976. Am. Rev. Respir. Dis. 113: 701–4.
4. ISHIZAKA, T., K. ISHIZAKA, D. H. CONRAD & A. FROESE. 1978. J. Allergy Clin. Immunol. 61: 320–30.
5. OGAWA, M., K. ISHIZAKA, T. ISHIZAKA, W. D. TERRY, T. A. WALDMANN & O. R. MCINTYRE. 1971. Am. J. Med. 51: 193–99.
6. SHEARD, P., P. KILLINGBACK & A. BLAIR. 1967. Nature (London) 216: 283–84.
7. ORANGE, R., M. VALENTINE & K. AUSTEN. 1968. J. Exp. Med. 127: 767–82.
8. KAY, A., D. STECHSCHULTE & K. AUSTEN. 1971. J. Exp. Med. 133: 602–19.
9. BENVENISTE, J. 1974. Nature (London) 249: 581–82.
10. SEHON, A. H. & L. GYENES. 1971. In Immunological Diseases, Vol. 2, 2nd edit. M. Samter, Ed.: 785–811. Little, Brown. Boston.
11. PARISH, W. E. 1973. In Asthma. K. D. and L. M. Lichtenstein, Eds.: 72–90. Academic Press. New York.
12. TADA, T., K. OKUMURA, B. PLATTEAU, A. BECKERS & H. BAZIN. 1975. Int. Arch. Allergy Appl. Immunol. 48: 116–31.
13. HENOCQ, E., M. GARCELON & L. BERRENS. 1973. Clin. Allergy 3: 461–69.
14. MARSH, D. G. 1975. In The Antigens, Vol. 3. M. Sela, Ed.: 271–359. Academic Press. New York.
15. PATTERSON, R., I. M. SUSZKO, C. R. ZEISS, J. J. PRUZANSKY & E. BACAL. 1978. J. Allergy Clin. Immunol. 61: 28–35.
16. TAKATSU, K. & K. ISHIZAKA. 1975. Cell. Immunol. 20: 276–89.
17. ISHIZAKA, K., H. OKUDAIRA & T. P. KING. 1975. J. Immunol. 114: 110–15.
18. LIU, T.-T., C. A. BOGOWITZ, R. F. BARGATZE, M. ZINNECKER, L. R. KATZ & D. H. KATZ. 1979. J. Immunol. 123: 2456–65.
19. FILION, L. G., W. Y. LEE & A. H. SEHON. 1980. Cell. Immunol. 54: 115–28.
20. USUI, M. & T. MATUHASI. 1979. J. Immunol. 122: 1266–72.
21. BENACERRAF, B. & R. N. GERMAIN. 1979. Fed. Proc. Fed. Am. Soc. Exp. Bio. 38: 2053–57.
22. CANTOR, H. & E. A. BOYSE. 1975. J. Exp. Med. 141: 1376–1389.
23. CANTOR, H. & R. K. GERSHON. 1979. Fed. Proc. Fed. Am. Soc. Exp. Biol. 38: 2058–64.
24. KATZ, D. H. 1977. Lymphocyte Differentiation, Recognition and Regulation. Academic Press. New York.
25. LOOR, F. & G. E. ROELANTS, Eds. 1977. B and T Cells in Immune Recognition. John Wiley and Sons. New York.
26a. MÖLLER, G. Ed. 1975. Suppressor T Lymphocytes, Transplantation Reviews, Vol. 26. Munksgaard. Copenhagen.
26b. MÖLLER, G., Ed. 1978. Role of Macrophages in the Immune Response, Immunological Reviews, Vol. 40. Munksgaard. Copenhagen.

27a. ABUCHOWSKI, A., T. VAN ES, N. C. PALCZUK & F. F. DAVIS. 1977. J. Biol. Chem. **252:** 3578–81.
27b. ABUCHOWSKI, A., J. R. MCCOY, N. C. PALCZUK, T. VAN ES & F. F. DAVIS. 1977. J. Biol. Chem. **252:** 3582–86.
28. LEE, W. Y. & A. H. SEHON. 1977. Nature (London) **267:** 618–19.
29. LEE, W. Y. & A. H. SEHON. 1978. Int. Arch. Allergy Appl. Immunol. **56:** 196–206.
30. LEE, W. Y. & A. H. SEHON. 1978. Immunol. Rev. **41:** 200–47.
31. WIE, S. I., C. W. WIE, W. Y. LEE, L. G. FILION, A. H. SEHON & E. ÅKERBLOM. 1981. Int. Arch. Allergy Appl. Immunol. **64:** 84–99.
32. LEE, W. Y. & A. H. SEHON. 1978. Int. Arch. Allergy Appl. Immunol. **56:** 159–70.
33. HOLFORD-STREVENS, V., W. Y. LEE, K. A. KELLY & A. H. SEHON. 1982. Int. Arch. Allergy Appl. Immunol. **67:** 109–16.
34. KING, T. P., L. KOCHOUMIAN & L. LICHTENSTEIN. 1977. Arch. Biochem. Biophys. **178:** 442–50.
35. KING, T. P., L. KOCHOUMIAN & N. CHIORAZZI. 1979. J. Exp. Med. **149:** 423–36.
36. SMORODINSKY, N., B. U. VON SPECHT, R. CESLA & S. SHALTIEL. 1981. Immunol. Lett. **2:** 305–9.
37. LEE, W. Y., A. H. SEHON & E. ÅKERBLOM. 1981. Int. Arch. Allergy Appl. Immunol. **64:** 110–14.
38. TAKATSU, K. & K. ISHIZAKA. 1977. J. Immunol. **118:** 151–58.
39. CHIORAZZI, N., D. A. FOX & D. H. KATZ. 1976. J. Immunol. **117:** 1629–37.
40. MICHAEL, J. G. & I. L. BERNSTEIN. 1973. J. Immunol. **111:** 1600–1.
41. URBAN, J. F. JR., T. ISHIZAKA & K. ISHIZAKA. 1977. J. Immunol. **118:** 1982–86.
42. ERB, P. & M. FELDMANN. 1975. J. Exp. Med. **142:** 460–72.
43. PIERCE, C. W., J. A. KAPP & B. BENACERRAF. 1977. Cold Spring Harbor Symp. Quant. Biol. **41:** 563–70.
44. SKIDMORE, B. J. & D. H. KATZ. 1977. J. Immunol. **119:** 694–701.
45. SHEVACH, E. & A. S. ROSENTHAL. 1973. J. Exp. Med. **138:** 1213–29.
46. LEE, W. Y. & A. H. SEHON. 1979. Immunol. Lett. **1:** 31–37.
47. HUBBARD, D. A., W. Y. LEE & A. H. SEHON. 1981. J. Immunol. **126:** 407–13.
48. LEE, W. Y. & A. H. SEHON. 1981. J. Immunol. **126:** 414–18.
49. LEE, W. Y., D. A. HUBBARD, V. CRIPPS & A. H. SEHON. 1980. Int. Arch. Allergy Appl. Immunol. **63:** 1–13.
50. LEE, W. Y. & A. H. SEHON. 1981. Immunol. Lett. **2:** 347–52.
51. PARISH, C. R. 1975. In Transplantation Reviews, Vol. 25. G. Möller, Ed.: 98–120.
52. KRUEGER, K. S., W. Y. LEE & A. H. SEHON. 1981. Fed. Proc. Fed. Am. Soc. Exp. Biol. **40:** 964.
53. KISHIMOTO, T., Y. HIRAI, M. SUEMURA, K. NAKANISHI & Y. YAMAMURA. 1978. J. Immunol. **121:** 2106–12.
54. LEE, W. Y., A. H. SEHON & B. U. VON SPECHT. 1981. Eur. J. Immunol. **11:** 13–17.
55. WIE, S. I., C. W. WIE, W. Y. LEE & A. H. SEHON. 1979. Proc. Annu. Meet. Can. Fed. Biol. Soc. **22:** 71.
56. SY, M.-S., M. H. DIETZ, R. N. GERMAIN, B. BENACERRAF & M. I. GREENE. 1980. J. Exp. Med. **151:** 1183–95.
57. WEINBERGER, J., B. BENACERRAF & M. DORF. 1980. J. Exp. Med. **151:** 1413–23.
58. WEINBERGER, J., R. GERMAIN, B. BENACERRAF & M. DORF. 1980. J. Exp. Med. **152:** 161–69.
59. EARDLEY, D., F. W. SHEN, H. CANTOR & R. K. GERSHON. 1979. J. Exp. Med. **150:** 44–50.

60. GERMAIN, R. N., J. THESE, J. A. KAPP & B. BENACERRAF. 1978. J. Exp. Med. 147: 123–36.
61. GERMAIN, R. N., J. THEZE, C. WALTENBAUGH, M. E. DORF & B. BENACERRAF. 1978. J. Immunol. 121: 602–7.
62. GERMAIN, R. & B. BENACERRAF. 1978. J. Immunol. 121: 608–12.
63. HARVEY, M. A., L. ADORINI, A. MILLER & E. SERCARZ. 1979. Nature (London) 281: 594–96.
64. HIRAI, Y. & A. NISONOFF. 1980. J. Exp. Med. 151: 1213–31.

DISCUSSION OF THE PAPER

E. DIENER (*University of Alberta, Edmonton, Alta.*): Alec, you said that you believe that your suppressor cells are idiotype-specific. Have you tried to inhibit them with the idiotype?

SEHON: No, I said that I suspect that they are. This experiment is being planned.

J. CHILLERS (*Scripps Clinic and Research Foundation, La Jolla, Calif.*): If I understand your model, you believe that PEG may be masking certain epitopes on your antigen. Yet you are inducing suppressor cells with PEG-OA. What is the specificity of these suppressor cells, and how are they working on other cells that may be recognizing those determinants?

SEHON: This question has been plaguing us for quite a while. However, this finding is reconcilable with the hypothesis, which is currently in vogue and which had been postulated by Benacerraf, that T cells may be able to recognize even short regions of the antigens, *i.e.,* three or four amino acids, and not necessarily the integral conformation of the antigenic determinants. The fact that tolerogenic conjugates induce a markedly reduced histamine release from sensitized mast cells *in vitro*, or have a reduced allergenicity *in vivo,* is interpreted as indicating that coupling of mPEG molecules to the antigen results in masking or distortion of the antigenic determinant(s) and hence in a reduced binding of the antigen to the IgE molecules fixed on the mast cells. However, this does not mean that the T cells may not be able to interact *in vivo* with a partially hidden determinant. As stated earlier, the main hypothesis for using nonimmunogenic mPEG conjugates was that the macrophages have to be bypassed in order to induce immunological suppression. To examine the validity of this hypothesis, we are studying the effects of pulsed macrophages with OA-PEG. However, this problem is not as simple as it appears at first sight, since even five times recrystallized OA does not consist of a single component, but has been shown to contain at least four constituents in addition to monomeric OA on gel fractionation. Hence, if any of these constituents is not converted to the corresponding tolerogenic PEG conjugates on reaction of the original OA preparation with mPEG, the administration of the complex OA-PEG reaction product would induce suppression only to some and not to all constituents. Moreover, it would be difficult to establish with a heterogenous antigenic mixture which of the constituents is(are) being recognized by the macrophages. Because of these complications, we are attempting to isolate conjugates of OA-PEG that combine neither with preformed anti-OA antibodies nor, presumably, with receptors on B cells by subjecting the crude OA-PEG preparations to solid phase immunoabsorption with anti-OA. Those OA-PEG preparations depleted of conjugated molecules which are still recognizable by anti-OA antibodies will be tested with respect to their tolerogenic capacity and the ability of the macrophages to process them.

D. W. SCOTT (*Duke University Medical School, Durham, N.C.*): That experiment is being done. There's evidence that, after you get to a certain point of PEG modification in the enzyme systems used by the Rutgers group, you no longer have antibody-binding capacity. These are essentially non-immunogenic at that point. Whether they are tolerogenic or "suppressorogenic" is under investigation. This is being studied at Rutgers and in my lab by Dr. Palczuk, who is on sabbatical from Rutgers.

J. A. BERZOFSKY (*National Institutes of Health, Bethesda, Md.*): Would a PEG-modified antigen be incorporated into a cell membrane and will the resulting antigen-modified cell serve as a tolerogen?

SEHON: We haven't tested this idea yet.

SCOTT: That would be a nice experiment.

QUESTION: Have you done it, David?

SCOTT: No.

G. W. SISKIND (*Cornell University Medical College, New York, N.Y.*): As we complete this morning's session, it occurs to me that, ever since tolerance was first described, investigators have been trying to do two things: obtain complete tolerance and place tolerance mechanisms under a single heading—find a unified, single-type mechanism for tolerance. It occurs to me that very few of the systems that we look at have complete or total tolerance. Tolerance is almost always a relative phenomenon, a down regulation, or a reduced production. Secondly, it occurs to me that efforts to put all forms of tolerance under a single rubric may very well be doomed to fail. We have a more complicated system than that.

THE ROLE OF THE T ACCEPTOR CELL
IN SUPPRESSOR SYSTEMS

ANTIGEN-SPECIFIC T SUPPRESSOR FACTOR ACTS VIA A T ACCEPTOR CELL; THIS RELEASES A NONSPECIFIC INHIBITOR OF THE TRANSFER OF CONTACT SENSITIVITY WHEN EXPOSED TO ANTIGEN IN THE CONTEXT OF I-J

Geoffrey L. Asherson

Division of Immunological Medicine
Clinical Research Centre
Watford Road, Harrow, Middlesex HA1 3UJ England

Marek Zembala

Division of Clinical Immunology
Institute of Paediatrics
Copernicus Medical School
Cracow, Poland

INTRODUCTION

The development of our knowledge of suppressor cell systems that influence contact and delayed hypersensitivity may be divided into five stages. The first stage was the recognition of suppressor cells[1, 2] and the realization that T suppressor cells limited contact and delayed hypersensitivity.[1, 3] The second stage was the observation that suppressor cells made antigen-specific factors.[4, 5] The other stages were the recognition of several types of suppressor cells, some of which only acted when given early in the immune response (Ts-aff) and others of which acted at the expression stage in a 24-h experiment (Ts-eff);[6-8] the recognition that some suppressor cells were antigen-driven, while others were anti-idiotype–driven; and the recognition of genetic restrictions in the action of suppressor cells and suppressor factors involving the major histocompatibility complex and, in the case of anti-idiotype suppressor cells, the Igh-V locus that controls the variable region of the immunoglobulin molecules and antigen-specific T cell factors.[11-13]

Recently, attention has shifted to the modes of interaction among the various T suppressor cells. In the idiotype-anti-idiotype link, either a T suppressor cell, variously called Ts_1, Ts^i, or Ts-aff, or an antigen-specific T suppressor factor gives rise to an anti-idiotype suppressor cell by a process of immunization. In the acceptor cell link, a nonspecific inhibitor is produced by an acceptor cell that has been armed with antigen-specific T suppressor factor and subsequently exposed to the corresponding antigen.

FIGURE 1 illustrates the observations on T suppressor cells that depress delayed hypersensitivity to the NP (4-hydroxy-3-nitrophenylacetyl) and the arsanil groups.[12] The injection of haptenized lymphoid cells gave rise to antigen-directed Ts (Ts_1) cells. These cells liberated an antigen-specific T suppressor factor (TSF). The cells or the factor then acted as an immunogen and induced the formation of Ts_2 (Ts^e) in the presence of more antigen. This Ts_2 is an anti-idiotypic suppressor cell; it is interesting to ask why the Ts_1 should act

71

0077–8923/82/0392–0071 $1.75/0 © 1982, NYAS

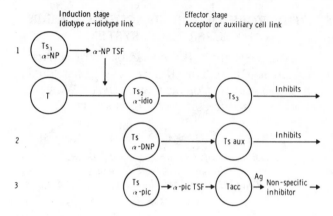

FIGURE 1. The linkages between the T suppressor cells involved in the suppression of contact and delayed hypersensitivity.

Schema 1 illustrates the idiotype-anti-idiotype link in which an anti-NP (4-hydroxy-3-nitrophenylacetyl) T suppressor cell produces an antigen-specific factor. Either the cell or the factor then acts as an immunogen to produce a suppressor anti-idiotypic Ts_2. This Ts_2 does not act directly on the transfer of contact sensitivity, but indirectly through Ts_3.[14, 12]

Schema 2 illustrates an anti-dinitrophenyl T suppressor cell that acts *via* an auxiliary T suppressor cell.[15]

Schema 3 illustrates the T acceptor cell link that is the subject of this paper. An anti-picryl T suppressor cell produces an anti-picryl T suppressor factor. This arms an acceptor T cell that, when exposed to an antigen corresponding in specificity to the TSF, liberates a nonspecific inhibitor of the transfer of contact sensitivity.

as an effective immunogen for its production and why the dominant response should be suppressive. The Ts_2 acted at the expression phase of the delayed hypersensitivity reaction and caused suppression in a 24-h experiment. However, it did not act directly, but indirectly through a Ts_3.[14]

FIGURE 1 also illustrates the auxiliary T suppressor cell of Sy *et al.*[15] The basic observation was that a T suppressor cell acting at the efferent or expression phase of contact sensitivity (Ts-eff) to dinitrofluorobenzene did not act directly, but indirectly through an auxiliary T suppressor cell (Ts-aux). This cell was characterized by the sensitivity of its precursors to cyclophosphamide and adult thymectomy.

THE ACCEPTOR CELL LINK

The concept of the acceptor cell is central to this paper and is illustrated in FIGURE 1. It occurs in the picryl (trinitrophenyl) and oxazolone (4-ethoxy-methylene-2-phenyloxazolone) systems. The injection of water-soluble, chemically reactive hapten gives rise to T suppressor cells, Ts-eff, which act at the expression phase of the contact sensitivity reaction. This cell, or another T cell in the same population, produces antigen-specific T suppressor factor *in vitro*.[16] This TSF has no direct effect on the transfer of contact sensitivity but acts indirectly by arming a cell that may be called an auxiliary or acceptor cell.

This cell, in turn, does not affect contact sensitivity, but releases, when exposed to antigen, a nonspecific inhibitor that may be the proximate cause of suppression.

In fact, there is a close formal analogy between the present schema and the IgE antibody–mast cell system. TABLE 1 illustrates that, in both systems, a specific B or T cell makes an antigen-specific product—IgE or TSF. This product then acts as a mobile receptor and arms an acceptor cell. IgE arms a mast cell or basophil, while TSF arms a T acceptor cell or macrophage.[17, 18] The armed cell can then be triggered by antigen. Mast cells liberate the pharmacological mediator histamine, while T acceptor cells and macrophages [18] liberate nonspecific inhibitors of the transfer of contact sensitivity.

EXPERIMENTAL DETECTION OF THE ACCEPTOR CELL

The detection of the T acceptor cell and of the nonspecific inhibitor is illustrated in FIGURE 2 and the protocol is summarized in TABLE 2. The acceptor cell population is produced by immunization with contact sensitizing agents and the lymph node and spleen cells are then armed by incubation in supernatants containing T suppressor factor. After washing, the cells are exposed to antigen, *i.e.,* haptenized spleen cells, and the supernatant is harvested at 2 h. Finally, this supernatant is tested for its ability to block passive transfer of contact sensitivity by immune cells incubated in it. The cells are injected into mice that are challenged with contact sensitizer on the ear immediately afterwards; contact sensitivity is assessed by the increment of ear thickness at 24 h.

In a typical experiment, the T acceptor cell population was produced by immunization with picryl chloride or oxazolone and either armed with anti-picryl TSF or left unarmed. Finally, the armed population was exposed to antigen. The nonspecific inhibitor was tested for its ability to block passive transfer by cyclo pic cells (four-day picryl immune cells from mice pretreated with cyclophosphamide). FIGURE 3 shows that pic-induced, nylon wool–purified T acceptor cells armed with anti-pic TSF and exposed to picryl antigen cause 69% suppression of contact sensitivity. This did not occur if either the TSF or the antigen were omitted. The lowest three lines show that comparable suppression occurred when the acceptor cell population was produced by immunization with oxazolone. It was concluded that the antigen used to generate the T acceptor cell population was unimportant. Other experiments using a

TABLE 1

ACCEPTOR CELL SYSTEMS

System	Antibody	T Cell Product	
Cell producing specific factor	B cell	T cell	T cell
Antigen-specific factor	IgE	TSF	TSF
Acceptor cell	Mast cell	Tacc	Macrophage
Triggering antigen	Sol. ag	Cell ag	Ag
Nonspecific mediator	Histamine	Nonsp. inhib.	Nonsp. inhib.

NOTE: This scheme illustrates the formal analogy between acceptor cells in the antibody and specific T suppressor factor systems.

Table 2

COMPONENTS OF THE T ACCEPTOR SYSTEM

Production of Ts-eff (cs)	7 d PSA/PCL cells *
Production of ag-specific TSF	48-h supernatant †
Production of Tacc population	4-d PCL or ox ‡ nylon wool T
Arming of Tacc population	Incubation in TSF for 1 h §
Triggering of armed Tacc	Addition of picrylated spleen ‖
Production of nonspecific inhibitor	Incubation for 2 h ¶
Testing of nonspecific inhibitor	4-d ox or cyclo ox cells **

* Picrylsulphonic acid 3.5 mg was administered intravenously on day 0 and day 3. A 5% solution of picryl chloride was painted on day 6. Regional lymph nodes and spleen were harvested on day 7.

† Cells were cultured at 10^7 ml^{-1} in RMPI 1640 with 2.5% inactivated fetal calf serum.

‡ Mice were painted with 5% picryl chloride or 3% oxazolone and regional lymph nodes and spleen were harvested on day 4. Nylon wool T cells were prepared.

§ The T acceptor population was incubated at 3×10^7 ml^{-1} in 0.75 ml TSF, diluted, spun down, and washed once.

‖ Spleen lymphoid cells were picrylated in 10 mM picrylsulphonic acid in pH 6.9 cacodylate buffer for 10 min at room temperature and washed three times. 10^7 cells were used for 3×10^7 armed acceptor cells.

¶ The cells were spun down and resuspended at 40×10^7 ml^{-1} in 2.5% inactivated fetal calf serum and incubated for 2 h.

** Normal mice, or mice given 150 mg kg^{-1} cyclophosphamide intraperitoneally two days beforehand, were painted with 3% oxazolone. Regional lymph node and spleen cells were taken at four days and incubated at 5×10^7 ml^{-1} ($37°$ C, 45 min) in nonspecific inhibitor. Finally, $4-5 \times 10^7$ viable cells were transferred to each of five mice and their ears were painted with 1% oxazolone. Contact sensitivity was assessed by the increment of ear thickness at 24 h in units of 10^{-3} cm $\pm$ s.d

similar protocol showed that normal (nonimmune) spleen and thymus cells lacked T acceptor cell activity and that the precursor of the T acceptor cell was sensitive to cyclophosphamide (150 mg kg^{-1}) and to adult thymectomy performed two weeks beforehand.

THE T ACCEPTOR CELL IS Cy^s, ATx^s, Lyt 1⁻2⁺, I-J⁺, AND Fc^+

The following experiments made use of a modified protocol for the demonstration of acceptor cell activity, which is illustrated in FIGURE 4. The nylon wool–purified T acceptor population was treated with anti-haptene TSF, washed, and then coincubated with immune cells whose specificity corresponded to the TSF. This immune population contains both antigen needed to trigger the release of nonspecific inhibitor [7] and the passive transfer population that is the target for the inhibition. After incubation, the cells were injected into normal mice and the contact sensitivity reaction read at 24 h. This protocol was used to confirm that the generation of, and perhaps the precursor of, the T acceptor cell was sensitive to cyclophosphamide and adult thymectomy (FIGURE 5).

The surface markers of the T acceptor cell were determined by treating the acceptor cell population with antiserum and then panning on $F(ab')_2$ rabbit anti-mouse IgG, as outlined in FIGURE 6. It may be important to use $F(ab')_2$, as the acceptor cell has receptors for Fc. The T acceptor cell was Lyt 1⁻2⁺, as judged by monoclonal antibody kindly provided by I. F. C. McKenzie and I-J⁺ using B10.A (3R) anti-5R serum (FIGURE 7). The cell had receptors for mouse serum immunoglobulin (ammonium sulphate precipitate) and Fc fraction prepared by pepsin digestion and gel filtration. It also had Fc receptors for anti-DNP myeloma IgA that had been purified by affinity chromatography on dinitrophenylated albumin linked to sepharose.

THE T ACCEPTOR CELL HAS RECEPTORS FOR ANTIGEN-SPECIFIC T SUPPRESSOR FACTOR

It is commonly assumed that receptors are on the cell surface, although, in some hormone systems, the receptors are cytoplasmic or nuclear.[19] The following experiment investigated whether the T acceptor cell had surface receptors for TSF and could be panned on haptenized albumin following arming with anti-haptene TSF. The protocol is shown in FIGURE 8. The acceptor cell population was produced by immunization with picryl chloride and armed with

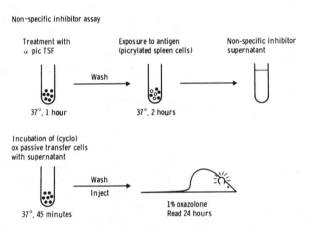

FIGURE 2. An assay for the nonspecific inhibitor of the passive transfer of contact sensitivity. This is a two step assay that detects T acceptor cell activity. In the first step, the nonspecific inhibitor is produced by arming T acceptor cells with TSF and exposing them to antigen. In the second step, the nonspecific inhibitor is assayed. In practice, the acceptor cell population (nylon wool T cells prepared from pooled four-day immune regional lymph node and spleen cells of CBA mice immunized with 0.15 ml 3% oxazolone or 5% picryl chloride) was incubated in anti-picryl TSF. After dilution, centrifugation, and one wash, the cells were mixed with picrylated spleen cells. After centrifugation the cells were resuspended in medium and incubated for 2 h. The inhibitor supernatant was stored at −20° C and tested by incubating passive transfer cells (four-day immune cells from normal mice or mice given cyclophosphamide two days before painting) in it for 45 min. Finally, the cells were washed and injected into groups of five mice. The ears of the recipients were challenged immediately afterwards with contact sensitizer and the increment of ear thickness was measured at 24 h with an engineer's micrometer and expressed in units of 10^{-3} cm ± S.D.[16, 7]

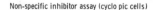

Non-specific inhibitor assay (cyclo pic cells)

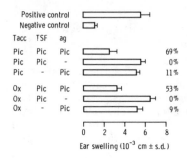

Tacc	TSF	ag		
Positive control				
Negative control				
Pic	Pic	Pic		69%
Pic	Pic	-		0%
Pic	-	Pic		11%
Ox	Pic	Pic		53%
Ox	Pic	-		0%
Ox	-	Pic		9%

0   2   4   6   8
Ear swelling (10⁻³ cm ± s.d.)

FIGURE 3. Production of nonspecific inhibitor of the passive transfer of contact sensitivity by arming T acceptor cell populations with anti-picryl T suppressor factor and exposing them to the corresponding antigen (picrylated spleen cells). The protocol is outlined in FIGURE 2 and TABLE 2. The graph shows contact sensitivity in groups of five recipient mice measured by the increment of ear thickness at 24 h in units of 10^{-3} cm ± S.D. The first-line (positive control) shows the transfer by four-day cyclophosphamide picryl immune cells incubated in medium. The second line (negative control) shows the nonspecific swelling in mice that received no cells. The remaining lines show the transfer by immune cells incubated in supernatants prepared, for instance (line 3), by arming T acceptor cells prepared by immunization with picryl chloride in anti-picryl T suppressor factor and then triggering the release of nonspecific inhibitor with picrylated spleen cells. The percentages refer to the percentage of inhibition of the transfer of contact sensitivity, regarding the differences between the positive and negative control as the greatest possible inhibition, *e.g.*, 0% refers to the absence of inhibition, *i.e.*, the transfer is at least as large as in the positive control.

Acceptor cell assay

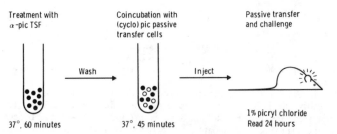

FIGURE 4. A one step assay for acceptor cell activity. This is an abridged version of the two step assay (FIGURE 2). After arming, the T acceptor population is mixed with picryl immune cells (passive transfer cells), preferably from mice pretreated with cyclophosphamide. These cells both provide picryl antigen to trigger the release of nonspecific inhibitor and the passive transfer cells that are the target of its action. In practice, a population of 1.5×10^8 armed T acceptor cells is incubated with 2.5×10^8 passive transfer cells in 10 ml medium. After 45 min, the cells are spun down and resuspended in 5 ml; 1 ml is injected into each of five mice.

Mice from cyclophosphamide-treated cells are preferable because they usually give better transfer and because they would not be affected by TSF, which might leach off the acceptor cell population despite washing.

Acceptor cell assay

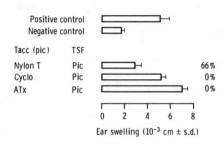

FIGURE 5. An acceptor cell assay illustrating that T acceptor cell activity does not occur in mice pretreated either with cyclophosphamide or by adult thymectomy. Cyclophosphamide (150 mg kg^{-1}) was given two days before painting with picryl chloride and the acceptor cells were taken four days after painting. The mice were thymectomized at five weeks and painted three weeks later.

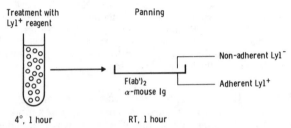

FIGURE 6. The separation of cells into marker positive and marker negative populations by panning. Nylon wool T acceptor cell populations were incubated in antisera such as monoclonal anti-Lyt 1 and anti-Lyt 2 and B10.A(3R) anti-5R at 50×10^7 ml^{-1} for one hour at $4°$ C. After dilution, centrifugation, and washing, 5×10^7 cells in 5% inactivated newborn calf serum were applied to 9-cm diameter bacteriological Petri dishes and allowed to adhere for one hour. The dishes had been coated with 20 μg ml^{-1} F(ab')$_2$ rabbit anti-mouse Ig for two hours and then "neutralized" with 50% inactivated newborn calf serum.

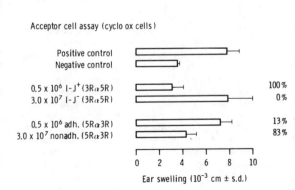

FIGURE 7. An acceptor cell assay illustrating that the T acceptor cell is I-J$^+$. The acceptor cell population was produced by painting CBA mice with picryl chloride and was treated with B10.A(3R) anti-5R (anti-I-J^k) serum at a dilution of 1 to 26. As a control, cells were treated with 5R anti-3R serum (irrelevant anti-I-J). The cells were then panned on Petri dishes coated with affinity purified F(ab')$_2$ rabbit anti-mouse immunoglobulin.

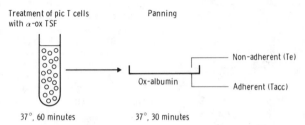

Isolation of T acceptor cell

FIGURE 8. Purification of T acceptor cells by panning. Four-day immune nylon wool T cells were armed under standard conditions with anti-picryl T suppressor factor and washed. Their ability to adhere to Petri dishes coated with oxazolonated albumin was then tested. The adherent cells showed T acceptor cell activity, while the nonadherent cells were inactive. The 9-cm diameter bacteriological Petri dishes were coated with oxazolonated albumin in phosphate buffered saline at 100 μg ml^{-1} for 2 h and "neutralized" with 50% inactivated newborn calf serum. Panning was undertaken under T cell conditions, i.e., centrifugation at 80 g followed by 30 min incubation at 37° C. See also the legend to FIGURE 6.

anti-oxazolone TSF. FIGURE 9 shows that acceptor cell activity was found in the initial population and the population adherent to ox-albumin and was virtually absent from the nonadherent population. It was concluded that there was a receptor for TSF on the surface of acceptor cells and that the antigen-binding site of the bound TSF was exposed and able to cause the acceptor cell to adhere to antigen. Further experiments showed that the acceptor cell did not behave as though it were armed with TSF *in vivo*.

ESTIMATE OF THE NUMBER OF T ACCEPTOR CELLS

An estimate can be formed of the percentage of T acceptor cells in nylon wool–purified T cells from pooled four-day immune lymph node and spleen cells. It is based on the percentage yield of live cells on panning and the observation that the nonadherent cells are depleted of T acceptor cell activity. The percentage of I-J$^+$ cells was 1–3%, of Fc$^+$ cells, 5%, and of cells which have receptors

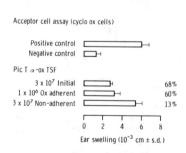

FIGURE 9. Purification of T acceptor cells by arming with anti-oxazolone T suppressor factor and panning on oxazolonated albumin. Nylon wool T, picryl immune cells were armed with anti-oxazolone TSF and then panned under T cell conditions on Petri dishes coated with oxazolonated bovine serum albumin (see FIGURE 8). The acceptor cell activity was then tested by coincubation with "cyclophosphamide" ox immune cells. To make allowances for losses, the 1×10^6 adherent cells were obtained from 4.2×10^7 armed nylon wool T (initial) cells.

for antigen-specific TSF, 2%. If it is assumed that the nonadherent population, which lacks acceptor cell activity, had been depleted of 80% of its acceptor cells, we get an upper limit of around 3%. The actual figure is probably lower, since nonspecific adherence of cells to control plates is 1–2%.

COMPARISON BETWEEN THE T ACCEPTOR CELL AND OTHER AUXILIARY CELLS

The distinctive feature of an acceptor cell is that it is passively armed by an antigen-specific molecule such as TSF and then liberates a nonspecific factor on exposure to antigen. It is not clear which of the auxiliary T cells described in the literature show this feature. TABLE 3 suggests that the acceptor cell in Tada's system, which depresses antibody production, is very similar to the present T acceptor cell.[20, 21] The auxiliary T suppressor cell of Sy et al., which is needed for the action of a T suppressor cell in the system of contact sensitivity to dinitrofluorobenzene, might be the same as the present cell, but the data are incomplete.[15] The fact that it adheres to nylon wool might be due to minor variations in technique. The Ts_3 of Benacerraf appears to be different, as specific immunization is required for its production.[11, 12] However, it is possible that the control mode of immunization was inappropriate for generating Ts_3.

The present system is different from the acceptor cell system in which anti-picryl and anti-oxazolone TSF act via a macrophage.[17, 18] In particular, the macrophage system is based on a plastic-adherent Thy 1⁻ cell while the present system is based on a nylon wool–nonadherent Lyt 2⁺ cell. Moreover, the nonspecific inhibitor in the macrophage system has a molecular weight on gel filtration of around 10 000–20 000, while the nonspecific inhibitor in the present system has a molecular weight of 30 000–40 000 daltons on Sephadex G-100 gel filtration.

It is puzzling that, although the T suppressor cell produced by painting with

TABLE 3

COMPARISON OF THE PROPERTIES OF THE T ACCEPTOR CELL
WITH THE Ts-AUXILIARY CELL OF SY et al.,[15] THE Ts₃ OF BENACERRAF'S GROUP,[14]
AND THE T ACCEPTOR CELL OF TADA'S GROUP [20, 21]

	Tacc (cs)	Ts-aux (cs)	Ts₃ (cs-dh)	Tacc (ab)
Immunization required for generation	yes	yes	yes	yes
Specific immunization required	no	—	—	—
Final nonspecific effect	yes	—	—	yes
Soluble nonspecific inhibitor	yes	—	—	—
Precursor sensitivity to cyclophosphamide	yes	yes	yes	yes
Precursor sensitivity to adult thymectomy	yes	yes	—	yes
Lyt 1⁻ 2⁺	yes	yes	Lyt 2⁺	yes
I-J⁺	yes	yes	yes	yes
Fc receptor	yes	—	—	—
Genetic restriction	I-J	—	Ia	I-J
Armed by specific T suppressor factor	yes	—	—	yes

supraoptimal doses of dinitrofluorobenzene acts *via* an auxiliary T cell, the anti-DNP TSF produced by cells from mice injected with dinitrobenzenesulphonic acid apparently acts directly on the passive transfer cell.[22] In particular, it has been reported to act on cells from mice treated with cyclophosphamide and not to cause suppression when peritoneal exudate cells are used as acceptor cells. Moorhead has also reported that the anti-DNP TSF, unlike the anti-picryl TSF, cannot be absorbed by haptenized albumin linked to sepharose, is K and D and not I-J restricted in its action[23] and in its absorption by four-day specifically immune cells, and has I-C and not I-J determinants.[22]

I-J Region Genetic Restriction between the Mouse Producing TSF and the Antigen Triggering the Release of Nonspecific Inhibitor

In the acceptor cell system, it is possible to vary the genotype of the mouse in which the TSF is produced, the genotype of the acceptor cell population, the genotype of the cells on which the triggering antigen is presented, and the genotype of the immune population on which the nonspecific inhibitor is tested. Analysis shows that the nonspecific inhibitor is not genetically restricted in its action and that the genotype of the acceptor cell is unimportant. However, there is a genetic restriction between the mouse used to produce the TSF and the haptenized cell used to trigger the acceptor cell. FIGURE 10 shows a typical experiment.

Further experiments using the congenic B10.A series in which TSF was prepared in B10.A and B10.A (3R) mice showed that genetic matching in I-J was both necessary and sufficient. In particular, haptenized 5R cells (I-J different, other loci identical) failed to trigger.

Structure of T Suppressor Factor: An Antigen-Combining Site and the I-J Gene Product Recognition Site Occur on the Same Molecular Complex

The question was asked whether there were two separate molecules in crude T suppressor factor supernatants: one that binds hapten and another that recognizes the I-J gene product. It is known that TSF binds to haptenized albumin on sepharose and can be eluted with hapten.[16] In the following experiment, diaminohexane was linked to microcrystalline cellulose using sodium periodate and reduction with sodium borohydride and then picrylated or oxazolonated.[25] After absorption, the TSF was eluted with the appropriate picryl or oxazolone-ϵ-aminocaproic acid. FIGURE 11 shows that both the crude and purified factors were genetically restricted. It was concluded that the molecular complex recognizing the I-J gene product also carried a binding site for the haptene.

FIGURE 12 shows the simplest structure for the antigen-specific T suppressor factor that embodies these features. The model shows two binding sites—one for the I-J product and one for the hapten. It is not known whether these form one large site or two separate domains, but the binding to the hapten site is strong enough to allow absorption to haptenized beads and subsequent elution. There is also a binding site for the acceptor cell. Finally, the model should allow for the fact that TSF is itself I-J$^+$ and there is evidence based on

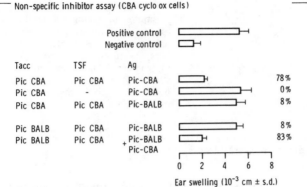

Non-specific inhibitor assay (CBA cyclo ox cells)

FIGURE 10. The genetic restriction between the source of the T suppressor factor and the antigen used to trigger the T acceptor cell. T acceptor cell populations were prepared in either CBA or Balb/c mice. They were then armed with anti-picryl TSF prepared in CBA mice and triggered by picrylated CBA or Balb/c spleen cells. Note that inhibitor supernatant was only produced when the genotypes of the source of both the TSF and the triggering antigen were the same. The last line shows that picrylated Balb/c spleen cells did not interfere with the ability of picrylated CBA cells to trigger acceptor cells armed with CBA TSF.

hybridoma TSF that the I-J site is a separate chain that is not covalently linked to the molecule bearing the antigen-combining site.[26] This model should be considered against the background of current knowledge of the structure of TSF. It has a molecular weight of around 70 000 daltons. Work based on binding to haptenized beads, radio-iodination *in situ* and specific elution with low-molecular-weight hapten followed by SDS polyacrylamide gel electrophoresis suggests that the antigen-binding molecule has two moieties. These are at

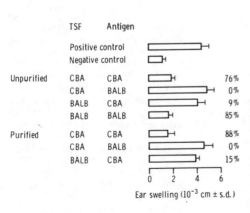

FIGURE 11. The genetic restriction in the action of crude and purified T suppressor factor: the restriction lies between the mouse in which the TSF was prepared and the antigen (haptenized spleen cell) used to trigger the release of nonspecific inhibitor. Picryl acceptor cells were armed with anti-picryl TSF prepared in CBA or Balb/c mice. The purified TSF was prepared by absorption onto pic-rylated microcrystalline cellulose and elution with 3 mg ml^{-1} picryl-ϵ-aminocaproic acid.[25, 16] Losses of 50% of the starting material were assumed. The triggering antigen was picrylated CBA or Balb/c spleen cells and the nonspecific inhibitor was tested on oxazolone passive transfer cells.

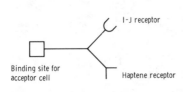

FIGURE 12. Diagram of the antigen-specific T suppressor factor. Note the binding site(s) for the acceptor cell, the hapten, and the I-J determinant. The hapten and the I-J binding sites are shown as separate, but the question of whether or not they form one large site is still very interesting. The suppressor factor bears I-J determinants, but this is not shown in the diagram.[22]

27 000 and 48 000 daltons and are distinct from γ and μ heavy chains and κ and λ light chains on fingerprinting.[25, 25a]

THE REQUIREMENTS FOR TRIGGERING THE T ACCEPTOR CELL

Monovalent antigen does not trigger mast cells coated with specific IgE. However, mast cells coated with IgE against two separate haptenic determinants can be triggered by simple synthetic molecules that bear both haptens univalently. This is interpreted as showing that cross-linking of IgE is required for the triggering of histamine release by mast cells.[28] A similar experiment, which asked whether cross-linking of the hapten-binding site and the I-J recognition site on different molecules of T suppressor factors leads to triggering of the acceptor cell, was undertaken in the present system. In practice, the CBA acceptor cell was armed with anti-oxazolone TSF from a CBA mouse and anti-picryl TSF from a Balb/c mouse. This cell is readily triggered to release nonspecific inhibitor by oxazolonated CBA cells or picrylated Balb cells but is unaffected by picrylated CBA cells (FIGURE 13). It may be inferred that occupancy or cross-linking of both the hapten and the I-J recognition site on a single molecule is required. This does not exclude the possibility that cross-linking of separate TSF molecules is required but that binding at the I-J site or the picryl site alone is readily reversible and hence too weak to allow stable cross-linking.

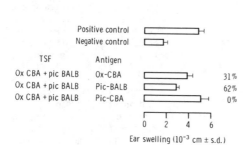

FIGURE 13. The failure of crossed antigen (picrylated CBA spleen cell) to liberate nonspecific inhibitor from a T acceptor cell armed with anti-oxazolone TSF from a CBA mouse and anti-picryl TSF from a Balb/c mouse. Four-day immune ox cells (15×10^8) served as a source of T acceptor cells and were armed with a mixture of 4 ml anti-oxazolone TSF (CBA) and 4 ml anti-picryl TSF (Balb/c). They were then triggered either with the appropriate antigen, *i.e.*, oxazolonated CBA spleen cells or picrylated Balb cells, or with crossed antigen, *i.e.*, picrylated CBA cells. The inhibitor supernatant was tested on picryl passive transfer cells.

THE ROLE OF THE I-J GENE PRODUCTS IN T SUPPRESSOR CELL SYSTEM

In considering the role of I-J gene products, it is important to remember that this is a complex locus and that the I-J antigen on T suppressor cells is different from the I-J antigen on acceptor cells and on antigen-presenting cells (macrophages).[29, 30] Hence, it is not clear that the products recognized by the sera are the same as the products responsible for genetic restriction.

TABLE 4 summarizes the involvement of I-J gene products in suppressor cell systems. The Ts-eff in the picryl system is I-J$^+$; this is true of some but not all suppressor T cells. Similarly, anti-picryl TSF, anti-idiotypic TSF, and some monoclonal TSF bear I-J determinants, but this is not true for anti-DNP TSF.[9, 22, 31, 32] The various acceptor cells (TABLE 3) are I-J$^+$. Moreover, in the present system and in an antibody suppressor system,[21] there is an I-J restriction between the TSF and the triggering antigen.

Ia restriction has been observed in the NP system.[33] Furthermore, I-J differences favor the occurrence of neonatal tolerance and inhibit the mixed lymphocyte reaction and the activation of macrophages,[34-36] and favor the differentiation of a primed T suppressor cell into an active cell.[37]

TABLE 4

THE I-J LOCUS AND SUPPRESSOR T CELL SYSTEMS

The T suppressor cell, the T suppressor factor, and the T acceptor and auxiliary T suppressor cells are I-J$^+$

I-J genetic restriction in the action of TSF
I-J differences favor neonatal tolerance
I-J differences limit mixed lymphocyte reaction
I-J differences limit activation of macrophages
I-J differences "activate" primed T suppressor cells

Mitchison suggested that antigen presented in the context of I-J was the induction signal for T suppressor cell responses.[35] This is shown diagrammatically in FIGURE 14. The antigen-presenting cell, which might be an I-J$^+$ macrophage [29] or a Langerhans cell or a T cell,[38] presents the antigen in the context of I-J. This is recognized by a virgin suppressor cell with receptors for both antigen and I-J that differentiates into a T suppressor cell. This Ts is I-J$^+$ and has receptors for both I-J and antigen and releases TSF bearing these two receptors. When this TSF arms the T acceptor cell, triggering requires occupancy of both the I-J and the antigen receptor sites. In other words, the genetic restriction between the TSF and the triggering antigen is a natural consequence of the induction of the Ts by an I-J$^+$ cell and the recognition of private (strain-specific) and not public (group-specific) determinants on the I-J molecule. In fact, the major histocompatibility (MHC) restriction in cytotoxic killing is explained in the same way, i.e., the virgin cytotoxic T cell is induced by hapten in the context of MHC by virtue of receptors for both MHC and hapten determinants and the cytotoxic T cell recognizes and kills targets with the same determinants. In support of this view there is now formal evidence for MHC-restricted antigen binding by a T hybridoma clone.[39]

The view that antigen in the context of I-J leads to a T suppressor cell response may explain the production of suppressor anti-idiotypic T cell responses. It is known that certain antigen-directed T suppressor cells and T suppressor factors induce an anti-idiotypic T suppressor response. The question arises as to why this is a suppressor and not a helper response. One possible explanation follows from the observation that the Ts_1 is I-J+ and that the TSF product is I-J+ and may attach to an I-J+ cell. Under these circumstances, the idiotype may be seen in the context of I-J. Following Mitchison's principle, this may induce a suppressor response. Similarly, the fact that the acceptor cell is I-J+ and has Fc receptors raises the question of whether or not immune complexes adhere to the acceptor cell that presents them in the context of I-J and generates anti-idiotypic T suppressor response.

The hypothesis that antigen in the context of I-J is an induction signal for the T suppressor cell response is well supported by the evidence. However, not all antigen presented in the context of I-J gives rise to an overt suppressor cell

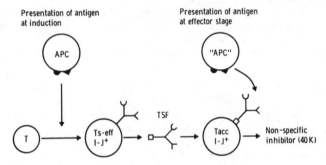

FIGURE 14. A diagram explaining the I-J genetic restriction in terms of the hypothesis that antigen in the context of I-J is the induction signal for a suppressor T cell response. The diagram shows an I-J+ antigen-presenting cell (APC), which may be a macrophage or T cell, with hapten on its surface. A virgin T cell with receptors for both I-J and the hapten sees the APC and differentiates into a Ts-eff cell with the same receptors. This cell makes the TSF that arms the T acceptor cell. Finally, the T acceptor cell is triggered to release nonspecific inhibitor when it meets an APC with hapten on its surface that can occupy both the hapten and the I-J receptor sites on the TSF. It is interesting that the initial antigen-presenting cell, the Ts-eff, the TSF, the T acceptor cell, and the final antigen-presenting cell are all I-J+.

response,[29] while some antigen-specific T suppressor factors are unrestricted, or K and D restricted, in their action [40, 41] and not I-J restricted. In fact, it may be necessary to determine which of the several I-J gene products provides the induction signal for T suppressor cells and it is likely that presentation in the context of I-J is only one of several ways of inducing suppressor cells. In any event, the hypothesis illustrates a possible role of major histocompatibility antigens in determining the class of the immune response.[35]

SUMMARY

Specific T suppressor factor works through a T suppressor cell. This cell, when armed with T suppressor factor, releases a nonspecific inhibitor of the passive transfer of contact sensitivity when exposed to hapten corresponding in specificity to the T suppressor factor and not to the acceptor cell.

The T acceptor cell is Lyt 1^-2^+, I-J$^+$, and Fc$^+$, and its generation is sensitive to cyclophosphamide and adult thymectomy. Immunization is needed for its genesis, but the precise antigen is not important.

There is a genetic restriction between the mouse used to produce the TSF and the haptenized cell used to trigger the release of the nonspecific inhibitor from the acceptor cell. The genotype of the acceptor cell is unimportant.

T suppressor factor adheres to the T acceptor cell; this can be used as a basis for purifying the cell by panning on antigen corresponding to the TSF. This provides an estimate of the number of T acceptor cells four days after immunization of 1–2% pooled lymph node and spleen T cells.

When an acceptor cell is armed with two different TSF, e.g., anti-oxazolone TSF from a CBA mouse and anti-picryl TSF from a Balb/c mouse, it cannot be triggered by crossed antigen, i.e., picrylated CBA spleen cells.

These findings lead to a model of T suppressor factor with a binding site for hapten, a second binding site for I-J, and a third site for binding to the acceptor cell. Triggering of the acceptor cell requires occupancy of the hapten and the I-J binding sites of a single molecule. Whether cross-linking between molecules is required is not known.

The I-J genetic restriction is explained on the basis of the recent hypothesis that antigen in the context of I-J is the induction signal for T suppressor cells and that the T suppressor cell and its products have recognition sites for both hapten and the private (i.e., strain-specific) sites of I-J gene products. This implies that the same I-J gene product must be present on the "antigen-presenting cell" that triggers the release of nonspecific inhibitor from the T acceptor cell armed with T suppressor factor and on the antigen-presenting cell that induces the production of T suppressor factor.

The idiotype-directed Ts$_2$ is known to result from immunization with antigen-specific T suppressor factor, which is I-J$^+$. The hypothesis that antigen in the context of I-J is the signal for the suppressor cell response offers a simple explanation of why the T suppressor factor generates a suppressor anti-idiotype response.

ACKNOWLEDGMENTS

We wish to thank the members of the department of Immunological Medicine who have helped in this work and, in particular, Vittoria Colizzi, Bridget James, Valerie Stein, and Madeleine Watkins. Marek Zembala thanks the Wellcome Trust and the Polish Academy of Sciences, grant no. 10.5, for financial support.

REFERENCES

1. GERSHON, R. K. & H. KONDO. 1971. Infectious immunological tolerance. Immunology 21: 903.
2. ASHERSON, G. L., M. ZEMBALA & R. M. R. BARNES. 1971. The mechanism of immunological unresponsiveness to picryl chloride and the possible role of antibody mediated depression. Clin. Exp. Immunol. 9: 111.
3. ZEMBALA, M. & G. L. ASHERSON. 1974. T cell suppression of the T cell phenomenon of contact sensitivity. Nature (London) 244: 227.

4. TADA, T., K. OKUMURA & M. TANIGUCHI. 1973. Regulation of homocyto-tropic antibody formation in the rat. VIII. An antigen specific T cell factor that regulates anti-haptene homocytotropic antibody response. J. Immunol. **111:** 952.

5. ZEMBALA, M. & G. L. ASHERSON. 1974. T cell suppression of contact sensitivity in the mouse: The role of soluble suppressor factor and its inter-action with macrophages. Eur. J. Immunol. **4:** 804.

6. MILLER, S. D., M. S. SY & M. W. CLAMAN. 1978. Suppressor T cell mecha-nisms in contact sensitivity. I. Efferent blockade by syninduced suppressor T cells. J. Immunol. **112:** 265.

7. ASHERSON, G. L., M. ZEMBALA, W. R. THOMAS & M. A. C. C. PERERA. 1980. Suppressor cells and the handling of antigen. Immunol. Rev. **50:** 3.

8. THOMAS, W. R., M. C. WATKINS & G. L. ASHERSON. 1981. Differences in the ability of T cells to suppress the induction and expression of contact sensitivity. Immunology **42:** 53.

9. GERMAIN, R. N. & B. BENACERRAF. 1980. Helper and suppressor T cell factors. Springer Sem. Immunopath. **3:** 93.

10. MOORHEAD, J. W. & H. N. CLAMAN. 1979. Regulation of cell mediated im-munity by antibodies: Possible role of anti-receptor antibodies in the regula-tion of contact sensitivity of DNFB in mice. J. Immunol. **123:** 2593.

11. CLAMAN, H. N. 1980. Control of experimental contact sensitivity. Adv. Im-munol. **30:** 151.

12. GERMAIN, R. N. & B. BENACERRAF. 1981. A single major pathway of T-lymphocyte interactions in antigen-specific immune suppression. Scand. J. Immunol. **13:** 1.

13. SY, M. S., A. BROWN, B. A. BACH, B. BENACERRAF, P. D. GOTTLIEB, A. NISONOFF & M. I. GREENE. 1981. Genetic and serological analysis of the expression of the crossreactive idiotypic determinants on anti-p-azobenzenearsonate anti-bodies and p-azobenzenearsonate-specific suppressor T cell factor. Proc. Nat. Acad. Sci. USA **78:** 1143.

14. SUNDAY, M. E., B. BENACERRAF & M. E. DORF. 1981. Hapten-specific T cell responses to 4-hydroxy-3-nitrophenylacetyl. VIII. Suppressor cell pathways in cutaneous sensitivity responses. J. Exp. Med. **153:** 811.

15. SY, M. S., S. D. MILLER, J. W. MOORHEAD & H. N. CLAMAN. 1979. Active suppression of 1-fluoro-2,4-dinitrobenzene immune T cells. Requirement for an auxiliary T cell induced by antigen. J. Exp. Med. **149:** 1197.

16. ASHERSON, G. L. & M. ZEMBALA. 1980. T suppressor cells and suppressor factor which act at the efferent stage of contact sensitivity reaction: Their production in mice injected with water soluble, chemically reactive deriva-tives of oxazolone and picryl chloride. Immunology **4:** 1005.

17. PTAK, W., M. ZEMBALA, G. L. ASHERSON & J. MARCINKIEWICZ. 1981. In-hibition of contact sensitivity by macrophages. Int. Arch. Allergy Appl. Immunol. **65:** 121.

18. PTAK, W., M. ZEMBALA, M. HANCZAKOWSKA-RECKLICKA & G. L. ASHERSON. 1978. Non-specific macrophage suppressor factor: Its role in the inhibition of contact sensitivity to picryl chloride by specific T suppressor factor. Eur. J. Immunol. **8:** 645.

19. BAXTER, J. D., N. L. EBERHARDT, J. W. APRILETTI *et al.* 1979. Thyroid hormone receptor and responses. Recent Prog. Horm. Res. **35:** 97.

20. TANIGUCHI, M., T. TADA & T. TAKUHISA. 1976. Properties of the antigen specific suppressive T-cell factor in the regulation of antibody response of the mouse. III. Dual gene control of the T-cell-mediated suppression of the antibody response. J. Exp. Med. **144:** 20.

21. TANIGUCHI, M. & T. TOKUHISA. 1980. Cellular consequences of the suppres-sion of antibody response by antigen specific T cell factor. J. Exp. Med. **151:** 517.

22. MOORHEAD, J. W. 1979. Soluble factors in tolerance and contact sensitivity to 2,4-dinitrofluorobenzene in mice. III. Histocompatibility antigens associated with the hapten dinitrophenyl serve as target molecules on 2,4-dinitrofluorobenzene immune T cells for soluble suppressor factor. J. Exp. Med. **150:** 1432.

23. MOORHEAD, J. W. 1977. Soluble factors in tolerance and contact sensitivity to PNFB in mice. II. Genetic requirements for suppression of contact sensitivity by soluble suppressor factor. J. Immunol. **119:** 1773.

24. ZEMBALA, M., G. L. ASHERSON & V. COLIZZI. 1982. Haptene-specific T suppressor factor recognises both haptene and I-J region products on haptenized spleen cells. Nature (London) **297.** In press.

25. SKIBINSKI, G., G. L. ASHERSON, B. JAMES, H. HOLLIMAN, N. RICHARDSON, A. FROGGATT, M. GLENNIE, D. SYMONS & M. TAUSSIG. Structural studies on specific antigen-binding molecules from T cells. Submitted.

25a. TAUSSIG, M. J., G. L. ASHERSON, A. HOLLIMAN, N. RICHARDSON & G. SKIBINSKI. 1982. Structural and functional studies on antigen-specific suppressor factors from T cells and T cell hybrids. Curr. Top. Microbiol. Immunol. **100:** 43.

26. TANIGUCHI, M., I. TAKEI & T. TADA. 1980. Functional and molecular organisation of an antigen-specific suppressor factor from a T cell hybridoma. Nature (London) **283:** 227.

27. ASHERSON, G. L., M. ZEMBALA, B. MAYHEW & J. KREJCI. 1975. *In vitro* absorption and molecular weight of specific T cell suppressor factor. Nature (London) **72:** 253.

28. SIRAGANIAN, R. P., W. A. HOOK & B. B. LEVINE. 1975. Histamine release from basophils. Activation by bivalent haptenes. Immunochemistry **12:** 149.

29. NIEDERHUBER, J. E., P. ALLEN & O. L. MAY. 1979. The expression of Ia antigenic determinants on macrophages required for the *in vitro* antibody response. J. Immunol. **122:** 1342.

30. HABU, S., K. YAMAUCHI, R. K. GERSHON & D. B. MURPHY. 1981. A non T:non B cell bears 1-A, 1-E, 1-J and Tla (Qa-1?) determinants. Immunogenetics **13:** 215.

31. NOONAN, F. P. & W. J. HALLIDAY. 1980. Genetic restrictions of the serum factor mediated tolerance in trinitrochlorobenzene hypersensitivity. Cell. Immunol. **50:** 41.

32. LIEW, F. Y., D. Y. SIA, C. R. PARISH & I. F. C. McKENZIE. 1980. Major histocompatibility gene complex (MHC) coded determinants on antigen specific suppressor factor for delayed-type hypersensitivity and surface phenotypes of cells producing the factor. Eur. J. Immunol. **10:** 305.

33. OKUDA, K., M. MINAMI, D. H. SHERR & M. E. DORF. 1981. Hapten-specific T cell responses to 4-hydroxy-3-nitrophenyl acetyl. XI. Pseudogenetic restrictions of hybridoma suppressor factor. J. Exp. Med. **154:** 468.

34. STREILEIN, J. W. & J. KLEIN. 1980. Neonatal tolerance of H-2 alloantigens. I. I region modulation of tolerogenic potential of K and D antigens. Proc. R. Soc. London **207:** 461.

35. CZITROM, A. A., G. H. SUNSHINE & N. A. MITCHISON. 1980. Suppression of the proliferative response to H-2D by I-J subregion gene products. Immunogenetics **11:** 97.

36. ZINKERNAGEL, R. M. 1980. Activation of suppression of bacteriocidal activity of macrophages during a graft-versus-host reaction against I-A and I-J region differences, respectively. Immunogenetics **10:** 373.

37. BROMBERG, J. S., B. BENACERRAF & M. H. GREENE. 1981. Mechanisms of regulation of cell-mediated immunity. VII. Suppressor T cells induced by suboptimal doses of antigen plus an I-J specific allogeneic effect. J. Exp. Med. **153:** 437.

38. THOMAS, W. R., A. J. EDWARDS, M. C. WATKINS & G. L. ASHERSON. 1980. Distribution of immunogenic cells after painting with the contact sensitizers— fluorescein isothiocyanate and oxazolone; different sensitizers form immunogenic complexes with different cells. Immunology **39:** 21.
39. LONAI, P., J. PURI & G. HAMMERLING. 1978. H-2 restricted antigen binding by a hybridoma clone that produces antigen specific helper factor. Proc. Nat. Acad. Sci. USA **78:** 549.
40. KONTIAINEN, S. & M. FELDMANN. 1978. Suppressor-cell induction in vitro IV. target of antigen-specific suppressor factor and its genetic relationships. J. Exp. Med. **147:** 116.
41. LIEW, F. Y. & W. L. CHAN-LIEW. 1978. Regulation of delayed-type hypersensitivity. II. Specific suppressor factor for delayed-type hypersensitivity to sheep erythrocytes in mice. Eur. J. Immunol. **8:** 167.

DISCUSSION OF THE PAPER

G. M. SHEARER (*National Cancer Institute, Bethesda, Md.*): Geoffrey, I want to congratulate you on a most beautiful piece of work, and am delighted that you are showing so clearly that the unkind view that I-J doesn't exist is not true. It's a restricting element for the suppressor cell as your data, as well as ours and others, have shown.

The other point of importance is a demonstration that the cell you call the acceptor cell, which I think would be identical to the auxiliary cell or the Ts_3 cell, could be coated with more than one specificity. Do you have any data on that point?

ASHERSON: Yes. You can arm the cell with anti-picryl and anti-oxazolone T suppressor factor *in vitro*, and then you can trigger it with either. You can't trigger it with what I might call a cross immunogen, with the I-J corresponding to one factor and the hapten corresponding to the other factor. *In vivo*, the T acceptor cell four days after immunization does not behave as though it's armed *in vivo* with factor. You can't pull it out on an antigen plate.

QUESTION: I wonder how you have dealt with the conundrum of a cell and a factor having a molecule or a determinant on it, and yet appearing to be specifically restricted by something coming from the same genetic region?

ASHERSON: I think this point needs further exploration. It's known from several people's work, probably dating back to Tada, that the antisera against the I-J locus behave as though they recognize two different antigenic determinants. Before speculating in this area, I would really like to know whether the I-J product on the T suppressor factor is the same I-J product as that on the acceptor cell.

J. R. BATTISTO (*Cleveland Clinic Foundation, Cleveland, Oh.*): Have you tried blocking the portion of TSF that attaches to the acceptor cell to see if the TSF is still active?

ASHERSON: No.

BATTISTO: For instance, one might put TSF on the acceptor cell and then lyse it so as to have portions of the membrane attached to the TSF. Would the TSF still be active?

ASHERSON: I think that's a very nice thought. We have done some immunochemical studies that consisted of binding the material to antigen and then labeling it; we found that the T suppressor supernatant contains an antigen-binding molecule that, on SDS, has 48 000 and 27 000 M.W. components with appropriate specificity controls, and that neither of these are immunoglobulin.[25, 25a] But, because we use SDS polyacrylamide, we haven't got products that have been suitable for back-testing to see if we could get an isolated part of the molecule that would bind onto the cell. But I think that this—in principle—could be done, and would be rather exciting.

H. N. CLAMAN (*University of Colorado Medical School, Denver, Col.*): John Moorhead, also, has similar data showing that the final common pathway for delivery of the negative signal is triggered by specific antigen, but acts nonspecifically in the end on the target. Do you know much about the nature of the link between the factor and the acceptor cell?

ASHERSON: Do I know anything about the conditions under which it will bind, for instance?

CLAMAN: Or inhibit binding?

ASHERSON: No, I've got no data on that whatsoever.

CLAMAN: You have not been able to or have not tried to block it with anything?

ASHERSON: No. Shearer and Zinkernagel's discussion of associative recognition has hitherto been a discussion of whether a cell has one or two receptors on its surface. Now, we've got one molecule that appears to give you genetic limitation. The question is now whether these recognition sites are on one or separate domains. So, obviously, one would very much like to dissect the T suppressor factor much as one dissects an immunoglobulin molecule into domains. That would answer the questions about the nature of the receptor that one finds on the acceptor cell, what inhibits it, and so on.

QUESTION: Geoff, you mentioned that your acceptor cell had a receptor for IgA. Have you prepared cells with receptors for the Fc portion of IgA, which Dick Lynch mentioned, and seen whether those will remove your suppressor factor?

ASHERSON: No. I'm afraid what we did was simply to take a myeloma, bind it on hapten, purify it so you get pure IgA, and do a panning experiment. So we haven't analyzed that further. The Fc was pepsin Fc from serum immunoglobulin.

SELF MOLECULES IN INDUCTION OF HYPERSENSITIVITY AND TOLERANCE IN DNCB CONTACT SENSITIVITY IN THE GUINEA PIG

Ladislav Polak

Pharma Research Department
F. Hoffmann-La Roche & Co. Ltd.
CH 4002 Basle, Switzerland

INTRODUCTION

Several authors have demonstrated that hapten-modified mononuclear cells, particularly macrophages, are capable of inducing both sensitization and tolerance in mice. The resulting effect of an application of haptenized macrophages was largely dependent upon the mode of administration. Haptenized macrophages injected intradermally induced contact sensitivity to the specific hapten,[1, 2] while their intravenous application resulted in tolerance.[3]

Furthermore, it has been demonstrated in the same experimental animals that the mechanism of tolerance induced with haptenized cells differs from that induced by intravenously injected hapten. The intravenously injected hapten activates specific suppressor cells, which, in turn, inhibit the development of sensitized memory and effector cells, *i.e.*, suppress the afferent limb of the immune response. The tolerance so induced is transferable by lymphoid cells, is of limited duration, and is reversible by cyclophosphamide treatment. On the other hand, tolerance induced by an intravenous injection of haptenized macrophages is not transferable by lymphoid cells and seems to be due to clonal deletion.[3]

In further experiments with mice, it has been demonstrated that hapten-modified Langerhans cells, known to play a decisive role in the induction of contact sensitivity, are capable of inducing tolerance under certain conditions. This is particularly true for uv-irradiated cells.[4] In contrast to haptenized macrophages, intravenously injected haptenized Langerhans cells induced contact sensitivity; not, as one would expect, tolerance.[2] This not-undisputed sensitizing effect was increased by cyclophosphamide pretreatment.[5]

However, contact sensitivity in mice is different in several respects from contact sensitivity in guinea pigs and humans. Both contact sensitivity and tolerance in mice are relatively short-lived,[6, 7] whereas, in guinea pigs and humans, they last a whole life.[8] Contact sensitivity in mice is transferable not only with lymphocytes but, unlike in guinea pigs, also with serum and serum-coated macrophages.[9] The eliciting reaction starts to appear as early as 4 h after challenge and the infiltrate consists mainly of polymorphonuclear granulocytes.[10, 11] Basophils, which are a typical constituent of infiltrates in contact sensitivity reactions in guinea pigs and humans, are almost entirely absent in mice.[12] Recent findings that delayed hypersensitivity in mice could be transferred with clones of either T helper cells, which are Lyt 1+,2,3-,[13] or T killer cells, which are Lyt 1-,2,3+,[14] make the definition of this reaction even more controversial.[15]

On the other hand, the close resemblance of contact sensitivity in guinea

0077–8923/82/0392–0090 $1.75/0 © 1982, NYAS

pigs to allergic contact dermatitis in man makes the investigation of the role of self components in the induction of contact sensitivity and tolerance in this experimental animal model particularly interesting, in spite of some technical difficulties.

In *in vitro* experiments with guinea pig cells it has been shown that both induction and elicitation of contact sensitivity is dependent upon the presence of a self component (Ia antigen) on the surface of stimulatory cells, *i.e.*, macrophages [16] or Langerhans cells.[17] Moreover, it has been demonstrated that the *in vitro* elicitation as expressed by an increased DNA synthesis by sensitized lymphocytes is strictly dependent upon the Ia homology of inducer and elicitor macrophages. Ia homology of T lymphocytes and inducer macrophages is, however, not an absolute requirement.[18]

In the present study, an attempt is made to verify *in vivo* the validity of the *in vitro* results for guinea pigs concerning the role of self components in the induction and elicitation of contact sensitivity. Dinitrophenylated macrophages injected intradermally induced contact sensitivity in syngeneic guinea pigs, while an intravenous application resulted in tolerance to the specific hapten. This tolerization was, unlike sensitization, not under genetic control. Furthermore, it has been demonstrated that, in contrast to *in vitro* results, the genetic restriction of sensitization was on the level of antigen recognition, where the presence of lymphocytes directed against the non-self Ia structures on histoincompatible macrophages seems to be of decisive importance.

MATERIAL AND METHODS

Animals

We used inbred strain 2 and strain 13, semi-inbred Rockefeller, and outbred Himalayan spotted white guinea pigs of both sexes weighing 400 to 600 g from the stock of the Institute for Biomedical Research, Füllinsdorf, Switzerland. They were fed on a pellet diet supplemented *ad libitum* with water containing vitamin C.

Antigens

DNCB (2,4-dinitrochlorobenzene) from Merck, Darmstadt, West Germany; DNFB (2,4-dinitrofluorobenzene) from Fluka A.G., Buchs SG, Switzerland; $DNBSO_3$ (2,4-dinitrobenzene sulfonic acid sodium salt) from Eastman Kodak, Rochester, New York; DNP-BGG (2,4-dinitrophenyl$_{16}$–bovine-γ-globuline) the stock of the Institute for Biomedical Research, Füllinsdorf, Switzerland. and DNP-GPA (2,4-dinitrophenyl$_{19}$–guinea pig serum albumin) were prepared by Dr. D. Gillessen, F. Hoffmann-La Roche, Basle, Switzerland, according to Little and Eisen.[19] DNP-GP skin (2,4-dinitrophenyl–guinea pig skin protein conjugate) prepared *in vivo* was kindly supplied by Dr. D. Parker, Royal College of Surgeons, London.[20] DNP-Mϕ (dinitrophenylated guinea pig peritoneal exudate cells) were prepared (1) for sensitization by reacting oil-induced peritoneal exudate cells (PEC) with a DNFB solution in Hanks BSS (Gibco, Europe, Glasgow, Scotland) (10×10^7 cells ml^{-1}; 10 μg DNFB ml^{-1}, 30 min, 37° C, pH 8.2) and (2) for tolerization according to Claman and Miller.[21]

Briefly, 93 mg DNFB dissolved in 0.5 ml ethanol was incubated overnight at 37° C in 99.5 ml Hanks BSS, pH 7.2. Peritoneal exudate cells (5×10^6 ml^{-1}) were reacted with 0.1 ml of this DNFB solution for 30 min at 37° C. DNP-SPL (dinitrophenylated guinea pig spleen cells) for tolerization were prepared by the same method. All cells were washed twice in Hanks BSS. FCA (Freund's complete adjuvant), was obtained from DIFCO Laboratory, Detroit, Michigan.

Sensitizing Methods

DNCB e.c. was an epicutaneous application of 25 μl of a 50% solution of DNCB in acetone on the nape of the neck. DNFB/FCA (5×0.1 ml of DNFB (total 500 μg) homogenized in FCA) was injected intradermally into foot pads and the nape of the neck. DNP-protein conjugates were injected in the same dose alone or homogenized in FCA. DNP-Mϕ (5×10^7 cells in 0.5 ml Hanks BSS divided into five aliquots) was injected into the foot pads and the nape of the neck. On some occasions, 0.1 ml Freund's complete adjuvant was injected into the same injection sites within 10 min. DNP-Mϕ membranes were prepared by Dr. B. J. Takacs.[22] A cell equivalent of 1.5×10^8 macrophages was injected in the same way as haptenized macrophages.

Guinea pigs were challenged 14 d later by an epicutaneous application of 25 μl of 0.09%, 0.05%, and 0.03% DNCB solutions in acetone on three shaved skin areas of 2 cm^2 each. The reactions were evaluated 24 h later as follows: [23] pink, spots—0.5, red, confluent—1.0, red, confluent, swollen—2.0. The degree of contact sensitivity of each animal is expressed as the total of all three reactions.

Induction of Tolerance

500 mg kg^{-1} DNBSO$_3$ dissolved in distilled sterile water (2 ml kg^{-1}) was injected intravenously on two occasions with a two week interval. An attempt at sensitization was always performed 14 d thereafter. DNP-Mϕ or DNP-SPL ($2/3 \times 10^8$ ml^{-1}) was injected intravenously into the veins of the legs. Sensitization was attempted 14 d after this injection.

Transfer of Contact Sensitivity

Donor guinea pigs were injected intraperitoneally with 20 ml sterile light paraffin oil (Drakeol 6-VR, Penn-Drake, Butler, Pennsylvania). Four days later, peritoneal exudate cells were obtained by washing out the peritoneal cavity with 150 ml Hanks BSS; 2×10^8 washed cells in 3 ml Hanks BSS were then injected into the veins of the legs.

Cyclophosphamide Treatment

250 mg kg^{-1} cyclophosphamide (Endoxan-Asta, Asta-Werke, Brackwede, West Germany) was injected intraperitoneally, dissolved in sterile distilled water, 3 d prior to sensitizing procedure.

Induction of Contact Sensitivity with Haptenized
(Dinitrophenylated) Macrophages and Its Genetic Restriction

The results of attempts to induce contact sensitivity with various dinitro-phenylated (DNP) proteins and haptenized macrophages are presented in FIGURE 1. When the contact sensitivity–inducing capacity of various DNP-protein conjugates and the capacity of hapten-modified macrophages (DNP-Mφ) was compared, it became evident that the latter are the most potent sensitizers. DNP bound to heterologous proteins such as bovine-γ-globuline (DNP-BGG) does not induce contact sensitivity to an epicutaneous challenge with dinitrochlorobenzene (DNCB), irrespective of whether or not FCA was used for sensitization. DNP conjugates with homologous proteins such as guinea

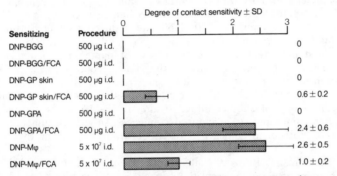

FIGURE 1. Induction of contact sensitivity with different DNP-conjugates. Groups of eight Rockefeller strain guinea pigs were sensitized by an intradermal injection either of 500 μg dinitrophenylated proteins alone or homogenized in FCA (DNP-GPA) or of 5×10^7 DNP-Mø. In separate groups, 0.1 ml FCA was injected into the sites of macrophage injections. Fourteen days later, animals were challenged epicutaneously with 25 μl of 0.09%, 0.05%, and 0.03% solutions of DNCB in acetone on the shaved flank and their reactions evaluated 24 h later, as described in Materials and Methods. The results are presented as the mean degree of contact sensitivity of each group ± S.D.

pig skin extract (DNP-GP skin) or guinea pig serum albumin (DNP-GPA) become sensitizers only when they are injected intradermally homogenized in FCA. Addition of FCA to hapten-modified macrophages decreases rather than increases the level of contact sensitivity. Furthermore, the degree of DNCB contact sensitivity induced by an intradermal injection of DNP-Mφ is higher than that achieved by unconjugated hapten applied epicutaneously and is of about the same degree as that achieved with the unconjugated hapten injected intradermally homogenized in FCA (TABLE 1).

It is noteworthy that, unlike all the other sensitizing methods using DNCB, induction of contact sensitivity with DNP-Mφ is not accompanied by produc-tion of anti-DNP-antibodies detectable by passive cutaneous anaphylaxis (PCA) reaction (TABLE 2).

Furthermore, it should be stressed that only minute amounts of the hapten bound to a very low number of macrophages are required for the induction of

TABLE 1

COMPARISON OF THE DEGREE OF CONTACT SENSITIVITY
INDUCED BY UNCONJUGATED HAPTEN AND HAPTEN-MODIFIED MACROPHAGES

Sensitizing Method	Dose of DNP	Degree of Contact Sensitivity ± s.d.
DNCB e.c.	1 mg	1.9 ± 0.5
DNFB/FCA i.d.	500 μg	3.8 ± 3.8
DNP-Mø i.d.	0.5 μg	4.0 ± 0.9

NOTE: All guinea pigs were challenged with DNCB epicutaneously 14 d after sensitizing procedures (see Material and Methods).

DNCB contact sensitivity with DNP-Mø. In fact, 1×10^6 DNP-Mø, containing about 8 ng bound hapten, was sufficient to induce a clearly positive contact sensitivity, whereas about 4×10^7 DNP-Mø induced contact sensitivity to a degree rarely achieved by other sensitizing methods (FIGURE 2).

The most important outcome of the use of hapten-modified macrophages was the evidence for the existence of the genetic control of the induction of contact sensitivity. In FIGURE 3, it is shown that DNP-Mø of inbred strain guinea pigs are capable of inducing contact sensitivity in syngeneic animals but not in guinea pigs of another inbred strain. DNP-Mø of the partially inbred Rockefeller guinea pig strain induced contact sensitivity in guinea pigs of the same strain, but not in guinea pigs of either strain 2 or strain 13 (results not shown).

Furthermore, DNP-Mø of both strain 2 (results not shown) and strain 13 guinea pigs induced contact sensitivity in all F_1 guinea pigs (2×13 animals) and in about 50% of the F_2 guinea pigs. On the other hand, when DNP-Mø of the outbred Himalayan spotted white strain were used for sensitization of guinea pigs of the same strain, only a fraction of the guinea pigs (about 35%) became contact sensitive, i.e., responded to an epicutaneous challenge with the hapten DNCB by a specific inflammatory skin reaction (FIGURE 4).

TABLE 2

ANTI-DNP PCA ANTIBODIES IN DNCB CONTACT–SENSITIVE GUINEA PIGS

Induction	Guinea Pig Strain	Mean Antibody Titer
DNCB e.c.	Rockefeller	1:19
DNFB/FCA i.d.	Rockefeller	1:687
DNP-Mø Rock	Rockefeller	0
DNP-Mø Rock	2	0
DNP-Mø Rock	13	0

NOTE: Guinea pigs were sensitized either epicutaneously with an application of 1 mg DNCB in acetone or intradermally with either 500 μg DNFB homogenized in 0.5 ml FCA or 5×10^7 DNP-Mø. The results are expressed as the antibody titer inducing a definite positive PCA reaction of 10 mm diameter to 1 mg DNP-BGG injected intravenously in 1% Evans blue in 0.15 M NaCl.

The Role of Self Components in Hapten Recognition

The failure of guinea pigs injected with allogeneic DNP-Mϕ to exhibit contact sensitivity reactions may be due either to lack of recognition of the antigenic complex by specific T cells or to the nonidentity of carriers used for induction and carriers formed by the challenge. In other words, guinea pigs injected with allogeneic DNP-Mϕ might be either sensitized to this antigenic complex but unable to exhibit contact sensitivity reactions to the unconjugated epicutaneously applied hapten or not at all hypersensitive because of the inability of specific T cells to recognize the hapten on non-self components.

To resolve this problem, an attempt was made to elicit a skin reaction in animals injected with allogeneic DNP-Mϕ by an intradermal injection of this antigenic complex.

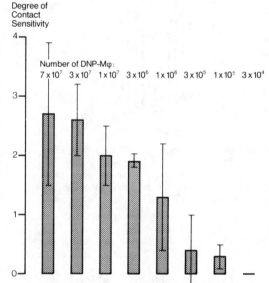

FIGURE 2. Effect of the number of DNP-Mø on the degree of contact sensitivity. Groups of eight Rockefeller guinea pigs were injected intradermally with different amounts of DNP-Mø and challenged 14 d later with DNCB, as described in Material and Methods. The results are expressed as in FIGURE 1.

However, the reaction to the hapten, if present, was completely masked by the reaction to the foreign cells. In order to overcome this difficulty, lymphocytes from DNP-Mϕ-treated guinea pigs were transferred to F_1 (2×13) recipients, which are unable to exhibit skin reactions to parental macrophages. The results of these experiments are presented in FIGURE 5.

Peritoneal exudate lymphocytes (Ly) from strain 2 guinea pigs that had been sensitized by intradermally injected syngeneic (strain 2) DNP-Mϕ were capable of transferring this contact sensitivity to F_1 (2×13) recipients. On the other hand, peritoneal exudate lymphocytes from strain 2 donors that had been injected 14 d previously with allogeneic (strain 13) DNP-Mϕ failed to transfer contact sensitivity to F_1 (2×13) recipients. This was in spite of the fact that complexes of DNP with macrophage components of both strain 2 and strain 13 determinants are formed by an epicutaneous application of DNCB.

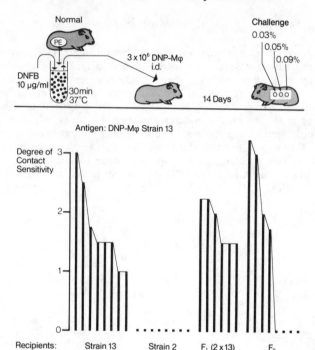

FIGURE 3. Genetic restriction of induction of contact sensitivity with DNP-Mø. Groups of eight guinea pigs of strain 13, strain 2, F₁ (2 × 13), and F₂ were injected intradermally with 3×10^6 DNP-Mø of strain 13 and challenged epicutaneously with DNCB 14 d later. The reactions were evaluated as described in Materials and Methods and expressed as the degree of contact sensitivity of individual animals.

We concluded from this result that strain 2 guinea pigs are not hypersensitive to the antigenic complex consisting of the hapten (DNP) and allogenic (strain 13) macrophages.

In order to establish whether the failure of hapten recognition is due to the rejection of the allogeneic DNP-Mφ, an attempt was made to sensitize parental strain guinea pigs with F₁ (2 × 13) DNP-Mφ that contain both strain 2 and 13 determinants but are rejected in parental recipients. From the results presented in FIGURE 5, it is evident that DNP-Mφ from F₁ (2 × 13) guinea pigs were, in fact, successful in inducing contact sensitivity in parental guinea pigs when injected intradermally. This result is not compatible with the hypothesis that the lack of recognition of a hapten on non-self macrophages is due to early rejection of these cells.

In further experiments, it is demonstrated (FIGURE 6) that preparations of dinitrophenylated membranes from DNP-Mφ are capable of inducing DNCB contact sensitivity, provided that they are injected intradermally together with normal macrophages of the syngeneic strain. Thus, membranes of DNP-Mφ from strain 13 guinea pigs induced DNCB contact sensitivity not only in strain 13 but also in strain 2 animals when applied together with syngeneic normal macrophages of the corresponding strains.

Dinitrophenylated membranes alone were capable of sensitizing only syngeneic guinea pigs, while allogeneic animals did not become contact sensitive.

Induction of Tolerance with Hapten-Modified Macrophages

In contrast to the intradermal application, intravenously injected DNP-Mϕ induced a state of tolerance, *i.e.*, guinea pigs injected intravenously failed to react to an epicutaneous challenge with a non-skin-irritating dose of this hapten (FIGURE 7). However, when the hapten was applied intradermally in FCA (DNFB/FCA), the tolerance was reversed and the guinea pigs reacted to an epicutaneous challenge with an inflammatory reaction. An intraperitoneal injection of 250 mg kg^{-1} cyclophosphamide (Cy) to tolerant guinea pigs 3 d before the sensitizing attempt with DNCB epicutaneously also reversed the tolerance (FIGURE 8).

In contrast to induction of contact sensitivity with DNP-Mϕ, this tolerization was not genetically restricted. Guinea pigs of both strain 2 and strain 13

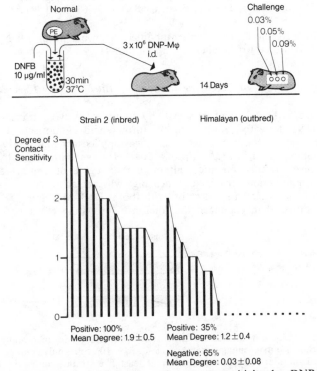

FIGURE 4. Comparison of induction of contact sensitivity by DNP-Mϕ in an inbred and in an outbred strain. Strain 2 (12 animals) and Himalayan spotted white (20 animals) guinea pigs were intradermally injected with DNP-Mϕ of the same strain and challenged epicutaneously with DNCB 14 d later. The reactions were evaluated and the results expressed as in FIGURE 3.

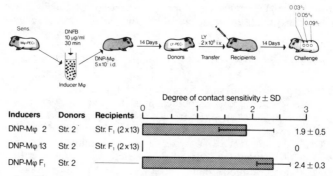

FIGURE 5. Attempts to transfer contact sensitivity from parental guinea pigs sensitized with syngeneic or allogeneic macrophages to F_1-recipients. Peritoneal exudate cells (2×10^8) from strain 2 guinea pigs, which had been injected i.d. 14 d previously with either strain 2 or strain 13 DNP-Mø (5×10^7), were injected i.v. into F_1 (2×13) recipients. Fourteen days later, these guinea pigs (five in each group) were challenged epicutaneously with DNCB and the results evaluated and expressed as in FIGURE 1. In a control group, strain 2 guinea pigs were injected i.d. with DNP-Mø of F_1 (2×13) and challenged with DNCB 14 d later.

were equally well tolerized by hapten-modified macrophages of either strain 13 or the partially inbred Rockefeller strain (FIGURE 9).

Reversal by DNP-Mφ of Tolerance Induced by Intravenously Injected Hapten

Tolerance to DNCB contact sensitivity induced by two intravenous injections of a DNP derivative, dinitrobenzenesulfonic acid sodium salt ($DNBSO_3$), was not reversed by the hapten whether it was applied epicutaneously or intradermally homogenized in FCA (FIGURE 10). However, intradermally injected DNP-Mφ reversed this tolerance, although the degree of contact sensitivity observed in nontolerant sensitized guinea pigs was not achieved. A simultaneously performed sensitizing attempt with both DNP-Mφ and DNFB/FCA eliminated rather than enhanced the tolerance-abrogating effect of DNP-Mφ.

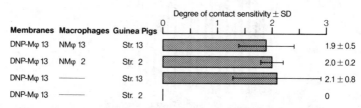

FIGURE 6. Induction of contact sensitivity with DNP-Mø membranes. DNP-modified strain 13 macrophage membranes (1.5×10^8 cell equivalent per animal) were injected intradermally into groups of at least five strain 2 or strain 13 guinea pigs, either alone or together with 5×10^7 normal macrophages syngeneic with the recipient strain. Strain 2 and strain 13 guinea pigs were injected i.d. with intact strain 13 DNP-Mø (5×10^7 per animal), together with 5×10^7 normal macrophages syngeneic with the recipient strain. All recipient animals were challenged 14 d later with DNCB e.c. and the results evaluated and expressed as in FIGURE 1.

FIGURE 7. Induction of tolerance to DNCB contact sensitivity by an intravenous injection of hapten-modified macrophages of peritoneal exudate or spleen cell origin. Groups consisting of eight Rockefeller strain guinea pigs were injected intravenously with 2×10^8 hapten-modified peritoneal exudate (DNP-Mø) or spleen (DNP-SPL) cells. Sensitization was attempted 14 d later with either DNCB e.c. or DNFB in FCA i.d. Guinea pigs were challenged epicutaneously with DNCB 14 d after the sensitizing attempt and the resulting reactions presented as in FIGURE 1. DNCB e.c. sensitized guinea pigs served as controls.

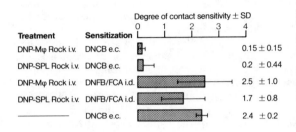

Treatment	Sensitization	Degree of contact sensitivity ± SD
DNP-Mφ Rock i.v.	DNCB e.c.	0.15 ± 0.15
DNP-SPL Rock i.v.	DNCB e.c.	0.2 ± 0.44
DNP-Mφ Rock i.v.	DNFB/FCA i.d.	2.5 ± 1.0
DNP-SPL Rock i.v.	DNFB/FCA i.d.	1.7 ± 0.8
———	DNCB e.c.	2.4 ± 0.2

FIGURE 8. Reversal by cylophosphamide (Cy) treatment of tolerance induced by intravenously injected DNP-Mø or DNP-SPL. Cyclophosphamide (250 mg kg⁻¹) was applied intraperitoneally into DNP-Mø or DNP-SPL intravenously tolerized animals 3 d before an attempt at sensitization with DNCB e.c. Guinea pigs were challenged and the results evaluated and presented as in FIGURE 7.

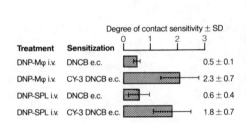

Treatment	Sensitization	Degree of contact sensitivity ± SD
DNP-Mφ i.v.	DNCB e.c.	0.5 ± 0.1
DNP-Mφ i.v.	CY-3 DNCB e.c.	2.3 ± 0.7
DNP-SPL i.v.	DNCB e.c.	0.6 ± 0.4
DNP-SPL i.v.	CY-3 DNCB e.c.	1.8 ± 0.7

Inducers	Recipients	Sensitization	Degree of contact sensitivity ± SD
DNP-Mφ 13 i.v.	GP 2	DNCB e.c.	0.25 ± 1.5
DNP-SPL 13 i.v.	GP 2	DNCB e.c.	0.08 ± 0.07
DNP-Mφ Rock i.v.	GP 13	DNCB e.c.	0
DNP-SPL Rock i.v.	GP 13	DNCB e.c.	0
DNP-SPL Rock i.v.	GP 2	DNCB e.c.	0.25 ± 0.5
———	GP 2	DNCB e.c.	2.1 ± 0.4
———	GP 13	DNCB e.c.	2.3 ± 0.3

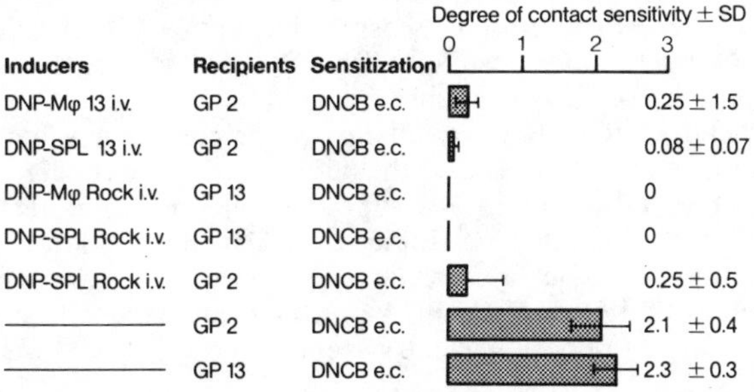

FIGURE 9. Genetic restriction of induction of tolerance to DNCB contact sensitivity with DNP-Mø or DNP-SPL. Hapten-modified peritoneal exudate (DNP-Mø) or spleen (DNP-SPL) cells of strain 13 or Rockefeller strain guinea pigs were injected intravenously into strain 2 or strain 13 animals. Sensitization was attempted with DNCB e.c. 14 d later and the results were assessed and presented as in FIGURE 7.

Discussion

Carrier Specificity

It is an established fact that the same antigenic complex (hapten-carrier conjugate) is required for elicitation of delayed hypersensitivity reactions as for its induction.[24] Since, in contact sensitivity, this complex is formed *in vivo* in the skin by an epicutaneous challenge with the hapten, the nature of the carrier(s) remains unknown, despite intense efforts.

The high efficiency with which DNP-Mϕ induces contact sensitivity indicates that the carrier might be a constituent of the membrane of macrophages or Langerhans cells.[25] This efficiency is evident from the following observations: For the induction of contact sensitivity with the hapten either alone or conjugated with homologous proteins, much higher amounts of DNP are required than in the case of macrophage-bound hapten. The actual difference is even more pronounced, since a high proportion of the hapten is bound to immuno-

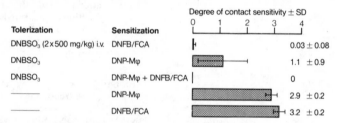

Tolerization	Sensitization	Degree of contact sensitivity ± SD 0 1 2 3 4	
DNBSO₃ (2×500 mg/kg) i.v.	DNFB/FCA		0.03 ± 0.08
DNBSO₃	DNP-Mφ		1.1 ± 0.9
DNBSO₃	DNP-Mφ + DNFB/FCA		0
———	DNP-Mφ		2.9 ± 0.2
———	DNFB/FCA		3.2 ± 0.2

FIGURE 10. Reversal by intradermally injected DNP-Mø of tolerance induced by i.v. injected hapten. Tolerance was induced in Rockefeller strain guinea pigs (groups of eight animals) by two intravenous injections of dinitrobenzenesulfonic acid sodium salt (DNBSO₃) with a 14 d interval. Two weeks after the second i.v. injection, guinea pigs were treated i.d. with either 500 μg DNFB in FCA, 5×10^7 DNP-Mø, or a combination of both. Challenge with DNCB e.c. was performed 14 d after the sensitizing attempt and the results were evaluated and expressed as in FIGURE 7.

logically irrelevant proteins of the macrophage membrane (Polak and Takacs, unpublished results). Furthermore, sensitization with DNP-protein conjugates failed in the absence of FCA, while, when DNP-Mϕ is used for sensitization, additional application of FCA is inhibitory.

There exists no unambiguous explanation of the contact sensitivity–inhibiting effect of FCA. One possibility is that the addition of FCA converts the optimal sensitizing effect of DNP-Mϕ into a supraoptimal one, resulting in a partial high zone tolerance. The other possibility is that the application of FCA simultaneously with DNP-Mϕ but not in a homogenized state resembles the effect of pretreatment with FCA. Such FCA-pretreatment caused a suppression of the following immune response in some systems.[26]

Genetic Restriction

The fact that contact sensitivity was induced with syngeneic DNP-Mϕ only indicates that the protein carrier must be a genetically controlled structure on macrophage membranes that differs from strain to strain. In extensive *in vitro* studies, it has been shown that the immune response associated (Ia) antigen could fulfill such a carrier function.[16, 18] The formation of a conjugate of the hapten and Ia antigen has, however, never been sufficiently documented and is still a matter of discussion.

The genetic control of the *in vivo* induction of contact sensitivity with DNP-Mϕ was confirmed in our experiments using F_1 (2 × 13) and F_2 guinea pigs as well as semi-inbred Rockefeller strain and outbred Himalayan spotted white animals for sensitization. The genetic restriction of induction also excludes the possibility that sensitization was induced by unconjugated hapten present in the macrophage suspension.

There are several possible ways to interpret the failure to elicit a contact sensitivity skin reaction in guinea pigs injected intradermally with allogeneic DNP-Mϕ.

Heterology of Carrier Proteins

Since contact sensitivity reactions are dependent upon the homology of the carriers involved in both the induction and the elicitation, the reason for a failure to respond might be the nonidentity of these carriers. In strain 2 animals challenged epicutaneously with the hapten, the antigenic complex formed in the skin consists of this hapten and the Ia structures of strain 2 macrophages. If such an animal is sensitized with DNP-Mϕ of strain 13, contact sensitivity could not be elicited either by DNP-Mϕ of strain 2 or by an epicutaneous application of the sole hapten. These animals may, however, respond to an intradermal challenge with DNP-Mϕ of strain 13. This has, in fact, been demonstrated *in vitro* when lymphocytes directed against non-haptenized allogeneic macrophages were eliminated by treatment with bromode oxyuridine (BUdR) and light.[18] It is, however, difficult to evaluate a skin reaction in strain 2 guinea pigs challenged intradermally with strain 13 DNP-Mϕ, since the hapten-specific reaction is masked by the reaction against allogeneic nonhaptenized macrophages.

Lack of Antigen Recognition

It was important to decide whether guinea pigs injected intradermally with allogeneic DNP-Mϕ become hypersensitive to this complex, as is the case with animals sensitized to hapten-heterologous protein conjugates (*e.g.*, DNP-BGG). In order to overcome the difficulties in evaluating hapten-specific reactions elicited with allogeneic DNP-Mϕ, an attempt was made to transfer the assumed sensitivity to allogeneic DNP-Mϕ from the parental strain to F_1 (2 × 13) animals and elicit the skin reaction in those recipients which do not develop histoincompatibility reactions to cells from parental strains.

Whereas F_1 (2 × 13) recipients adoptively sensitized with lymphocytes from parental guinea pigs, sensitized previously with syngeneic DNP-Mϕ, reacted positively to an epicutaneous challenge with the hapten, recipients of lymphocytes from parental guinea pigs injected intradermally with allogeneic DNP-Mϕ failed to exhibit an inflammatory skin reaction to an epicutaneous challenge.

From these results it may be concluded that guinea pig T cells do not recognize the hapten presented on allogeneic macrophages. One reason for this lack of recognition might be the rejection of allogeneic DNP-Mϕ. However, the positive outcome of the attempt to sensitize parental strain animals with F_1 (2 × 13) DNP-Mϕ refutes this possibility, since parental recipients reject F_1 cells the same way they reject allogeneic cells. The *in vitro* evidence of recognition of allogeneic haptenized macrophages was achieved by prior elimination of T cells directed against nonhaptenized allogeneic cells.[18] The discrepancy between these results and our *in vivo* results could not be explained on the basis of the experiments described.

Membrane Proteins as Carriers

The reason why DNP bound to allogeneic macrophages behaves differently from DNP bound to other foreign proteins, *e.g.*, BGG, has yet to be explained. It seems that, in this respect, an intact macrophage behaves like a "nonmetaboliz-able carrier" that cannot be processed and consequently does not form immuno-genic complexes that might be presented by the host macrophages. Similar situations have been described for dextran, sephadex, and other high molecular sugars, as well as for the copolymer of D-glutamine and D-lysine (D-GL). However, in contrast to these nonmetabolizable carriers, allogeneic DNP-macrophages do not induce tolerance when injected intradermally. Moreover, pretreatment with cyclophosphamide did not render allogeneic DNP-Mϕ im-munogenic (Polak, unpublished). These results could be considered evidence that the failure of allogeneic DNP-Mϕ to induce contact sensitivity is due to genetic incompatibility rather than to activation of specific suppressor cells. Only intact macrophages lack both immunogenicity and tolerogenicity. Hap-tenized macrophage membranes are immunogenic for both syngeneic and allo-geneic guinea pigs, provided that they are administered in the presence of normal syngeneic macrophages. This has been demonstrated both *in vitro*[27] and *in vivo*. In this respect, haptenized membranes behave like other foreign proteins. Haptenized membranes alone do not sensitize allogeneic but only syngeneic guinea pigs. This may be due to the involvement of the animals' own macrophages. In *in vitro* experiments, macrophage-depleted sensitized T cell suspensions do not respond to stimulation with only haptenized macrophage membranes.[27]

Induction of Tolerance with Haptenized Macrophages

The phenomenon of tolerance induced by hapten-modified cells has been extensively studied in mice. Claman and his coworkers have demonstrated that, in this system, tolerance was induced with both allogeneic[28] and syngeneic[29] hapten-modified cells. According to some of these studies, specific suppressor cells were activated in both cases. However, in the former case, suppressor cells affected only the very early stages of sensitization whereas, in the latter case, the efferent limb of the immune response was inhibited. According to some other studies, intravenously injected haptenized lymphoid cells were able to induce tolerance by clonal inhibition (abortion or blockade). This tolerance, in contrast to the previously mentioned suppressor cell–mediated types, was cyclophosphamide resistant[30] and not transferable.

In guinea pigs, tolerance induced with haptenized peritoneal exudate or spleen cells is not genetically restricted, *i.e.*, it can be induced with allogeneic as well as syngeneic intravenously injected DNP-Mφ and DNP-SPL. However, the tolerance thus induced was unlike the tolerance induced by feeding or by intravenous injections of the hapten; it was reversed by repeated challenges with DNCB as well as by sensitization with the hapten homogenized in FCA. Pretreatment with cyclophosphamide also abrogated the state of tolerance. From these results, one may assume that the tolerance induced by DNP-Mφ in guinea pigs is suppressor cell–mediated and not due to clonal abortion or blockade. However, further experiments are required to obtain a final answer.

Reversal by DNP-Mφ of Tolerance Induced by Intravenously Injected Hapten

On the other hand, it has been clearly demonstrated that, in guinea pigs, tolerance to DNCB contact sensitivity induced by either intravenous injections or feeding of the hapten is mediated by the activation of specific suppressor cells.[31, 32] This tolerance is complete and permanent, transferable with both lymphoid cells [33] and parabiosis [34] and reversible by cyclophosphamide treatment.[31] Suppressor cells in this system mainly affect the afferent limb of the immune response;[34] they thus resemble allo-induced suppressor cells in mice.

It is remarkable that a tolerance that could not be reversed either by repeated challenge or by resensitizing attempts with or without the use of FCA was at least partially abrogated by an intradermal injection of syngeneic DNP-Mφ.

There are several possible explanations of this reversal of tolerance.

Contact sensitivity is considered a complex phenomenon directed against several DNP-protein determinants.[35] In order to achieve complete tolerance, the response to all determinants formed by the sensitizing process has to be suppressed. This is apparently achieved by intravenously injected hapten when sensitization is attempted by epicutaneous application of DNCB or by an intradermal injection of the hapten homogenized in FCA. However, when the hapten is applied conjugated to macrophages, the spectrum of determinants may partially differ from those formed by an application of the unconjugated hapten and inhibited by specific suppressor cells. In that case, contact sensitivity could be elicited by lymphocytes reacting to the nonsuppressed determinants. Reversal by DNCB in FCA of tolerance induced by DNP-Mφ could be similarly explained. It has been shown that a larger number of determinants are formed by sensitization with hapten homogenized in FCA than by epicutaneous application of the hapten.[37]

The development of complete and permanent tolerance is dependent upon the activation of a sufficient number of specific suppressor cells. One may speculate that i.v. injected hapten induces only a fraction of the required suppressor cells. Through sensitization with the hapten either alone or homogenized in FCA, additional suppressor cells,[36] necessary for achieving a complete tolerance, are activated. DNP-Mφ injected intradermally may, however, not have the ability to activate enough suppressor cells to complete the tolerogenic process. Consequently, the effect of DNP-Mφ can not be called a reversal of tolerance, but rather an insufficient contribution to its full induction. This hypothesis is supported by the fact that an additional intradermal injection of DNCB in FCA simultaneously with sensitization with DNP-Mφ did not enhance the tolerance-abrogating effect of DNP-Mφ; on the contrary, the partial reversal of tolerance was abolished and the animals became completely unresponsive.

There is, however, a third possible way that DNP-Mϕ could have reversed tolerance. It is possible that suppressor cells induced tolerance by preventing the processing of the hapten by macrophages with the result that the antigenic complex cannot be formed. If macrophages are haptenized *in vitro*, suppressor cells are no longer capable of preventing antigen recognition and development of hypersensitivity. This hypothesis is, however, unable to explain the tolerance-reconstituting effect of an additional application of DNFB/FCA.

The results presented in this study clearly demonstrate the crucial importance of genetically controlled membrane proteins in the induction of contact sensitivity. The relationship between these proteins and the carriers in contact sensitivity reactions and the reason hapten-modified macrophages are capable of reversing tolerance have yet to be elucidated.

SUMMARY

Dinitrophenylated macrophages are efficient inducers of contact sensitivity and of tolerance to dinitrochlorobenzene, depending on the mode of application. Contact sensitivity induced by an intradermal injection of DNP-Mϕ is genetically restricted, whereas tolerance induced by an intravenous injection is, in guinea pigs, not under genetic control. This tolerance is complete in the majority of animals, but is reversed by DNCB in Freund's complete adjuvant and prevented by pretreatment with cyclophosphamide. Tolerance induced by an intravenous injection of the unconjugated hapten is not reversed by DNCB in FCA, but is abrogated by an intradermal injection of DNP-Mϕ. This abrogation does not occur, however, when DNCB in FCA is applied simultaneously with the DNP-Mϕ. In further experiments, it is demonstrated that the genetic restriction of induction of contact sensitivity by DNP-Mϕ is on the level of antigen recognition and is not due to the nonidentity of the Ia structures on macrophages used for induction and the Ia structures involved in elicitation of contact sensitivity.

REFERENCES

1. MOTTRAM, P. L. & J. F. A. MILLER. 1980. Delayed-type hypersensitivity induced by antigen-pulsed, bone marrow-derived macrophages. Eur. J. Immunol. **10:** 165–70.
2. PTAK, W., D. ROZYCKA, P. W. ASKENASE & R. K. GERSHON. 1980. Role of antigen-presenting cells in the development and persistence of contact hypersensitivity. J. Exp. Med. **151:** 362–75.
3. CLAMAN, H. N., S. D. MILLER, M. S. SY & J. W. MOORHEAD. 1979. Two pathways for tolerance to contact sensitivity. *In* Immunologic Tolerance and Macrophage Function. J. F. Baram, J. R. Battisto, and C. W. Pierce, Eds.: 223–43. Elsevier/North-Holland. Amsterdam.
4. GREENE, M. I., M. S. SY, M. KRIPKE & B. BENACERRAF. 1979. Impairment of antigen-presenting cell function by ultraviolet radiation. Proc. Nat. Acad. Sci. USA **76:** 6591–95.
5. IKEZAWA, Z., M. SATO, R. NAGAI & K. OKUDA. 1981. Cell surface expression of I-A products is required for contact sensitivity induction by trinitrophenyl-coupled epidermal cells. Eur. J. Immunol. In press.
6. GREEN, J. A., J. WILLIAMS & H. B. LEVY. 1977. Specific restoration of delayed hypersensitivity by lymphoid tissue extracts. J. Immunol. **118:** 1936–43.
7. CLAMAN, H. N., P. PHANUPHAK & J. W. MOORHEAD. 1974. Tolerance to contact sensitivity—A role for suppressor T-cells? *In* Immunological Tolerance.

Mechanisms and Potential Therapeutic Applications. D. H. Katz and B. Benacerraf, Eds.: 123–28. Academic Press. New York.

8. POLAK, L. & C. RINCK. 1978. Persisting activity of suppressor cells in T-cell mediated immune response. J. Immunol. **121:** 762–66.

9. ASHERSON, G. L. & M. ZEMBALA. 1970. Contact sensitivity in the mouse. IV. The role of lymphocytes and macrophages in passive transfer and the mechanism of their interaction. J. Exp. Med. **132:** 1–15.

10. DE SOUSA, M. A. B. & D. M. V. PARROTT. 1969. Induction and recall in contact sensitivity. Changes in skin and draining lymph nodes of intact and thymectomized mice. J. Exp. Med. **130:** 671–90.

11. PARROTT, D. M. V., M. A. B. DE SOUSA & J. FACHET. 1970. The response of normal, thymectomized and reconstituted mice on contact sensitivity. Clin. Exp. Immunol. **7:** 287–393.

12. DVORAK, H. F. & A. M. DVORAK. 1974. Cutaneous basophil hypersensitivity. *In* Progress in Immunology II, Vol. 3. L. Brent and J. Holborow, Eds.: 171–81. Elsevier/North Holland. Amsterdam.

13. BIANCHI, A. T. J., H. HOOIJKAAS, R. BENNER, R. TEES, A. A. NORDIN & M. H. SCHREIER. 1981. Clones of helper T cells mediate antigen-specific, H-2 restricted DTH. Nature (London) **290:** 62–63.

14. WEISS, S. & G. DENNERT. 1981. T cell lines active in the delayed-type hypersensitivity reaction (DTH). J. Immunol. **126:** 2031–35.

15. NASH, A. A. & P. G. H. GELL. 1981. The delayed hypersensitivity T cell and its interaction with other T cells. Immunol. Today **2:** 162–65.

16. THOMAS, D. W. & E. M. SHEVACH. 1976. Nature of the antigenic complex recognized by T lymphocytes. I. Analysis with an in vitro primary response to soluble protein antigens. J. Exp. Med. **144:** 1263–73.

17. STINGL, G., S. I. KATZ, L. CLEMENT, I. GREEN & E. M. SHEVACH. 1978. Immunologic functions of Ia-bearing epidermal Langerhans cells. J. Immunol. **121:** 2005–13.

18. THOMAS, D. W., U. YAMASHITA & E. M. SHEVACH. 1977. The role of antigens in T cell activation. Immunol. Rev. **35:** 97–120.

19. LITTLE, J. R. & H. N. EISEN. 1967. Preparation of immunogenic 2,4-dinitrophenyl proteins. *In* Methods in Immunology and Immunochemistry, Vol. 1, Preparation of Antigens and Antibodies. C. A. Williams and M. W. Chase, Eds: 128–33. Academic Press. New York.

20. PARKER, D. & J. L. TURK. 1970. Studies on the ability of the subcellular fractions of epidermis, painted in vivo with DNFB, to cause contact sensitization in the guinea pig. Int. Arch. Allergy Appl. Immunol. **37:** 440–48.

21. CLAMAN, H. & S. E. MILLER. 1976. Requirements for induction of T cell tolerance to DNFB: Efficiency of membrane-associated DNFB. J. Immunol. **117:** 480–85.

22. TAKACS, B. J. & T. STAEHELIN. 1981. Biochemical characterization of cell surface antigens using monoclonal antibodies. *In* Immunological Methods, Vol. 2. I. Lefkovits and B. Pernis, Eds.: 27–56. Academic Press. New York.

23. FREY, J. R. & P. WENK. 1957. Experimental studies on the pathogenesis of contact eczema in the guinea-pig. Int. Arch. Allergy Appl. Immunol. **11:** 81–100.

24. GELL, P. G. H. & B. BENACERRAF. 1961. Studies on hypersensitivity. IV. The relationship between contact and delayed sensitivity: a study on the specificity of cellular immune reactions. J. Exp. Med. **113:** 571–85.

25. TAMAKI, K., FUJIWARA, H. & S. I. KATZ. 1981. The role of epidermal cells in the induction and suppression of contact sensitivity. J. Invest. Dermatol. **76:** 275–78.

26. JANKOVIC, B. C. 1962. Impairment of immunological reactivity in guinea pigs by prior injection of adjuvant. Nature (London) **193:** 789–90.

27. HEBER-KATZ, E. & E. M. SHEVACH. 1980. TNP-coupled membranes stimulate T cell proliferation via the macrophage. J. Immunol. **124:** 1503–5.

28. MILLER, S. D., M. S. SY & H. N. CLAMAN. 1978. Suppressor T cell mecha-

nisms in contact sensitivity. I. Efferent blockade by syninduced suppressor T cells. J. Immunol. **121:** 265–73.

29. MILLER, S. D., M. S. SY & H. N. CLAMAN. 1978. Suppressor T cell mechanisms in contact sensitivity. II. Afferent blockade by alloinduced suppressor T cells. J. Immunol. **121:** 274–80.

30. MILLER, S. D., M. S. SY & H. N. CLAMAN. 1977. The induction of hapten-specific T cell tolerance using hapten-modified lymphoid membranes. II. Relative roles of suppressor T cells and clone inhibition in the tolerant state. Eur. J. Immunol. **7:** 165–70.

31. POLAK, L. 1975. Suppressor cells in different types of unresponsiveness to DNCB contact sensitivity in guinea pigs. Clin. Exp. Immunol. **19:** 543–49.

32. POLAK, L., H. GELEICK & J. L. TURK. 1975. Reversal by cyclophosphamide of tolerance in contact sensitization. Immunology **28:** 939–42.

33. POLAK, L. 1976. Studies on the role of suppressor cells in specific unresponsiveness to DNCB. Immunology **31:** 425–32.

34. POLAK, L. 1975. The transfer of tolerance to DNCB-contact sensitivity in guinea pigs by parabiosis. J. Immunol. **114:** 988–91.

35. POLAK, L., A. POLAK-WYSS & J. R. FREY. 1974. Development of contact sensitivity to DNCB in guinea pigs genetically differing in their response to DNP skin protein conjugates. Int. Arch. Allergy Appl. Immunol. **46:** 417–26.

36. POLAK, L. & C. RNICK. 1977. Effect of the elimination of suppressor cells on the development of DNCB contact sensitivity in guinea pigs. Immunology **33:** 305–11.

37. POLAK, L. & R. J. SCHEPER. 1981. In vitro DNA synthesis in lymphocytes from guinea pigs epicutaneously sensitized with DNCB. J. Invest. Dermatol. **76:** 133–36.

DISCUSSION OF THE PAPER

H. N. CLAMAN (*University of Colorado Medical School, Denver, Col.*): Would you tell us a little about what sort of macrophages these are? Where do you get them and how do you induce them?

POLAK: We used peritoneal exudate cells, which were induced by oil and then irradiated, in almost all our experiments. We also used spleen cells with the same effect in some control experiments. We never purify the cells. But, as you know, it's difficult to completely rid macrophage suspensions of lymphocytes.

CLAMAN: In the experiments where haptenated macrophages seem to interfere with the tolerant state, and where this state was blocked by an injection of hapten in FCA, how do you know that you didn't produce some antibody with the latter injection that interfered with the effectiveness of the haptenated macrophages?

POLAK: We looked at the production of antibodies after giving DNP-Mϕ and after epicutaneous sensitization and, measured by PCA, we never induced antibodies at all. We also used the tolerogenic carrier DNP-DGL. These animals had no trace of antibodies to DNP. Despite that, these animals could be tolerized and the tolerance was as firm and as complete as in animals that did have this antibody. So I think that this excludes the role of antibodies in the induction of tolerance in this system.

REGULATION OF CONTACT ALLERGY IN THE B CELL–DEFICIENT MOUSE

Henry C. Maguire, Jr.

Department of Medicine
Division of Dermatology
Hahnemann Medical College and Hospital
Philadelphia, Pennsylvania 19102

INTRODUCTION

In dealing with the immunological response to nonreplicating antigens, it has been proposed that B cells or their products modulate T cell reactions.[1-10] A number of mechanisms for such regulation have been proposed, including the masking of antigenic sites by antibody or antigen-antibody complexes, and the reaction of specific T cell receptors with antigen-antibody complexes or with anti-idiotypic antibody. We have investigated the role of B cells in allergic contact dermatitis (ACD) in the mouse. In particular, a number of ACD phenomena have been evaluated for their dependence on B cells, *viz.*, (1) the induction and expression of ACD, (2) the spontaneous waning of ACD in conventionally sensitized mice, (3) the specific immunological tolerance to contact allergens induced by pretreatment with parenteral hapten or haptenated spleen cells, (4) immunopotentiation by cyclophosphamide or by the local administration of a suspension of killed *C. parvum* (*P. acnes*), (5) the flare-up of previous test sites following the local administration of parenteral allergen, and (6) the acquisition and expression of photoallergic contact dermatitis (photo ACD). Our model is ACD in mice made B cell deficient by the chronic administration from birth of a goat antisera to mouse IgM. We have found that all ACD reactions that we have so far studied are well expressed in B cell–deficient mice. When a direct comparison has been made between matched intact and B cell–deficient mice, no significant differences have been discerned, as might be expected were there substantial B cell regulation of these T cell reactions. We conclude that B cell participation is not required in the diverse ACD phenomena that we have so far examined; an optional or minor subsidiary function of B cells cannot be excluded, nor can we exclude a decisive role for B cells in aspects of ACD not yet examined.

MATERIALS AND METHODS

Animals. C57B1/6 males and CBA females were periodically purchased from the Jackson Laboratories and served as breeding stock. Breeding pairs were set up in individual cages. The mice were housed in plastic cages, with wood shavings for bedding; the cages were individually covered with glass wool bonnets. The mice were fed fresh Purina Mouse Chow and had unlimited access to acidified water (pH about 3.0). Antibiotics were not used. The colony was kept in a temperature-controlled, light-cycled room. Other strains of mice were obtained from the Jackson Laboratory or from the Institute for

107

0077-8923/82/0392-0107 $1.75/0 © 1982, NYAS

Cancer Research (Fox Chase, Pennsylvania) and kept under similar conditions. Unintentional losses of experimental animals were extremely rare.

B Cell Suppression. A male adult goat was immunized subcutaneously at intervals of 2–3 weeks with a mouse myeloma protein, MOPC 104-E (λ ,μ; Litton Bionetics) emulsified in complete Freund's adjuvant (Difco, Detroit, Michigan). Stock antisera was derived from several pooled bleedings that were first taken about two years after the start of immunization. The antisera was heat inactivated and absorbed with erythrocytes of the mouse strain in which it was ultimately used. Breeding pairs were inspected five days a week. Offspring that could be positively identified as having been born within 24 h were injected intraperitoneally with the absorbed goat antisera to mouse IgM, and continued to receive this antisera three times per week indefinitely. The putatively B cell–deficient mice had the following characteristics: (1) their sera, as determined by precipitation in gel, lacked mouse IgM and contained goat antimouse IgM, (2) their spleen cells, as determined by direct immunofluorescence, all lacked surface immunoglobulin, in contrast to the spleen cells from control mice, (3) their spleen cells failed to respond in culture to the B cell mitogen lipopolysaccharide (LPS) but did respond normally to the T cell mitogen concanavalin-A (Con A) and, (4) in contrast to normal mice who developed high titers of specific antibody, they failed to make any detectable antibody response to sheep red blood cells (hemagglutination, hemolysis in gel) or to DNP-KLH (radioimmune assay using protein A) (TABLE 1). These findings relative to this B cell–deficient model are in accord with reports from other laboratories that study mice made B cell deficient in this way.[11, 12]

Chemicals. DNFB (1-fluoro 2,4-dinitrobenzene; Eastman Chemicals, Rochester, N.Y.), oxazolone (4-ethoxy methylene-2-phenyl-oxazolone; BDH Chemicals, Ltd., Poole, England), DNBSO$_3$, (1-sulfonate 2,4-dinitrobenzene; Eastman Chemicals, Rochester, N.Y.), cyclophosphamide (Cy, Sigma Chemicals, St. Louis, Mo.), and 3,3′,4′,5-tetrachlorosalicylanilide (TCSA; Research Institute for Fragrance Materials, Englewood Cliffs, N.J.) were obtained. A preparation of heat-killed *C. parvum* (*P. acnes*), originating from cultures derived from strain #11827 of the American Type Culture Collection, was a gift from Dr. Irving Millman.[13]

Sensitization and Challenge. Mice were sensitized by the application daily for 2 d of 0.02 ml 0.5% DNFB or 5% oxazolone in a solvent consisting of four parts acetone and one part corn oil. Challenge was made by the application of 0.01 ml 0.2% DNFB (or 0.1% oxazolone) in the same solvent on the external aspect of the distal portion of a normal ear.[14] Baseline and subsequent readings were made with an engineer's micrometer equipped with a rachet.

Photosensitization. Test mice were anesthetized with pentabarbital, photoallergen was pipetted onto a clipped site on the flank, and the site was then irradiated with medium wave ultraviolet light (UVB, 0.1 J cm^{-2}) followed by long wave ultraviolet light (UVA, 5.0 J cm^{-2}). Challenge was made on an ear with 0.01 ml of test chemical followed by UVA (5.0 J cm^{-2}). The UVB source was a bank of four fluorescent sunlamp tubes (FS-20); their spectrum extends from about 280 nm to 380 nm with a peak at approximately 313 nm. The UVA source was a bank of four fluorescent blacklight tubes (F-20 BL); their spectrum extends from 310 nm to about 400 nm, peaking at 360 nm. The method is basically that used for the study of classical ACD in mice, the extra steps being those required for the activation of the process by ultraviolet light.[15]

Histology. Ear specimens were secured at the end of an experiment, preserved in 10% neutral buffered formalin, and processed to hematoxylin-eosin slides by routine procedures.

Statistics. The significance of differences between study groups in particular experiments was analyzed by a one-tailed Mann-Whitney U Test.[16]

Preparation of DNFB-Reacted Cells. A single-cell suspension of spleen cells was made and washed in RPMI 1640. The red cells were lysed with ammonium chloride and the cell suspensions washed and resuspended in RPMI 1640 to a concentration of 5×10^6 ml^{-1}; 0.1 ml of a 5 mM solution of DNFB was then added for every ml of cells. The cells were incubated at room temperature for 30 min with occasional gentle mixing. The suspension was then pelleted and resuspended in RPMI 1640.[17]

TABLE 1

SERUM ANTIBODY TITERS TO DNP IN NORMAL MICE
AND IN ANTI-IgM TREATED MICE

Control Mouse	Anti-DNP Antibody	α-Igm Mouse	Anti-DNP Antibody
1	1:10 935 *	1	< 1:5
2	1:3645	2	< 1:5
3	1:10 935	3	< 1:5
4	1:98 415	4	< 1:5
5	1:98 415	5	< 1:5
6	1:3645	6	< 1:5
7	1:10 935	7	< 1:5
8	1:295 245	8	< 1:5

* Highest serum dilution with binding of DNP-HSA $\geq$ 50%.
NOTE: Groups of eight control and eight anti-IgM treated mice received 200 μg DNP-KLH in complete Freund's adjuvant subcutaneously on day 0 and a further 20 μg DNP-KLH in saline on day 10. All mice were bled on day 16. By radio-immune assay, using Staph protein A (Kessler, S.W. 1976. J. Immunol. **117:** 1482–90), there were high titers of anti-DNP antibody in each of the eight controls and no anti-DNP antibody activity detected in any of the eight mice that were chronically treated with anti-IgM.

RESULTS

ACD in B Cell–Deficient Mice

Allergic contact dermatitis can readily be induced in B cell–deficient mice. The degree of the contact hypersensitivity, as assessed by challenge on the ear, parallels that of allergic contact dermatitis induced by similar means in normal intact mice of the same strain. The results of a typical experiment can be seen in TABLE 2. The histology of the ACD challenge reaction in the B cell–deficient mouse (different experiment), as evaluated by routine hematoxylin-eosin sections, is similar to that seen in normal mice (FIGURE 1). It is interesting that, in our experience, the ACD challenge reactions in B cell–deficient mice are not

TABLE 2

DNFB Contact Sensitivity in Normal and B Cell–Deficient Mice

Group	Day 0	Day 1	Day 5	Day 6
Normal	0.5% DNFB 0.02 ml left flank	0.5% DNFB 0.02 ml left flank	0.2% DNFB 0.01 ml left ear	12.4 ± 3.3 *
α-IgM				12.6 ± 2.7

* Increase in ear thickness ± s.d., mm × 10⁻².

(* Increase in ear thickness ± S.D., mm $\times 10^{-2}$.)

NOTE: Groups of normal and B cell–deficient mice were sensitized by the application of DNFB to a clipped area on the left flank on day 0 and day 1. On day 5, they were challenged on the left ear. The induced inflammation at 24 h, as estimated by the increase in ear thickness, is shown. The ear reaction of the toxicity control group at 24 h was 1.1 ± 0.7.

TABLE 3

Spontaneous Loss of Allergic Contact Dermatitis Reactivity in B Cell–Depleted Mice

α-IgM Group	Day 0,1 (all groups)	Day 5 (group I)	Day 6	Day 10 (group II)	Day 11	Day 15 (group III)	Day 16
I	DNFB Sensitization	DNFB Challenge	11.6 ± 4.6*	—	—	—	—
II	—	—	—	DNFB Challenge	5.5 ± 1.2	—	—
III	—	—	—	—	—	DNFB Challenge	2.1 ± 1.3

* Increase in ear thickness ± s.d., mm $\times 10^{-2}$.
I > II, p < 0.01.
II > III, p < 0.01.

NOTE: Three groups of B cell–depleted mice received 0.02 ml of 0.5% DNFB on a clipped site on the left flank on day 0 and day 1. The mice of each group were challenged once, on the days indicated, in parallel with a group of toxicity control mice. The net increase in ear thickness at 24 h is tabulated.

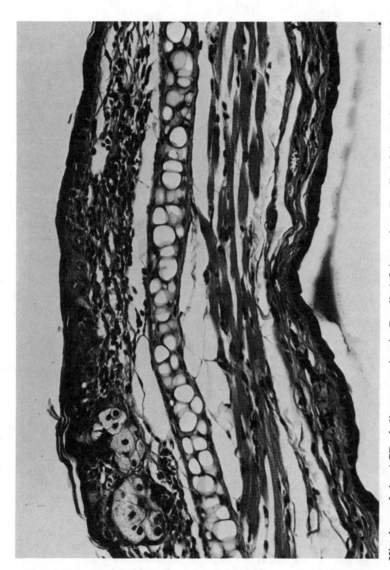

FIGURE 1. Histology of the ACD challenge reaction in B cell–deficient mice. B cell–deficient mice were sensitized to DNFB on day 0 and day 1. They were challenged on the left ear with DNFB on day 5 and biopsies made of the challenge sites two days later. A hematoxylin-eosin section from a representative specimen is shown. There is edema and a dermal infiltrate consisting of histiocytes and lymphocytes. (Magnification ×170.)

prolonged, as might be expected if there were a deficiency in pertinent suppressor cells resulting from their B cell deficiency.[28]

Rapid Waning of ACD in B Cell–Deficient Mice

In mice, a spontaneous loss of T cell hypersensitivity soon after sensitization has been observed following immunization both with sheep red blood cells (SRBC) and with contact allergens.[19, 10] This waning of hypersensitivity is seen with conventional sensitization and can be abrogated if immunological adjuvants are used.[19] It has been attributed to antibodies.[19, 10] We have contact sensitized normal and B cell–deficient mice using, in different experiments, DNFB and oxazolone. A consistent finding has been that the ACD reactions of both normal and B cell–deficient mice peak at 5 to 7 d and then rapidly decline. The results of a typical experiment with B cell–deficient mice is shown in TABLE 3. It is curious that a similar rapid falloff in reactivity does not occur with ACD in humans, rats, hamsters, or chickens sensitized in a comparable way.

Immunological Tolerance

Specific immunological tolerance to simple chemical allergens has been induced with parenteral hapten in both man and a variety of experimental animals.[20-23] It has been suggested that this tolerance might be mediated by antibody.[3] We have studied the induction of immunological tolerance in B cell–depleted mice. Such mice can be as readily tolerized to DNFB contact sensitization by the prior intravenous injection of $DNBSO_3$ as normal mice of the same strain.[24] We have found no evidence that antibody contributes to immunological tolerance induced by parenteral hapten.

Immunological tolerance to contact allergens can also be induced with haptenized cells. This was first demonstrated by Battisto and Bloom in their classic guinea pig experiments.[25] The intravenous administration of haptenated cells has also been used to induce immunological tolerance in other rodent species, including mice.[26] We have found that B cell–deficient mice can become tolerized following an intravenous injection of spleen cells reacted with DNFB (TABLE 4). This finding suggests that neither B cells nor antibody mediate the induction of specific immunological tolerance by haptenated lymphoid cells.

Immunopotentiation of ACD

Treatment with cyclophosphamide before sensitization markedly increases the resultant contact hypersensitivity, as evidenced by an increase in the intensity and duration of the challenge reaction. We first described this phenomenon in guinea pigs sensitized to DNCB; it has since been observed in a variety of species and with a wide range of immunogens.[27] Recently, immunopotentiation of delayed-type hypersensitivity to DNFB and to keyhole limpet hemocyanin (KLH) as a result of cyclophosphamide pretreatment has been observed in man.[28] Cyclophosphamide immunopotentiation has been attributed to the inhibition by that drug of B suppressor cells.[5, 8, 9] We have studied cyclophosphamide immunopotentiation in B cell–depleted mice and found that such mice respond to immunopotentiation by cyclophosphamide pretreatment as readily as normal mice.[29] In accordance with other lines of evidence, it appears that the mechanism of cyclophosphamide immunopotentiation of delayed-type hypersensitivity reactions is primarily through its effect on T suppressor cells (and, in particular, on their precursors).[30, 31]

The acquisition of ACD can be heightened in rodents by treatment of the sensitization site with killed *C. parvum*.[32, 33] The immuno-adjuvant effect with the *C. parvum* resembles that seen with complete Freund's adjuvant. Since *C. parvum* can be a potent stimulator of B cell reactions, we wondered whether *C. parvum* immunopotentiation of allergic contact dermatitis in mice might depend on B cell mediation. In fact, ACD can readily be immunopotentiated in B cell–depleted mice by the administration of *C. parvum* into the sensitization

TABLE 4

SPECIFIC IMMUNOLOGICAL TOLERANCE INDUCED WITH DNP SPLEEN CELLS
IN B CELL–DEFICIENT MICE

α-Igm Group	Day -7	Day 0,1	Day 5	Day 6
I	DNP-spleen cells i.v.	DNFB sensitization	DNFB challenge	1.4 ± 1.3 * 14.2 ± 2.9
II	—			
III	DNP-spleen cells i.v.	Oxazolone sensitization	Oxazolone challenge	8.6 ± 2.1
IV	—			7.0 ± 0.8

* Increase in ear thickness ± s.d., mm × 10^{-2}.
II > I, p < 0.01.
NOTE: Two groups of CBA X C57B1/6 B cell–deficient mice received 10^8 syngeneic DNP-spleen cells intravenously on day -7. One group, in parallel with a further group of untreated B cell–deficient mice, was sensitized to and challenged with DNFB. The second DNP-spleen cell–injected group, in parallel with a second B cell–deficient control group, was sensitized to oxazolone. On day 5, the different groups were ear challenged with either DNFB or oxazolone as shown. The net (experimental minus toxicity control) 24 h reactions are tabulated.

site (TABLE 5). The degree of immunopotentiation was comparable to that obtained with ACD in normal mice. We believe that *C. parvum* immunopotentiation is probably mediated by macrophages in the lymph nodes regional to the sensitization site, although there is no direct evidence for this thesis.

The Flare Reaction

A reinflammation of old faded test sites of allergic contact dermatitis is seen following the injection of parenteral allergen in experimental animals; it has been clinically observed in man. An antibody basis for this phenomenon has been suggested.[34] In initial experiments, we found that the flare reaction could readily be induced in normal mice sensitized to DNFB and later injected with

$DNBSO_3$. The reaction was specific, in that test sites in mice sensitized to and challenged with oxazolone did not flare following intravenous $DNBSO_3$. The flare in the normal mouse is often evident at 4 h; this suggested that the phenomenon is mediated by antibody. Would the flare reaction appear in B cell–deficient mice? We have tested this in six different experiments and have found that the flare could readily be produced in the B cell–deficient mouse in every case (TABLE 6). It is interesting that the flare often appears at 4 h in the B cell–deficient mice, as it does in normal mice. This suggests that an assay at 4 h of challenge sites does not necessarily discriminate against T cell reactions. Positive contact challenge reactions at 4 h have been observed in allergic contact dermatitis in B cell–deficient chickens.[35]

TABLE 5

LOCAL *Corynebacterium Parvum* HEIGHTENS THE ACQUISITION
OF ALLERGIC CONTACT DERMATITIS IN B CELL-DEPLETED MICE

α-IgM Group	Day 0 (groups I–III)	Day 1	Day 5 (all groups)	Day 6
I	DNFB	*C. parvum* (30 μg) right flank	DNFB ear challenge	11.8 ± 3.5 *
II	right	*C. parvum* (30 μg) left flank		5.6 ± 0.9
III	flank	Saline right flank		5.4 ± 1.8
IV	—	—		0.5 ± 0.5

* Increase in ear thickness, mm $\times$ 10^{-2}.
I > II, p < 0.01.
I > III, p < 0.02.
NOTE: Three groups of B cell–deficient mice were sensitized to DNFB on day 0. The next day, group I was injected with *C. parvum* in the sensitization site, group II received a similar injection on the opposite flank, and group III mice, in parallel, were given saline in the sensitization site. All mice were challenged on day 5; the reactions at 24 h for the 3 groups and a toxicity control group are shown.

Photo-ACD

In recent studies, we have induced photoallergic contact dermatitis in mice.[15] Photo-ACD to compounds such as 3,3′,4′,5-tetrachlorosalicylanilide, chlorpromazine, and 6-methylcoumarin are readily induced in a variety of strains of mice. Ordinarily, such compounds do not induce ACD; however, if the sensitization and the challenge sites are irradiated with long wave ultraviolet light (UVA) following the application of a photoallergen, a delayed-type hypersensitivity reaction develops. The induced hypersensitivity is specific and can be adoptively transferred with cells derived from the lymph nodes regional to the sensitization site.[15] In order to evaluate the role of B cells in the expression and regulation of photo-ACD in mice, we attempted to induce photo-ACD in B cell–depleted mice. Indeed, such mice can readily be photo contact sensitized. The results of one such experiment are outlined in TABLE 6. The histology of the reactions are comparable to those seen in normal mice photosensitized to TCSA or sensitized to contact allergens such as dinitrochlorobenzene or oxazolone (FIGURE 2). These findings provide additional evidence that photo-ACD is a T cell phenomenon and is not decisively regulated by B cells.

TABLE 6

THE FLARE REACTION IN NORMAL AND IN B CELL–DEFICIENT MICE

Group	Both Groups			+ 4 h		+ 24 h	
	Day 0,1	Day 5	Day 13	Left Ear	Right Ear	Left Ear	Right Ear
I (normal)	DNFB sensitization	DNFB challenge Left ear	DNBSO$_3$ 750mg i.p.	3.8 ± 2.4 *	0.1 ± 1.0	3.7 ± 1.7	0.8 ± 1.3
II (α-IgM)				4.3 ± 2.6	0.3 ± 0.9	3.8 ± 2.9	1.1 ± 1.2

* Increase in ear thickness ± S.D., mm × 10^{-2}.
Left > right: I (4 h) $p < 0.01$; (24 h) $p < 0.03$
II (4 h) $p < 0.01$; (24 h) $p < 0.01$

NOTE: Normal and B cell–deficient mice were sensitized on the flank and challenged on one ear with DNFB. Eight days post-challenge, all mice were injected i.p. with DNBSO$_3$ after a baseline reading of ear thickness. The increase in ear thickness (± S.D.) is shown for each group.

Discussion

We have studied the development of allergic contact dermatitis and related phenomena in mice rendered B cell deficient by the chronic administration of a heterologous antisera to mouse IgM. The model of the B cell–deficient mouse has been used by a number of investigators for different purposes and the effectiveness of the B cell immunosuppression has been confirmed by measurement of a variety of independent parameters.[11, 12, 36]

The reaction of ACD and of tuberculin hypersensitivity can be mimicked by antibody.[37] We have failed to find a discernible contribution of possible

TABLE 7

PHOTOALLERGIC CONTACT DERMATITIS TO 3,3', 4',5 TETRACHLOROSALICYLANILIDE
INDUCED IN B CELL–DEFICIENT MICE

α-IgM Group	Day 0 (group I)	Day 1	Day 6 (both groups)	Day 7	
				TCSA-UVA Left Ear	UVA-TCSA Right Ear
I	TCSA UVB-UVA	TCSA UVB-UVA C. parvum	TCSA + UVA	11.5 ± 2.3	2.5 ± 1.4
II	—	C. parvum		2.5 ± 0.5	1.7 ± 1.2

Left ear: I > II, $p < 0.001$

NOTE: A group of B cell–deficient mice received 0.02 ml 1% TCSA on a clipped area of the flank followed by UVB and UVA on day 0 and day 1. The photosensitization site was injected intradermally with 30 μg C. parvum on day 1; an untreated group of B cell–deficient mice was similarly injected with C. parvum. On day 6, mice of both groups were photochallenged on the ear by the application of 0.01 ml TCSA followed by UVA on the left ear. The right ear received 0.01 ml of 1% TCSA after the UVA; the reactions at 24 h are shown.

effector antibody in the ACD challenge reactions of routinely sensitized mice when comparing normal with B cell–deficient mice. This is not surprising since, following conventional sensitization of mice with hapten, the anti-hapten specific antibody response is negligible at a time when the ACD reaction is well expressed.[38]

There is considerable precedent in the case of tissue transplantation for the suppression of T cell reactions by antibody with specificity for surface antigen.[39] Our results suggest that such antibody does not account for the rapid spontaneous loss of ACD in the mouse or for the induction of specific immunological tolerance by parenteral hapten or haptenized cells. Autoantibody with specificity for idiotype would appear to play a significant role in the regulation of B cell responses.[40] The cross-reactivity of T cell and B cell idiotypes has been demonstrated with haptens such as azobenzene arsonate.[41] This suggests a mechanism for the physiological B cell regulation of ACD reactions by means

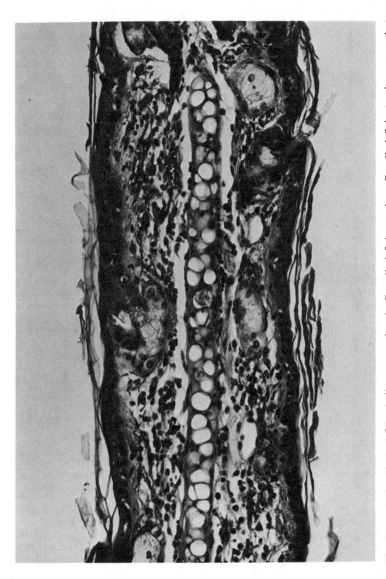

FIGURE 2. Histology of the photo-ACD challenge reaction in B cell–deficient mice. B cell–deficient mice were photosensitized to TCSA on day 0 and day 1. On day 5, the mice were photochallenged with TCSA and biopsies taken at 48 h. A hematoxylineosin section from a representative specimen is shown. There is a dermatitis characterized by edema and a dermal infiltrate consisting primarily of lymphocytes and histiocytes. (Magnification ×170.)

of specific antibody to pertinent idiotype.[10] In our B cell-deficient mice exhibiting ACD, we have not yet observed a lacuna that would imply the absence of regulation by anti-idiotypic antibody.

A number of lines of evidence suggest that cyclophosphamide immunopotentiates T cell reactivity by means of its ultimate effect on T suppressor cells. Our findings argue against cyclophosphamide modulation of B suppressor cells as a significant mechanism in this immunopotentiation. Local heat-killed *C. parvum* immunopotentiates ACD in mice, rats, guinea pigs, and hamsters. Phenomenologically, its heightening of the acquisition of ACD in mice resembles the immunoadjuvant effect of complete Freund's adjuvant on ACD in guinea pigs.[32, 42] A similar mechanism may be involved.

Recently, with Dr. K. Kaidbey, we have developed a mouse model for the study of photo contact allergens.[15] The mouse provides an advantageous experimental model, since its genetic and immunological parameters are well defined and, for purposes of comparison, there is much recent work dealing with ACD in that species. Our finding that photo-ACD is well expressed in B cell–deficient mice provides evidence that, like conventional ACD, it is a T cell phenomenon.

SUMMARY

We have examined the obligate role of B cells in the regulation of allergic contact dermatitis. Our model is ACD in mice made B cell deficient by the chronic administration from birth of a goat antisera to mouse IgM. The following ACD phenomena are well demonstrated in these mice: (1) acquisition and expression of ACD, (2) spontaneous waning of ACD soon after sensitization, (3) immunological tolerance induced by pretreatment with either parenteral hapten or haptenated spleen cells, (4) immunopotentiation by means of either cyclophosphamide or the local administration of a suspension of killed *C. parvum* (*P. acnes*), (5) the flare-up of previous test sites following the local administration of parenteral allergen, and (6) acquisition and expression of photo-ACD. We conclude that B cell participation is not required for these ACD phenomena, although an optional or subsidiary function for B regulatory cells is not excluded.

REFERENCES

1. POLAK, L., J. L. FREY & J. L. TURK. 1970. Studies on the effect of systemic administration of sensitizers to guinea pigs with contact sensitivity to inorganic metal compounds. V. Studies on the mechanism of the "flare-up" reaction. Clin. Exp. Immunol. 7: 739–44.

2. ASHERSON, G. L., M. ZEMBALA & R. M. R. BARNES. 1971. The mechanism of immunological unresponsiveness to picryl chloride and the possible role of antibody mediated depression. Clin. Exp. Immunol. 9: 111–21.

3. HALLIDAY, W. J. & B. A. J. WALTERS. 1974. The mechanism of tolerance in contact hypersensitivity to DNFB in guinea pigs. Clin. Exp. Immunol. 16: 203–12.

4. TURK, J. L. & D. PARKER. 1974. B-cell modulation of T cell function in delayed hypersensitivity with special reference to contact sensitivity. Monogr. Allergy 8: 44–53.

5. KATZ, S. I., D. PARKER & J. L. TURK. 1974. B-cell suppression of delayed hypersensitivity reactions. Nature (London) 251: 550–51.

6. MACKANESS, G. B., P. H. LAGRANGE, T. E. MILLER & T. ISHIBASHI. 1974. Feedback inhibition of specifically sensitized lymphocytes. J. Exp. Med. **139:** 543–59.
7. LANGRANGE, P. H., G. B. MACKANESS & T. E. MILLER. 1974. Potentiation of T-cell mediated immunity by selective suppression of antibody formation with cyclophosphamide. J. Exp. Med. **139:** 1529–39.
8. NETA, R. & S. B. SALVIN. 1974. Specific suppression of delayed hypersensitivity: The possible presence of a suppressor B cell in the regulation of delayed hypersensitivity. J. Immunol. **113:** 1716–25.
9. ZEMBALA, M., G. L. ASHERSON, J. NOWOROLSKI & B. MAYHEW. 1976. Contact sensitivity to picryl chloride: The occurrence of B-suppressor cells in the lymph nodes and spleen of immunized mice. Cell. Immunol. **25:** 266–78.
10. SY, M.-S., J. W. MOORHEAD & H. N. CLAMAN. 1979. Regulation of cell mediated immunity by antibodies: Possible role of anti-receptor antibodies in the regulation of contact sensitivity to DNFB in mice. J. Immunol. **123:** 2593–98.
11. GORDON, J. 1979. The B lymphocyte deprived mouse as a tool in immunobiology. J. Immunol. Methods **25:** 227–38.
12. COOPER, M. D., J. F. KEARNEY, W. E. GOTHINGS & A. R. LAWTON. 1980. Effects of anti-Ig antibodies on the development and differentiation of B cells. Immunol. Rev. **52:** 29–53.
13. MILLMAN, I., A. W. SCOTT & T. HALBHERR. 1977. Antitumor activity of propionibacterium acnes (C. parvum) and isolated cytoplasmic fractions. Cancer Res. **37:** 4150–55.
14. ASHERSON, G. L. & W. L. PTAK. 1969. Contact and delayed hypersensitivity in the mouse. I Active sensitization and passive transfer. Immunology **15:** 405–16.
15. MAGUIRE, H. C., JR. & K. KAIDBEY. 1982. Experimental photoallergic contact dermatitis: A mouse model. J. Invest. Derm. In press.
16. SIEGAL, S. 1956. Nonparametric Statistics. McGraw Hill. New York.
17. MILLER, S. D. & H. N. CLAMAN. 1976. The induction of hapten-specific T cell tolerance by using hapten-modified lymphoid cells. I. Characteristics of tolerance induction. J. Immunol. **117:** 1519–26.
18. POLAK, L. & C. RINCK. 1977. Effect of the elimination of suppressor cells on the development of DNFB contact sensitivity in guinea pigs. Immunology **33:** 305–11.
19. LAGRANGE, P. H. & G. B. MACKANESS. 1975. A stable form of delayed type hypersensitivity. J. Exp. Med. **141:** 82–96.
20. FREI, W. 1928. Über willkürliche Sensibilisierung gegen chemischedefinierte Substanzen I. Untersuchungen mit Neosalvarsan am Menschen. Klin. Wochenschr. **7:** 539–42.
21. SULZBERGER, M. D. 1929. Hypersensitiveness to neoarsphenamine in guinea pigs. Arch. Dermatol. **20:** 669–97.
22. CHASE, M. W. 1946. Inhibition of experimental drug allergy by prior feeding of the sensitizing agent. Proc. Soc. Exp. Biol. Med. **61:** 257–59.
23. LOWNEY, E. D. 1973. Suppression of contact sensitization in man by prior feeding of antigen. J. Invest. Dermatol. **61:** 90–93.
24. MAGUIRE, H. C., JR., W. P. WEIDANZ & S. J. SCHUSTER. 1980. Tolerance to a contact allergen in the mouse does not require antibody. Fed. Proc. Fed. Am. Soc. Exp. Biol. **39:** 2122.
25. BATTISTO, J. R. & B. R. BLOOM. 1966. Dual immunological unresponsiveness induced by cell membrane coupled hapten or antigen. Nature (London) **212:** 156–57.
26. CLAMAN, H. N. & S. E. MILLER. 1976. Requirements for induction of T cell tolerance to DNFB: efficiency of membrane-associated DNFB. J. Immunol. **117:** 480–85.

27. MAGUIRE, H. C., JR. & V. L. ETTORE. 1967. Enhancement of dinitrochloro-benzene (DNCB) contact sensitization by cyclophosphamide in the guinea pig. J. Invest. Dermatol. **48:** 39–43.
28. MAGUIRE, H., D. BERD, P. ENGSTROM, A. PAUL & M. MASTRANGELO. 1981. Cyclophosphamide (Cy) increases the acquisition of T-cell immunity in patients with melanoma or colo-rectal cancer. Proc. Am. Assoc. Cancer Res. **22:** 279.
29. MAGUIRE, H. C., JR., L. FARIS & W. WEIDANZ. 1979. Cyclophosphamide intensifies the acquisition of allergic contact dermatitis in mice rendered B-cell deficient by heterologous anti-IgM antisera. Immunology **37:** 367–72.
30. ASKENASE, P. W., B. J. HAYDEN & R. K. GERSHON. 1975. Augmentation of delayed-type hypersensitivity by doses of cyclophosphamide which do not affect antibody responses. J. Exp. Med. **141:** 697–702.
31. DIAMANTSTEIN, T., M. KIOS, H. HAHN & S. KAUFMAN. 1981. Direct *in vitro* evidence for different susceptibilities to 4-hydroperoxycyclophosphamide of antigen-primed T cells regulating humoral and cell-mediated immune responses to sheep erythrocytes: A possible explanation for the inverse action of cyclophosphamide on humoral and cell-mediated immune responses. J. Immunol. **126:** 1717–19.
32. CIPRIANO, D. & H. C. MAGUIRE, JR. 1981. Specific T-cell immunopotentiation by C. parvum. Proc. Am. Assoc. Cancer Res. **22:** 280.
33. MAGUIRE, H. C., JR. 1981. Immunopotentiation of allergic contact dermatitis in the guinea pig with C. parvum (P. acnes). Acta Derm. Venereol. **61:** 565–67.
34. POLAK, L. & J. L. TURK. 1968. Studies on the effect of systemic administra-tion of sensitizers in guinea pigs with contact sensitivity to inorganic metal compounds. II. The flare-up of previous test sites of contact sensitivity and the development of a generalized rash. Clin. Exp. Immunol. **3:** 253–62.
35. WEIDANZ, W. P., W. T. WEBER & H. C. MAGUIRE, JR. 1976. Allergic contact dermatitis in the B cell deficient chicken. Int. Arch. Allergy Appl. Immunol. **50:** 755–58.
36. GRUN, J. L. & W. P. WEIDANZ. 1981. Immunity to plasmodium chabaudi adami in B cell deficient mouse. Nature (London) **290:** 143–45.
37. CHASE, M. W. 1970. Can plasma transfer tuberculin or hapten hyper-sensitivity? Fed. Proc. Fed. Am. Soc. Exp. Biol. **92:** 701 (#2576).
38. TAKAHASHI, C., S. NISHIKAWA, Y. KATSURA & T. IZUMI. 1977. Anti-DNP antibody response after topical application of DNFB in mice. Immunology **33:** 589–96.
39. KALISS, N. & A. A. KANDUTSCH. 1956. Acceptance of tumor homograft by mice injected with antiserum. I. Activity of serum fractions. Proc. Soc. Exp. Biol. Med. **91:** 118–121.
40. JERNE, N. 1976. The immune system: a web of V domains. Harvey Lect. **70:** 93–110.
41. SY, M.-S., A. R. BROWN, B. BENACERRAF & M. I. GREEN. 1980. Antigen and receptor dimer regulatory mechanisms. III. Induction of delayed-type hyper-sensitivity to azobenzene-arsonate with anti-cross-reactive idiotypic antibodies. J. Exp. Med. **151:** 896–909.
42. MAGUIRE, H. C., JR. & M. W. CHASE. 1970. Studies on the sensitization of animals with simple chemical compounds. XIII. Sensitization of guinea pigs with picric acid. J. Exp. Med. **135:** 357–75.

DISCUSSION OF THE PAPER

J. W. MOORHEAD (*University of Colorado Medical School, Denver, Col.*): Did you pretreat your animals with cyclophosphamide also in the experiments where you show transient contact sensitivity in B cell–deficient mice? Does the response stay up any longer in Cy-pretreated animals than in non-Cy-pretreated animals, both of which are B cell deficient?

MAGUIRE: I believe it does. I can't think of the particular experiment.

H. N. CLAMAN (*University of Colorado Medical School, Denver, Col.*): Dr. Moorhead asks that because we have investigated the phenomenon of the falloff of contact sensitivity in Balb/c mice—were those Balb/c mice? It's important because our conclusions were that this falloff was due to the presence of an anti-idiotypic antibody, which obviously depends upon the presence of B cells. Maybe we're going to have to have another look at that.

J. CHILLER (*Scripps Clinic and Research Foundation, La Jolla, Calif.*): Once made deficient, do mice show any B cell activity following one of those regimens which induce T cell activity? That is, is it possible that, by inducing T cell activity, particularly T helper cell activity in some of these cases, you finally do break through into B cell activity? In other words, at the end of some of your experiments did you look for the possibility that you do, in fact, have specific antibody in deficient animals?

MAGUIRE: I can't recall that we ever looked for specific antibody.* The mice we tested were immunized with sheep cells and with DNP-KLH and were not in an experiment. This can and should be done.

CLAMAN: As a dermatologist, do you doubt that antibody is an important factor in contact dermatitis, which has gone on for a period of time, perhaps with repeated sensitizations, rather than in the somewhat artificial and limited form of contact dermatitis that you and I and a lot of other people look at in mice? As you know, if you keep painting mice with DNFB, (as shown by Merrill Chase with injections with Freund's adjuvant) you get perfectly respectable antibody titers. So what do you think would be the behavior of your B cell–deficient mice if you prolonged your sensitization regimen or looked at regulatory phenomena sometime later on?

MAGUIRE: Certainly you can have antibody in contact allergy to poison ivy. There are some people who get almost immediate symptoms. Certainly you can get skin reactions from high titers of antibody, as Dr. Chase showed some years ago. This is pseudo-contact allergy, a reaction that people can confuse with genuine contact T cell reactions. If you look way down the line after repeated immunizations, you might begin to see B cell regulation. My experiments do not exclude the possibility.

---

* [Note added in proof: In a published experiment that I overlooked, we studied the antibody response to SRBC in groups of B cell–depleted mice that had been sensitized to NDMA (*p*-nitrosodimethylaniline), with or without cyclophosphamide pretreatment.[29] In contrast to intact mice sensitized in parallel, the anti-IgM-treated mice made no detectable antibody response following SRBC immunization.]

THE ROLE OF SUPPRESSOR T CELL NETWORKS IN THE REGULATION OF DNFB CONTACT SENSITIVITY

RECEPTOR–ANTI-RECEPTOR INTERACTIONS IN EFFERENT SUPPRESSION *

Stephen D. Miller,[†] Larry D. Butler,[‡] and Henry N. Claman [‡]

† Department of Microbiology and Immunology
Northwestern University Medical School
Chicago, Illinois 60611

‡ Division of Clinical Immunology
Departments of Medicine and of Microbiology and Immunology
University of Colorado Health Sciences Center
Denver, Colorado 80262

INTRODUCTION

Intravenous injection of hapten- or antigen-mediated lymphoid cells is an efficient means of inducing specific unresponsiveness of both cellular and humoral immune responses.[1-6] Our laboratory has been studying the regulation of the T cell–mediated phenomenon of 2,4-dinitro-1-fluorobenzene (DNFB) contact sensitivity, in which tolerance is induced by prior i.v. injection of dinitrophenyl-modified syngeneic lymphoid cells (DNP-LC).[2] This unresponsive state has been separated into two distinct antigen-specific mechanisms: clone inhibition and the action of suppressor T cells (Ts). This distinction is based on kinetic experiments and the susceptibility of Ts induction to pretreatment with either cyclophosphamide (Cy) or splenectomy.[7]

Injection of syngeneic DNP-LC induces Ts in two mechanically distinct waves.[8] Three to seven days after tolerization, both spleen and lymph nodes of tolerant mice contain specific Ts_1 that bear receptors for DNP [8, 9] and are active in suppressing the expression (efferent limb) of DNFB immune T cells (T_{DH}, which passively transfer delayed contact hypersensitivity).[10] At 14 d after tolerization, a second-order Ts (Ts_2) is found that acts by suppressing the induction (afferent) phase of the contact sensitivity response.[8] The efferent suppression mediated by Ts_1 is non-MHC (major histocompatibility) restricted,[9, 10] as demonstrated by the inhibition of the passive transfer of DNFB contact sensitivity by both syngeneic and allogeneic T_{DH} cells. More detailed examination of this non-MHC restricted suppression has revealed that it is polyclonal in nature, i.e., composed of a collection of distinct MHC-restricted Ts, some of which are directed against DNP-syngeneic and others against DNP-allogeneic determinants.[9, 11]

We have also described an antigen-specific Ts auxiliary (Ts-aux) cell that is integrally involved in efferent suppression of T_{DH} by efferent-acting Ts raised by supraoptimal doses of antigen.[12] A similar cell has recently been shown in efferent suppression of delayed-type hypersensitivity (DTH) to the haptens azobenbene arsonate (ABA) and nitroiodophenyl (NIP).[13, 14] The Ts-aux is

* This research was supported, in part, by grants from the National Institutes of Health of the United States Public Health Service, nos. AI–18755 and AI–12685.

122

a Cy-sensitive, I-J$^+$ T cell that arises during the course of contact sensitization concomitantly with T_{DH} and serves as the instrument for the efferent regulation of those T_{DH} in conjunction with Ts_1.

This report examines the cellular interactions between Ts_1 and Ts-aux in the mediation of efferent suppression in terms of antigen (hapten), MHC, and allotype specificity and the receptor nature of the cells. Receptor-bearing Ts_1 appear to focus on the effector immune cells *via* passively bound DNP-MHC complexes on the T_{DH} surface and subsequently activate Ts-aux cells *via* receptor–anti-receptor interactions, resulting in the delivery of the final suppressive signal.

MATERIALS AND METHODS

Animals. Balb/c mice were purchased from Cumberland View Farms, Clinton, Tenn. CBA/J, C3H/HeJ, and B10.BR mice were purchased from the Jackson Laboratory, Bar Harbor, Me. Balb.Ig^b allotype congenic mice were the gift of Dr. Noel Warner, University of New Mexico School of Medicine, and were bred in our laboratory.

Antigens. 2,4-dinitro-1-fluorobenzene was obtained from Sigma Chemical Co., St. Louis, Mo. 2,4,6-trinitro-1-chlorobenzene (TNCB) was obtained from Matheson, Coleman & Bell, East Rutherford, N.J.

Cyclophosphamide Treatment. Mice were injected with 150–200 mg kg^{-1} Cy (Mead Johnson & Co., Evansville, Ind.) diluted in sterile distilled water two days before contact sensitization with DNFB.

Induction of Suppressor T Cells. Erythrocyte-free spleen cells were dinitrophenylated exactly as previously described.[2] 5×10^7 DNP-modified lymphoid cells were injected i.v. into syngeneic mice seven days before transfer. Single cell suspensions were prepared from lymph nodes (pooled peripheral and mesenteric) of tolerant mice and used as the source of Ts.

Induction and Passive Transfer of Contact Sensitivity. DNFB immune delayed hypersensitivity T cells were obtained from donors sensitized with 25 μl of 0.5% DNFB in 4:1 acetone : olive oil on the shaved abdomen and 5 μl on each ear on days 0 and 1. They also received 5 μl on each front paw on day 0. TNCB immune T_{DH} were obtained from mice sensitized with 100 μl of 7% TNCB on the shaved abdomen and 5 μl on the ears and front paws on day 0. Draining (inguinal, axillary, brachial, and cervical) lymph nodes were removed from the DNFB-sensitized mice on day 4 and from TNCB-sensitized mice on day 5. Single cell suspensions were prepared in balanced salt solution (BSS) and 5×10^7 cells were transferred i.v. to syngeneic recipient mice. Within one hour of transfer, recipient mice and uninjected controls were challenged on the dorsal surface of each ear with 20 μl of 0.2% DNFB, and increased ear swelling was measured with an engineer's micrometer 24 h later.[10] The increment in ear thickness is termed "ear swelling" and is expressed in units of micrometers.

Efferent Ts Assay—Inhibition of Passive Transfer of Contact Sensitivity. 5×10^7 tolerant lymph node cells (Ts) were cotransferred with 5×10^7 DNFB immune T_{DH} derived from either normal or Cy-pretreated donors to normal, syngeneic recipients. Recipients were ear challenged within 1 h of transfer.

Positive control mice received only T_{DH} cells and negative controls were ear challenged only. The percentage of suppression was calculated according to the following formula, using ear swelling values:

$$\% \text{ Suppression} = \left[\frac{\text{Positive Control} - \text{Experimental}}{\text{Positive Control} - \text{Negative Control}} \right] \times 100\%$$

Antiserum Preparation. Monoclonal IgM anti-Thy 1.2 ascitic fluid was obtained from New England Nuclear Corp., Boston, Mass. Monoclonal IgM anti-Lyt 2.2 ascitic fluid was obtained from Dr. Phillipa Marrack, National Jewish Hospital and Research Center, Denver, Col. Anti-DNP serum was obtained from either Balb/c mice or rabbits immunized three times with DNP_{20}-rabbit gamma globulin emulsified in complete Freund's adjuvant (CFA) and the serum was absorbed extensively with mouse spleen and thymocytes. Anti-T_{DH} idiotypic autoantiserum was prepared by Dr. John Moorhead, University of Colorado Medical Center, Denver, Col., from Balb/c mice immunized repeatedly with purified Balb/c DNFB immune T_{DH} cells emulsified in CFA. Its specificity and characteristics are described elsewhere (J. W. Moorhead, manuscript submitted for publication).

Antiserum Treatment. 10^8 lymph node cells per ml were treated with a 1:200 dilution of monoclonal anti-Thy 1.2 or anti-Lyt 2.2 serum or with a 1:20 dilution of anti-DNP or anti-T_{DH} serum for 1 h at 4° C. The cells were then washed once in BSS, resuspended in guinea pig (1:6) or rabbit (1:10) complement containing 10 μg ml^{-1} DNAse, and incubated for 30 min at 37° C. The cells were washed twice in BSS and resuspended in BSS at the appropriate concentration for cell transfer.

Statistical Analyses. The statistical significance of differences in ear swelling reactions between experimental groups was calculated using the student's *t* test.

RESULTS

The Auxiliary Cell Is Required for Efferent Suppression of Syngeneic, but Not Allogeneic Immune Lymph Node Cells

We first asked if Ts-aux was required for efferent suppression of immune T_{DH} that were syngeneic or allogeneic to the Ts_1 population. Therefore, Ts_1 were prepared from lymph node cells (LN) of Balb/c or CBA/J mice tolerized seven days previously with syngeneic DNP-LC. These Ts were cotransferred with DNFB immune LN cells derived from normal or Cy-pretreated Balb/c or CBA/J mice to recipients that were syngeneic to the T_{DH} donors. The results are shown in TABLE 1. Balb/c Ts_1 were able to suppress T_{DH} derived from normal (group A), but not Cy-pretreated (group B) Balb/c donors. However, these same Balb/c Ts_1 were able to fully suppress the passive transfer of immunity mediated by allogeneic T_{DH} derived from either normal (group C) or Cy-pretreated (group D) donors. Groups E and F show that CBA Ts_1 are able to suppress normal or Cy T_{DH} derived from Balb/c donors. Thus, it appears that a Cy-sensitive auxiliary cell derived from an immunogenic regimen is required for efferent suppression of syngeneic, but not allogeneic, T_{DH} by non-MHC restricted Ts_1.

TABLE 1

EFFERENT-ACTING Ts_1 SUPPRESS ALLOGENEIC
BUT NOT SYNGENEIC T_{DH} CELLS FROM Cy-PRETREATED DONORS

| | Cells Transferred to Recipient Mice Syngeneic to T_{DH} Donors * | | | |
Group	Ts_1 (5×10^7)	Cy T_{DH} (5×10^7)	Normal T_{DH} (5×10^7)	Suppression $\pm$ SEM (%)
A	Balb/c	—	Balb/c	78.1 ± 4.0 †
B	Balb/c	Balb/c	—	3.6 ± 3.0
C	Balb/c	—	CBA/J	89.8 ± 5.3 †
D	Balb/c	CBA/J	—	92.4 ± 3.6 †
E	CBA/J	—	Balb/c	78.2 ± 6.6 †
F	CBA/J	Balb/c	—	86.4 ± 5.1 †

* The indicated cell suspensions were mixed *in vitro* and injected immediately into recipients syngeneic to the T_{DH} donors.
† Significant suppression, $p < 0.05$.

Cellular Nature of the Auxiliary Cell

To confirm that the Cy-sensitive cell required for efferent suppression of T_{DH} by Ts_1 was similar to the Ts-aux cell that we had previously described,[12] we determined its cellular nature. As seen in TABLE 2, Balb/c Ts_1 were able to suppress T_{DH} derived from normal (group A), but not from Cy-pretreated (group B), syngeneic Balb/c donors. Cotransfer of normal T_{DH} treated with BSS + C' (group C) or anti-Lyt 2.2 + C' (group D) along with Ts_1 and Cy

TABLE 2

CELLULAR NATURE OF THE ANTIGEN-ACTIVATED AUXILIARY CELL ACTIVE
IN EFFERENT SUPPRESSION

| | Balb/c Cells Transferred to Normal Balb/c Recipients | | | | | |
Group	Ts_1 (5×10^7)	Cy T_{DH} (5×10^7)	Normal T_{DH} (5×10^7)	Antiserum Treatment of Normal T_{DH}	Δ Ear Swelling * $(\mu m \pm SEM)$	Suppression (%)
A	+	—	+	BSS+C'	10.4 ± 7.9 †	87.0
B	+	+	—	—	66.8 ± 5.6	15.5
C	+	+	+	BSS+C'	13.5 ± 4.1 †	83.0
D	+	+	+	α Lyt 2.2+C'	20.3 ± 3.3 †	74.3
E	+	+	+	α Thy 1.2+C'	69.9 ± 11.9	11.6
F	+ (α Ly-2.2+C')	—	+	—	84.6 ± 8.1	−7.1

* Ear swelling in recipients minus ear swelling in negative controls (ear challenged only).
† Significant suppression, $p < 0.05$.

T_{DH} restored suppression, but prior treatment of the normal T_{DH} with anti-Thy 1.2 + C′ (group E) did not. We thus conclude that the auxiliary cell is a Cy-sensitive, Thy 1.2+, Lyt 2.2- cell. In contrast, Group F shows that Ts_1 is sensitive to lysis with anti-Lyt 2.2 + C′.

Antigen Specificity of Ts-aux

As we had previously reported that the Ts-aux activity was contained in DNFB immune T cell populations,[12] we were next interested in determining the antigen specificity of the activity. Therefore, Balb/c Ts_1 and T_{DH} derived from Cy-pretreated Balb/c donors were transferred to syngeneic recipients along with DNFB immune T_{DH} derived from normal, syngeneic Balb/c or allogeneic CBA/J mice or along with TNCB immune T_{DH} derived from syngeneic Balb/c mice. The results (TABLE 3) show that cotransfer of Balb/c DNFB immune T_{DH} along with Balb/c Ts_1 and Cy T_{DH} restores suppression to an 81% level (group B), but cotransfer of syngeneic Balb/c TNCB immune T_{DH} (group C)

TABLE 3

ANTIGEN SPECIFICITY OF Ts-AUX ACTIVTIY

	Balb/c Cells Transferred to Normal Balb/c Recipients			Δ Ear Swelling * (μm $\pm$ SEM)	Suppression (%)
Group	Ts_1 (5×10^7)	Cy T_{DH} (5×10^7)	Normal T_{DH} (5×10^7)		
A	+	+	−	65.5 ± 5.3	0
B	+	+	+ (Balb/c DNFB)	12.4 ± 3.8 †	81.0
C	+	+	+ (Balb/c TNCB)	56.6 ± 4.3	9.4
D	+	+	+ (CBA/J DNFB)	62.7 ± 2.5	4.2

* Ear swelling in recipients minus ear swelling in negative controls (ear challenged only).
† Significant suppression, p < 0.01.

or allogeneic CBA/J DNFB immune T_{DH} (group D) does not. We conclude that the Ts-aux cell must come from syngeneic DNFB immune lymph node cell populations, and thus appears to be antigen specific and possibly MHC restricted.

Ts-aux Activity is Both MHC and Allotype Restricted

To test whether the interaction of Ts_1 and Ts-aux in efferent suppression was MHC restricted, the ability of normal T_{DH} from various H-2^k strains to restore suppression on cotransfer with CBA Ts-1 and CBA Cy$_{DH}$ was assessed. As seen in TABLE 4, CBA Ts_1 suppress the passive transfer of sensitivity mediated by normal CBA T_{DH} to an approximately 80% level (group A), but fail to suppress CBA Cy T_{DH} (group B). The addition of either normal CBA T_{DH} (group C) or C3H T_{DH} (group D) results in suppression, but the addition of B10.BR normal DNFB immune T_{DH} (group E) does not. This result was somewhat surprising, but could be explained if the interaction between Ts_1 and

TABLE 4

MHC RESTRICTION OF Ts-AUX ACTIVITY

Group	Cells Transferred to Normal CBA/J Recipients			Δ Ear Swelling * (μm $\pm$ SEM)	Suppression (%)
	Ts_1 (5×10^7)	Cy T_{DH} (5×10^7)	Normal T_{DH} (5×10^7)		
A	CBA	—	CBA	30.7±6.6 †	79.5
B	CBA	CBA	—	149.4±9.7	0
C	CBA	CBA	CBA	43.9±6.4 †	70.6
D	CBA	CBA	C3H	28.2±10.2 †	81.1
E	CBA	CBA	B10.BR	150.9±6.4	−0.9

* Ear swelling in recipients minus ear swelling in negative controls (ear challenged only).

† Significant suppression, $p < 0.01$.

Ts-aux was MHC and allotype restricted, since both CBA and C3H mice are H-2^k, Igh-1^j, while B10.BR mice are H-2^k, Igh-1^b.

We next used allotype congenic Balb/c (H-2^d, Igh-1^a) and Balb.Ig^b (H-2^d, Igh-1^b) mice to test this hypothesis. As seen in TABLE 5, Balb/c Ts_1 can suppress the passive transfer of normal, isogeneic Balb/c T_{DH} (group A), but do not suppress the passive transfer of allotype-disparate Balb.Ig^b (group B) T_{DH}. However, Groups H and J show that passive transfer of contact sensitivity is not allotype restricted, since normal and Cy-pretreated Balb.Ig^b T_{DH} both transfer high levels of sensitivity to Balb/c recipients. In restoration experiments, cotransfer of normal Balb/c T_{DH} (group D) with Balb/c Ts_1 and Cy T_{DH} restores suppression to a level of 65%, but cotransfer of normal Balb.Ig^b

TABLE 5

Ts_1–Ts-AUX INTERACTION IS ALLOTYPE RESTRICTED

Group	Cells Transferred to Normal Balb/c Recipients			Δ Ear Swelling * (μm $\pm$ SEM)	Suppression (%)
	Ts_1 (5×10^7)	Cy T_{DH} (5×10^7)	Normal T_{DH} (5×10^7)		
A	Balb/c	—	Balb/c	12.4±2.5 †	92.5
B	Balb/c	—	Balb.Ig^b	75.2±5.6	6.4
C	Balb/c	Balb/c	—	78.5±5.3	0.3
D	Balb/c	Balb/c	Balb/c	31.5±4.3 †	65.5
E	Balb/c	Balb/c	Balb.Ig^b	85.6±5.1	0
F	Balb/c	Balb.Ig^b	Balb/c	18.3±2.3 †	84.7
G	—	Balb/c	—	78.5±6.6	—
H	—	Balb.Ig^b	—	80.3±7.6	—
I	—	—	Balb/c	83.6±3.0	—
J	—	—	Balb.Ig^b	79.8±2.5	—

* Ear swelling in recipients minus ear swelling in negative controls (ear challenged only).

† Significant suppression, $p < 0.01$.

T_{DH} (group E) does not. Interestingly, group F, in which Balb/c Ts_1 were shown to suppress Balb.Ig^b Cy T_{DH} when cotransferred with normal Balb/c T_{DH} (as the Ts-aux source), shows that the final suppression is not allotype restricted. These data indicate that Ts_1 and Ts-aux must share both MHC and Igh-1 encoded gene products to achieve efferent suppression, but that, once activated, the final suppression is not allotype restricted.

Receptor Nature of Ts-aux

The allotype restriction of the Ts_1–Ts-aux interaction shown above suggested the possibility that these cells may interact *via* receptor-antireceptor (idiotype–anti-idiotype) pathways. To more firmly establish this possibility, the effects of treatment with anti-T_{DH} serum + C' and affinity-purified rabbit anti-DNP serum + C' on Ts-aux activity were both investigated. As shown in TABLE 6, cotransfer of normal T_{DH} cells treated with either NMS + C' (group B) or

TABLE 6

RECEPTOR NATURE OF TS-AUX

Group	Balb/c Cells Transferred to Normal Balb/c Recipients			Antiserum Treatment of Normal T_{DH}	Δ Ear Swelling * (μm$\pm$SEM)	Suppression (%)
	Ts_1 (5×10^7)	Cy T_{DH} (5×10^7)	Normal T_{DH} (5×10^7)			
A	+	+	−	—	82.8$\pm$15.7	0
B	+	+	+	NMS+C'	22.4$\pm$12.7 †	73.0
C	+	+	+	$\propto$ DNP+C'	75.2$\pm$11.9	9.4
D	+	+	+	$\propto$ T_{DH}+C'	21.1$\pm$11.7 †	74.4
E	+	−	+	—	11.9$\pm$6.4 †	85.7

* Ear swelling in recipients minus ear swelling in negative controls (ear challenged only).

† Significant suppression, $p < 0.05$.

anti-T_{DH} serum + C' (group D), but not anti-DNP serum + C' (group C), along with Ts_1 and Cy T_{DH} led to significantly greater levels of suppression than the transfer of Ts_1 and Cy T_{DH} alone (group A). Thus, Ts-aux activity is apparently susceptible to lysis with a subset of anti-DNP antibodies (*i.e.*, DNP idiotypes) and C', suggesting that Ts-aux is antireceptor (anti-idiotypic) in nature.

Target Molecules of Efferent Suppression

In order to explain how DNP-specific Ts_1 can suppress DNP-specific T_{DH} cells with the cooperation of Ts-aux, two relevant observations have to be noted. First, we have reported that the efferent suppressive activity of Ts_1 can be blocked in suspension by incubating tolerant cells with DNP-modified lymphoid cell membrane preparations that are H-2D region compatible, but not by monovalent DNP-lysine or polyvalent DNP-protein conjugates.[9] Second, a DNP-specific soluble suppressor factor (SSF) active in suppressing DNFB immune T_{DH} cells has been shown to be H-2K/D restricted [15, 16] and uses passively bound DNP-modified K/D region products on the T_{DH} cells as its target molecule.[17] Thus, we were interested in knowing if DNP-specific Ts_1 also used passively bound DNP-MHC products on T_{DH} cells to focus the suppression and lead to Ts-aux activation. We took advantage of the fact that DNFB immune T_{DH} cells cultured overnight *in vitro* are able to transfer sensitivity at levels comparable to freshly prepared lymph node cells, but are not suppressed by SSF, due to shedding of passively bound DNP-H-2 K/D complexes.[17] Thus, we asked if cotransfer of Ts_1 with T_{DH} cultured overnight would lead to efferent suppression. As shown in TABLE 7, Ts_1 suppressed the passive transfer of sensitivity mediated by freshly prepared T_{DH} cells by 96% (group B), but failed to suppress T_{DH} cells cultured overnight (group C). This lack of suppression was not due to the loss of Ts-aux activity; cotransfer of

TABLE 7

FAILURE OF Ts_1 TO SUPPRESS DNFB IMMUNE T_{DH} CELLS CULTURED OVERNIGHT IS NOT DUE TO LOSS OF TS-AUX ACTIVITY

| | Balb/c Cells Transferred to Normal Balb/c Recipients | | | | |
Group	Ts_1 (5×10^7)	Cy T_{DH} (5×10^7)	Normal T_{DH} (5×10^7)	Δ Swelling * (μm±SEM)	Suppression (%)
A	+	+	−	63.2±7.1	0
B	+	−	+ (Fresh)	2.5±7.4 †	96.1
C	+	−	+ (Cultured)	63.2±8.1	0
D	+	+	+ (Fresh)	6.1±1.5 †	90.4
E	+	+	+ (Cultured)	5.8±4.3 †	90.6

* Ear swelling in recipients minus ear swelling in negative controls (ear challenged only).
† Significant suppression, $p < 0.01$.

freshly prepared T_{DH} (group D) and T_{DH} cultured overnight (group E) along with Ts_1 and Cy T_{DH} both led to levels of suppression significantly greater than those due to transfer of Ts_1 and Cy T_{DH} alone (group A). Thus, the failure of Ts_1 to suppress T_{DH} cultured overnight appears to be due to the loss of passively bound DNP-MHC complexes from the T_{DH} surface, resulting in a lack of a target for Ts_1 focusing.

DISCUSSION

The experiments reported in this paper serve to extend our previous observations on T cell–T cell interactions in efferent suppression of DNFB contact sensitivity.[12] The major findings are as follows: (1) DNP-specific, Lyt 2+, efferent-acting Ts_1 cells suppress both the passive transfer of sensitivity mediated by syngeneic and that mediated by allogeneic DNFB immune T_{DH} cells, (2)

Ts_1 fail to suppress the passive transfer of sensitivity mediated by DNFB immune T_{DH} cells from Cy-pretreated syngeneic donors, (3) suppression of syngeneic Cy T_{DH} by Ts_1 can be restored by the addition of a Cy-sensitive, Thy 1+, Lyt 2-, I-J+ Ts-auxiliary cell derived from normal immune T_{DH} populations, but not by normal unsensitized lymph node cells [12] (TABLES 1 and 2; also unpublished results), (4) the interaction between Ts_1 and Ts-aux in mediating efferent suppression appears to be both antigen specific and allotype restricted, (5) Ts-aux is sensitive to lysis with anti-DNP (idiotype) + C′ and thus appears to be antireceptor (anti-idiotypic) in nature, and (6) there appears to be a requirement for passively bound DNP-MHC complexes on the T_{DH} surface to serve as a focus for DNP-specific Ts_1. These results are consistent with reports demonstrating T cell–T cell interactions in the activation of both helper and suppressor circuits.[18-22]

It is clear that an important subset of T cells (Ts-aux) necessary for the mediation of efferent suppression of primed T_{DH} cells arise comcomitantly with the immune T_{DH} cells. Thus, perturbation of the immune system by topical application of DNFB, which leads to strong DNP-specific DTH reactivity, also leads to the generation of Ts-aux cells that are integrally involved in the down regulation of the T_{DH} cells when efferent-acting Ts_1 are introduced into the system. Ts_1–Ts-aux cooperation is apparently not necessary for the suppression of allogeneic T_{DH} cells by non-MHC restricted Ts_1, since DNFB immune T_{DH} cells from normal and Cy-pretreated allogeneic donors are both fully suppressed. We feel that this may be related to the polyclonal nature of the Ts_1 population. We have reported previously,[9] based on blocking experiments with soluble DNP membranes, that the Ts_1 population is composed of a collection of distinct MHC-restricted Ts, some of which are directed against DNP-syngeneic and others against DNP-allogeneic determinants. MHC-restricted Ts_1 are obtained if the animal is tolerized with syngeneic DNP-LC labeled with limiting amounts of DNFB (S. Miller, in preparation). Those directed against DNP-allogeneic determinants appear to be of much higher affinity than those directed against DNP-syngeneic determinants, as Ts_1 suppression of allogeneic T_{DH} cells can be inhibited with much lower (100-fold) concentrations of allogeneic DNP membranes. Thus, inhibition of allogeneic T_{DH} cells may be able to be mediated directly by Ts_1 due to the high affinity of binding, but suppression of syngeneic T_{DH} cells requires amplification by Ts-aux due to the lower affinity of binding.

It is apparent that Ts-aux generation requires immunogenic stimulation by the correct route. Thus, topical application of DNFB leads to Ts-aux activation, while the i.v. injection of syngeneic DNP-LC favors activation of Ts_1 without apparent Ts-aux activation. Ts-aux generation was shown to be antigen specific, since only DNFB-sensitized syngeneic lymph node cells could restore suppression of transfers of Balb/c Ts_1 and Balb/c Cy T_{DH}. In addition, the interaction of Ts_1 and Ts-aux in the delivery of efferent suppression appears to be both MHC-and Igh-1 allotype-restricted (TABLES 4 and 5), since MHC-compatible, allotype-compatible, normal T_{DH} cells are required for the restoration of suppression. The present data also suggest that, once allotype-matched Ts_1 and Ts-aux have interacted, the final suppressive signal is not allotype restricted. This was shown by data wherein Balb/c Ts failed to suppress allotype-disparate Balb.Ig^b normal T_{DH} (containing Balb.Ig^b T_{DH} and Ts-aux populations), but did suppress Balb.Ig^b Cy T_{DH} (containing only Balb.Ig^b T_{DH}) when normal T_{DH} from Balb/c DNFB-immune donors were cotransferred. These data strongly suggest, but do not prove, that Ts-aux is the actual effector Ts subset in efferent suppression. Thus, the final phase of efferent suppression appears to be similar to that in the ABA and NIP DTH systems, where the final suppression is also not allotype restricted [13, 14] and similar to the feedback suppression system of Eardley *et al.*,[23] where allotype-linked interactions have been described. The Igh-1 allotype compatibility requirement between Ts_1 and Ts-aux in the present system suggested that receptor-antireceptor interactions were involved in efferent suppression. Also, the fact that Ts-aux activity is eliminated by treatment with rabbit anti-DNP serum (DNP idiotype) and complement is strong evidence that Ts-aux is antireceptor (anti-idiotypic) in nature. If Ts-aux is indeed anti-idiotypic, it must arise as a result of recognition of an idiotype-bearing cell induced by contact sensitization. The restrictions noted in this system are also similar to the ABA system,[24] in that successful efferent suppression is restricted by both MHC and Igh-1 gene products. It is possible that the restrictions noted in efferent suppression of DNFB contact sensitivity may be contributed independently by Ts_1 and Ts-aux. The H-2 restriction may be the property of the requirement that Ts_1 recognize passively bound DNP-H-2 determinants on the target T_{DH} cell (see below), while the Igh-1 restriction is related to the receptor nature of the Ts_1 (DNP receptor-bearing) and Ts-aux (antireceptor bearing) cells.

The final point brought out in these studies is the observation that Ts_1 do not suppress T_{DH} cells from normal mice that have been cultured *in vitro* overnight (TABLE 7). This failure to suppress is not related to loss of Ts-aux activity following *in vitro* incubation; both fresh T_{DH} and T_{DH} cultured overnight can restore suppression when cotransferred with Ts_1 and Cy T_{DH}. Rather, we feel that it is related to the loss of passively bound DNP-modified H-2 determinants from the surface of the target T_{DH} cells. Moorhead has described a DNP-specific soluble suppressor factor active in suppressing purified DNFB-immune T_{DH} cells.[15] The SSF suppresses and is absorbed by H-2K/D compatible DNFB immune T_{DH} cells. The absorption is blocked by pretreating the cells with either anti-DNP or anti-H-2K/D specific antisera, showing that the targets of the SSF molecule are DNP-K/D determinants on the T_{DH} surface, which are apparently picked up from antigen-presenting cells.[17] DNFB immune T_{DH} cultured overnight, although able to transfer contact sensitivity at levels comparable to freshly prepared T_{DH}, are not suppressed by or able to absorb SSF, due to shedding of the passively bound DNP-MHC complexes. Thus, the failure of Ts_1 to suppress cultured T_{DH} appears to be due to the loss of target complexes from target T_{DH} cells, resulting in a lack of focus of Ts_1. Experiments are now in progress to determine if the addition of small amounts of antigen, in the form of soluble DNP membranes, to cultured T_{DH} cells will render them sensitive to efferent suppression.

It is relevant to compare the present efferent suppressor circuit to those which have been described in the ABA and NIP DTH systems.[25] In those systems, i.v. injection of hapten-coupled spleen cells leads to the induction of idiotype-positive, I-J+ Ts_1 cells that bind antigen and inhibit the induction (afferent) phase of the DTH response. Ts-F_1 factors from these cells induce anti-idiotypic second-order Ts_2 cells that inhibit the efferent phase of the DTH response. These anti-idiotypic Ts_2 cells interact with allotype-matched idiotype-positive Ts_3 cells that are present in ABA immune lymph node populations and suppress the response in an idiotype-nonspecific manner. The present data indicate that an antigen-binding Ts_1 cell can serve as an effector suppressor cell through cooperation with antireceptor Ts-aux cells; alternatively, Ts_1 also induce second-order Ts_2 cells that inhibit the induction phase of DNFB contact sensitivity.[8] The differences between this and the ABA and NIP systems may be related to a number of points: (1) the fact that the ABA and NIP systems are characterized by a major idiotype response may make them different from the heterogeneous DNFB system, (2) induction of DTH by the s.c. injection of ABA-LC may not be a good inducer of anti-idiotypic Ts-aux (Ts_3) cells, and (3) induction of DTH by the s.c. injection of ABA-LC, as opposed to skin painting large amounts of DNFB, may not result in sufficient quantities of passively bound antigen on the T_{DH} surface to provide a target for idiotype-positive Ts_1 cells. At any rate, these and other results indicate the complexity of suppressor circuits and suggest that the circuits may vary depending on the antigenic system, the assays employed to dissect the systems, and the point at which the circuit is entered.

FIGURE 1 shows a proposed model of efferent suppression in the DNFB contact sensitivity system based on the results reported herein. We propose that DNP-specific Ts_1 recognize passively bound DNP–H-2 complexes on the T_{DH} surface. This step serves to focus the suppression on the relevant T_{DH} target cells and then allows Ts-aux activation *via* receptor-antireceptor (idiotype–anti-idiotype) interactions with the receptor on the appropriate allotype-matched Ts_1. Following Ts-aux activation, the final efferent suppressive signal appears to be non-allotype-restricted (TABLE 5) and preliminary data indicate that it may also be antigen nonspecific (S. D. Miller, unpublished results). Whether the final suppressor signal is delivered directly by the Ts_1 cell, by the Ts-aux cell, by a soluble suppressor factor from these cells, or indirectly *via* other undefined cellular intermediates is not clear at this time. Also, the precise nature and mechanism of delivery of the final phase of the efferent suppressor signal have yet to be determined. At present, experiments are in progress to develop T cell hybridomas of the various Ts subsets to help answer some of these questions.

In conclusion, it is clear that Ts subsets involved in efferent suppression arise concomitantly with effector T_{DH} cells. It is also apparent from this and other systems that the cellular circuits involved in immune suppression are varied and complex.[13, 14] These circuits appear to consist of complementary subsets of T cells bearing idiotypic or anti-idiotypic receptors. Depending on the system employed, the nature and state of the target cell of the suppression, etc., the circuit can be entered at different points and employ different sets of cells to achieve the final phase of the pathway, *i.e.*, suppression. Thus, a hypothesis unifying the methods of achieving suppression in various model systems must await more experimentation.

SUMMARY

T cell interactions involved in efferent suppression of DNFB contact sensitivity have been investigated. DNP-specific, Lyt 2^+ Ts_1 cells were shown to suppress the passive transfer of contact sensitivity mediated by syngeneic or allogeneic DNFB immune T_{DH} cells. However, Ts_1 fails to suppress the passive transfer of sensitivity mediated by DNFB immune T_{DH} cells from Cy-pretreated syngeneic donors. Suppression of the Cy T_{DH} by Ts_1 can be restored by the addition of a Thy 1^+, Lyt 2^- cell derived from normal DNFB immune donors. Thus, an antigen-activated Ts-auxiliary (Ts-aux) cell is required for efferent suppression of T_{DH} by Ts_1. The interaction between Ts_1 and Ts-aux was shown to be both antigen-specific and allotype-restricted, as only the addition of DNFB immune, allotype-compatible normal T_{DH} cells to Ts_1 and Cy T_{DH} resulted in restoration of suppression. The Ts-aux was also sensitive to treatment with anti-DNP serum and C', indicating that it is anti-receptor (anti-idiotypic) in nature. In addition, it was shown that Ts_1 fails to suppress normal T_{DH} cultured overnight *in vitro*. The data do not suggest that this lack of suppression is due to loss of Ts-aux activity from the cultured T_{DH} preparation, but rather that Ts_1 focuses upon passively bound DNP-MHC complexes on the target T_{DH} population that are shed *in vitro*. Following Ts_1 focusing to the T_{DH}, it appears that Ts-aux is activated *via* receptor-anti-receptor interactions, resulting in the delivery of the final efferent suppressive signal.

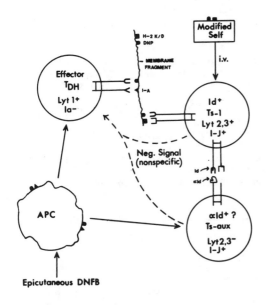

FIGURE 1. A proposed model of efferent suppression in DNFB contact sensitivity.

ACKNOWLEDGMENTS

The authors wish to thank Helen Lind and Robbie Dustin for their excellent technical assistance.

REFERENCES

1. BATTISTO, J. R. & B. R. BLOOM. 1966. Nature (London) **212:** 156–57.
2. MILLER, S. D. & H. N. CLAMAN. 1976. J. Immunol. **117:** 1519–26.
3. LONG, C. A. R. & D. W. SCOTT. 1977. Eur. J. Immunol. **7:** 1–5.
4. BACH, B. A., L. SHERMAN, B. BENACERRAF & M. I. GREENE. 1978. J. Immunol. **121:** 1460–68.
5. MILLER, S. D., R. P. WETZIG & H. N. CLAMAN. 1979. J. Exp. Med. **149:** 758–73.

6. SHERR, D. H., N. K. CHEUNG, K. M. HEGHINIAN, B. BENACERRAF & M. E. DORF. 1979. J. Immunol. **122:** 1899–904.
7. MILLER, S. D., M. S. SY & H. N. CLAMAN. Eur. J. Immunol. **7:** 165–70.
8. MILLER, S. D., L. D. BUTLER & H. N. CLAMAN. 1982. J. Immunol. In press.
9. MILLER, S. D. 1979. J. Exp. Med. **150:** 676–92.
10. MILLER, S. D., M. S. SY & H. N. CLAMAN. 1978. J. Immunol. **121:** 265–73.
11. CLAMAN, H. N., S. D. MILLER & M. S. SY. 1977. J. Exp. Med. **146:** 49–58.
12. SY, M. S., S. D. MILLER, J. W. MOORHEAD & H. N. CLAMAN. 1979. J. Exp. Med. **149:** 1197–207.
13. SY, M. S., A. NISONOFF, R. N. GERMAIN, B. BENACERRAF & M. I. GREENE. J. Exp. Med. **153:** 1415–25.
14. SUNDAY, M. E., B. BENACERRAF & M. E. DORF. 1981. J. Exp. Med. **153:** 811–22.
15. MOORHEAD, J. W. 1977. J. Immunol. **119:** 315–21.
16. MOORHEAD, J. W. 1977. J. Immunol. **119:** 1773–77.
17. MOORHEAD, J. W. 1979. J. Exp. Med. **150:** 1432–47.
18. FELDMANN, M., D. G. KILBURN & J. LEVY. 1975. Nature (London) **256:** 741–43.
19. CANTOR, H. & R. ASOFSKY. 1972. J. Exp. Med. **153:** 764–73.
20. HOWE, M. L. & L. COHEN. 1975. J. Immunol. **115:** 1227–33.
21. TURKIN, D. & E. E. SERCARZ. 1977. In The Immune System: Regulatory Genetics. E. Sercarz, L. A. Herzenberg and C. F. Fox, Eds.: 539–50. Academic Press. New York.
22. TADA, T., M. TANIGUCHI & T. TOKUHISA. 1978. In Ir Genes and Ia Antigens. H. O. McDevitt, Ed.: 517–27. Academic Press. New York.
23. EARDLEY, D. D., F. W. SHEN, H. CANTOR & R. K. GERSHON. 1979. J. Exp. Med. **150:** 44–50.
24. DIETZ, M. H., M. S. SY, B. BENACERRAF, A. NISONOFF, M. I. GREENE & R. N. GERMAIN. 1981. J. Exp. Med. **153:** 450–63.
25. GERMAIN, R. N. & B. BENACERRAF. 1981. Scand. J. Immunol. **13:** 1–16.

DISCUSSION OF THE PAPER

B. BENACERRAF (*Harvard Medical School, Boston, Mass.*): The data you presented is in every way in agreement with that which has been gathered in our laboratory except for one point. That is, in the initiation of the system, your first cell is already a cell that functions in the efferent mode.

MILLER: Correct.

BENACERRAF: The first cell, as identified in the ABA and NP systems in our laboratory, functions as an inducer cell, and, at least in the ABA system, is an Lyt 1 cell. So some systems may be even more rapid than others in development. For instance, in the ABA system, which is a very slow system, we can stop at the Ts_1 cell and never get to a Ts_2 unless we reimmunize. In the NP system, Ts_1 and Ts_2 of our system are concomitant. We have to go to isolation on plates to show that they were both present and distinguish them from each other. I wonder whether you did not have an inducer Lyt 1 Ts_1 in your system that could, quite possibly, have been antigen specific, being present before the one that you actually identified as your Ts_1. If that were the case, by treating your population with an Lyt 2 serum, you would end up with an

Lyt 1 population that could act as an inducer in an untreated animal. I wonder if you've done the experiment.

MILLER: That's a very good point. No, we haven't looked soon after tolerization. As I mentioned, we can identify the efferent Ts_1 at three days. Whether an Lyt 1 inducer population is present before three days is not known, but certainly possible. A difference between the ABA system and this system is that, when you induce delayed-type hypersensitivity with ABA-coupled cells, you're actually using very small amounts of antigen. I wonder whether this antigenic complex on the immune cell surface, which seems to be an important focus for an antigen-binding suppressor cell, may not be present in sufficient amounts in the ABA system and that an antigen-binding suppressor cell in that system may have an effector function if that antigen focus is there.

J. A. BERZOFSKY (*National Institutes of Health, Bethesda, Md.*): I'd like to ask two questions with regard to your killing the T auxiliary cell activity with anti-DNP and complement. First, since the T auxiliary cell is induced by antigen priming, is it possible that there's enough DNP on the surface of that cell for the anti-DNP and complement to kill it? This would differ from recognition of the idiotype by the anti-DNP antibody. Second, if, in fact, the killing is by recognition of the anti-DNP idiotype on the anti-DNP antibodies, can you inhibit this with DNP lysine? That is, is it a site-specific anti-idiotypic recognition?

J. W. MOORHEAD (*University of Colorado Medical School, Denver, Col.*): I think that the fact that the anti-idiotype and complement does not reverse the effect of the suppressor cells and anti-DNP does speaks against the theory that there is DNP complex on the cell's surface. And just a point of correction: it is mouse anti-DNP antibodies we're using, not rabbit. In answer to your second question—we haven't done that as yet.

L. A. HERZENBERG (*Stanford University Medical School, Stanford, Calif.*): We've been working with an antibody suppression system, the suppression of anti-DNP IgG antibody. It parallels the system that you're dealing with in so many ways that I wonder whether you see one of the features that we see. We have an induction system and then an effector mechanism as you do. If we work *in vivo* with an animal and simply prime him in a way in which the animal begins to produce antibody, we then have to use a substantially stronger stimulus to induce suppression in that animal than if we started out initially with an untreated animal. Conversely, if we induce suppression, we have to use a stronger stimulus to induce antibody production after that time. We characterize this as a bistable system, since it's the classical definition for such. Does your system do the same thing?

MILLER: We have never looked at the primed animals.

CLAMAN: Let me rephrase the question, as I think I understand it. Dr. Miller and other people have been discussing the induction of tolerance in normal animals that were later sensitized. It's not very difficult these days (after the leads that Merrill Chase gave us) to induce tolerance in normal animals. After that, it's difficult to sensitize. The reverse, the induction of tolerance or unresponsiveness in previously sensitized animals is, I believe, one of the things you're talking about. Once you prime the system and get it going, how easy is it to turn it off? And the results in the contact system, done by deWeck and Frey and tried by us some years ago, are, in fact, that, once you've primed the animal, it's extremely difficult to induce desensitization. So, in that case, there are either quantitative or qualitative differences between trying to induce tolerance in an untreated animal and trying to produce unresponsiveness in a sensitized animal.

HERZENBERG: My question is, Can you make the animals go in the opposite direction if you push hard enough, and will they go in either opposite direction if you push hard enough?

CLAMAN: You can desensitize primed mice for about forty-eight to seventy-two hours, at which time the sensitized state bounces right back, which is exactly what was found in the guinea pig. My guess is that you could probably desensitize more firmly if you tried harder. But we don't yet know what the molecular nature of trying hard is.

G. L. ASHERSON (*Clinical Research Centre, Harrow, Midd.*): In the picryl system, there aren't any idiotypic antibodies that upset the T suppressor effector cell and this may explain the difficulty of producing unresponsiveness involving that mechanism after immunization.

SELECTIVE EXPANSION OF H-2 RESTRICTED CYTOTOXIC T LYMPHOCYTES TO TNP-SELF BY INJECTION OF TRINITROBENZENE SULFONATE

Gene M. Shearer and Robert B. Levy

Immunology Branch
National Cancer Institute
Bethesda, Maryland 20205

A better understanding of the immune system's ability to distinguish its own from foreign immunogenic determinants is of central importance in addressing the issue of tolerance to self and non-self. The demonstration that major histocompatibility complex (MHC)-encoded self determinants are recognized in association with foreign antigens has emphasized the significance of recognition of self. The cytotoxic T lymphocyte (Tc) response of both mouse and human leukocytes to foreign antigens, including viruses,[1-3] minor transplantation antigens,[4, 5] and haptens [6-9] has provided some of the most extensively studied immune systems for investigating MHC restriction and self recognition. The hapten-modified self Tc models, many of which have been presented in reports in this volume, provide certain advantages compared to Tc models involving viral infection or expression of complex minor transplantation antigens, since (1) *in vivo* priming is not required (but is required in most other models), (2) well-defined chemical antigens can be covalently linked to cell surface proteins, and (3) haptens can be directed to particular amino acid residues, depending on the haptenic reactive group.[10, 11] However, the hapten-self Tc model is complex; in some respects, even more complex than other models. Tc responses to trinitrophenyl (TNP)-modified self,[12] as well as to all haptens that couple to amino groups of proteins,[11] are not as restricted as the virus-self and the minor antigen-self Tc responses. Thus, populations of hapten-specific Tc can be generated that recognize hapten-modified MHC-mismatched targets. It has been suggested that this cross-reactive lysis does actually involve self recognition, but that there are self determinants that are (1) expressed by some but not all individuals or strains within a species (shared self determinants) and (2) common to all individuals within the species (monomorphic).[9, 13] Such cross-reactive lysis on TNP-modified H-2-mismatched targets has been reported to be controlled by H-2-linked immune response (Ir) genes, with the H-2b and H-2k strains representing the high and low responder haplotypes, respectively.[14] This is the reverse of the H-2-linked Ir gene patterns for Tc activity against TNP-modified, H-2-matched targets, in which the H-2k and the H-2b are the high and low haplotypes, respectively.[15] In the context of self recognition, effector cells that are MHC restricted (*i.e.*, those which lysis only MHC-matched targets) have been thought to use unique or polymorphic self determinants. A final element of the complexity of the TNP Tc system is illustrated by the fact that effector cells specific for hapten-self can be generated by *in vitro* stimulation with MHC alloantigenic cells.[16]

Since the virus-self and minor antigen-self systems, which are more restricted than TNP-self, all require either *in vivo* immunization or *in vivo* priming followed by *in vitro* sensitization, the point was raised that *in vivo* immunization

137

0077–8923/82/0392–0137 $1.75/0 © 1982, NYAS

may influence the extent of H-2 restriction detected in these Tc assays.[9] However, *in vivo* priming of mice to the TNP-hapten either by injecting TNP-modified syngeneic spleen cells or by skin painting with trinitrochlorobenzene (TNCB) [17] did not result in a selective increase in Tc responses that were more H-2 restricted than the primary *in vitro* response. The present report summarizes recent studies in which the injection of soluble trinitrobenzene sulfonate (TNBS) did result in selective priming of TNP-Tc that recognize polymorphic self determinants.

In the present study, C57BL/10 (H-2^b) and B10.BR (H-2^k) mice were injected with 5 or 10 mg soluble TNBS. At weekly intervals thereafter, we compared the ability of the spleens of these mice with that of uninjected control mice to generate enhanced secondary TNP-specific Tc responses *in vitro*. This was done by culturing the spleen cells with syngeneic cells modified with various concentrations of TNBS (see TABLES 1–4). Five days later, the effectors generated were assayed on unmodified and TNBS-modified syngeneic and allogeneic splenic blast target cells.[10]

The injection of C57BL/10 mice with 5 and 10 mg TNBS resulted in priming and suppression, respectively, for Tc to TNP-self (TABLE 1). This was observed both in cultures stimulated with 5 mM TNP-self (high dose) and with 0.5 mM TNP-self (low dose). Neither priming nor suppression was observed for an allogeneic Tc response to B10.D2 (H-2^d). Results from the same experiment using B10.BR mice are summarized in TABLE 2. In contrast to the results of TABLE 1, the injection of both 5 and 10 mg TNBS into B10.BR mice resulted in suppressed Tc potential to TNP-self whether the cultures were stimulated with 5 mM TNP-self (high dose) or with 0.1 mM TNP-self (low dose). Again, no effect of TNBS injection was detected on the allogeneic Tc response to

TABLE 1

THE EFFECT OF INJECTING C57BL/10 MICE WITH SOLUBLE TNBS
ON THE SECONDARY *in Vitro* TC RESPONSE TO TNP-SELF

		Specific Lysis on Targets at Effector:Target Ratio Shown (%)					
		C57BL/10–TNP (5 mM)			B10.D2		
TNBS Injection	Stimulated *in Vitro* with	40	20	10	10	5	2.5
None	C57BL/10–TNP (5 mM)	17	17	5			
	C57BL/10–TNP (0.5 mM)	10	2	0			
	B10.D2				73	48	32
5 mg	C57BL/10–TNP (5 mM)	49	41	26			
	C57BL/10–TNP (0.5 mM)	22	22	10			
	B10.D2				67	49	36
10 mg	C57BL/10–TNP (5 mM)	0	0	0			
	C57BL/10–TNP (5 mM)	0	0	0			
	B10.D2				77	47	33

NOTES: TNBS was injected intravenously seven days before the *in vitro* stimulation.

All experiments were run using a pool of 2–4 spleens as a source of responding cells.

TABLE 2

THE EFFECT OF INJECTING B10.BR MICE WITH SOLUBLE TNBS
ON THE SECONDARY *in Vitro* Tc RESPONSE TO TNP-SELF

TNBS Injection	Stimulated *in Vitro* with	Specific Lysis on Targets at Effector:Target Ratio Shown (%)					
		B10.BR–TNP (5 mM)			B10.D2		
		40	20	10	10	5	2.5
None	B10.BR–TNP (5 mM)	60	55	51			
	B10.BR–TNP (0.1 mM)	46	39	24			
	B10.D2				57	46	26
5 mg	B10.BR–TNP (5 mM)	59	55	38			
	B10.BR–TNP (0.1 mM)	18	16	6			
	B10.D2				54	46	26
10 mg	B10.BR–TNP (5 mM)	48	51	25			
	B10.BR–TNP (0.1 mM)	25	19	7			
	B10.D2				57	45	30

NOTES: TNBS was injected intravenously seven days before the *in vitro* stimulation.

B10.D2 (H-2^d). These H-2 linked, strain-related differences in TNP-self Tc potential after TNBS injection are probably related to the fact that B10.BR and C57BL/10 mice are high and low Tc responders to TNP-self, respectively,[15] and may reflect the effects of these Ir genes on the induction of tolerance and priming.

TNP-self Tc from the C57BL/10 strain exhibit a high degree of cross-reactive lysis on TNP-modified H-2-mismatched targets.[12] Since the data of TABLE 1 indicate that this strain was primed by 5 mg TNBS, the effects of priming were further investigated. The spleens of C57BL/10 mice injected with 5 mg TNBS 22 d earlier were tested for primed Tc potential by *in vitro* sensitization against 5 mM or 0.5 mM TNP-self or against Balb/c (H-2^d) allogenic cells. The effectors generated were assayed on TNP-self and Balb/c targets. The data summarized in TABLE 3 indicate that priming was detected for TNP-self activity but not for allogeneic Tc activity. Particularly noteworthy is the observation that allogeneic stimulated effectors that lyse TNP-self targets[16] did not exhibit enhanced Tc activity in mice primed with TNBS. This last result raised the possibility that the priming observed may have mainly affected those clones of Tc which recognize TNP in association with polymorphic self determinants (*i.e.*, highly restricted clones).

To test the possibility that TNBS injection can induce priming selective for Tc clones that recognize polymorphic self determinants, spleen cells from C57BL/10 mice primed 18 d earlier with 5 mg TNBS were sensitized with 10 mM and 1 mM TNP-self, and the effectors generated were assayed on unmodified and TNBS-modified syngeneic (C57BL/10) and allogeneic (B10.BR and B10.D2) targets. These effectors were also assayed on unmodified and TNBS-modified targets from the intra-H-2 recombinant mouse strains B10.A (5R) (which shares K, I-A, and I-B with C57BL/10), and HTG (which shares the D region with C57BL/10). The results shown in TABLE 4 indicate that (1) an enhanced secondary Tc response was detected on TNBS-modified

TABLE 3

PRIMING FOR SECONDARY Tc POTENTIAL IN C57BL/10 MICE
DOES NOT AFFECT TNP-SELF SPECIFIC CLONES STIMULATED BY H-2 ALLOANTIGENS

		Specific Lysis on Targets at Effector:Target Ratio Shown (%)					
		C57BL/10-TNP (5 mM)			Balb/c		
TNBS Injection	Stimulated *in Vitro* with	40	20	10	20	10	5
None	C57BL/10–TNP (5 mM)	28	23	23			
	C57BL/10–TNP (0.5 mM)	5	0	0			
	Balb/c	20	13	10	64	62	54
5 mg	C57BL/10–TNP (5 mM)	50	38	37			
	C57BL/10–TNP (0.5 mM)	36	28	21			
	Balb/c	17	15	10	60	60	57

NOTE: TNBS was injected intravenously 22 d before the *in vitro* stimulation.

syngeneic targets, (2) no enhanced secondary cross-reactive lysis was detected, although the level of cross-reactive lysis usually observed in a primary Tc was detected, and (3) the enhanced Tc activity was detected on TNBS-modified H-2D region-matched (HTG), but not H-2K end-matched (B10.A(5R)) targets. These findings indicate that the mode of *in vivo* priming for a hapten in a mouse strain that has been reported not to exhibit extensive H-2 restriction can influence the pattern of restricted effectors detected. This observation raises a number of points that should be discussed.

First, H-2 restriction has been shown to be influenced by the thymic environment in which T lymphocytes mature,[18, 19] and probably also by the extrathymic environment.[20] The results summarized here suggest that there are also peripheral mechanisms (manipulated by priming) that can influence the extent of MHC restriction for polymorphic self determinants. It should be noted, however, that immunization to TNP-self by skin painting with TNCB or by injecting TNBS-modified syngeneic lymphocytes does not selectively prime for

TABLE 4

PRIMING FOR SECONDARY Tc POTENTIAL TO TNP-SELF
IN C57BL/10 MICE IS SELECTIVE FOR H-2D^b-RESTRICTED CLONES

Stimulated *in Vitro* with:	Effector:Target Ratio	C57BL/10		B10.BR		B10.D2		B10.A(5R)		HTG	
		N *	I *	N	I	N	I	N	I	N	I
C57BL/ 10–TNP (10 mM)	40	28	40	19	19	20	18	30	32	24	46
	20	24	32	8	11	12	10	24	19	17	31
	10	11	22	6	1	6	6	14	11	12	19
C57BL/ 10–TNP (1 mM)	40	11	32	16	12	10	14	16	20	11	37
	20	3	23	2	4	6	6	11	13	8	23
	10	1	16	0	2	0	6	7	5	4	13

* N indicates the Tc responses of normal mice; I indicates the Tc responses of mice injected with 5 mg TNBS 18 d before the *in vitro* stimulation. The maximum lysis detected on unmodified targets from all five strains was less than 5%.

the more restricted Tc clones. Thus, it may be that only particular immunizing signals result in priming for polymorphic self recognition. This could be due to the selective expansion of restricted Tc precursors and helpers, or to the prevention of expansion (*via* suppression) of the unrestricted populations.

Second, it should be noted that the detection of restricted and unrestricted Tc populations is not limited to hapten-self models, since both HLA-restricted [21, 22] and -unrestricted [23, 24] lytic activity has been reported for human Tc responses to Epstein-Barr virus. It is noteworthy that whether restricted or unrestricted Tc were detected depended on the mode of immunization.

Third, it was surprising that the restricted secondary response detected in the C57BL/10 mice was specific for TNP recognized in association with H-2D^b self, but not for TNP recognized in association with H-2K^b, since the Tc of unprimed mice do not exhibit such preferential self recognition. Thus, although H-2^b mice are H-2-linked genetic low responders to all haptens that modify amino groups of proteins,[11, 15] this H-2-restricted secondary response exhibited an all-or-none pattern identical to the H-2^b responses reported for the H-Y antigen,[25] influenza virus,[26] and Murine Sarcoma virus.[27] These findings emphasize the complex nature of the self determinants that can be recognized by cytotoxic T lymphocytes, and underscores the similarities of Ir gene control for a number of unrelated and non-cross-reacting foreign antigens.

In the context of recognition of self and non-self, and hence of tolerance to self and non-self, the contributors to this volume should be aware that self recognition is a complex phenomenon. Although the most dramatic effects of determining self from non-self have been demonstrated to occur before T cells enter the peripheral lymphoid pool, post-thymic events may also play a regulatory role in self recognition. Such a system might provide a fail-safe mechanism that would function to prevent autoimmune reactions, and might be regulated by anti-idiotypic antibodies or MHC-restricted antibodies that recognize self plus foreign antigen.

The cytotoxic T lymphocyte response of mice to trinitrophenyl-modified syngeneic cells is under H-2-linked Ir gene control and exhibits partial H-2 restriction. Mice of the H-2^b haplotype (C57BL/10) are genetic low responders but show extensive cross-reactive lysis on TNP-modified H-2 unmatched targets (these Tc are unrestricted). In this study, we injected C57BL/10 mice intravenously with trinitrobenzene sulfonate and tested the Tc potential at weekly intervals thereafter by *in vitro* sensitization of spleen cells to TNP-self. The results indicate that (1) the mice injected with TNBS were primed to generate enhanced secondary Tc to TNP-self, (2) the enhanced component of this response was H-2 restricted, in contrast to unprimed Tc, and (3) the restricted Tc recognized TNP-D^b self but not TNP-K^b self. The results indicate that the mode of immunization can affect the H-2 restriction and Ir-controlled response patterns of T cells, and emphasizes the complexity of self recognition.

REFERECES

1. ZINKERNAGEL, R. M. & P. C. DOHERTY. 1979. Adv. Immunol. **27:** 32.
2. MCMICHAEL, A. J., A. TING, H. J. ZWEERINK & B. A. ASKONAS. 1977. Nature (London) **270:** 524.
3. BIDDISON, W. E., S. M. PAYNE, G. M. SHEARER & S. SHAW. 1980. J. Exp. Med. **152:** 204s.
4. GORDON, R. D., E. SIMPSON & L. E. SAMELSON. 1975. J. Exp. Med. **142:** 1108.

142   Annals New York Academy of Sciences

5. GOULMY, E., A. TERMIJTELEN, B. A. BRADLEY & J. J. VAN ROOD. 1977. Nature (London) **266:** 544.
6. SHEARER, G. M. & A.-M. SCHMIT-VERHULST. 1979. Adv. Immunol. **25:** 55.
7. FRIEDMAN, S. M., N. NEYHARD & L. CHESS. 1977. J. Immunol. **120:** 630.
8. SHAW, S., D. L. NELSON & G. M. SHEARER. 1978. J. Immunol. **121:** 281.
9. SHAW, S. & G. M. SHEARER. 1978. J. Immunol. **121:** 290.
10. LEVY, R. B., G. M. SHEARER, J. C. RICHARDSON & P. A. HENKART. 1981. J. Immunol. **127:** 523.
11. LEVY, R. B., P. A. HENKART & G. M. SHEARER. 1981. J. Immunol. **127:** 529.
12. BURAKOFF, S. J., R. N. GERMAIN & B. BENACERRAF. 1976. J. Exp. Med. **144:** 1609.
13. LEVY, R. B., P. E. GILHEANY & G. M. SHEARER. 1980. J. Exp. Med. **152:** 405.
14. BILLINGS, P., S. J. BURAKOFF, M. E. DORF & B. BENACERRAF. 1978. J. Exp. Med. **148:** 341.
15. SHEARER, G. M., A.-M. SCHMITT-VERHULST, C. B. PETTINELLI, M. W. MILLER & P. E. GILHEANY. 1979. J. Exp. Med. **149:** 1407.
16. LEMMONIER, F., S. J. BURAKOFF, R. N. GERMAIN & B. BENACERRAF. 1977. Proc. Nat. Acad. Sci. USA **74:** 1229.
17. FUJIWARA, H., R. B. LEVY & G. M. SHEARER. 1981. Immunobiology **160:** 472.
18. BEVAN, M. J. 1977. Nature (London) **269:** 417.
19. ZINKERNAGEL, R. M., G. N. CALLAHAN, A. ALTHAGE, S. COOPER, P. A. KLEIN & J. KLEIN. 1978. J. Exp. Med. **147:** 897.
20. KRUISBEEK, A., S. SHARROW, B. MATHEISON & A. SINGER. 1981. J. Immunol. **127:** 2168.
21. MISKO, I. S., D. J. MOSS & J. H. POPE. 1980. Proc. Nat. Acad. Sci. USA **77:** 4247.
22. TSOUKAS, C. D., R. I. FOX, S. F. SLOVIN, D. A. CARSON, M. PELLEGRINO, S. FONG, J.-L. PASQUALI, S. FERRONE, D. KUNG & J. H. VAUGHN. 1981. J. Immunol. **126:** 1724.
23. LIPINSKI, M., W. H. FRIDMAN, T. TURSZ, C. VINCENT, D. PIOUS & M. FELLOWS. 1979. J. Exp. Med. **150:** 1310.
24. SEELEY, J., E. SVEDMYR, O. WEILAND, G. KLEIN, E. MOLLER, E. ERIKSSON, K. ANDERSSON & L. VAN DER WAAL. 1981. J. Immunol. **271:** 298.
25. VON BOEHMER, H., H. WERNER & N. K. JERNE. 1978. Proc. Nat. Acad. Sci. USA **75:** 2439.
26. HERME, M., C. M. HETHERINGTON, P. R. CHANDLER & E. SIMPSON. 1978. J. Exp. Med. **147:** 758.
27. DOHERTY, P. C., W. E. BIDDISON, J. R. BENNICK & B. B. KNOWLES. 1978. J. Exp. Med. **148:** 534.
28. GOMARD, E., V. DUPREZ, T. REME, M. J. K. COLOMBANI & J. P. LEVY. 1977. J. Exp. Med. **146:** 909.

DISCUSSION OF THE PAPER

J. A. BERZOFSKY (*National Institutes of Health, Bethesda, Md.*): You used two methods of priming. One was i.v. injection and the other was skin painting. You also used two reagents. One was TNBS and the other was TNCB. I wonder whether you can distinguish which of these differences is critical in causing these effects because the two reagents can react with different groups on proteins. As to routes, skin painting and i.v. immunization may preferentially affect different groups of macrophages or Langerhan's cells.

SHEARER: We haven't studied that at all. You may be right; these different factors may be responsible for the differences we see.

L. D. BUTLER (*University of Colorado Health Sciences Center, Denver, Col.*): Scott was unable to suppress the Tc response by injecting TNP in cells. I wonder whether you have been able to suppress the Tc response by injecting TNP in cells, or by coupling the hapten to the cell, or whether you must always present it i.v. in a soluble form whereby it can complex with some molecule in the host.

SHEARER: Our experience has been that, if we inject TNP-modified syngeneic cells—depending on the H-2 control of the response—we either get priming or no augmentation of the Tc response. We have not yet been able to detect a diminution of the response.

G. L. ASHERSON (*Clinical Research Centre, Harrow, Midd.*): You commented that one of the strains of mice responds very poorly to hapten on amino groups but responds very well to hapten on sulfhydryl groups. One would then expect picryl sulfonic acid to combine with both amino and sulfhydryl groups under physiological conditions. What happens to one of your high responders if you haptenate the sulfhydryl groups and then picrylate the cell so as to occupy the amino groups? Is there a complex interreaction? Is the critical issue here the occupation of the amino groups or of the sulfhydryl groups?

SHEARER: I don't know that we've done that exact experiment. Bob Levy has studied this extensively. He finds that he can, in fact, apparently identify, at least by a chemical definition, two types of self-reactive sites; those that preferentially or exclusively bind to amino groups and those that bind to sulfhydryl groups. So if you take two haptens that don't cross-react at the killer level, but that will presumably home in on the same amino group, you can cross-compete to some extent.

J. FORMAN (*Dallas, Tex.*): The cross-reactive Tc that are raised in the B haplotype strain—are they restricted to the K^b rather than the D^b determinants?

SHEARER: I would say that they're not restricted to any polymorphism. We haven't done any cold target inhibition studies yet.

LEVY: In response to your question, Dr. Asherson, I actually did those experiments. The answer is that you can't raise the response to an amino-reactive group of haptens by first modifying the sulfhydryls.

IN VIVO REGULATION OF THE PRIMARY RESPONSE OF CYTOLYTIC T CELLS TO HAPTEN-ALTERED SELF ANTIGENS BY AN INDUCIBLE SUPPRESSOR T CELL *

J. R. Battisto and H. L. Wong

Department of Immunology
Cleveland Clinic Foundation
and
Case Western Reserve University
Cleveland, Ohio 44106

INTRODUCTION

In view of the likelihood that cytolytic T lymphocytes (Tc) with specificity for altered self-antigens may be made protective by eliminating cells that are virally infected or cancerous, or possess unwanted immunological capabilities, several investigative groups have directed considerable attention to their induction *in vitro* and *in vivo*.[1-18] The *in vivo* Tc response to hapten-conjugated syngeneic splenic cells has presented investigators with several formidable problems because certain aspects of its induction and regulation have not been precisely reflected *in vitro*. Early on, for instance, Tc with haptenated-self specificity were seen to be readily inducible *in vitro*,[1-3] but not at all *in vivo*.[4] The inability to generate Tc *in vivo* was shown to be due to the presence of a naturally occurring suppressor T cell that is cyclophosphamide sensitive but apparently nonfunctional in the *in vitro* experimental situation.[16, 17] Recently, this Lyt 2, 3+ T cell has been shown to regulate the presence of an interleukin 2 (IL-2) inhibitor *in vivo*.[19]

To add to the problems, a tolerance protocol that induces suppressor T cells active on delayed-type hypersensitivity (DTH) *in vivo* has been shown to have no suppressive effect upon *in vitro* Tc responses.[8-10] On the contrary, spleen cells of mice exposed to derivatized spleen cells actually develop augmented primary hapten-specific Tc reactions *in vitro*.[8-10] The enhancement has been attributed to priming a radio-resistant helper T cell.[10]

Furthermore, Finberg *et al.* have shown that the suppressor T cells induced by intravenously administered soluble hapten or syngeneic cell-coupled hapten are able to suppress *in vitro* the augmented response caused by subcutaneous priming.[11] Thus, the hapten-conjugated spleen cells given intravenously result in the generation of suppressor cells that are apparently directed to the helper T cells induced by *in vivo* priming.

Using a system capable of circumventing the naturally occurring suppressor cell without the use of cyclophosphamide, we have been able to examine the developmental and regulatory aspects of the primary Tc response to hapten-altered syngeneic cells conducted entirely *in vivo*.[12] The host's helper T cells

* This work was supported by a grant from the National Institute of Allergy and Infectious Diseases, National Institutes of Health, no AI 18305.

144

are stimulated with a minor histocompatibility locus (Mls)–disparate auxiliary cell at the same time that hapten-derivatized syngeneic cells trigger precursor Tc (pre-Tc).

We have reported that initiating tolerance for DTH with cell membrane-coupled hapten does not reduce the primary in vivo Tc response. On the other hand, tolerance induced with soluble hapten prevented hapten-specific DTH and primary Tc. Although hapten-specific suppressor T cells that depress DTH arise in this system, they have no regulatory effect upon in vivo generation of primary Tc when given adoptively.[20, 21] Furthermore, the soluble hapten method for inducing tolerance apparently has no detrimental effect upon either helper cells or pre-Tc. Our results using mice with an H-2^k histocompatibility background showed that both of these sets of cells derived from hapten-injected hosts were fully functional in in vitro tests.[22] Recently, Butler et al. have reported that unresponsiveness in Tc induced with soluble hapten is H-2 linked.[23] H-2^d mice that were made unresponsive with hapten in vivo demonstrated the inability to make Tc in a primary response both in vivo and in vitro. On the other hand, mice of the H-2^k strain showed this inability only in vivo. The tolerance of H-2^d mice demonstrable in vitro was shown to be controlled by a cyclophosphamide-sensitive cell and the unresponsiveness was reversed by the addition of supernatants from Concanavalin A (Con A)–stimulated spleen cells.[23] Thus, at least in certain strains of mice, the induction of tolerance with soluble hapten appears to generate suppressor cells that are directed at the level of helper T cells.

In DTH, tolerance brought about by hapten-coupled spleen cells induces the appearance of two suppressor T cells: Ts$_1$, which is active on the efferent limb, and Ts$_2$, which is directed toward the afferent phase. Since, in our earlier work, we had shown that Ts$_1$ were unable to prevent the appearance of primary in vivo Tc, we next wished to determine whether tolerance procedures that might cause the appearance of idiotype-specific Ts$_2$ would be effective in that regard.

Here we show for the first time that tolerance induced with hapten-derivatized syngeneic spleen cells can prevent Tc directed toward hapten-altered self antigens from being generated in vivo. Furthermore, the tolerance is adoptively transferable using splenic T cells of tolerized hosts.

MATERIALS AND METHODS

Mice

The animals used in these experiments were, for the most part, female C3H/HeN (H-2^k, Mls^c) mice (eight weeks old), purchased from Charles River Breeding Laboratories, Wilmington, Mass., and female CBA/J (H-2^k, Mls^d) mice (eight weeks old), purchased from the Jackson Laboratory, Bar Harbor, Me.

In Vivo Generation of Hapten-Specific Tc

In vivo sensitization was accomplished as described elsewhere.[12] Briefly, 20×10^6 CBA/J spleen cells and 20×10^6 TNP-coupled C3H/HeN spleen cells were injected into both hind footpads of all experimental C3H/HeN mice.

For TNP modification, 60×10^6 C3H/HeN spleen cells were resuspended in 1 ml of 10 mM trinitrobenzene sulfonic acid (TNBS, Eastman Kodak, Rochester, N.Y.), after removing all red cells with 0.83% NH$_4$Cl, and incubated at 37° C for 10 min. Afterwards, the cells were washed twice with medium and then used for the injections. After five days, the draining popliteal lymph nodes were removed and used in the *in vitro* chromium release effector assay.

In Vitro *Chromium Release Effector Assay*

The *in vitro* chromium release assay was a slight modification of the procedure used by Simpson *et al.*[24] Normally, the target cells were splenic cells treated with Concanavalin A for 48 to 72 hours (10×10^6 cells per 10 μg Con A) in supplemented RPMI 1640 medium (Gibco, Grand Island, N.Y.). Following blastogenesis, these cells were labeled with Na$_2^{51}$CrO$_4$ (100–200 μCi per 30×10^6 blast cells in 1 ml medium for 90 min at 37° C). The labeled cells were then washed twice and those cells to be TNP-modified (20×10^6) were resuspended in 0.5 ml medium to which 1 ml of 10 mM TNBS was added. The cells were allowed to incubate at 37° C for 10 min. Once they were TNP modified, the cells were washed twice with medium and used, along with unmodified cells, as targets in the actual assay. Graded numbers of effector cells (draining popliteal lymph node cells from experimtntal and control mice) were added to 2.5×10^4 target cells in each well of a 96-well round bottom microtiter plate (Microbiological Associates), centrifuged for 5 min at 45 g and incubated for 3 h at 37° C in 5% CO$_2$. Maximum release of chromium was determined by adding 1% sodium dodecyl sulfate (SDS) to the appropriate number of target cells alone, and spontaneous release was determined by incubating targets with medium alone. The average maximum release for all experiments in this report was 3547.0 cpm. The spontaneous release was always no greater than 25% of the maximum release. After incubating for 3 h, the plates were centrifuged for 10 min at 17 g, and 100 μl of supernatant was taken off and assayed for ^{51}Cr in a Beckman 310 gamma counter. Results were expressed as the percentage of specific lysis, (cpm experimental − cpm spontaneous release) ÷ (cpm maximum release − cpm spontaneous release) $\times$ 100.

Preparation of Cells to be Injected I.V.

Cells to be injected i.v. were hapten modified in the following manner. Single cell suspensions were obtained from the spleens of mice; red cells were then removed by treatment with 0.83% NH$_4$Cl, followed by washing. Afterwards, the cells were resuspended in Earle's Balanced Salt Solution (EBSS, Gibco, Grand Island, N.Y.) to a concentration of 20×10^6 ml^{-1}. To each ml of cells, 1 ml of either 1 mM or 10 mM TNBS was added; the suspension was then allowed to stand at room temperature for 30 min with continuous shaking, followed by washing twice with EBSS.

Membrane-coupled hapten-exposed spleen cells were obtained from mice that had been injected one week earlier with 50×10^6 (10 mM) TNP-modified syngeneic spleen cells.

Each of these cells was used as described in the Results section.

Treatment of Cells with Anti-Thy 1.2

Monoclonal anti-thy 1.2 was purchased from New England Nuclear (Boston, Mass.), diluted to the appropriate strength, and added (0.5 ml) to 100×10^6 cells with 0.5 ml of agarose-absorbed guinea pig complement (Gibco, Grand Island, N.Y.). This suspension was then incubated at 37° C in 5% CO_2 for 45 min, after which the cells were washed, counted, and used as described.

RESULTS

Control of Tc Induction by Tolerance—Earlier Findings

We have shown in earlier publications that Tc directed toward hapten-altered self antigens can be controlled by inducing tolerance toward two antigenic stimuli: (1) the Mls antigen(s) on the auxiliary cell that stimulates helper T cells, and (2) the hapten used to alter self antigens.[12, 20, 21] This information is summarized in TABLE 1. We had found that, even when tolerance

TABLE 1

CONTROL OF TC INDUCTION *in Vivo*

At the Mls level

By tolerance toward the Mls antigen
    MLR is decreased by 50%
    CML is decreased by 70%

At the hapten level

By tolerance toward the hapten
    a. Induced by soluble hapten (TNBS); DTH is decreased by 75%, CML is decreased by 80%
    b. Not induced by membrane-coupled hapten alone; DTH decreased by 75%, CML remains intact

for the mixed lymphocyte reaction (MLR) toward the Mls antigen was induced only partially (50%) by injecting C3H host animals with (C3H × CBA) F_1 splenic cells intravenously, the cell mediated lympholysis (CML) response toward hapten-altered self was markedly reduced.

Regulation of the Tc response at the hapten level was demonstrable only when soluble hapten was injected intravenously. By this method, both hapten-specific DTH and CML were reduced by at least 75%. A dichotomy between regulation of the two responses appeared when adoptive transfer of tolerance for the CML response was unsuccessful, despite the fact that it effectively suppressed hapten-specific DTH. We have noted that the precursors of Tc in animals made tolerant with soluble hapten are fully competent when tested for hapten-specific Tc generation *in vitro*.[22] Furthermore, the helper cells from such animals were functional *in vitro* when stimulated with Mls antigen.[22]

An additional divergence in regulation of DTH and CML became apparent when tolerance induced by hapten-derivatized syngeneic spleen cells was seen to be incapable of controlling the CML system in spite of the fact that DTH was readily down regulated (TABLE 1). Neither the suppressor cells that arise by this method of tolerance induction nor the soluble supernatant suppressor factor from the induced cells suppressed CML either in the sensitization (afferent) or effector phase.[21] Thus, the efferent suppressor T cell controlling DTH (Ts_1 (DTH)) showed no regulatory activity over CML.

Prevention of Tc Appearance by Tolerance Induced with Membrane-Coupled Hapten

Efforts were directed towards determining whether hapten coupled to syngeneic spleen cells would be tolerogenic for the CML system by using several other regimens. The first regimen tried consisted of intravenously injecting TNP-coupled spleen cells (50×10^6) mixed with spleen cells (50×10^6) from mice that had received TNP-coupled syngeneic spleen cells one week earlier. Spleen cells from the latter mice are referred to as "membrane-coupled hapten–exposed" (MCH-exposed). After one week, the mice were injected in the rear paws with the appropriate mixture of cells in an attempt to induce appearance of the Tc. Five days later, cells of the popliteal lymph nodes were examined for the presence of cytolytic effector cells. As can be seen in TABLE 2, control mice that had been exposed only to the sensitization procedure developed the level of hapten-specific lysis ordinarily achieved. In contrast, lymph node cells from mice receiving MCH-exposed plus hapten-coupled spleen cells one week earlier displayed markedly reduced specific lysis. This was true no matter whether 1 mM or 10 mM TNP had been used to conjugate the syngeneic spleen cells. When 10 mM hapten-derivatized spleen cells alone were injected one week before sensitization, no diminution in the capability to generate Tc was observed. Furthermore, mice that were sensitized immediately following the receipt of MCH-exposed spleen cells showed no diminution in the degree of specific lysis (TABLE 2). Thus, generation of hapten-specific Tc can be eliminated by intravenously injecting MCH-exposed spleen cells mixed with hapten-derivatized spleen cells one week before attempting sensitization.

Mechanism for Tolerance Induced by This Method

The question that naturally arises is, Is the tolerance induced in this manner adoptively transferable? This was answered affirmatively when mice that had received spleen cells (100×10^6) from tolerized donors immediately before sensitization for Tc displayed half the development of Tc of control mice (TABLE 3). Furthermore, when spleen cells from tolerized donors were treated with anti-thy 1.2 antibodies plus complement for one hour before being transferred, the suppressive effect was lost (TABLE 3). In this way, the cells mediating suppression of the generation of primary Tc in vivo were identified as T cells.

Additional Regimens Using Membrane-Coupled Hapten That Achieve Tolerance for the CML System

Tolerance for DTH as achieved with hapten-derivatized spleen cells was originally described as best induced by two intravenous injections spaced a week

TABLE 2

GENERATION OF HAPTEN-SPECIFIC TC CAN BE CONTROLLED BY INTRAVENOUS INJECTION OF SPLEEN CELLS EXPOSED TO MCH PLUS HAPTEN-DERIVATIZED SPLEEN CELLS

Mice Injected I.V. with	Days Elapsed between I.V. Injections and Sensitization for Tc *	Percentage of Specific Lysis of TNP-C3H T Cell Blasts	
		25:1	100:1
Nothing	N.A.†	14.7	33.1
MCH-exposed spleen cells ‡ + 1 mM TNP-C3H spleen	7	1.9	7.3
MCH-exposed spleen cells + 10 mM TNP-C3H spleen	7	1.3	4.9
10 mM TNP-C3H spleen	7	N.D.	31.0
MCH-exposed spleen cells	0	N.D.	29.4

* TNP-C3H + CBA/J spleen cells in hind paws.

† Not applicable; this positive control group received only sensitization for Tc.

‡ From mice injected with syngeneic membrane–coupled hapten on one occasion seven days earlier.

apart, followed by a rest interval before attempting sensitization.[25] We decided to use this method, since it had not been tried for the CML system. Mice were intravenously injected on one or two occasions with syngeneic spleen cells that had been conjugated at a 10 mM TNBS concentration. When two injections were given, they were spaced one week apart and sensitization for Tc was initiated one week after the second injection. Animals receiving the single injection were sensitized for Tc either after one week or after two weeks.

As may be seen in FIGURE 1, lymph node cells from animals that had been sensitized for Tc one week after a single injection of tolerogen displayed the full capability to develop Tc. This observation corroborates our earlier re-

TABLE 3

TC CAN BE PREVENTED in Vivo BY AN INDUCIBLE SUPPRESSOR T CELL

Immediately Before Sensitization for Tc, Mice Were Injected with	Treatment of Transferred Cells	Percentage of Specific Lysis of TNP-C3H T Cell Blasts	
		25:1	100:1
Nothing	—	21.1	46.7
Spleen cells from tolerized mice *	None	7.5	23.8
Spleen cells from tolerized mice *	α-θ + C'	19.5	45.1

* Injected i.v. with MCH-exposed spleen cells + hapten-derivatized spleen cells.

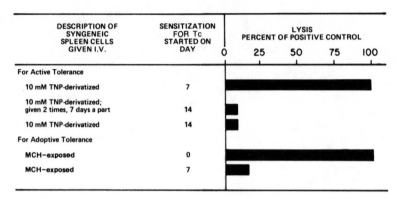

DESCRIPTION OF SYNGENEIC SPLEEN CELLS GIVEN I.V.	SENSITIZATION FOR Tc STARTED ON DAY	LYSIS PERCENT OF POSITIVE CONTROL			
		0 25 50 75 100			
For Active Tolerance					
10 mM TNP-derivatized	7				
10 mM TNP-derivatized; given 2 times, 7 days a part	14				
10 mM TNP-derivatized	14				
For Adoptive Tolerance					
MCH—exposed	0				
MCH—exposed	7				

FIGURE 1. Prevention of the appearance of Tc by tolerance induced through hapten-coupled syngeneic spleen cells.

ports.[20, 21] In marked contrast, animals that had been sensitized for Tc two weeks following the initial tolerogen injection (no matter whether or not they received a second injection of tolerogen at one week), displayed only 10% of the positive control lytic response. Thus, a two-week interval between administering tolerogen and attempting sensitization appears to be essential to the down regulation of the CML system.

As a consequence of this finding, we wondered whether an adoptive transfer of spleen cells from animals that had been injected with hapten-coupled cells for one week would succeed in tolerizing recipients if an additional week were permitted to elapse before attempting sensitization. As may be seen in FIGURE 1, when spleen cells of mice that had received hapten-coupled syngeneic spleen cells were transferred to mice and sensitization was started immediately, the recipients, as well as the positive controls, developed Tc fully. When, however, sensitization was initiated one week after cell transfer, the recipients were incapable of developing Tc. Thus, the necessity for a two-week interval between the administration of the initial tolerogen and the beginning of sensitization was again demonstrated by these data.

DISCUSSION

We have reported in the past that tolerance induced by hapten-derivatized syngeneic spleen cells, while fully capable of preventing hapten-specific DTH, is unable to control the Tc response.[20, 21] In those experiments, one week was allowed to elapse between the administration of tolerogen and the initiation of sensitization for each of the immunological parameters. Here we show that the primary *in vivo* immunization for Tc directed to hapten-altered self can, indeed, be prevented through tolerance induced by hapten-coupled syngeneic spleen cells. This was first observed when MCH-exposed spleen cells were mixed with hapten-coupled spleen cells and injected intravenously one week before sensitization for Tc was initiated. Thus, two weeks intervened between the original injection of tolerogen and the attempt to sensitize for Tc. The down regulation of Tc was adoptively transferred to new mice with splenic cells from tolerized animals. T cells within the tolerant spleens were shown to mediate the suppression. While these suppressor cells were induced by a method that parallels those used to induce idiotype-specific suppressor T cells for DTH,[26, 27] their specificity is still unknown (TABLE 4). Furthermore, from the manner in which our experiments have been conducted, their activity would appear to be directed toward the afferent limb of the CML response. This has yet to be definitively established. Since the suppressor cells are inducible, this characteristic would tend to differentiate them from the naturally occurring suppressor cell (Ts_0) that is also known to be active on the primary CML in vivo (TABLE 4).

Although this is the first reported description of an induced suppressor T cell for the primary CML system oriented to altered self, we refer to the cell as Ts_2 ($CML^{1°}$). In this way, it can readily be discriminated from Ts_0 ($CML^{1°}$) and from the induced suppressor T cell that has been shown by Finberg et al. to be operative on the secondary CML conducted in vitro, Ts_1 ($CML^{2°}$).[11] The latter has been shown to be hapten-specific and oriented to a radiation-resistant helper T cell. More recently, Butler et al. have reported that unresponsiveness can be induced in vivo using soluble TNBS that is demonstrable by the primary in vitro generation of Tc. This unresponsiveness, mediated by suppressor T cells, appears to be H-2-linked, since it was seen in H-2^d mice but not H-2^k mice. Furthermore, the suppression may be directed to helper T cells because it was reversed by Con A–stimulated splenic cell supernatants.[23]

We have also described here three other ways by which tolerance induced by hapten-coupled syngeneic spleen cells could prevent the appearance of primary Tc in vivo. These were discovered as a consequence of control experiments. We found that tolerance was achievable with MCH-exposed spleen cells alone and that there was no necessity to incorporate hapten-derivatized spleen cells. However, when MCH-exposed spleen cells alone were used to induce tolerance, it was essential that a week elapse before sensitization for Tc was attempted. We had reported earlier and show again here that, when sensitization for Tc is initiated immediately following adoptive transfer of the MCH-exposed spleen cells, no reduction in the response is observed. In the other two methods, hapten-derivatized spleen cells injected intravenously twice, seven days apart, and once, followed by a two-week rest, achieved tolerance for the CML system. In both of these methods, the additional week may be essential to the induction of Ts_2 ($CML^{1°}$). However, the adoptive transfer experiments necessary to seek the evidence for suppressor cells have yet to be performed.

Common to all four methods reported here for inducing tolerance with hapten-derivatized syngeneic spleen cells is the fact that two weeks elapse

TABLE 4

CHARACTERISTICS OF SOME SUPPRESSOR T CELLS AFFECTING DTH AND CML

Characteristics	Cell Subpopulations				
	Ts_1(DTH)	Ts_2(DTH)	Ts_0($CML^{1°}$)	Ts_1($CML^{2°}$)	Ts_2($CML^{1°}$)
Specificity	Antigen	Idiotype	Altered self	Antigen	Idiotype(?)
Limb where active	Efferent	Afferent	Afferent	Afferent (helper cell)	Afferent(?)
Other	Inducible	Inducible	Naturally occurring Cy-sensitive	Inducible	Inducible

between their administration intravenously and the initiation of sensitization for Tc. Since injecting the hapten-derizatized cells induces the appearance of several types of hapten-oriented cells, a question that arises is, Which are important to the appearance of Ts_2 (CML[1°])?

Still another query provoked by these experiments is, Does soluble hapten evoke unresponsiveness in H-2[k] mice that is demonstrable by adoptive transfer of suppressor cells? Thus far, this has not been achieved in the primary *in vivo*[21] or primary *in vitro*[23] systems.

SUMMARY

Tc directed toward hapten-altered self antigens have been prevented from appearing *in vivo* by inducing tolerance with hapten-derivatized syngeneic spleen cells. When the latter cells were coinjected intravenously with hapten-tolerized spleen cells one week before attempting sensitization for Tc, the hapten-specific Tc were not generated. Tolerance induced in this manner was adoptively transferable to untreated hosts using spleen cells of tolerized animals. The cell responsible for down regulating the CML response was identified as a theta antigen–bearing cell. Three additional methods have been described in which induction of Tc could be prevented by tolerance initiated through the use of hapten-derivatized syngeneic spleen cells. Common to all four methods is a two-week interval between the initial administration of tolerogen and the start of sensitization for Tc formation.

ACKNOWLEDGMENTS

The authors thank Dr. Subhash Gautam for lively discussions as well as editing this manuscript and Ms. Michael Hart for her expert typing.

REFERENCES

1. SHEARER, G. M. 1974. Cell mediated cytotoxicity to trinitrophenyl-modified syngeneic lymphocytes. Eur. J. Immunol. **4:** 527.
2. FORMAN, J. 1974. On the role of the H-2 histocompatibility complex in determining the specificity of cytotoxic effector cells sensitized against syngeneic trinitrophenyl-modified targets. J. Exp. Med. **142:** 403.
3. HODES, R. J., K. S. HATHCOCK & G. M. SHEARER. 1975. Synergy between subpopulations of normal mouse spleen cells in the *in vitro* generation of cell-mediated cytotoxicity specific for "modified self" antigens. J. Immunol. **115:** 1122.
4. STARZINSKI-POWITZ, A., K. PFIZENMAIER, M. RÖLLINGHOFF & H. WAGNER. 1976. *In vivo* sensitization of T cells to hapten-conjugated syngeneic structures of the major histocompatibility complex. I. Effect of *in vitro* culture upon generation of cytotoxic T lymphocytes. Eur. J. Immunol. **6:** 799.
5. SCOTT, D. W. & C. A. LONG. 1976. Role of self carriers in the immune response and tolerance. I. B-cell unresponsiveness and cytotoxic T-cell immunity induced by haptenated syngeneic lymphoid cells. J. Exp. Med. **144:** 1369.
6. SCHMIDT-VERHULST, A.-M. & G. M. SHEARER. 1976. Multiple H-2 linked immune response gene control of H-2 D associated T-cell–mediated lym-

pholysis to trinitrophenyl-modified autologous cells: Ir-like genes mapping to the left of I-A and within the I region. J. Exp. Med. **144:** 1701.

7. BILLINGS, P., S. J. BURAKOFF, M. E. DORF & B. BENACERRAF. 1978. Genetic control of cytolytic T lymphocyte response. I. Ir gene control of the specificity of cytolytic T lymphocyte responses to trinitrophenyl-modified syngeneic cells. J. Exp. Med. **148:** 341.

8. FUJIWARA, H., R. B. LEVY, G. M. SHEARER & W. P. TERRY. 1979. Studies on *in vivo* priming of the TNP-reactive cytotoxic effector cell system. I. Comparison of effects of intravenous inoculation with TNP-conjugated cells on the development of contact sensitivity and cell-mediated lympholysis. J. Immunol. **123:** 423.

9. LAKE, J. 1979. Enhanced *in vitro* TNP-specific cytotoxic T lymphocyte responses by cells from mice rendered tolerant for contact sensitivity by TNP-conjugated lymphoid cells. Fed. Proc. Fed. Am. Soc. Exp. Biol. **38:** 1214.

10. FINBERG, R., M. I. GREENE, B. BENACERRAF & S. J. BURAKOFF. 1979. The cytolytic T lymphocyte responses to trinitrophenyl modified syngeneic cells. I. Evidence for antigen specific helper T cells. J. Immunol. **123:** 1205.

11. FINBERG, R., S. J. BURAKOFF, B. BENACERRAF & M. I. GREENE. 1979. The cytolytic T lymphocyte response to trinitrophenyl-modified syngeneic cells. II. Evidence for antigen-specific suppressor T cells. J. Immunol. **123:** 1210.

12. BUTLER, L. D. & J. R. BATTISTO. 1979. *In vivo* generation of hapten-specific killer T cells without elimination of suppressor cells. J. Immunol. **122:** 1578.

13. LEVY, R. B. & G. M. SHEARER. 1979. Regulation of T cell mediated lympholysis by the murine major histocompatibility complex. I. Preferential *in vitro* responses to trinitrophenyl-modified self K- and D-coded gene products in parental and F_1 hybrid mouse strains. J. Exp. Med. **149:** 1379.

14. SHEARER, G. M., A.-M. SCHMITT-VERHULST, C. B. PETTINELLI, M. W. MILLER & P. E. GILHEANY. 1979. H-2-linked genetic control of murine T cell-mediated lympholysis to autologous cells modified with low concentrations of trinitrobenzene sulfonate. J. Exp. Med. **149:** 1407.

15. WAGNER, H., M. RÖLLINGHOFF, K. PFIZENMAIER, C. HARDT & G. JOHNSCHER. 1980. T-T cell interactions during *in vitro* cytotoxic T lymphocyte responses. II. Helper factor from activated Lyt 1+ T cell is rate limiting (i) in T cell responses to non-immunogenic allo-antigen, (ii) in thymocyte responses to allogeneic stimulator cells; and (iii) recruits alloreactive or H-2 restricted CTL precursors from the Lyt 123+ T cell subset. J. Immunol. **124:** 1059.

16. RÖLLINGHOFF, M., A. STARZINSKI-POWITZ, K. PFIZENMAIER & H. WAGNER. 1977. Cyclophosphamide-sensitive T lymphocytes suppress the *in vivo* generation of antigen-specific cytotoxic T lymphocytes. J. Exp. Med. **145:** 455.

17. TAGART, V. V., W. R. THOMAS & G. L. ASHERSON. 1978. Suppressor T cells which block the induction of cytotoxic T cells *in vivo*. Immunology **34:** 1109.

18. HALE, A. H. & M. P. MCGEE. 1981. H-2 haplotype specificity of molecular requirements for TNP recognition by anti-hapten cytotoxic T lymphocytes. Cell. Immunol. **58:** 147.

19. HARDT, C., M. RÖLLINGHOFF, K. PFIZENMAIER, H. MOSMANN & H. WAGNER. 1981. Lyt-23+ cyclophosphamide-sensitive T cells regulate the activity of an interleukin 2 inhibitor *in vivo*. J. Exp. Med. **154:** 262.

20. BUTLER, L. D. & J. R. BATTISTO. 1979. *In vivo* generation and regulation of killer T cells directed towards hapten-coupled syngeneic cells. Ann. N.Y. Acad. Sci. **332:** 524.

21. BUTLER, L. D., H. L. WONG & J. R. BATTISTO. 1980. Use of immunotolerance to dissect the mechanisms regulating appearance of hapten-specific killer T cells *in vivo*. J. Immunol. **124:** 1245.

22. WONG, H. L. & J. R. BATTISTO. 1981. *In vivo* development and regulation of cytolytic T cells specific for altered self antigens. *In* Proceedings of the

International Workshop on Lymphokines and Thymic Factors, A. L. Goldstein, Ed.: 227–37. Raven Press. New York.

23. BUTLER, L. D., S. D. MILLER & H. N. CLAMAN. 1981. Unresponsiveness in hapten-specific cytotoxic T lymphocytes. I. Characteristics of tolerance induction in adult mice. J. Immunol. 127: 1383.

24. SIMPSON, E., R. GORDON, M. TAYLOR, J. MERTIN & P. CHANDLER. 1975. Micromethods for induction and assay of mouse mixed lymphocyte reaction and cytotoxicity. Eur. J. Immunol. 5: 451.

25. BATTISTO, J. R. & B. R. BLOOM. 1966. Mechanisms of immunologic unsponsiveness: A new approach. Fed. Proc. Fed. Am. Soc. Exp. Biol. 25: 152.

26. SY, M.-S., M. H. DIETZ, R. N. GERMAIN, B. BENACERRAF & M. I. GREENE. 1980. Antigen-and receptor-driven regulatory mechanisms. IV. Idiotype-bearing I-J+ suppressor T cell factors induce second-order suppressor T cells which express anti-idiotypic receptors. J. Exp. Med. 151: 1183.

27. WEINBERGER, J. Z., R. N. GERMAIN, B. BENACERRAF & M. E. DORF. 1980. Hapten-specific T cell responses to 4-hydroxy-3-nitrophenyl acetyl. V. Role of idiotypes in the suppressor pathway. J. Exp. Med. 152: 161.

DISCUSSION OF THE PAPER

G. L. ASHERSON (*Clinical Research Centre, Harrow, Midd.*): Is it possible that the Ts_0 on the left-hand side of your table and the Ts_2 on the right-hand side could be the same cell? In that case, what you're calling a naturally occurring suppressor is really just a precursor that's immunized *in vivo*.

BATTISTO: While that's possible, we don't think so because we immunize in the hind paw with both the hapten-coupled syngeneic cells and the Mls-disparate cell; this circumvents that naturally occurring suppressor cell.

L. D. BUTLER (*University of Colorado Health Sciences Center, Denver, Col.*): In the original scheme, does IL-2 expand the pre-Tc population? The IL-2 should also be produced here with the M locus difference. How do you think the efferent suppressor cell is working in that case?

BATTISTO: In other words, your question is: Is the induced suppressor cell directed against the IL-2? Is it making suppressor factor that would interact with interleukin-2? I don't think so, because there's plenty of interleukin-2 inhibitor in the serum of mice, as Wagner has shown. That inhibitor is there for some five days after treatment with 950 rads. Therefore, that inhibitor is constant. It's absent in the athymic mouse, as you know. Therefore, the question, How do you circumvent that inhibitor? is a good one. We don't know the answer. We think the induced suppressor cell that we have described here may be anti-idiotypic. But we have no data on that point as yet.

J. CHILLER (*Scripps Clinic and Research Foundation, La Jolla, Calif.*): Are any of the cells you're talking about making IL-2 inhibitors like those which are found in normal mouse serum? I'm not doubting the existence of such molecules. In fact, however, we know that animals do make T cell responses. So there must be something within various lymphoid organs causing a certain reduction in their net activity below that magical (let's say) five percent level. Do you have any evidence that any of your suppressor cells are making a molecule that counteracts IL-2?

BATTISTO: We have tried the SSF that comes from Ts_1. It is inactive on both the *in vivo* and the *in vitro* primary Tc response. We have not been able to inhibit the primary *in vivo* or the primary *in vitro* Tc response at either limb with SSF. That is the only factor that we've worked with, thus far.

QUESTION: Can I ask the same question of Dr. Asherson or anybody else? That is, Is there any evidence that the nonspecific entity in these various populations of suppressor lymphocytes, particularly those which are in the category of "nonspecific in their mode of action," is an anti-interleukin or anti-T-expanding factor?

ASHERSON: The auxiliary suppressor, or the acceptor cell, works within 24 h, and the passive transfer cell is probably a nondividing population, according to the work of Moorhead and Miller. So I assume that, in that system, it's rather unlikely to be working through interleukin-2. I presume that the suppressor cells that act at the afferent limb can interfere with DNA synthesis. We don't know whether there's a final nonspecific mediator. If there were, it might well work on interleukin-2. But that's speculation for the moment.

ACTIVATION OF DISTINCT SUBSETS OF T SUPPRESSOR CELLS WITH TYPE III PNEUMOCOCCAL POLYSACCHARIDE COUPLED TO SYNGENEIC SPLEEN CELLS *

Helen Braley-Mullen

Departments of Medicine and Microbiology
University of Missouri School of Medicine
Columbia, Missouri 65212

INTRODUCTION

Antigens coupled to autologous lymphoid cells and injected by the i.v. route have been shown to be very effective tolerogens.[1-7] In most instances, tolerance induced by antigen-coupled cells has been shown to be mediated, at least in part, by antigen-specific suppressor T cells (Ts).[1-7] Previous studies from this laboratory have shown that the thymus-independent (TI) antigen type III pneumococcal polysaccharide (S3) coupled to syngeneic spleen cells (S3-SC) can induce tolerance in euthymic but not in athymic mice.[6] Although this observation suggested that tolerance induced by S3-SC might be mediated by Ts, spleen cells from tolerant mice did not suppress the antibody response to S3 after transfer to normal mice.[8] Subsequent studies, however, revealed that mice made tolerant with S3-SC did produce S3-specific Ts that could be demonstrated upon adoptive transfer to normal mice if tolerant spleen cells were first cultured *in vitro* in the presence of S3 and a soluble membrane component of S3-SC (S3-SC SM).[8] The present studies were undertaken in an effort to characterize these S3-specific Ts to determine if they had properties similar to Ts that are activated by conventional T cell–dependent (TD) antigens.[1-5, 9] During the course of these studies, we also found that the *in vitro* subculture step required to obtain detectable Ts could be circumvented if mice were pretreated with cyclophosphamide (Cy). The Ts induced in Cy-treated mice were also characterized and were found to differ from the Ts induced *in vitro*.

MATERIALS AND METHODS

Mice. CAF$_1$ mice were obtained from the Jackson Laboratory, Bar Harbor, Me. Female mice, 8–12 weeks old, were used for all experiments.

Preparation of Tolerogen. S3 was coupled to CAF$_1$ spleen cells as previously described.[6] Mock-SC were treated with the coupling agent (chromic chloride) alone. Soluble membrane components of Mock-SC (Mock-SC SM) or S3-SC (S3-SC SM) were prepared as previously described.[8] Mice were injected i.v. with Mock-SC SM or S3-SC SM in an amount equivalent to 5×10^7 SC.[6, 8]

* This research was supported by a grant from the National Institutes of Health, no. CA–25054. The author is the recipient of a National Institutes of Health Research Career Development Award, no. AI–00322.

Induction and Assay of Ts Induced in Vitro. Mice were injected i.v. with S3-SC SM. Four or five days later, spleen cells from these mice were cultured *in vitro* for 48 h with Mock-SC SM (positive control) or with S3 and S3-SC SM (experimental). Cells were harvested, washed four times in balanced salt solution (BSS), counted and injected i.v. (3–5 × 10^6 cells per recipient) into normal CAF$_1$ mice, which were immunized one day later with an optimal dose of 0.6 μg S3. IgM plaque-forming cells (PFC) were counted five days later. The culture conditions and requirements for Ts induction by this method were described in detail previously.[8]

Induction and Assay of Ts Induced in Cy-Treated Mice. Mice were given 100 mg kg^{-1} Cy i.p. and were injected i.v. with Mock-SC SM (control) or S3-SC SM (experimental) two days later. Seven or eight days later, spleen cells were removed and cell suspensions were prepared in BSS. Cells were washed in BSS, counted, and injected i.v. into normal CAF$_1$ recipients, which were immunized 4–6 h later with 0.6 μg S3. IgM PFC were determined five days later.

Antiserum Treatment. In some experiments, spleen cells were depleted of T cells or T cell subsets by treatment with various antisera and complement as described previously.[7, 8] The antisera used were anti-Thy 1.2 (AKR anti-C$_3$H), anti-Lyt 1.2 (C$_3$H anti-C$_3$H.CE), anti-Lyt 2.2 (C$_3$H × B62.1 F$_1$ anti-B6), anti-I-J^k (Balb/c × B10.A (3R) F$_1$ anti-B10.A (5R)), and anti-I-J^b (B10.A (5R) anti-B10.A (3R)). They were prepared as previously described and their activity and specificity have also been described.[7]

Separation of Ts on Antigen- and Antibody-Coated Plates. A modification of the method of Mage *et al.* was used to deplete spleen cell populations of cells with binding affinity for S3 or anti-S3.[10] Either tissue culture grade petri plates were coated with 5 ml of 100 μg ml^{-1} S3, S3–bovine gamma globulin (BGG), or S3-tyrosine[6] or polystyrene plates were coated with 100 μg ml^{-1} of affinity purified anti-S3 antibody at 4° C overnight. Plates were washed extensively with saline and then with BSS containing 2% fetal calf serum (FCS). Spleen cells (50 × 10^6 per plate) were then added to plates in 5 ml BSS-FCS. After 60 min at 4° C, nonadherent cells were removed by gently swirling and washing the plates with BSS. Plates were rinsed additionally one or twice with BSS, then adherent cells were removed by gently scraping the plates with a plastic policeman. Cells were centrifuged, washed twice in BSS, and counted before being transferred to mice. In general, 70–80% of the cells were recovered in the nonadherent fractions and 5–10% in the adherent fractions.

Adult Thymectomy (ATx). For some experiments, mice were thymectomized at 4–5 weeks of age and used as cell recipients 10–12 weeks later.

RESULTS

Surface Phenotype of in Vitro–Induced Ts

In order to determine the T cell subset of the Ts induced after being cultured *in vitro,* spleen cells from tolerant mice were cultured with Mock-SC SM or S3 and S3-SC SM, as described in Materials and Methods. Cells were then treated with various antisera and complement prior to transfer to normal CAF$_1$ mice. As seen in TABLE 1, spleen cells cultured with S3 and S3-SC SM sup-

TABLE 1

EFFECT OF ANTI-I-J SERUM ON *in Vitro*–INDUCED SUPPRESSOR CELLS

Cells Cultured with *	Treatment †	IgM PFC per Spleen ‡
Mock-SC SM	None	$11\,367 \pm 1361$
S3 + S3-SC SM	C′	4375 ± 932
S3 + S3-SC SM	Anti-Thy 1.2 + C′	$14\,100 \pm 2186$
S3 + S3-SC SM	Anti-I-J^k + C′	9375 ± 2009
S3 + S3-SC SM	Anti-I-J^b + C′	5138 ± 925

* See Materials and Methods.
† Cells were treated as indicated and 2×10^6 cells were transferred i.v. to normal CAF$_1$ recipients, which were then immunized with S3. CAF$_1$ spleen cells are Thy 1.2$^+$ and I-J^{k+}.
‡ Mean PFC per spleen $\pm$ SEM (4–5 mice per group).

pressed the antibody response to S3 after transfer to normal mice. The suppressive activity of these cells was eliminated after treatment with anti-Thy 1.2 or anti-I-J^k and complement, but was not affected by the control anti-I-J^b serum. In addition, absorption of the anti-I-J^k serum with B10.A (5R) spleen cells (which should remove anti-I-J reactivity) eliminated the ability of the antiserum to remove suppressor cell activity (data not shown). Thus, the suppressor cells induced after being cultured *in vitro* are T cells that bear I-J encoded antigens on their surface. As seen in TABLE 2, suppressor activity was also eliminated when spleen cells were treated with anti-Lyt 2.2 but not after treatment with anti-Lyt 1.2 and complement. Thus, these Ts belong to the Lyt 1$^-$2$^+$ cell subset. The increased suppression observed in this experiment with anti-Lyt 1.2–treated cells did not occur in all experiments of this type. The possible significance of this observation will be discussed below.

In Vitro–*Induced Ts are Removed on Antibody-Coated Plates*

To begin to determine the receptor specificity of the Ts induced *in vitro*, spleen cells cultured with S3 and S3-SC SM were separated on S3 or anti-S3 coated plates, as described in Materials and Methods. As seen in TABLE 3, unseparated spleen cells (group B) again suppressed the antibody response to S3. Elimination of antigen (S3) binding cells (group C, *i.e.*, S3 nonadherent)

TABLE 2

EFFECT OF ANTI-LYT ANTISERA ON *in Vitro*–INDUCED SUPPRESSOR CELLS

Cells Cultured with	Treatment *	IgM PFC per Spleen †
Mock-SC SM	None	$17\,775 \pm 2596$
S3 + S3-SC SM	C′	4475 ± 892
S3 + S3-SC SM	Anti-Lyt 1.2 + C′	750 ± 50
S3 + S3-SC SM	Anti-Lyt 2.2 + C	$11\,750 \pm 1311$

* See second footnote, TABLE 1.
† Mean PFC per spleen $\pm$ SEM (4–5 mice per group).

TABLE 3

In Vitro–Induced Ts are Removed on Anti-S3 Plates

Group	Cells Cultured with	Source of Cells *	No. of Cells Transferred	IgM PFC per Spleen †
A	Mock-SC SM	Unfractionated	5×10^6	17 820 ± 1663
B	S3 + S3–SC SM	Unfractionated	5×10^6	7825 ± 349
C	S3 + S3–SC SM	S3 nonadherent	5×10^6	5840 ± 968
D	S3 + S3–SC SM	S3 adherent	2×10^6	12 083 ± 2460
E	S3 + S3–SC SM	Anti-S3 nonadherent	5×10^6	13 700 ± 2732
F	S3 + S3–SC SM	Anti-S3 adherent	2×10^6	5225 ± 687
G	S3 + S3–SC SM	Unfractionated	2×10^6	6912 ± 264

* Cultured cells were separated on S3- or anti-S3-coated plates (see Materials and Methods) before transfer.

† Mean PFC per spleen ± SEM (4–5 mice per group).

had no effect on the degree of suppression obtained, while removal of anti-S3 binding cells (group E, anti-S3 nonadherent) resulted in the elimination of suppressor activity. The suppressor cells could be eluted from the anti-S3 plates (group F, anti-S3 adherent). Thus, the *in vitro*–induced Ts may have anti-idiotypic-type receptors, in accordance with previous studies by others.[9]

In Vitro–*Induced Ts Cannot Suppress Responses in ATx or Cy-Treated Recipients*

To determine whether Ts induced during culture act by directly suppressing S3-specific B cells or whether they act on another T cell in the recipient to mediate suppression, cells were transferred to normal recipients, ATx recipients, or recipients pretreated with 20 mg kg⁻¹ Cy (TABLE 4). Whereas cells cultured with S3 and S3-SC SM suppressed the S3 response when transferred to normal mice, the same cells had no effect on the S3 response of ATx or Cy-treated

TABLE 4

In Vitro–Induced Ts Act on an ATx- and Cy-Sensitive Recipient Cell

Cells Cultured with	Treatment of Recipients *	IgM PFC per Spleen †
Mock-SC SM	None	14 690 ± 1720
S3 + S3–SC SM	None	2795 ± 406
Mock-SC SM	ATx	10 975 ± 1543
S3 + S3–SC SM	ATx	12 675 ± 1253
Mock-SC SM	20 mg kg⁻¹ Cy	8888 ± 2472
S3 + S3–SC SM	20 mg kg⁻¹ Cy	9600 ± 1137

* CAF₁ recipients were either normal mice or mice that had been ATx ten weeks earlier or treated two days earlier with 20 mg kg⁻¹ Cy.

† Mean PFC per spleen ± SEM (4–5 mice per group).

recipients. These results suggest that these Ts act on another T cell in the recipient to mediate the final suppression of S3-specific B cells.

Precursors of Ts are Cy Resistant

To further characterize the Ts induced *in vitro*, donor mice were given 100 mg kg^{-1} Cy two days before injection of S3-SC SM. Since Ts precursors have often been shown to be Cy sensitive,[2, 4, 7, 9] we expected to find that Cy-treated mice would possess cells that, when cultured *in vitro*, would not develop Ts. However, as shown in TABLE 5, spleen cells from Cy-pretreated tolerant mice did develop Ts after culture with S3 and S3-SC SM. Indeed, in most experiments (*e.g.*, exp. 2, TABLE 5), cells from Cy-treated mice even suppressed the S3 response after culture with Mock-SC SM, suggesting that the *in vitro* subculture step might not be needed to induce S3-specific Ts, provided that the donors were treated with Cy before the induction of tolerance *in vitro*.

TABLE 5

S3-SPECIFIC TS PRECURSORS ARE CY RESISTANT

Treatment of Donors *	Cells Cultured with	IgM PFC per Spleen †	
		Exp. 1	Exp. 2
S3-SC SM	Mock-SC SM	7100 ± 742	7475 ± 269
S3-SC SM	S3 + S3-SC SM	3408 ± 669	2544 ± 483
S3-SC SM + Cy	Mock-SC SM	10 675 ± 3546	4075 ± 739
S3-SC SM + Cy	S3 + S3-SC SM	2669 ± 640	3600 ± 876

* Donors were either normal mice or mice given 100 mg kg^{-1} Cy two days before injection of S3-SC SM (see Materials and Methods).

† Mean PFC per spleen ± SEM (3–4 mice per group).

Induction of Ts in Cy-Treated Mice

In order to determine if Ts could be induced entirely *in vivo* in Cy-treated mice, both normal and Cy-treated CAF$_1$ mice were injected with Mock-SC SM or S3-SC SM. One week later, spleen cells from these mice were transferred to normal CAF$_1$ mice, which were then immunized with S3 (TABLE 6). As noted previously,[8] spleen cells from normal mice made tolerant with S3-SC SM did not suppress the S3 response upon transfer. However, when mice were treated with Cy prior to injection of S3-SC SM, their spleen cells suppressed the S3 response after transfer. These suppressor cells were T cells, since suppression was eliminated if cells were treated with anti-Thy 1.2 and complement before transfer (last line, TABLE 6). These Ts were specific for S3, since Cy-treated mice given Mock-SC SM did not have detectable suppressor cells (TABLE 6). Moreover, when Ts were transferred to mice that had been immunized with S3 together with other antigens, *i.e.*, polyvinylpyrrolidone (PVP) or horse erythrocytes, only the response to S3 was suppressed (manuscript in preparation).

TABLE 6

INDUCTION OF Ts IN CY-TREATED TOLERANT MICE

Treatment of Donors	Cy *	IgM PFC/Spleen ‡
Mock-SC SM	—	13 000 ± 1518
S3-SC SM	—	13 375 ± 1750
Mock-SC SM	+	14 700 ± 1315
S3-SC SM	+	5600 ± 1793
S3-SC SM	+ †	10 725 ± 1012

* Mice received 100 mg kg^{-1} Cy two days before Mock- or S3-SC SM. Seven days later, 5×10^6 cells were transferred to normal recipients.
† Cells treated with anti-Thy 1.2 + C' before transfer.
‡ Mean PFC per spleen ± SEM (4 mice per group).

Surface Phenotype of Ts in Cy-Treated Mice

In order to determine if the Ts induced in Cy-treated mice were similar to the Ts induced after *in vitro* culture, Ts were induced as in TABLE 6 and spleen cells were treated with anti-I-J^k or anti-Lyt 1.2 or 2.2 and complement before transfer (TABLE 7). As before, spleen cells from donors given Cy and S3-SC SM suppressed the S3 response after transfer. Suppression was eliminated when spleen cells were treated with anti-Thy 1.2, anti-Lyt 2.2, or anti-I-J^k, but not when they were treated with anti-Lyt 1.2 and complement (TABLE 7). Thus, the Ts induced in Cy-treated mice are Lyt 1$^-$2$^+$ and I-J$^+$ and, as such, are similar to the Ts induced after *in vitro* culture (TABLES 1 and 2).

Ts Induced in Cy-Treated Mice Differ from Ts Induced During *in* Vitro *Culture*

Since the Ts induced *in vitro* could be removed on anti-S3-coated plates (TABLE 3), it was of interest to determine if the Ts induced in Cy-treated mice had similar receptor specificity. As shown in TABLE 8, Ts induced in Cy-treated mice were not removed on anti-S3-coated plates. These Ts also could not be effectively absorbed on plates coated with various forms of antigen, *i.e.* S3,

TABLE 7

I-J AND LYT PHENOTYPE OF Ts INDUCED IN CY-TREATED MICE

Donor Treatment	Treatment of Cells	IgM PFC per Spleen †
Mock-SC SM + Cy *	None	14 753 ± 3139
S3-SC SM + Cy	C'	5163 ± 683
S3-SC SM + Cy	Anti-Thy 1.2 + C'	12 425 ± 1025
S3-SC SM + Cy	Anti-Lyt 1.2 + C'	6500 ± 1365
S3-SC SM + Cy	Anti-Lyt 2.2 + C'	19 825 ± 4672
S3-SC SM + Cy	Anti-I-J^K + C'	18 300 ± 3063

* 100 mg ky^{-2} Cy two days before Mock- or S3-SC SM.
† Mean PFC per spleen ± SEM (4–5 mice per group).

TABLE 8

Ts Induced in Cy-Treated Mice are not Removed on Anti-S3 Plates

Donor Treatment *	Source of Cells †	IgM PFC per Spleen ‡	
		Exp. 1	Exp. 2
Mock-SC SM + Cy	Unfractionated	14 840 ± 2993	23 340 ± 3200
S3-SC SM + Cy	Unfractionated	4568 ± 433	7440 ± 1527
S3-SC SM + Cy	Anti-S3 nonadherent	4110 ± 608	8754 ± 1230
S3-SC SM + Cy	S3 nonadherent	7150 ± 433	N.D.
S3-SC SM + Cy	S3-tyrosine nonadherent	N.D.	9850 ± 549
S3-SC SM + Cy	S3-BGG nonadherent	N.D.	11 633 ± 1128

* See first footnote, TABLE 8.
† Spleen cells were separated on anti-S3- or S3-coated plates before transfer. 5×10^6 cells were transferred per recipient.
‡ Mean PFC per spleen ± SEM (4–5 mice per group).

S3-tyrosine, or S3-BGG (TABLE 8). Thus, the receptor specificity of Ts induced in Cy-treated mice is unknown (see Discussion) but clearly differs from that of the Ts induced *in vitro* (TABLE 3).

The Ts induced *in vitro* were shown to require an ATx and Cy-sensitive recipient cell to mediate suppression (TABLE 4). To determine if Ts induced in Cy-treated mice had a similar requirement, spleen cells from donors given Cy and Mock- or S3-SC-SM were transferred to normal or Cy-treated recipients (TABLE 9). A similar degree of suppression was observed in both groups of recipients, suggesting that these Ts might act by directly suppressing S3-specific B cells.

DISCUSSION

Previous studies have shown that antigens coupled to autologous lymphoid cells activate antigen-specific Ts when injected into mice by the i.v. route.[1-8] Activation of Ts by antigen-coupled cells occurs with simple haptens,[1-3] complex proteins,[4, 5] and with TI antigens such as PVP.[7] The TI antigen S3 coupled to

TABLE 9

Ts Induced in Cy-Treated Mice Suppress Responses in Cy-Treated Recipients

Donor Treatment *	Recipient Treatment †	IgM PFC per Spleen ‡
Mock-SC SM + Cy	None	16 880 ± 716
S3-SC SM + Cy	None	4305 ± 474
Mock-SC SM + Cy	20 mg kg^{-1} Cy	22 940 ± 1852
S3-SC SM + Cy	20 mg kg^{-1} Cy	7145 ± 1197

* See first footnote, TABLE 7.
† Recipients were either not treated or given 20 mg kg^{-1} Cy two days before transfer of 5×10^6 cells per recipient.
‡ Mean PFC per spleen ± SEM (5 mice per group).

spleen cells (S3-SC) can also activate S3-specific Ts, although these Ts can be demonstrated only if spleen cells from mice made tolerant with S3-SC are subcultured *in vitro* with antigen (S3) and a soluble form of the tolerogen, S3-SC SM.[8] Because of the unusual activation requirements for these S3-specific Ts, it was of interest to further characterize these cells in order to determine their relationship to Ts described in other systems.[2-5, 7, 9]

The results presented here indicate that S3-specific Ts induced *in vitro*[8] are I-J+ (TABLE 1), Lyt 1-2+ (TABLE 2), and derived from Cy-resistant precursors (TABLE 5). These Ts could be removed on plates coated with anti-S3 antibody (TABLE 3), suggesting that the Ts receptors may be anti-idiotypic in nature (see below). It was also noted that these *in vitro*–induced Ts were unable to suppress the S3 response in recipients that had been ATx or pretreated with Cy (TABLE 4), suggesting that they act on a recipient T cell to mediate the final suppression of S3-specific B cells.[11-13] The *in vitro*–induced Ts described here thus appear to be similar to the so-called second-order Ts, or Ts$_2$. Thus, Ts$_2$ precursors are not Cy-sensitive,[9] Ts$_2$ are usually I-J+ and Lyt 1-2+,[9, 14] bear anti-idiotypic receptors,[9, 14, 15] and act on recipient T cells, *i.e.*, Ts$_3$ to mediate the final suppression of effector cells.[11-13] However, Ts$_2$ are usually capable of suppressing ongoing delayed hypersensitivity (DTH) responses[9, 15] or antibody responses,[14] whereas the *in vitro*–induced Ts described here are effective only if they are injected prior to immunization with S3 (unpublished observations).

The results presented here also demonstrate that S3-SC SM can activate Ts directly, *i.e.*, without the requirement for *in vitro* subculture, if donor mice are pretreated with Cy (TABLE 6). Although previous studies have shown that Cy alone can sometimes activate antigen-nonspecific suppressor cells,[16, 17] this report is, to our knowledge, the first indication that the induction of antigen-specific Ts can be augmented in Cy-treated mice. Indeed, in most cases it has been found that the precursors of Ts induced by antigen-coupled cells are Cy-sensitive.[2, 4, 7] Since the *in vitro*–induced Ts described above also derive from Cy-resistant precursors (TABLE 5), it was anticipated that the Ts induced *in vivo* in Cy-treated mice (TABLE 6) would have the same characteristics as the *in vitro*–induced Ts. Although Ts induced *in vitro* and in Cy-treated mice are both I-J+ and Lyt 1-2+ (TABLES 1, 2, and 7), they appear to differ in their receptor specificity and in the mechanism by which they suppress S3 responses. Thus, Ts induced *in vitro* can be removed on anti-S3 coated plates (TABLE 3), while the Ts induced in Cy-treated mice cannot (TABLE 8). Moreover, the Ts induced in Cy-treated mice may directly suppress S3-specific B cells, since suppression occurs in both normal and Cy-treated recipients (TABLE 9). Therefore, S3-SC SM can apparently activate two distinct Ts subsets, both of which act to suppress primary IgM responses to S3. One of the Ts subsets (induced *in vitro*) is apparently similar to that designated Ts$_2$ in other systems.[9, 14, 15] The Ts induced in Cy-treated mice differ from Ts$_2$ in receptor specificity and by the fact that suppression does not require a Cy-sensitive recipient T cell (TABLES 8 and 9). The fact that the precursors of the Ts are Cy-resistant also suggests that they are not identical to either the Ts$_1$ or Ts$_3$ subsets described by others.[9, 11-13] Further studies will be required to determine the role of these cells in the regulation of antibody responses to S3.

Although the studies described here indicate that the two Ts we have described differ from each other in their receptor specificity (TABLES 3 and 8), it should be emphasized that further studies are needed to fully define the receptor specificity of both cells. The ability to remove *in vitro* activated Ts on antibody-coated plates suggests that these cells may have anti-idiotypic receptors.[9, 14, 15] However, it is possible that these cells might instead have idiotypic receptors that bind antigen during the *in vitro* subculture and that it is this bound antigen that has affinity for the antibody-coated plates. Studies are currently in progress to differentiate between these two possibilities. Moreover, the receptor specificity of the Ts induced in Cy-treated mice is as yet unknown, since these cells could not be removed on either S3 or anti-S3 coated plates (TABLE 8). These cells may have antigen-binding receptors that were not detected because the amount or configuration of S3 on the plates was insufficient to absorb them. Alternatively, these cells may have very low affinity receptors (either antigen or antibody binding) so that it is just not possible to absorb them to the plates efficiently. Finally, both antibody- and antigen-binding Ts populations could exist in spleens of Cy-treated tolerant mice so that sequential absorption on both S3 and anti-S3 coated plates is needed to absorb Ts activity. Studies are currently in progress to examine these possibilities and to definitively determine the receptor specificity of these Ts.

Finally, it is apparent that both of the Ts subsets induced by S3-SC SM have unusual activation requirements. The induction of tolerance with S3-SC (or S3-SC SM) is T cell dependent,[8] yet it is not possible to demonstrate the presence of Ts in tolerant spleen cells unless the cells undergo a second activation step *in vitro* [8] or the tolerant mice are pretreated with Cy (TABLE 6). This suggests that another cell type present in S3-SC tolerant mice can interfere with the expression or activation of S3-specific Ts. Although the identity of this cell is not yet known, previous studies suggest that it is a T cell [8] that, as shown here, is apparently Cy-sensitive (TABLE 6). This cell may also be Lyt 1+, since treatment of *in vitro*–induced Ts with anti-Lyt 1.2 and complement in some cases results in increased suppressor activity in the remaining cells (TABLE 2). The relationship of the cell that interferes with Ts detection in this system to amplifier T cells,[18] contrasuppressor T cells,[19] or abrosuppressor T cells [20] remains to be determined.

ACKNOWLEDGMENTS

The author thanks Patra Mierzwa for skilled technical assistance and Jean Rinacke for typing the manuscript.

REFERENCES

1. BATTISTO, J. R. & B. R. BLOOM. 1966. Nature (London) **212:** 156.
2. MILLER, S. D., M. S. SY & H. N. CLAMAN. 1977. Eur. J. Immunol. **7:** 165.
3. SCOTT, D. W. 1978. Cell. Immunol. **37:** 327.
4. MILLER, S. D., R. P. WETZIG & H. N. CLAMAN. 1979. J. Exp. Med. **149:** 758.
5. SHERR, D. H., N. K. CHEUNG, K. M. HEGHINIAN, B. BENACERRAF & M. E. DORF. 1979. J. Immunol. **122:** 1899.
6. BRALEY-MULLEN, H. 1980. Cell. Immunol. **52:** 132.
7. FRASER, V. & H. BRALEY-MULLEN. 1981. Cell Immunol. **63:** 177.
8. BRALEY-MULLEN, H. 1980. J. Immunol. **125:** 1849.
9. GERMAIN, R. N. & B. BENACERRAF. 1981. Scand. J. Immunol. **13:** 1.

10. MAGE, M. F., L. L. McHUGH & T. L. ROTHSTEIN.   1977.   J. Immunol. Methods **15**: 47.
11. SY, M. S., S. D. MILLER, J. W. MOOREHEAD & H. N. CLAMAN.   1979.   J. Exp. Med. **149**: 1197.
12. SY, M. S., A. NISONOFF, R. N. GERMAIN, B. BENACERRAF & M. I. GREENE. 1981.   J. Exp. Med. **153**: 1415.
13. SHERR, D. H., B. BENACERRAF & M. E. DORF.   1981.   J. Immunol. **125**: 1862.
14. SHERR, D. H. & M. E. DORF.   1981.   J. Exp. Med. **153**: 1445.
15. SY, M. S., M. H. DIETZ, R. N. GERMAIN, B. BENACERRAF & M. I. GREENE.   1980. J. Exp. Med. **151**: 1183.
16. McINTOSH, K., M. SEGRE & D. SEGRE.   1979.   Immunopharmacology **1**: 165.
17. BRACIALE, V. & C. R. PARISH.   1980.   Cell. Immunol. **51**: 1.
18. MARKHAM, R. B., N. D. REED, P. W. STASHAK, B. PRESCOTT, D. F. AMSBAUGH & P. J. BAKER.   1977.   J. Immunol. **119**: 1163.
19. GERSHON, R. K., D. D. EARDLEY, S. DURUM, D. R. GREEN, F. W. SHEN, K. YAMAUCHI, H. CANTOR & D. B. MURPHY.   1981.   J. Exp. Med. **153**: 1533.
20. DE KRUYFF, R. H., B. G. SIMONSON & G. W. SISKIND.   1981.   J. Exp. Med. **154**: 1188.

DISCUSSION OF THE PAPER

F. L. ADLER (*St. Jude Children's Research Hospital, Memphis, Tenn.*): I may have missed your evidence for your conclusion that the suppressors in both cases are antigen specific. What were your controls for antigen specificity?

MULLEN: I didn't show those data, but what we have done is transfer the suppressor cells and then doubly immunize the recipients with S3 and another T cell–independent antigen, PVP. In all cases, the response to the specific antigen is suppressed and the response to the other antigen is not.

D. R. GREEN (*Yale University, New Haven, Conn.*): You have two ways to produce suppressor cells in this system. But if you take cells right out of an animal that's just been injected with the tolerogen, you don't have any detectable suppressor cells. Have you ever attempted to look to see if there were suppressor cells there that were somehow masked? For instance, you show that they're Lyt 2+. If you remove Lyt 1 cells, does that have any effect on the appearance of suppression in these nonsuppressive mixtures?

MULLEN: We haven't looked at that for a long time, but it didn't appear to. We do know that, when the cells are cultured *in vitro,* there is a cell that can counteract the suppressive cell. In many cases, if we treat those cultured cells with anti-Lyt 1 and complement, we actually increase the degree of suppression. I think, indeed, that the reason we don't detect the cell in the original situation is that there is something in there that's masking the suppressor cell.

GREEN: We've detailed a cell circuit that has this activity, which we call the contrasuppressor circuit. It has the characteristics you describe, in that the effector cell is an Lyt 1+ cell, and, therefore, removal of that cell should increase suppression. Also, the evidence that you've shown is that it's Cy-sensitive. I think that this is important in explaining some of the differences that you point out between the Cy-induced suppressor cell and the cell that appears upon culture, in that the Cy-induced suppressor cell is being produced in an environment depleted of contrasuppressors. The culture-induced suppressor cell is produced where these cells are present. This can account for the differences in the suppressor cells. I'm a little surprised that you say the Cy-induced suppressor is I-J+. We didn't see the data for that. Some of our evidence suggests that the suppressor cells induced in the absence of contrasuppression tend to be I-J-. But that may not be a consistent finding. You gave some evidence for that.

J. CHILLER (*Scripps Clinic and Research Foundation, La Jolla, Calif.*): Could you give us an insight as to how either one of these suppressor mechanisms or both work in suppressing B cell activity? Do you think that there is, in fact, a direct focusing by specific B cells, which presumably have seen antigen, of such suppressor cells or factors from them? Do you have any evidence, for example, that you can actually rosette out such suppressor cells with B cells that have been incubated with antigen?

MULLEN: No, we have no evidence like that at all.

CHILLER: Do you know how they work? Do they work *via* B cells or *via* macrophages? What can you tell us in terms of mechanisms?

MULLEN: I can't tell you much because we really haven't begun to look at that, as yet. I think that the suppressor cell induced in the Cy-treated mice may very well act directly on the B cell. But certainly we can't exclude other mechanisms of action at this point. The other one clearly acts through another cell in the recipient, which is Cy-sensitive.

DELAYED-TYPE HYPERSENSITIVITY AND UNRESPONSIVENESS TO NUCLEIC ACID ANTIGEN

The Role of the Epitope Density and Crossreactivity between Nucleoside Coupled to Cell *

Yves Borel

Department of Medicine
Division of Immunology
Children's Hospital Medical Center
Boston, Massachusetts 02115

Mark I. Greene

Departments of Pediatrics and Pathology
Harvard Medical School
Boston, Massachusetts 02115

INTRODUCTION

The modification of cell surface antigens by haptens has been used to explore the mechanism of self recognition as well as to analyze the induction of cellular immunity and unresponsiveness.[1-5] This principle can be applied to potential autoantigens, since the covalent binding of autoantigens to self molecules could be useful for the immunoregulation of autoimmunity. For example, linking nucleoside to isogeneic spleen cells and linking nucleoside to isologous IgG are two different means of manipulating the immune systems.[6, 7] Unresponsiveness induced by nucleoside-coupled spleen cells is mediated by suppressor T cells, in contrast to unresponsiveness induced by nucleoside-coupled IgG,[8, 9] which is not. In addition, the specificity of the suppression of antibody formation induced by nucleoside-coupled spleen cells is broader than that induced by nucleoside-coupled IgG, which is exquisitely hapten specific.[7, 10]

In this paper, we will examine (1) whether one can elicit both cellular immunity and unresponsiveness to nucleoside-modified cells and (2) the role of the epitope density in these immune responses. It was found that nucleoside-specific cellular immunity can be elicited by either guanosine or adenosine coupled to syngeneic spleen cells in Balb/c mice. The epitope density, as measured by radiolabeled cell-bound nucleoside, was found to be a decisive factor in the induction of immunity. In addition, both guanosine and adenosine —which do not crossreact as immunogens or tolerogens when bound to soluble carrier proteins [19]—were found to crossreact when coupled to spleen cells in terms of both delayed hypersensitivity and unresponsiveness. These results are relevant to the mechanism of antigen recognition as well as to the regulation of autoimmunity.

* This research was supported by grants from the United States Public Health Service, nos. AM 16392, AI 13867–05, and AI 16396–02, and from the American Cancer Society, nos. IM–178 and IM–277.

167

MATERIALS AND METHODS

Animals

Six- to eight-week-old male Balb/c mice purchased from the Jackson Laboratory (Bar Harbor, Me.) and Charles River Breeding service (Boston, Mass.) were used as spleen cell donors and recipients.

Nucleosides

Adenosine (A) and guanosine (G) were obtained from Sigma Chemicals, (St. Louis, Mo.). (8-^{3}H)guanosine (^{3}H-G) (specific activity 5–15 mCi μmol^{-1}) and (2,8-^{3}H)adenosine (^{3}H-A) (specific activity 30–50 mCi μmol^{-1}) were purchased from New England Nuclear (Boston, Mass.).

Preparation of Nucleoside-Coupled Spleen Cells

G and A were each coupled to spleen cells by the method previously described,[7, 11] with slight modifications for greater precision. The procedure was as follows: Balb/c spleens were mashed in a glass tissue grinder filled with minimal Eagle's Medium (MEM), pH 7–8. The cells were washed three times in MEM, then counted and resuspended in MEM at a concentration of 250×10^6 white blood cells (WBC) per ml. Varying amounts of nucleoside (2, 10, or 20 mg) were suspended in 0.15 M NaHCO$_3$. Twenty to thirty μl of radionucleoside was added to this suspension and the mixture was oxidized with 0.1 M sodium periodate in saline. After stirring for 20 min at room temperature, the reaction was stopped with 15 μl of ethylene glycol. A 25 μl aliquot was taken in duplicate from this solution for an initial count of β activity. An equal volume of 0.15 M NaHCO$_3$ was added to the cell suspension (as above); the resulting suspension was added through tantalum gauze to the oxidized nucleoside solution. Binding was stopped after 15 min of stirring at room temperature with 100 mg of t-butylamine borane in 5 ml of 0.15 M NaHCO$_3$. After 2–3 min at room temperature, the reaction tube was filled with MEM and centrifuged for 10 min at 1200 rpm. After the conjugated cells were washed once more, they were resuspended at a concentration of 10–30×10^6 WBC per ml. Aliquots of 2 ml were placed in glass scintillation vials for scintillation counting; an aliquot was also set aside for determination of cell concentration.

Measurement of Radioactivity

Radioactivity was measured using a modification of the method of Kobayashi and Harris.† MEM was added to the cell aliquots and the cells were spun down

---

† This procedure is a modification of the procedure outlined by Y. Kobayashi and W. G. Harris in LSC Applications Notes #16 (NEN LSC Applications Lab). See also D. M. Weir, Ed. 1973. *Handbook of Experimental Immunology*, 2nd ed. Blackwell Scientific Publications. 25.6–25.7.

at 2000 rpm for 15–20 min. After removal of the supernatant, 0.5 ml of a solution containing about 2.5 mg ml^{-1} of bovine serum albumin in 0.15 M saline was added to each vial, and the cells were precipitated with 10% tri-chloracetic acid in distilled water. The vials were placed at 4° C overnight. The next day, the vials were centrifuged at 2400 rpm for 20–25 min and the supernatant TCA was removed. 1.5 ml of Protosol Tissue and Gel Solubilizer (New England Nuclear, Boston, Mass.) was added to each sample. Protosol and Econofluor were also added to the initial aliquots before counting. Beta counts were done in a Packard 3255 Tri-Carb Scintillation Counter, using a preset ^{3}H channel.

Calculation of the Epitope Density

As noted above, we obtained both initial samples (aliquots of 25 μl each taken from radiolabeled nucleoside solutions after oxidation) and final samples (aliquots containing approximately 25–50 $\times$ 10^6 radiolabeled cells per ml) for counting. All initial aliquots were taken in duplicate; all final aliquots were taken at least in triplicate. After precipitation of the cell suspensions with TCA, Protosol and Econofluor were added to all samples.

In order to calculate the number of bound molecules per cell (epitope density), the mean cpm per vial from both initial and final aliquots were related by the following straightforward formulae:

$$\frac{\text{Initial cpm per vial} \times \text{dilution factor}}{\text{initial moles nucleoside}} = \text{initial cpm per mole of nucleoside}$$

$$\frac{\text{Final cpm per vial}}{\text{initial cpm per mole of nucleoside}} = \text{moles of bound nucleoside}$$

$$\frac{\text{moles of bound nucleoside} \times \text{Avogadro's number}}{\text{number of white cells per final aliquot}} = \text{bound molecules of nucleoside per white cell}$$

Preparation of Antigens and Tolerogens

Murine IgG$_1$ was obtained through starch block electrophoresis from sera of Balb/c mice bearing the RPC$_5$ tumor, as previously described.[12] Keyhole limpet hemocyanin (KLH) (Pacific Biomarine Supply Co., Venice, Calif.) was prepared as described elsewhere.[12] 2,4-Dinitrobenzenesulfonic acid sodium salt (DNP) was obtained from Eastman Kodak Co. (Rochester, N.Y.), 2,4,6-tri-nitrobenzenesulfonic acid (TNP) was supplied by ICN/K & K Laboratories (Plainview, N.J.), and sheep red blood cells (SRBC) in Alsever's solution were purchased from Colorado Serum (Denver, Col.).

A and G were conjugated to protein by the method of Erlanger and Beiser.[11] DNP-protein conjugates were prepared as described previously.[12] Adenosine$_{27}$-IgG (A-IgG), and dinitrophenyl$_{16}$-IgG$_{2a}$ (DNP-IgG) were used as tolerogens at a dose of 0.2 mg i.v. We used guanosine$_{176}$-KLH (G-KLH) and adenosine$_{100}$-KLH (A-KLH) as immunogens.

All immunogens were given i.p. in complete Freund's adjuvant, except for sheep red blood cells, which were suspended in 0.15 M saline for i.p. administration. In every case, subscripts indicate the total molar ratio of hapten substitution on the carrier protein.

Experimental Protocol

The experimental groups consisted of 5–8 mice each. The basic experimental design was as follows, unless stated otherwise in the text. 30×10^6 G-SC or A-SC were injected subcutaneously in two sites on the dorsal flanks of the mice. Five days later, the mice were challenged with 10×10^6 G-SC or A-SC in a 25 μl volume in the left footpad. Control mice were either uninjected mice or mice injected with sham-treated spleen cells.

To induce DTH to azobenzene arsonate (ABA), 30×10^6 ABA-coupled cells were injected subcutaneously into two separate sites on the dorsal flanks of mice, as previously described.[5] The challenge was performed five days later by injecting 25 μl of 10 mM diazonium salt of p-arsanilic acid into the left footpad.

DTH reactivity was assessed 24 h after the footpad challenge by measuring the swelling of the footpad using a Fowler micrometer (Schlesinger's Tool, Brooklyn, N.Y.). The magnitude of the DTH reaction was expressed as the increment of the thickness of the challenged left footpad as compared with the untreated right footpad. Responses are given in units of 10^{-2} mm $\pm$ s.e.

For induction of unresponsiveness to DTH or plaque-forming cells (PFC), mice were injected with 80×10^6 A-SC or G-SC intravenously in the tail vein. Together with untreated mice they were immunized either for DTH or for antibody response, as described above. In one experiment, 0.2 mg A-IgG was given intravenously as a tolerogen. Five days after immunization, the immune response of each group was assayed five days before immunization either by footpad swelling or nucleoside-specific plaque-forming cells, as previously described.[5, 13] In other experiments, animals immunized with DNP-KLH or SRBC were assayed for PFC against TNP or SRBC.

RESULTS

Cellular Immunity to Guanosine-Coupled Spleen Cells

We initially investigated whether cellular immunity to guanosine-coupled spleen cells (G-SC), as measured by footpad swelling, could be elicited in Balb/c mice. Balb/c mice were immunized subcutaneously with a total of 3×10^7 G-SC in two sites; five days later, along with nonimmunized controls, they were challenged with 1×10^7 G-SC in the footpad (see Materials and Methods). Footpad swelling was measured 24 h after challenge.

The results of a typical experiment are shown in TABLE 1. Immunized animals did, indeed, have a greater response to G-SC than nonimmunized controls. The antigen specificity of this response was demonstrated in two ways: (1) mice immunized with sham-treated spleen cells failed to respond to challenge with G-SC and (2) mice immunized with G-SC failed to respond to challenge with ABA-coupled cells (ABA-SC). (In contrast, mice immunized with ABA-SC exhibited cellular reactivity to challenge with ABA-SC.) Thus, cellular immunity to G-SC is not induced by sham-treated SC or by SC modified with an unrelated hapten but requires both sensitization and challenge with G-SC.

To support the supposition that the immunity induced with G-SC is a form of delayed hypersensitivity (DTH), we examined whether lymph node (LN) cells taken from sensitized animals could adoptively transfer immunity into untreated animals. Donor animals were sensitized with G-SC five days before transfer; the immune LN cells were then treated with either anti-Thy 1.2 serum and complement or complement alone before injection.

While the animals receiving complement-treated LN cells showed immunity, treatment with anti-Thy 1.2 serum plus complement abrogated the response (data not shown). Therefore, cellular immunity to G-SC can be adoptively transferred, and requires the presence of thymus-derived cells. Moreover, no responses were seen at 4–6 h after challenge, and were only significantly apparent at 24 h.

TABLE 1

GUANOSINE NUCLEOSIDE-COUPLED SPLEEN CELLS INDUCE
SPECIFIC DELAYED-TYPE HYPERSENSITIVITY

Group	Immunization	Challenge	DTH (mean footpad response) (10^{-2} mm)	p
1	G-SC	G-SC	22	
2	Sham-SC	G-SC	12	< 0.01
3		G-SC	13	< 0.01
4	ABA-SC	ABA-SC	28	
5	G-SC	ABA-SC	11	< 0.01
6		ABA-SC	10	< 0.01

NOTE: Balb/c mice were immunized intracutaneously with a total of 3×10^7 haptenized spleen cells in two sites on their dorsal flanks. Five days later, the mice were challenged with 1×10^7 haptenized spleen cells in 25 μl in the footpad. The increase in footpad thickness was measured 24 h after challenge.

Cellular Immunity to Adenosine-Coupled Spleen Cells

Our next series of experiments was aimed at eliciting cellular immunity to adenosine, another nucleoside, again by the use of hapten-coupled isogeneic spleen cells. We were consistently unable to obtain a positive cellular response to adenosine-coupled spleen cells (A-SC) (for a representative result, see groups 1 and 2 of TABLE 2). In contrast, A-SC prepared according to the same prodecure were perfectly able to induce unresponsiveness to adenosine-specific PFC.

Two alternative explanations for these intitial findings were considered. First, Balb/c mice were simply unable to mount a cellular response to A-SC as detected by footpad swelling. Second, our preparation of hapten-modified SC resulted in differential amounts and quality of ligand on the cell surface, which was influential in the successful induction of T cell immunity to nucleosides. We reasoned that a difference in the binding efficiency of G and A might

TABLE 2

ROLE OF THE EPITOPE DENSITY AND CROSSIMMUNITY FOR DTH
BETWEEN A AND G NUCLEOSIDES-SC

Group	Immunization	Challenge	DTH (mean footpad response) (10^{-2} mm)	p
1	A_{42}-SC	A_{58}-SC	11	
2		A_{58}-SC	8	N.S.
3	A_{42}-SC	A_{310}-SC	19	
4		A_{310}-SC	5	< 0.005
5	G_{140}-SC	G_{390}-SC	16	
6		G_{390}-SC	7	< 0.01
7	G_{140}-SC	A_{310}-SC	30	
8		A_{310}-SC	12	< 0.01

NOTE: Mice were immunized and challenged and footpad swelling was measured as in TABLE 1. As explained in the text, group 1 and 2 animals received A-SC with a low epitope density for immunization and challenge; all other groups received haptenized spleen cells with epitope densities 4–6 times greater for immunization. All groups were challenged with haptenized spleen cells of high epitope density. In all instances, the subscript number reflects the number of molecules of nucleoside ($\times 10^6$) bound per cell.

lead to differing epitope densities (in terms of number of molecules of hapten bound per cell) for spleen cell suspensions of the two nucleosides. The availability of radiolabeled nucleosides enabled us to examine this possibility. Indeed, we found, in four experiments using the same binding protocol, a four-fold difference in terms of binding efficiency between the number of G and A molecules bound per cell (170×10^6 for G and 48×10^6 for A).

Our next task was to equalize the amounts of A and G bound to cell surfaces. As one would expect, we found that the degree of binding of G could be decreased by reducing the starting amount of hapten. In contrast, A-SC with an average epitope density equivalent to our standard preparation of G-SC could be obtained simply by keeping the molar amount of A constant, but increasing the molarity of the starting nucleoside-bicarbonate solution.

When high epitope density A-SC were used *in vivo*, we found that a positive cellular immune response to A-SC could indeed be detected (TABLE 2). In addition to illustrating a positive cellular response to A-SC, TABLE 2 demonstrates that Balb/c mice will also respond to challenge with high epitope A-SC when they have been immunized with G-SC. Thus, it appears that there is crossimmunity between G-SC and A-SC as detected by a T cell–dependent DTH response.

Crossunresponsiveness of G-SC and A-SC for DTH to G-SC

Groups of Balb/c mice were injected intravenously in the tail vein with 8×10^7 spleen cells coupled to either A or G five days before immunization with 3×10^7 G-SC intradermally; challenge with 1×10^7 G-SC occurred on day 10. Twenty-four hours later, the footpad swelling of these mice was compared to control mice similarly immunized and challenged with G-SC and to unimmunized mice receiving challenge alone. The results in TABLE 3 illustrate that intravenous administration of either G-SC or A-SC can abolish the DTH response elicited by G-SC. It is important to note that the epitope density of G-SC used for immunization and challenge was high (210×10^6 molecules per cell for immunization; 245×10^6 molecules per cell for challenge), while the A-SC administered i.v. had a relatively low amount of binding (85×10^6 molecules per cell).

In a parallel experiment, A-SC from the same haptenized cell preparation were used to reduce a B cell response. Six mice were given 8×10^7 A-SC five days before immunization with 0.4 mg A-KLH; control mice received A-KLH alone. Five days later, A-specific PFC were assayed. The results (controls—29 693 ± 6060 PFC per spleen; experimentals—11 838 ± 1859 PFC per spleen, $p < 0.005$) show that a low epitope density preparation of A-SC (indeed, cells from the same suspension) can induce unresponsiveness as detected by both PFC and DTH assays.

Dichotomy between Unresponsiveness Induced by Nucleoside Bound to Cells and Tolerance Induced by Nucleoside Bound to Isologous IgG

Next, we sought to determine whether crossunresponsiveness could also occur for a B cell immune response. TABLE 4 shows that G-specific antibody-forming cells produced following immunization with guanosine–keyhole limpet hemocyanin (G-KLH) are diminished by intravenous administration of either G-SC or A-SC. Thus, crossunresponsiveness appears to occur for both T and B cell immune responses when the hapten is presented on spleen cells.

In contrast, when adenosine is linked to isologous IgG (A-IgG) to make a tolerogen, its administration resulted in unresponsiveness specific for A. Moreover, administration of A-IgG enhanced rather than suppressed the response to G-KLH, confirming our previous observation.[10] Thus, nucleoside coupled to

TABLE 3

CROSSUNRESPONSIVENESS BETWEEN A-SC AND G-SC
TO SUPPRESS DTH TO G-SC

Tolerogen	Immunization	Challenge	DTH (mean footpad response) (10^{-2} mm)	p
—	G_{210}-SC	G_{245}-SC	44	
G_{445}-SC	G_{210}-SC	G_{245}-SC	17	< 0.005
A_{85}-SC	G_{210}-SC	G_{245}-SC	14	< 0.001
—	—	G_{245}-SC	11	

NOTE: On day 0, the indicated groups were pretreated with i.v. administration of 8×10^7 spleen cells haptenized as appropriate. Immunization on day 5, challenge on day 10, and measurement of footpad swelling increase on day 11 were all performed as in TABLE 1. The subscript represents the number of molecules of nucleoside $\times 10^6$ coupled per cell.

isologous IgG is more selective in its ability to induce unresponsiveness than the same ligand on cell surfaces.

DISCUSSION

Here we demonstrate cellular immunity as well as unresponsiveness to nucleoside-modified cells. The importance of the epitope density of cell-bound ligand in eliciting this cellular reaction is emphasized by the present observation. Perhaps of greater significance is the finding that crossreactivity at the T cell level or at the level of induction of unresponsiveness can occur between two related ligands, such as adenosine and guanosine, when these antigenic determinants are cell linked.

TABLE 4

DICHOTOMY BETWEEN THE SPECIFICITY OF UNRESPONSIVENESS INDUCED BY THE SAME LIGAND COUPLED EITHER TO CELLS (SC) OR IgG (γ1)

Tolerogen	Immunogen	PFC per Spleen ($\pm$ s.e.)	p
None	G-KLH	16 000 (5000)	
80×10^6 G-SC	G-KLH	5000 (1000)	0.05
80×10^6 G-SC	G-KLH	5000 (900)	0.05
None	A-KLH	19 000 (9000)	
80×10^6 A-SC	A-KLH	3000 (900)	0.01
None	G-KLH	15 000 (2000)	
A_{23}-γ1	G-KLH	22 000 (3000)	0.05
None	A-KLH	9000 (100)	
A_{23}-γ1	A-KLH	2600 (700)	0.001

NOTE: The experiments shown in the upper panel used the following protocol: on day 0, the indicated group received 8×10^7 haptenized WBC i.v. in the tail vein. Five days later, all groups were immunized with 0.4 mg of nucleoside-KLH in CFA i.p. PFC were assayed five days after immunization. Groups in the lower panel received 0.2 mg A-IgG$_1$ i.v. in the tail vein on day 0; the immunization on day 5 and PFC assay five days later were as in the upper panel.

The specificity of delayed hypersensitivity to guanosine-coupled spleen cells as measured by increased footpad swelling in Balb/c mice is shown in two ways: sham-treated spleen cells failed to sensitize mice challenged with G-SC and mice sensitized with G-SC failed to respond to an unrelated hapten-modified cell ABA-SC. Thus, both sensitization and challenge with nucleoside-modified cells is necessary to obtain increased footpad swelling. This cellular response appears to be T cell dependent because it can be adoptively transferred with immune lymph node cells to untreated animals; moreover, the increase in footpad swelling is abrogated by treatment of the LN cells with anti-Thy 1.2 and complement. Finally, the kinetics of the response indicate minimal swelling at 4 h and maximum at 24 h collectively. All these results taken together suggest a typical DTH reaction.

The study of the role of the epitope density in eliciting cellular immunity was prompted by our unexpected observation that intravenous administration of A-SC was perfectly able to induce unresponsiveness in terms of either a T cell (DTH) or B cell (PFC) immune response, while subcutaneous administration of A-SC failed to elicit cellular immunity to A-SC. In contrast, G-SC induced both types of immune response under the same experimental conditions. Since, among the four nucleosides, guanosine had been shown to be immunodominant for immunity,[14] the question arose as to whether Balb/c mice were unable to respond in terms of one type of immune response (DTH) but were still capable of generating suppressor T cells to the same ligand-modified cells. Alternatively, perhaps the epitope density of adenosine on cells was sufficient for tolerogenicity but not for immunogenicity. The availability of radiolabeled nucleosides allowed us to examine and resolve this issue. We found that, under the same binding conditions, the efficiency of covalent binding was four times higher for guanosine than for adenosine. By increasing the concentration of adenosine we were able to obtain a relatively high epitope density of adenosine bound per cell (in the same range as the standard amount of guanosine bound per cell), and subsequently induce DTH to A-SC. Furthermore, using a high epitope density A-SC in the challenging injection of mice sensitized with a relatively low epitope density of A-SC, we were able to elicit an increase in the foot pad swelling. In contrast, mice sensitized and challenged with low epitope density A-SC consistently failed to demonstrate delayed hypersensitivity, demonstrating that the epitope density at challenge is critical to a positive cellular response. In addition, our studies have revealed that the same suspension of A-SC with a relatively low epitope density was able to (1) sensitize the animals for subsequent challenge with high epitope density A-SC, yielding a positive DTH response, and (2) induce unresponsiveness in terms of either a T (DTH) or a B (PFC) cell immune response. This suggests that, above a certain threshold of cell-bound antigen, the same suspension of antigen-modified cells can stimulate several subsets of T cells.

Perhaps the most provocative finding of the above results is crossimmunity and crossunresponsiveness between guanosine and adenosine when presented on cells. Animals sensitized with G-SC can express delayed hypersensitivity not only if challenged with G-SC but also if challenged with A-SC. Similarly, A-SC can induce unresponsiveness to either a T cell immune response (DTH) or a B cell response (PFC) to G.

In contrast, neither A nor G linked to soluble carrier proteins crossreact in terms of both humoral immunity and tolerance in mice immunized with A-KLH or G-KLH.[10] Tolerance induced by either guanosine linked to isologous IgG or adenosine linked to isologous IgG is exquisitely hapten specific.[10] In fact, tolerance to adenosine seems to augment the response to guanosine. These results indicate that the specificity of unresponsiveness induced by a nucleoside coupled to cells is broader than the specificity of tolerance induced by the same nucleoside coupled to gamma globulin. How can we explain crossreactivity to cell-bound ligands in terms of the induction of both immunity and unresponsiveness? In other systems, it has been observed that the administration of ligand-coupled cells intravenously stimulates a first set of suppressor cells (Ts_1), which have been phenotyped to be Lyt 1+, I-J+.[5, 15] One might think that both Lyt 1 subsets of ligand-activated cells would have the same type of receptor repertoire. Crossreactions would be observed because some shared part of the adenosine and guanosine would be recognized by the Lyt 1+ DTH and Ts_1 sets. But it remains to be established in the nucleoside system that such Lyt 1 Ts_1 cells exist. Alternatively, it is conceivable that these two purine nucleosides coupled to isogeneic spleen cells crossreact not in the induction but in the expression of either DTH or T and B cell unresponsiveness, as has been shown for different antigenic determinants on the same polypeptide.[16]

Whatever the correct explanation for the above phenomenon, it emphasizes once again the dichotomy not only in the cellular mechanism but also in the specificity of unresponsiveness induced by the same ligand coupled to two different self molecules. The finding that both crossimmunity and crossunresponsiveness occur between two unlike ligands only when they are coupled to cells is relevant both in terms of the difference in antigenic recognition by T and B cells and in terms of the expression of cellular immunity to nucleic acid antigens. Cellular immunity to nucleic acid antigens is known to play a critical role in the pathogenesis of systemic lupus, but the role of cellular immunity is unknown. Thus, it appears that autoantigens bound to cells are able to elicit either Ts or TDTH responses specific to nucleic acid antigens; this might provide a powerful tool for specific immunoregulation of systemic lupus.

SUMMARY

Here we describe a new model to elicit cellular immunity and induce unresponsiveness to nucleic acid antigens. Delayed-type hypersensitivity could be elicited by immunizing and challenging Balb/c mice with either guanosine-coupled spleen cells (G-SC) or adenosine-coupled spleen cells (A-SC) measured by footpad swellings. The epitope density was critical for immunization.

This cellular reaction was specific to nucleosides, and crossimmunity was observed between A-SC and G-SC. In addition, crossunresponsiveness was observed between these two nucleosides. In contrast, soluble carrier proteins coupled with either guanosine or adenosine did not induce crossreactive immunity or unresponsiveness. This emphasizes the dichotomy in both the mechanism and the specificity of unresponsiveness induced by the same ligand bound to two different self molecules (such as cell or IgG). Finally, cellular immunity to nucleic acid antigens might be useful in ascertaining its involvement in experimental systemic lupus.

REFERENCES

1. BATTISTO, J. R. & B. R. BLOOM. 1966. Dual immunological unresponsiveness induced by cell membrane coupled hapten or antigen. Nature (London) **212:** 156.
2. LONG, C. A. R. & D. W. SCOTT. 1977. Role of self-carriers in the immune response and tolerance. II. Parameters of tolerance induced by haptenated lymphoid cells. Eur. J. Immunol. **7:** 1.
3. SHEARER, G. M., T. G. REHN & C. A. GURBURNO. 1975. Cell-mediated lympholysis of surface components controlled by the H-2K and H-2D serologic regions of the murine major histocompatibility complex. J. Exp. Med. **141:** 1348.
4. CLAMAN, H. N., S. D. MILLER & M. S. SY. 1977. Suppressor cells in tolerance to contact sensitivity against hapten-syngeneic and hapten-allogeneic determinants. J. Exp. Med. **146:** 49.
5. BACH, B. A., L. SHERMAN, B. BENACERRAF & M. I. GREENE. 1978. Mechanisms of regulation of cell-mediated immunity. II. Induction and suppression of delayed type hypersensitivity to azobenzearsonate coupled syngeneic cells. J. Immunol. **121:** 1460.

6. BOREL, Y., R. M. LEWIS & B. D. STOLLAR. 1973. Prevention of murine lupus nephritis by carrier-dependent induction of immunologic tolerance to denatured DNA. Science 182: 76.
7. BOREL, Y. & M. C. YOUNG. 1980. Nucleic acid–specific suppressor T cells. Proc. Nat. Acad. Sci. USA 77: 1593.
8. BOREL, Y., L. KILHAM, S. E. KURZ & C. L. REINISCH. 1980. Dichotomy between the induction of suppressor cells and immunologic tolerance by adult thymectomy. J. Exp. Med. 151: 743.
9. RAPS, E. C., B. P. GIROIR & Y. BOREL. 1981. The fine specificity of immune suppression of individual nucleosides. J. Immunol. 126: 1542.
10. MANTZOURANIS, E. C., B. D. STOLLAR & Y. BOREL. 1980. The fine specificity of tolerance to simple haptens (nucleosides and DNP): Induction of immunologic tolerance to one ligand may prime the animal to an analogous ligand. J. Immunol. 124: 2474.
11. ERLANGER, B. F. & S. M. BEISER. 1964. Antibody specific for ribonucleoside and ribonucleotide and their reaction to DNA. Proc. Nat. Acad. Sci. USA 52: 68.
12. BOREL, Y., D. T. GOLAN, L. KILHAM & H. BOREL. 1976. Carrier determined tolerance with various subclasses of murine myeloma IgG. J. Immunol. 116: 854.
13. STOLLAR, B. D. & Y. BOREL. 1977. Nucleoside specific tolerance suppresses antinucleoside antibody forming cells. Nature (London) 267: 158.
14. STOLLAR, B. D. & Y. BOREL. 1975. Carrier-induced tolerance to nucleic acid antigens. J. Immunol. 115: 1095.
15. WEINBERGER, J. Z., M. I. GREENE, B. BENACERRAF & M. E. DORF. 1979. Hapten specific T cell responses to 4-hydroxy-3-nitrophenyl acetyl. I. Genetic control of delayed type hypersensitivity by V_H and I-A region genes. J. Exp. Med. 149: 1336.
16. ADORINI, L., A. MILLER & E. E. SERCARZ. 1979. The fine specificity of regulatory T cells. I. Henn egg-white lysosome-induced suppressor T cells in a genetically nonresponder mouse strain do not recognize a closely related immunogenic lysozyme. J. Immunol. 122: 871.

DISCUSSION OF THE PAPER

M. W. CHASE (*Rockefeller University, New York, N.Y.*): I was glad to hear that the epitope density is of importance in eliciting cellular immunity and unresponsiveness by hapten-modified cells. This was well demonstrated by your presentation.

H. N. CLAMAN (*University of Colorado Medical School, Denver, Col.*): The observation that two unlike purine nucleosides linked to cells crossreact and do not when linked to soluble proteins is most fascinating. This demonstration suggests that there may be a difference between B and T cell recognition of antigen.

G. M. SHEARER (*National Cancer Institute, Bethesda, Md.*): Dr. Borel, have you examined whether strains of mice oriented to autoimmunity could elicit cellular immunity to nucleic acid–modified cells?

BOREL: Thus far, we have not examined this aspect, which is undoubtedly of great importance.

CONTROL OF AUTOIMMUNE RESPONSES INDUCED WITH MODIFIED SELF ANTIGENS *

David Naor and Nora Tarcic

Lautenberg Center for General and Tumor Immunology
Hadassah Medical School
Hebrew University
Jerusalem, Israel 91 010

INTRODUCTION

Structural changes in the self components of a multicellular organism might constitute a threat to its very existence, and therefore it is likely that there is a control mechanism programmed to detect such modified objects and eliminate them. It was suggested that the high vertebrates use the immune system for such a purpose: cells infected by a virus [1] or, perhaps, transformed to a malignant state [2] are recognized as modified self antigens and eradicated. The effector elements of the immune system that are stimulated by the altered cells must discriminate between the modified self antigenic structures and non-modified innocent bystanders; otherwise, a new threat, this time of self-destruction, will challenge the biological integrity of the animal. However, mistakes are always happening, and effector cells or antibodies stimulated by modified self antigens may cause damage to innocent cells as well. Those effector elements which have a broad recognition capacity obviously express a greater autoimmune threat than those effectors which have restricted specificity.

An alternative possibility is that modified self antigens may stimulate helper cells that recognize the modified structure, and that these cells may, in turn, activate both effector cells that detect and kill altered cells and effector cells that detect and cause damage to normal cells. In any case, it has been predicted that another control system would recognize the threatening effector elements, their precursors or cooperators, and inactivate them. It has been assumed that such a "censorship mechanism" [3] is mediated by suppressor cells programmed to detect autoimmune reactive cells, perhaps by recognizing idiotypic markers on their receptors in line with the idiotype network theory. [4]

If the above premise is correct, modified self antigens will not induce an autoimmune response under normal conditions. However, impairment of the suppressor cell function will confer on the animal a strong sensitivity to modified self antigens, and an autoimmune response may result. We have tested this hypothesis by injecting mice with a defective suppressor cell function with trinitrophenyl (TNP)-modified syngeneic cells and examining their autoimmune response. The main findings are briefly summarized in this paper.

* This research was supported by the Ahmanson Foundation.

178

0077–8923/82/0392–0178 $1.75/0 © 1982, NYAS

Mice

(NZB $\times$ NZW)F_1 female mice (NZB/W) of different ages were obtained from the Division of Rhematology, UCLA School of Medicine. Two- to three-month old nude (nu/nu) mice and their normal heterozygous (nu/+) and homozygous (+/+) littermates were kindly donated by Dr. D. Zipori and Prof. N. Trainin of the Weizmann Institute of Science, Rehovot, Israel. (C57BL/10Sn $\times$ C3H/HeDiSn)F_1 male mice ((B10C3)F_1) of different ages were obtained from the Department of Pathology, UCLA. Eight- to ten-week-old female A mice and C57BL/6 mice were obtained from the animal colony of the Hadassah Medical School of the Hebrew University, Jerusalem.

Preparation of Antigens

Trinitrophenylation of Erythrocytes. Sheep red blood cells (SRBC), mouse red blood cells (MRBC), or horse red blood cells (HRBC), in 1 ml packed-cell volumes were washed three times with phosphate-buffered saline (PBS), pH 7.2, and then incubated for 20 min at room temperature with 60 mg 2,4,6-trinitro-benzene sulfonic acid (TNBS) in 7 ml cacodylate buffer (0.28 M; pH 6.9). The cells were washed four times before being injected into the mice. Trinitro-phenylation of donkey red blood cells (DRBC) was performed as described by Rittenberg and Pratt.[5]

Bromelain Treatment. The technique of Linder and Edgington was used,[6] with minor modifications. Equal volumes of washed, packed (0.5 ml) MRBC or DRBC and reconstituted (0.5 ml) bromelain (Bromelase, Dade Reagents, Inc., Miami, Fla.) were incubated at 37° C for 60 min and then washed twice with 50–100 ml PBS containing 1% bovine serum albumin (BSA).

Trinitrophenylation of Spleen Cells. Spleen cells were removed from the mice and washed twice in Hank's balanced salt solution (HBSS). The splenocytes (120–180 $\times$ 10^6) were added to foil-wrapped flasks, each containing 10^{-4} M TNBS (Nutritional Biochemicals Corporation, Cleveland, Oh.) in 10 ml HBSS. The flasks were rocked gently at 37° C for 1.5 h. At the end of the incubation period, the cells were washed once in HBSS and twice in HBSS containing 0.06% glycylglycin (Merck, Darmstadt, W. Ger.), and finally irradiated with 3000 rad by a gamma cell 220 (Atomic Energy of Canada).

Hemolytic Plaque Assay

Four days after immunization the mice were killed, and the spleens of each group of mice were removed and pooled. Cell suspensions were prepared in Gey's solution, and immune responses were assayed by the hemolytic plaque-forming cell (PFC) assay.[7] It was found in our preliminary experiments that the four-day anti-SRBC and anti-TNP responses were mostly direct PFC responses. However, in order to avoid the minor possibility of missing indirect PFC, the plaques were developed in the presence of anti-mouse IgG (Cappel Laboratories, Downingtown, Penn.). The anti-mouse IgG diluted to 1:1000 failed to demonstrate any inhibitory effect on direct PFC but maximally facilitated the appearance of indirect secondary anti-SRBC and TNP-PFC. SRBC, MRBC, TNP-DRBC and bromelain-treated MRBC (B-MRBC) were used for indicating the hemolytic plaques. DRBC and B-DRBC indicator cells failed to detect PFC in spleens of mice injected with TNP-SRBC or TNP-MRBC.

The PFC assay was performed four days after immunization, since we found in previous experiments (unpublished data) that the immune response of mice to TNP-MRBC is very short-lived: the response peaked on the fourth day after immunization, declined dramatically on the fifth day, and disappeared completely by the seventh day.

Delayed-Type Hypersensitivity Assay

The delayed-type hypersensitivity assay (DTH) was performed 14 d after the immunization of the mice, unless otherwise indicated. The left footpad of the tested mouse was injected with 10^7 irradiated blast cells (3000 rad) suspended in 50 μl HBSS. The blast cells were prepared by incubating 2×10^8 spleen cells with 0.2 mg concanavalin A (con A) in 100 ml RPMI 1640 (GIBCO, Grand Island, N.Y.) for one or two days in a CO_2 incubator. The swelling of the footpad was measured 24 h later with a micrometer (Mitutoyo, Japan). A 0.01 mm difference in thickness between the injected and noninjected footpad was taken as one unit of DTH.

Immunization

As a standard procedure, 0.1 ml of a 20% (4×10^8 RBC) suspension of TNP-MRBC (syngeneic to the injected mouse) or TNP-SRBC in PBS was injected into the tail vein of the mouse (3–4 mice per group). Mice were injected s.c. with 10^7 TNP modified spleen cells (TNP-SC) suspended in 0.2 ml HBSS.

Procedures Used to Impose T Cell Deficiency

Adult Thymectomy (ATx). Eight- to ten-week old mice were thymectomized two to three weeks before immunization with TNP-SC. Those mice with thymic lobes or remnants were discarded from the study.

X-Irradiation. Mice were exposed to total body irradiation of 250 rad generated by a Phillips Ortho Voltage Machine on the day of immunization with TNP-SC.

Cyclophosphamide (Cy) Treatment. Mice were injected i.p. with 20 mg kg^{-1} Cy (Taro Ltd., Haifa, Israel) two days before immunization with TNP-SC.

Cell Transfer

Spleen cells from normal mice were prepared as a single cell suspension. Spleen cells deprived of T cells were obtained by treating 6×10^8 spleen cells with anti-Thy 1 serum (diluted 1:20 000) and guinea pig complement (diluted

1:10) in a final volume of 60 ml RPMI 1640. The anti-Thy 1 serum was generously provided by Dr. P. Lake, University College, London. The characterization of this antiserum has recently been published in detail elsewhere.[8] The complement was not cytotoxic to cells when tested alone at the dilution used to kill T cells in the presence of anti-Thy 1 serum. Thymus-derived enriched spleen cell populations were obtained by filtering 2×10^8 spleen cells through a nylon wool column.[9]

X-irradiated mice were injected i.v. with 5×10^7 normal spleen cells, nylon wool–passed cells, or cells treated with anti-Thy 1 serum and complement.

RESULTS

TNP-Modified Syngeneic RBC Induce Humoral Autoimmune Response in Old NZB/W Mice but not in Young NZB/W Mice

It has been previously shown that the anti-TNP immune response of mice to their TNP-syngeneic cells is not dependent on the presence of thymus-derived (T) cells, whereas the anti-TNP immune response to TNP-allogeneic or TNP-xenogeneic cells is T cell dependent. Furthermore, while the presence of T cells enables immune responses to TNP-allogeneic and TNP-xenogeneic cells, it markedly reduces the immune responses to TNP-syngeneic cells.[3, 10, 11] For example, irradiated C3H/HeJ mice reconstituted with bone marrow cells generated a stronger anti-TNP PFC response four days after the injection of TNP-MRBC than similarly treated mice reconstituted with bone marrow cells and thymocytes.[12] Similarly, C3H/HeJ mice injected with TNP-MRBC and anti-thymocyte serum (ATS) generated a stronger anti-TNP PFC response four days after the injection of TNP-MRBC than mice injected with TNP-MRBC and normal rabbit serum.[12] It was suggested that suppressor T cells are more sensitive to ATS than other subpopulations of thymus origin.[13]

These findings are supported by the fact that nude mice injected with TNP-MRBC generated, four days later, a stronger anti-TNP PFC response than nude mice injected with TNP-SRBC, whereas, under the same conditions, normal heterozygous mice injected with TNP-MRBC generated a markedly weaker anti-TNP PFC response than similar mice injected with TNP-SRBC (TABLE 1, groups A and B). Dividing the number of PFC per spleen generated four days after immunization with TNP-MRBC by the number of PFC per spleen generated four days after immunization with TNP-SRBC gives the immune balance (IB) index, which illustrates the immunoregulatory status of the animal.[14] Mice with an IB index of less than one have a normally functioning immunoregulation system (*e.g.,* TABLE 1, group A), whereas mice with an IB index greater than one have a defective suppressor cell function (*e.g.,* nu/nu mice, TABLE 1, group B; for further details see Reference 3).

In agreement with this conclusion, it was also found that young (5-week-old) NZB/W mice generated a stronger anti-TNP PFC response after injection of TNP-SRBC than after injection with anti TNP-MRBC, whereas old (35-week-old) NZB/W mice generated a stronger anti-TNP PFC response after injection of TNP-MRBC than after injection of TNP-SRBC (TABLE 1, groups C and D). Old NZB/W mice have an IB index greater than one, which suggests defective suppressor T cell function.[14] According to our prediction, mice with a defective suppressor T cell function should generate an autoimmune response after

TABLE 1

THE IMMUNE BALANCE AND THE AUTOIMMUNE RESPONSE OF NORMAL AND
T CELL–DEFICIENT MICE

Group	Mice	Number of Anti-TNP PFC per Spleen 4 d after Injection of TNP-MRBC ‡	Number of Anti-TNP PFC per Spleen 4 d after Injection of TNP-SRBC or TNP-HRBC ‡	IB Index	Number of Antiauto-MRBC PFC per Spleen 4 d after Injection of TNP-MRBC §
A	nu/ + heterozygous mice, 10 weeks of age *	1600	8900	0.18	—
B	nu/nu nude mice 10 weeks of age *	5500	1300	4.23	—
C	NZB/W mice, 5 weeks of age †	10 000	18 000	0.60	0
D	NZB/W mice 35 weeks of age †	1500	320	4.69	6200 ‖

* Injected with TNP-SRBC.
† Injected with TNP-HRBC.
‡ Detected in the PFC assay with TNP-DRBC.
§ Detected in the PFC assay with B-MRBC.
‖ Noninjected NZB/W mice 35 weeks of age generated 466 PFC per spleen.

injection with a modified self antigen. Indeed, TABLE 1 indicates that old NZB/W mice (IB index 4.69) generated a considerable antiauto-MRBC PFC response after injection of TNP-MRBC (6200 PFC per spleen, TABLE 1, group D). In contrast, young NZB/W mice (IB index 0.60) did not generate an antiauto-MRBC PFC response after similar treatment.

Similar findings were obtained after injecting aged normal (B10C3)F_1 mice (32 months old) with syngeneic TNP-MRC. These aged mice—in contrast to the young mice (2–9 months old)—generated a strong anti-TNP PFC response after an injection of TNP-MRBC and a very weak anti-TNP PFC response after an injection of TNP-SRBC. Once again, the high IB index suggests defective suppressor T cell function. Indeed, the aged (B10C3)F_1 mice generated antiauto-MRBC PFC response after an injection of TNP-MRBC, whereas the young mice failed to generate a like response when treated in a similar manner.[15]

TNP-Modified Syngeneic Spleen Cells Induce Autoimmune Response in A Mice with a Defective Suppressor T Cell Function

Our subsequent studies were extended to the field of DTH, where we perform a more accurate analysis of the cellular mechanism controlling the autoimmune response to modified self antigens. We set out to investigate whether "crippled" mice with a defective T cell function would generate auto-DTH after confrontation with syngeneic modified self antigens.

FIGURE 1 proves that mice deficient in suppressor T cell function generate an auto-DTH response after injection with modified self antigens, whereas normal mice are resistant to such treatment. Normal A mice injected with syngeneic TNP-SC and subsequently challenged with syngeneic blast cells exhibited the same background level of footpad swelling as normal mice injected with nonmodified spleen cells and challenged with syngeneic blast cells (FIGURE 1, group A vs. group B). In contrast, ATx, x-irradiated (250 rad), and Cy-treated mice generated a stronger DTH response after injection of syngeneic TNP-SC and subsequent challenge with blast cells (FIGURE 1, groups C to E) than similarly treated normal mice (FIGURE 1, group B).

Further insight into this response was obtained in the experiment whose results are presented in FIGURE 2. Both x-irradiated and ATx A mice generated a considerable DTH response after injection with TNP-SC and challenge with syngeneic blast cells (FIGURE 2, groups B and E). In contrast, crippled mice injected with nonmodified syngeneic spleen cells and challenged with syngeneic blast cells generated the same low background of footpad swelling as crippled mice that had been subjected to the footpad challenge only (FIGURE 2, groups C, D and F, G). The normal mice (FIGURE 2, group A) manifested the background level of the footpad swelling generated after the injection of syngeneic blast cells into their footpads.

FIGURE 3 demonstrates the auto-DTH response of A mice at different times after the injection of syngeneic TNP-SC. The mice generated a significant DTH response to the footpad challenge of syngeneic blast cells 7 and 14 d after injection of syngeneic TNP-SC, but not 21 d after the injection of syngeneic TNP-SC.

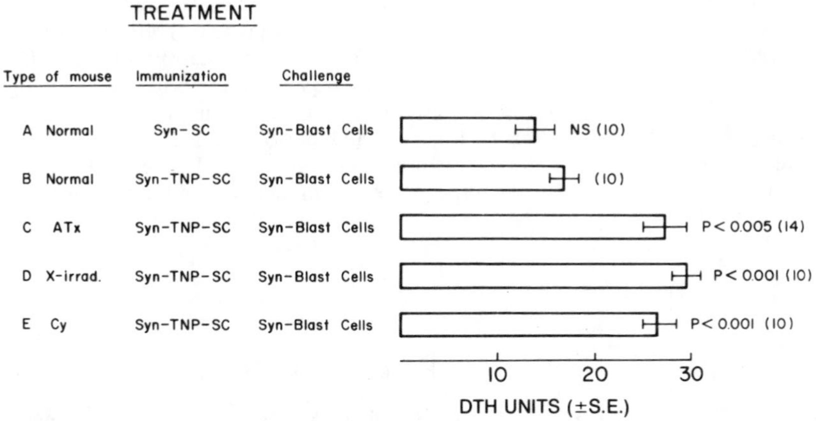

FIGURE 1. Generation of an auto-DTH response by mice with deficient suppressor T cell functions. The various types of A mice (as indicated in the figure) were injected with syngeneic TNP-SC and footpad challenged with syngeneic blast cells 14 d later. Footpad swelling was measured 24 h after the challenge. The p values were calculated by the Student's t test, examining the hypothesis that group B is identical with the other groups. The number of mice in each group is indicated in parentheses.

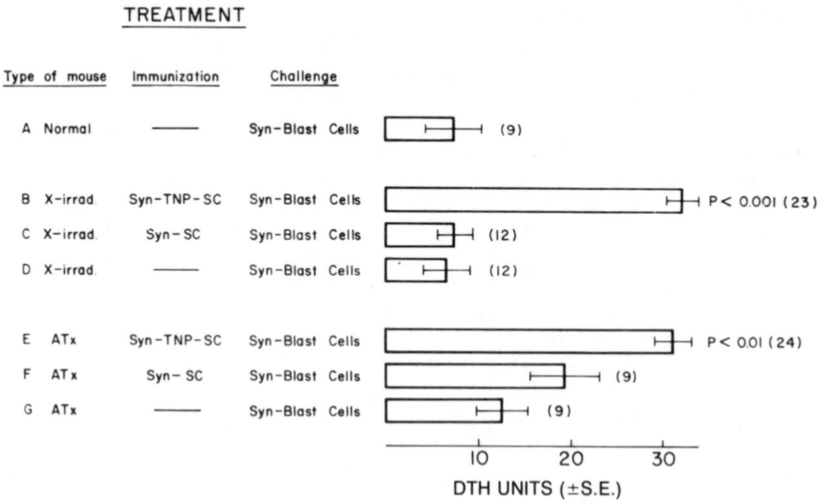

TREATMENT

Type of mouse	Immunization	Challenge		
A Normal	——	Syn–Blast Cells		(9)
B X–irrad.	Syn–TNP–SC	Syn–Blast Cells		P < 0.001 (23)
C X–irrad.	Syn–SC	Syn–Blast Cells		(12)
D X–irrad.	——	Syn–Blast Cells		(12)
E ATx	Syn–TNP–SC	Syn–Blast Cells		P < 0.01 (24)
F ATx	Syn–SC	Syn–Blast Cells		(9)
G ATx	——	Syn–Blast Cells		(9)

10   20   30
DTH UNITS (±S.E.)

FIGURE 2. Induction of an auto-DTH response by syngeneic TNP-SC in x-irradiated and adult thymectomized mice. A mice were treated as described in FIGURE 1. The p values were calculated by the Student's t test, examining the hypothesis that groups B and C and groups E and F are identical. The number of mice in each group is indicated in parentheses.

The strain restriction of the auto-DTH response is illustrated in TABLE 2. X-irradiated A mice injected with syngeneic TNP-SC responded to the footpad challenge of blast cells derived from syngeneic A mice but not to the footpad challenge of blast cells derived from allogeneic C57BL/6 mice (TABLE 2, group C). Furthermore, A mice injected with syngeneic TNP-SC cells and challenged with syngeneic blast cells generated a significantly stronger DTH response than A mice injected with allogeneic C57BL/6 TNP-SC and challenged in a similar manner (TABLE 2, group C vs. group E). This last group of mice (group E), however, generated the expected allogeneic DTH response after challenge with blast cells derived from C57BL/6 mice. This experiment suggests, therefore, that the DTH response of T cell–deficient mice to TNP-SC is,

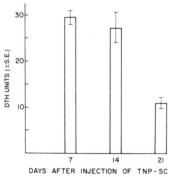

FIGURE 3. Development of the auto-DTH response induced with syngeneic TNP-SC. X-irradiated mice were injected with syngeneic TNP-SC and their DTH responses were assayed at different times after immunization. Each group contained three mice.

in fact, an autoimmune response, even though it was detected with syngeneic blast cells and not with normal syngeneic spleen cells (TABLE 2, group C).

The analysis of the cell population responsible for the suppression of this auto-DTH response is described in FIGURE 4. X-irradiated A mice injected with syngeneic TNP-SC generated the expected DTH response after a footpad challenge with syngeneic blast cells (FIGURE 4, group B). However, if the x-irradiated TNP-SC-injected mice were simultaneously transplanted with syngeneic normal spleen cells (FIGURE 4, group C) or syngeneic splenocytes that had been passed through a nylon wool column (FIGURE 4, group D), the DTH response to syngeneic blast cells was abrogated. In contrast, simultaneous transplantation of normal splenocytes previously treated with anti-Thy 1 serum and complement did not abrogate the auto-DTH response of the x-irradiated and TNP-SC-injected mice challenged with syngeneic blast cells (FIGURE 4, group E). Thus, this experiment indicated that suppressor T cells are programmed to control the auto-DTH response to modified self antigens.

TABLE 2

THE STRAIN RESTRICTION OF THE DTH RESPONSE TO TNP-SC

Group	The source of the Immunizing Spleen Cells (strain of mice)	Mice Were Immunized with *	DTH units ($\pm$ s.e.) Measured after Challenge with		
			Normal Spleen Cells (A mice)	Blast Cells (A mice)	Blast Cells (C57BL/6 mice)
A	A	Nothing	2.7 ± 1.8	2.0 ± 2.0	11.7 ± 1.7
B	A	Normal spleen cells	1.3 ± 0.9	9.0 ± 4.6	7.7 ± 4.3
C	A	TNP-SC	7.7 ± 4.0	35.3 ± 2.9	7.0 ± 3.5
D	C57BL/6	Normal spleen cells	3.7 ± 1.9	13.3 ± 1.75	35.3 ± 3.2
E	C57BL/6	TNP-SC	6.0 ± 2.1	17.0 ± 3.5	30.3 ± 6.7

* A mice (three per group) were immunized with various types of spleen cells and footpad challenged 14 d later. Footpad swelling was assessed 24 h after challenge.

DISCUSSION

The fact that the anti-hapten immune response to haptenated syngeneic cells is controlled by suppressor T cells has been established.[11, 16-19] However, since haptenated syngeneic cells can also potentiate autoimmune responses,[20] we postulated that the biological role of suppressor cells is the control of those cellular or humoral elements which threaten innocent bystander cells. If this hypothesis is correct, then mice with a deficient suppressor T cell function would generate an autoimmune response after the injection of haptenated syngeneic spleen cells or erythrocytes. Our experimental findings have shown that this premise is indeed correct. Severe suppressor T cell deficiency was found in old NZB/W mice[14] and aged normal (B10C3)F_1 mice;[15] such mice generated an antiauto-MRBC PFC response after the injection of TNP-MRBC. In addition, suppressor T cells were eliminated to a greater extent than other subpopulations of T cells by ATx,[21] x-irradiation,[22] and Cy injection.[22, 23] In agreement with our hypothesis, these treatments caused an auto-DTH response in mice injected with syngeneic TNP-SC. Moreover, reconstitution of the x-irradiated mice with T cells (FIGURE 4) abrogated the induction of the auto-DTH response in mice injected with TNP-SC. We can therefore conclude that suppressor cells control the potential autoimmune response to modified self-antigens.

The classification of the DTH response induced with syngeneic TNP-SC as an autoimmune response is justified in the light of the results described in TABLE 2. Mice with a deficient suppressor T cell function immunized with

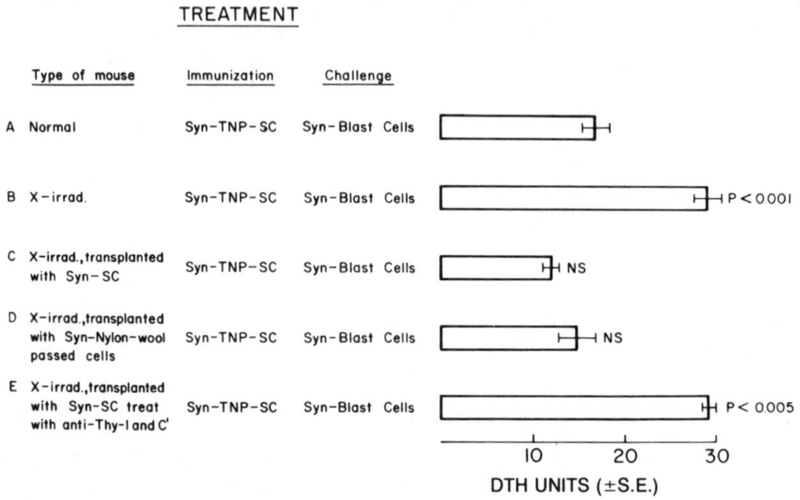

TREATMENT

Type of mouse	Immunization	Challenge	
A Normal	Syn-TNP-SC	Syn-Blast Cells	
B X-irrad.	Syn-TNP-SC	Syn-Blast Cells	P<0.001
C X-irrad.,transplanted with Syn-SC	Syn-TNP-SC	Syn-Blast Cells	NS
D X-irrad.,transplanted with Syn-Nylon-wool passed cells	Syn-TNP-SC	Syn-Blast Cells	NS
E X-irrad.,transplanted with Syn-SC treat with anti-Thy-I and C'	Syn-TNP-SC	Syn-Blast Cells	P< 0.005

DTH UNITS (±S.E.)

FIGURE 4. A characterization of the suppressor cells controlling the auto-DTH response induced with syngeneic TNP-SC. X-irradiated A mice were simultaneously injected with syngeneic TNP-SC plus normal spleen cells, normal spleen cells that had been passed through a nylon wool column, or normal spleen cells that had been treated with anti-Thy 1 serum and complement. The recipient mice were footpad challenged 14 d after the cell transfer, and the footpad swelling was measured 24 h later. Each group consisted of three mice. The p values were calculated by the Student's t test, examining the hypothesis that group A is identical with the other groups. (N.S.: not significant.)

syngeneic TNP-SC, but not with allogeneic TNP-SC, generated a DTH response after challenge with syngeneic blast cells but not after challenge with allogeneic blast cells. However, no DTH response was detected after challenge with normal spleen cells. The DTH response is, therefore, activated by antigens shared by TNP-SC and con A–induced blast cells, both of which are derived from the same strain of mouse. Since the inducer cells, but not the challenger cells, contain TNP groups, and the challenger cells, but not the inducer cells, may contain con A residues, the only antigens that are shared by both types of cell are self antigens that are expressed more extensively after blastogenesis. We can therefore conclude that the DTH response induced with modified self antigens is an autoimmune response.

An alternative explanation is that such a genetically restricted immune response is directed against shared antigenic specificities of TNP and con A, or of new antigens created by these reagents. However, the facts that TNP-MRBC and TNP-SC induce similar responses (compare TABLE 1 with FIGURE 1) under entirely different experimental conditions and that these responses are detected by different types of cell (B-MRBC and con A–stimulated blast cells) provide support for the former suggestion that modified self antigens induce autoimmunity.

SUMMARY

Our previous studies suggested that TNP-modified syngeneic red blood cells induced a humoral autoimmune response in mice with a defective T cell function but not in normal mice. This report describes the continuation of these studies in which we elucidated the auto–delayed-type hypersensitivity response of mice with a defective T cell function. The mice were immunized with syngeneic TNP-modified spleen cells and challenged 14 d later by injecting syngeneic nonmodified con A–stimulated spleen cells into the footpad. The DTH response was assessed 24 h later. Adult thymectomized, x-irradiated (250 rad), and Cy-treated mice injected with syngeneic TNP-SC generated a DTH response when subsequently challenged with syngeneic blast cells but not when challenged with allogeneic blast cells. In contrast, normal mice treated in a similar manner did not exhibit a significant DTH response. The auto-DTH response of x-irradiated mice injected with TNP-SC was abrogated when they were simultaneously transplanted with syngeneic spleen cells or nylon wool–passed syngeneic spleen cells. If the transplanted splenocytes had been treated with anti-Thy 1 serum and complement, they failed to abrogate the auto-DTH response of the above-mentioned mice. These results suggest that suppressor cells are programmed to control the autoimmune response induced with modified self antigens.

NOTE ADDED IN PROOF

In a few control experiments that were performed after the conference we found that four different types of syngeneic lymphoblasts elicited the immunological activity of the x-irradiated TNP-SC immunized A mice, *i.e.*, lymphoblasts induced by con A diluted in fetal calf serum (FCS)–containing media, lymphoblasts induced by con A diluted in normal mouse serum–containing media, lymphoblasts induced by lipopolysaccharide diluted in FCS-containing media and lymphoblasts induced *in vivo* by T cell growth factor (TCGF). In contrast, normal spleen cells that were incubated three hours with con A failed to elicit the DTH response of the above-mentioned mice. We transferred the DTH response of irradiated, TNP-SC-injected mice into untreated recipients with T cells, but not with serum.

REFERENCES

1. DOHERTY, P. C., R. V. BLANDEN & R. M. ZINKERNAGEL. 1976. Specificity of virus-immune effector T cells for H-2K or H-2D compatible interactions: Implications for H-antigen diversity. Transplant. Rev. **29:** 89.
2. BURNET, F. M. 1970. The concept of immunological surveillance. Prog. Exp. Tumor Res. **13:** 1.

3. NAOR, D. 1980. Unresponsiveness to modified self-antigens—A censorship mechanism controlling autoimmunity? Immunol. Rev. 50: 187.
4. JERNE, N. K. 1974. Towards a network theory of the immune system. Ann. Immunol. (Paris) 125C: 373.
5. RITTENBERG, M. B. & K. L. PRATT. 1969. Antitrinitrophenyl (TNP) plaque assay. Primary response of BALB/C mice to soluble and particulate immunogen. Proc. Soc. Exp. Biol. Med. 132: 575.
6. LINDER, E. J. & T. S. EDGINGTON. 1971. Ultramicro assay for anti-erythrocyte antibodies and erythrocyte antigens. Vox Sang. 21: 222.
7. JERNE, N. K., A. A. NORDIN & C. HENRY. 1963. The agar plaque technique for recognizing antibody-producing cells. In Cell-Bound Antibodies. B. Amos and H. Koprowsky, Eds.: 109. Wistar Institute Press. Philadelphia.
8. LAKE, P., E. A. CLARK, M. KORSHIDI & G. H. SUNSHINE. 1979. Production and characterization of cytotoxic Thy-1 antibody-secreting hybrid cell lines. Detection of T cell subsets. Eur. J. Immunol. 9: 875.
9. JULIUS, M. H., E. SIMPSON & L. A. HERZENBERG. 1973. A rapid method for the isolation of functional thymus-derived murine lymphocytes. Eur. J. Immunol. 3: 645.
10. KOSKIMIES, S. & O. MAKELA. 1976. T-cell-deficient mice produce more anti-hapten antibodies against syngeneic than against allogeneic erythrocyte conjugates. J. Exp. Med. 144: 467.
11. RAMOS, T., E. MOLLER & G. MOLLER. 1980. Induction of immunity and suppression by haptenated self structures. Immunol. Rev. 50: 227.
12. NAOR, D., R. SALTOUN & F. FALKENBERG. 1975. Lack of requirement for thymocytes for efficient antibody formation to trinitrophenylated mouse red cells in mice: Role of thymocytes in suppression of the immune response. Eur. J. Immunol. 5: 220.
13. TADA, T., M. TANIGUCHI & T. TAKEMORI. 1975. Properties of primed suppressor T cells and their products. Transplant. Rev. 26: 106.
14. NAOR, D., B. BONAVIDA, R. A. ROBINSON, I. N. SHIBATA, D. E. PERCY, D. CHIA & E. BARNETT. 1976. Immune response of New Zealand mice to trinitrophenylated syngeneic mouse red cells. Eur. J. Immunol. 6: 783.
15. NAOR, D., B. BONAVIDA & R. L. WALFORD. 1976. Autoimmune and aging: The age-related response of mice of a long-lived strain to trinitrophenylated syngeneic mouse red blood cells. J. Immunol. 117: 2204.
16. BOREL, Y. 1980. Haptens bound to self IgG induce immunologic tolerance, while when coupled to syngeneic spleen cells they induce immune suppression. Immunol. Rev. 50: 71.
17. CLAMAN, H. N., S. D. MILLER, M. S. SY & J. W. MOORHEAD. 1980. Suppressive mechanisms involving sensitization and tolerance in contact allergy. Immunol. Rev. 50: 105.
18. GREENE, M. I. & B. BENACERRAF. 1980. Studies on hapten specific T cell immunity and suppression. Immunol. Rev. 50: 163.
19. SCOTT, D. W., C. LONG, J. J. JANDINSKI & J. T. C. LI. 1980. Role of self MHC carriers in tolerance and the immune response. Immunol. Rev. 50: 275.
20. WEIGLE, W. O. 1973. Immunological unresponsiveness. Adv. Immunol. 16: 61.
21. BASTEN, A., J. F. A. P. MILLER & P. JOHNSON. 1975. T cell–dependent suppression of an anti-hapten antibody response. Transplant. Rev. 26: 130.
22. CHIORAZZI, N., D. A. FOX & D. H. KATZ. 1976. Hapten-specific IgE antibody responses in mice. VI. Selective enhancement of IgE antibody production by low doses of X-irradiation and by cyclophosphamide. J. Immunol. 117: 1629.
23. DARIENPARKER, J., M. DWYER & J. L. TURK. 1981. The effect of cyclophosphamide and role of suppressor cells in the desensitization of delayed hypersensitivity. Immunology 43: 191.

W. O. WEIGLE (*Scripps Clinic and Research Foundation, La Jolla, Calif.*):
Were the con A–activated blast cells being injected at the time that they were
producing interleukin-2 (IL-2)? Is it possible that a lot of your responses are
due to IL-2 acting on effector cells, expanding them, and that your suppression
is due to a suppressor factor that's neutralizing interleukin-2?

NAOR: Yes, it is possible. But we have an independent experimental protocol that also shows that TNP-syngeneic red blood cells can generate an autoimmune response. Comparing these two types of experimental protocols, I can
only stand by my conclusion.

P. LEVINE (*Ortho Diagnostic Systems, Raritan, N.J.*): My entire career
has been devoted to individual differences in human red blood cells. Now, all
these studies deal with inbred strains of animals, so each strain is equivalent
to one individual. But, in my experience, especially recent experience in
malignancies and so-called autoimmunization in man, we have developed a
concept of self and non-self. The evidence for this is very clear-cut. The first
of it came in 1951, when I described a case of malignancy, gastrocarcinoma,
which, by a serologic means, was shown to absorb antibody from the patient's
serum. The antibody was increased as a result of many transfusions of incompatible blood. Later on, it was shown that this was part of the P system. As
you know, there are four major blood group systems: A, B, O and P, and
their determinants are carbohydrates, sugars. And there are only two determinants; namely, galactose and acetyl galactosamine, with or without fructose,
and they explain the A, B, O, and P systems. There are natural antibodies to
these because these determinants are present in bacteria and in food. So there
is an active response to explain the origin of normal iso-agglutinins.

Only recently did we find out that the M and N determinants are a chain
of amino acids, and that the first and the fifth amino acids are the determinants.
Several years ago, we found that the Rh antigens, Duffy and Kell, are large
molecules and that they're closely associated with the membrane itself. So they
are lipoproteins. I mention this because only the A, B, O, and P antigens are
involved in adenocarcinoma. Twenty-five years later I sent that tumor to
Hakemori and we now have biochemical findings on this tumor. We find there
a large quantity of a hybrid antigen with a determinant; that is, beta-*N*-acetyl-
galactosamine. We find minute quantities of that in P-1, which I described
serologically, and also in "little P," the genotype of the patient. This would
correspond to what we now know about what's happening in cancer. We know
that a great many genes are produced and that most of them later seem to
disappear. But, in the case of malignancy, they remain in very minute quantities, and then they are activated in the course of adenocarcinoma. I want to
point this out to this group because we are, after all, interested very much in
human cancer investigations.

WEIGLE: Thank you very much.

G. M. SHEARER (*National Institutes of Health, Bethesda, Md.*): I'd like to
focus briefly on the addition of unmodified spleen cells to your system, which
illustrated suppressor cells, and point out the fact that, based on those observa-

tions, trinitrophenylated spleen cells, which you also inject, abrogate the suppressor function.

NAOR: Thank you very much.

F. L. ADLER (*St. Jude Children's Research Hospital, Memphis, Tenn.*): Your data convincingly answers the question that I had asked of Dr. Borel; namely, whether or not there is a distinct possibility that the injection of haptenated isologous or autologous cells may not set off a state of delayed sensitivity or other form of immunity. This is what one would expect on the basis of older data dealing with the altered self concept. My question is: have you found this delayed sensitivity to be restricted to blast cells, or are there other cells that will elicit the footpad swelling after the sensitization procedure that you used?

NAOR: As I indicated, normal cells cannot elicit this delayed-type sensitivity response. So, in order to elicit the immune response, you must expose some antigens, which appear during blastogenesis. I didn't try thymus or other types of cells.

D. W. SCOTT (*Duke University Medical Center, Durham, N.C.*): This is a related technical question. Several years ago, you pointed out the importance of the epitope density in modifying the spleen cells in order to elicit a positive "turn-on" for the immune response in a tumor system. How critical is the epitope density in this phenomenon? Also, have you tried only con A blasts? Have you tried, for example, lipopolysaccharide blasts? I think it might be important to know the cell type that is being recognized.

NAOR: No, so far we haven't tried LPS blasts. But with regard to the induction of the autoimmune delayed response, we studied the concentration of the TNP epitopes on the spleen cells. We found that a certain optimum concentration of TNBS is required in order to modify the spleen cells and thus obtain an efficient immunogen.

J. A. BERZOFSKY (*National Institutes of Health, Bethesda, Md.*): What is the nature of the change in the blast cells that made them able to elicit this response? And have you mapped its genetic restriction? Does it map to the I region or a particular subregion of the I region?

. NAOR: The experimental protocol that I presented to you started to be productive only about four months ago, so we are just beginning the process of doing the kinds of experiments that you mention.

TOLERANCE TO THYROGLOBULIN
BY ACTIVATING SUPPRESSOR MECHANISMS *

Y. M. Kong, I. Okayasu, A. A. Giraldo, K. W. Beisel,
R. S. Sundick, and N. R. Rose

Department of Immunology and Microbiology
Wayne State University School of Medicine
Detroit, Michigan 48201

C. S. David

Department of Immunology
Mayo Medical School
Rochester, Minnesota 55901

F. Audibert and L. Chedid

Immunothérapie Expérimentale
Institut Pasteur
75015 Paris

INTRODUCTION

The studies of Vladutiu and Rose demonstrated that the induction of autoimmune thyroiditis with emulsified mouse thyroglobulin (MTg) in good responder mice is linked to the *H-2* complex and requires T cells.[1,2] Subsequent studies in *H-2* congenic mice with the same B10 background [3,4] confirmed the *H-2* linkage of the gene controlling the immune response to thyroglobulin (the *Ir-Tg* gene). Similar segregation of good and poor responder strains on Balb/c and C3H backgrounds according to the *H-2* haplotype [5] further solidified the major role of the MHC in autoimmune thyroiditis. Both the *H-2* linkage and the need for T cells are found despite the use with MTg of different adjuvants— which have included complete Freund's adjuvant (CFA),[1,2] lipopolysaccharide (LPS),[3] and polyadenylic-polyuridylic acid complex (poly A:U).[4] LPS and poly A:U are both soluble adjuvants and have enabled investigators to study autoimmune responses induced by aqueous, unmodified MTg.

Self tolerance or the lack of autoimmunity in genetically susceptible, un-immunized mice cannot be attributed to the absence of antigen, inasmuch as thyroglobulin circulates in ng amounts in the natural host.[6,7] Nor can it be attributed to the lack of autoreactive T cells, since we have recently shown that autoreactive T cells exist in good responder mice.[8] The presence of MTg-reactive T cells was revealed by repeated injections (16 times in four weeks) of syngeneic MTg in the absence of adjuvant. IgG production reached high levels in all animals and 50% showed infiltration of the thyroid by mono-

* This research was supported by the William Beaumont Research Foundation and by a grant from the National Institutes of Health, no. AM 20023. YMK's sabbatical leave at the Institut Pasteur was supported by the NSF and CNRC (INT-7921278 and ATPA 651–6018, respectively) and by an NCI-INSERM fellowship, U.S.-France Cooperative Science Programs.

191

nuclear cells. In contrast, poor responder mice showed minimal, if any, antibody production and no thyroid lesions. Thus, autoreactive T cells can be activated to overcome regulatory controls that normally prevent autoimmune responses. That regulatory influences are strong is suggested by the cessation of antibody production in these animals when MTg was no longer given. To determine if regulation was mediated by suppressor cells, a tolerogenic regimen of MTg was devised and given to good responder mice. Preliminary data indicate that raising the *in vivo* level of MTg with two doses of exogenous MTg resulted in unresponsiveness.[9] The experimental findings are detailed in this report. To simulate physiological conditions of thyroid stimulation that would lead to the release of endogenous MTg,[7, 10, 11] thyroid-stimulating hormone (TSH) and thyrotropin-releasing hormone (TRH) were administered to good responder mice. Our findings show that suppression was induced by both the tolerogenic and hormonal regimens.

MATERIALS AND METHODS

Mice

CBA/J and C3H/Anf strains of the *k* haplotype were purchased from the Jackson Laboratory, Bar Harbor, Me. and Cumberland View Farms, Clinton, Tenn., respectively. Some CBA/ca mice were supplied by IFFA-Crédo Les Oncins L'Arbresle in France. Balb/c (*H-2*^{d}) mice were obtained from our colonies, which originated from the Jackson Laboratory. Only 8–10-week-old female mice were used.

Antigens

MTg was prepared from frozen mouse thyroids (Pel-Freez Biologicals, Inc., Roger, Ark.), as previously described.[12] Its concentration was determined spectrophotometrically at 280 nm and its purity verified by immunoelectrophoresis at a concentration of 10–15 mg ml^{-1} with both rabbit hyperimmune antiserum to thyroid extract and rabbit antiserum to mouse serum (Miles Laboratories, Inc., Elkhart, Ind.). MTg was stored in aliquots at $-20°$ C until use. Liver extract, used for control, was prepared similarly. Ovalbumin was purchased from Pentex, Inc., Kankakee, Ill.

Adjuvants

Escherichia coli LPS (Boivin) was purchased from Difco Laboratories, Detroit, Mich. *Salmonella enteritidis* LPS was prepared by precipitation with trichloroacetic acid and either obtained from Difco Laboratories or kindly supplied by Dr. C. D. Jeffries of our department. CFA containing *Mycobacterium tuberculosis*, H$_{37}$Ra (Difco Laboratories) was also used at a 1:1 ratio. Poly A:U was prepared by admixing equal amounts of poly A and poly U (Miles Laboratories, Inc., Elkhart, Ind.) 1 h before injection.

Tolerance Induction and Challenge

MTg was diluted in nonpyrogenic saline (McGaw Laboratories, Glendale, Calif.). Except as otherwise indicated in the text, tolerance induction was by injection of 200 μg MTg i.v. on days -10 and -3. Control groups were pretreated with saline or 200 μg of liver extract. Challenge was carried out with an immunizing regimen of 20 μg MTg i.v. on days 0 and 7 followed by 20 μg LPS i.v. 3 h later.[3] To facilitate the lymph node proliferation assay, challenge was also carried out with 60 μg MTg in CFA injected into the hind footpads on day 0.[13] The capacity of poly A:U to prevent tolerance induction by MTg was assessed as described previously with bovine gamma globulin (BGG).[14] Poly A:U was injected i.v. at a concentration of 300 μg in 0.2 ml nonpyrogenic saline 3 h after each dose of 200 μg MTg. The animals were then challenged as above.

Treatment with Thyroid-Regulating Hormones

Bovine TSH and synthetic TRH were purchased from Sigma Chemical Co., St. Louis, Mo. TSH and TRH at concentrations of 0.25 U and 1 μg, respectively, were administered i.p. either on days 0, 7, and 14 or daily from days 0 to 13. In some groups, 20 μg LPS was also given i.v. on days 1, 8, and 15. The animals were bled weekly and challenged 7 to 14 d after the completion of hormonal treatment with MTg plus LPS, as indicated in the tables.

Assay Procedures

Weekly serum samples were obtained from the tail artery from day 7 until the termination of the experiment. Antibody titers (with or without treatment with 0.1 M 2-mercaptoethanol) to MTg were determined with human group O erythrocytes coupled to MTg (1.0 mg ml^{-1}) with chromium chloride.[15] Antibodies to ovalbumin and TSH were similarly determined after conjugation at the same concentration. The animals were killed on days 24–28 after immunization with MTg plus LPS and the entire thyroid was sectioned for histological examination. Mice immunized with MTg in CFA were killed on day 8 or 14. The numbers of animals that had definite focal areas of infiltration in the thyroid were tabulated in the tables. The degree of mononuclear cell infiltration and destruction of thyroid follicles was also graded on a scale from 0 to 4 and expressed as a pathology index.[16]

The *in vitro* lymphocyte proliferative response to MTg was measured as described earlier.[13] Briefly, 4 $\times$ 10^5 popliteal lymph node cells from mice given MTg in CFA with or without MTg pretreatment were cultured for 72 or 96 h in 0.2 ml RPMI 1640 medium containing 1% normal mouse serum and 50 μM 2-mercaptoethanol. Cultures were pulsed with 1.2 μCi ^{3}H-thymidine (2 Ci mmol^{-1}, New England Nuclear, Boston, Mass.) for the final 16 h of culture. Cultured cells were harvested on glass fiber filters (Otto Hiller Co., Madison, Wis.) and washed with saline. Thymidine uptake was determined by counting in a liquid scintillation counter. Antigens used for stimulation were MTg (25 or 50 μg ml^{-1}) and PPD (25 μg ml^{-1}) (Parke Davis Co., Detroit, Mich.). Concanavalin A (con A) (2.5 μg ml^{-1}) (Difco Laboratories) was used as a polyclonal stimulator of T cells.

Transfer of Tolerance

Spleen and serum were obtained 3 d after the second MTg injection. Single cell suspensions were prepared by dispersion through 100-mesh stainless steel screens and washed twice. The cells (5×10^7 in 0.4 ml) were injected i.v. into normal syngeneic recipients. In some studies, spleen cells at a concentration of 10^7 ml^{-1} were separated into adherent and nonadherent fractions by sequential incubation in plastic dishes for one hour at 37° C. Cell fractions were washed twice and adjusted to 5×10^7 per 0.4 ml for transfer into recipient mice. Positive controls received no cell transfer or an equal number of normal spleen cells. In two experiments, 0.2 ml serum obtained from tolerized mice was injected i.v. into normal syngeneic recipients. Immunization with MTg in CFA into the hind footpads (day 0) was carried out immediately after cell transfer.

Anti-Thy 1 Serum Treatment

Spleen cells (5×10^7) were treated with 1 ml normal mouse serum (1:10) or monoclonal anti-Thy 1.2 serum (1:1000) New England Nuclear, Boston, Mass.) for 20 min at 37° C, washed once in RPMI and incubated with 1 ml rabbit complement (1:10) (Grand Island Biological Co., Grand Island, N.Y.) for 40 min at 37° C. The cells were then washed twice with RPMI and readjusted to 5×10^7 per 0.4 ml for cell transfer.

Statistical Analysis

All data were averaged and presented with standard error of the mean. The statistical significance of the differences between control and experimental groups was determined by the nonparametric Mann-Whitney U test as detailed by Siegel.[17]

RESULTS

Tolerance Induction in Good and Poor Responder Mice

Good responder C3H mice were given either two doses of 200 μg MTg on days −10 and −3 or a single dose on day −3 and challenged with MTg plus LPS on days 0 and 7. As shown in TABLE 1, the saline control group showed a rise to high antibody levels (averaging 13.8) by day 28 and mononuclear cell infiltration in 100% of the thyroids. In contrast, both antibody titers to MTg and thyroid pathology were negligible in mice pretreated with two doses of MTg. A single dose of MTg given 3 d before challenge was less efficacious than two doses commencing 7 d earlier, although both mean antibody titer and pathology index in the single-dose group were significantly lower than in the control group.

When three groups of poor responder Balb/c mice were similarly pretreated and challenged, antibody titers of 4.5–7.0 were found only in the saline-injected mice (TABLE 1). Thyroiditis was absent in all but one animal, as expected in poor responder mice.

TABLE 1

INDUCTION OF TOLERANCE IN GOOD RESPONDER C3H MICE AND POOR RESPONDER BALB/C MICE BY PRETREATMENT WITH MTg

Mouse Strain	Pretreatment		Mean Log$_2$ Titer ± s.e. After Challenge†			Thyroiditis	
	Day −10	Day −3	Day 14	Day 21	Day 28	Mean Index ± s.e.	No. Positive/Total
C3H (*H-2^k*)	MTg 200 µg	MTg 200 µg	1.6* ± 0.2	2.3 ± 0.2	1.3 ± 0.2	0.1 ± 0.1 ‡	1/6
		MTg 200 µg	1.4* ± 0.6	2.4 ± 0.9	4.3 ± 1.2	0.5 ± 0.1 §	5/7
		Saline	7.3 ± 0.7	12.2 ± 0.6	13.8 ± 1.1	1.1 ± 0.2	5/5
			< 1.0	< 1.0	< 1.0	0.0	0/7
Balb/c (*H-2^d*)	MTg 200 µg	MTg 200 µg	1.0* ± 0.3	< 1.0	< 1.0	0.0	0/5
		Saline	4.5 ± 0.6	7.0 ± 0.4	6.8 ± 0.5	0.1 ± 0.2	1/6

* Mercaptoethanol-sensitive.
† 20 µg MTg i.v. on days 0 and 7, 20 µg LPS i.v. 3 h later.
‡ p = 0.002 when compared to group pretreated with saline.
§ p = 0.005 when compared to group pretreated with saline.

Dose Dependency and Specificity of Tolerance

TABLE 2 presents data obtained when graded doses of MTg were used to induce tolerance in good responder CBA mice. Again, 200 μg MTg suppressed both antibody production and cellular infiltration. Incomplete tolerance was induced by 20 μg, although antibody levels and thyroid disease was significantly reduced. In contrast, two doses of 5 μg were not efficacious; autoimmune responses paralleled those in the saline-treated mice. TABLE 2 also shows that 200 μg of liver extract did not induce tolerance to a challenge with MTg and LPS; both antibody titers and thyroid pathology were similar to those in control mice.

To assess the capacity of lymph node cells from tolerant mice to proliferate upon MTg stimulation *in vitro,* mice were challenged with 60 μg MTg in CFA into the hind footpads. The data in TABLE 3 show that lymph node cells obtained on day 8 from MTg-pretreated and challenged mice did not respond to MTg *in vitro,* displaying background levels of thymidine uptake, whereas cells from mice without MTg pretreatment incorporated high levels of thymidine. Lymphocytes of both groups responded similarly to stimulation by con A and PPD. The lymphocytic proliferation expressed by MTg-tolerant mice to PPD demonstrates that their response to another antigen is not impaired. As reported previously, the proliferative responses in untreated mice were abrogated by treatment with anti-Thy 1.2 serum and complement.[13]

The assay of tolerance by T cell proliferation *in vitro* correlated well with assays by hemagglutination and thyroid pathology. After challenge with MTg in CFA into the hind footpads, 8 to 17 mice from untreated and MTg-pretreated groups were killed on days 8 and 14 and their autoimmune responses compared in three assays (TABLE 4). MTg-pretreated mice displayed minimal, if any, antibody titer, thyroid pathology and *in vitro* thymidine uptake. In contrast, immunized control mice showed an increase in antibody production and cellular infiltration but a decrease in *in vitro* thymidine uptake from days 8 to 14, as observed earlier.[13]

Duration of Tolerance and Mediation by Suppressor T Cells

The duration of tolerance was examined by varying the interval between the second injection of MTg and the immunizing regimen from 1 to 28 d. FIGURE 1 shows that, when the second injection of MTg preceded challenge by 3 to 28 d, antibody levels and thyroid pathology were markedly suppressed. An interval of 1 d did not suppress thyroiditis as efficaciously as longer intervals.

To determine if suppressor cells played a role in mediating tolerance, 5×10^7 spleen cells or 0.2 ml of serum from mice pretreated with 200 μg MTg on days -10 and -3 were transferred on day 0 to normal syngeneic recipients (FIGURE 2). Unfractionated spleen cells, but not serum, markedly suppressed the subsequent induction of thyroiditis with MTg in CFA. The suppressor cells were nonadherent to plastic and susceptible to the cytotoxic action of anti-Thy 1.2 serum and complement. Thus, suppressor T cells (Ts) are present in tolerant mice and may mediate tolerance for at least 28 d.

TABLE 2

INDUCTION OF TOLERANCE IN GOOD RESPONDER CBA MICE BY PRETREATMENT WITH MTG: DOSE DEPENDENCY AND SPECIFICITY OF INDUCTION

Pretreatment		Mean Log_2 Titer ± s.e. After Challenge †			Thyroiditis	
Day −10	Day −3	Day 14	Day 21	Day 28	Mean Index ± s.e.	No. Positive/ Total
MTg 200 µg	MTg 200 µg	2.3 * ± 0.3	1.5 ± 0.2	1.6 ± 0.3	0.2 ± 0.1 ‡	3/10
MTg 20 µg	MTg 20 µg	3.4 * ± 0.4	4.4 ± 0.8	6.7 ± 0.9	1.4 ± 0.2 §	6/6
MTg 5 µg	MTg 5 µg	7.0 ± 0.9	9.8 ± 0.9	12.5 ± 1.2	1.5 ± 0.3 ‖	5/6
Liver extract 200 µg	Liver extract 200 µg	8.2 ± 0.5	11.2 ± 0.7	13.3 ± 0.5	2.2 ± 0.2 ‖	6/6
Saline	Saline	6.7 ± 0.8	9.9 ± 0.9	11.6 ± 1.1	1.8 ± 0.3	8/9

* Mercaptoethanol-sensitive.
† 20 µg MTg i.v. on days 0 and 7, 20 µg LPS i.v. 3 h later.
‡ $p < 0.001$ when compared to group pretreated with saline.
§ $p = 0.05$ when compared to group pretreated with saline.
‖ Not significant when compared to group pretreated with saline.

TABLE 3

SPECIFICITY OF TOLERANCE IN GOOD RESPONDER CBA MICE AS MEASURED BY
LYMPHOCYTE PROLIFERATIVE RESPONSE TO *in Vitro* STIMULATION

	[³H]-Thymidine Uptake (mean cpm ± s.e.) after Challenge *	
Antigen Added	Untreated	MTg-Pretreated
None	2400 ± 90	1200 ± 90
MTg 25 μg ml⁻¹	45 200 † ± 1700	1300 ± 40
MTg 50 μg ml⁻¹	48 800 † ± 2400	1500 ± 200
PPD 25 μg ml⁻¹	84 500 † ± 4000	62 500 ± 3800
Con A 2.5 μg ml⁻¹	102 000 ± 5400	110 500 ± 6100

* Mice were given 200 μg MTg i.v. on days −10 and −3 and challenged with 60 μg MTg in CFA into hind footpads on day 0. Lymph node cells were cultured on day 8 and assayed 4 d later.

† The response was abrogated by treatment with anti-Thy 1.2 + C.

Interference with Tolerance Induction by Poly A:U

Poly A:U has been shown by Kong and Capanna to interfere with tolerance induction to BGG in mice.[14] Esquivel *et al.* also reported its ability to activate MTg-reactive T cells in good responder mice.[4] The effect of poly A:U on tolerance induction with MTg was therefore investigated. Poly A:U was given either on days −10 and −3 or only on day −3 after the injection of 200 μg MTg. Serum titers to MTg were assayed on day 0, just before challenge with MTg in CFA. The animals were killed on day 14; antibody titers and thyroid pathology were determined. As shown in TABLE 5, mice pretreated with two injections of poly A:U 3 h after 200 μg MTg formed antibodies at high levels.

TABLE 4

EXPRESSION OF TOLERANCE (MTG-PRETREATED) AND AUTOIMMUNITY (UNTREATED)
MICE IN THREE DIFFERENT ASSAYS AFTER CHALLENGE *

	Day 8		Day 14	
	Untreated	MTg-Pretreated	Untreated	MTg-Pretreated
Hemagglutination				
Mean log₂ titer ± s.e.	6.0 ± 0.5	1.6 ± 0.4	9.8 ± 0.6	< 1.0
Lymphocyte proliferation †				
Mean cpm × 10⁻³ ± s.e.	48.0 ± 2.4	1.6 ± 0.2	19.9 ± 0.2	1.0 ± 0.06
Thyroid Pathology				
Mean index ± s.e.	1.3 ± 0.2	0.1 ± 0.1	2.3 ± 0.2	0.0
No. positive/total	15/17	1/14	8/8	1/10

* Mice were pretreated with 200 μg MTg i.v. on days −10 and −3 and challenged with 60 μg MTg in CFA into the hind footpads on day 0.

† Uptake of [³H]-thymidine after 4 d incubation with MTg at 50 μg ml⁻¹.

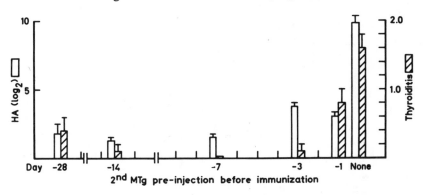

FIGURE 1. The duration of tolerance in good responder mice. Six groups (5–8 mice each) of CBA mice were given no treatment or pretreated with MTg 200 μg i.v. on days −35 and −28, −21 and −14, −14 and −7, −10 and −3, or −8 and −1. They were then immunized with 20 μg MTg and 20 μg LPS on days 0 and 7 and assayed for antibody production and thyroid pathology on day 28. Antibodies from pretreated mice were 2-mercaptoethanol sensitive.

The levels approached those seen in mice without pretreatment and in animals pretreated with poly A:U alone. Cellular infiltration was observed in six of seven animals. Poly A:U injected only on day −3 with the second dose of MTg was much less efficacious in preventing tolerance induction; antibody titers and incidence of infiltration were both reduced. Mice given MTg plus poly A:U but not the challenge dose displayed similarly low levels of responses, as reported earlier.[4]

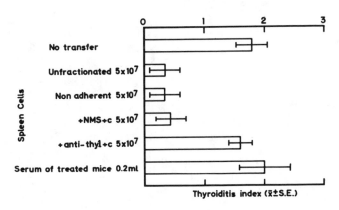

FIGURE 2. Transfer of tolerance with spleen cells from MTg-pretreated CBA mice to normal syngeneic recipients. After injection with 200 μg MTg i.v. on days −10 and −3, 5×10^7 spleen cells, treated with anti-Thy 1.2 serum or normal serum + C, were transferred i.v. on day 0 to normal recipients (6–7 per group). Other groups were given unfractionated spleen cells, plastic-nonadherent cells or 0.2 ml serum from the same MTg-pretreated mice. Recipient mice were then immunized in the hind footpads with 60 μg MTg in CFA and killed on day 14.

TABLE 5

INTERFERENCE WITH TOLERANCE INDUCTION BY POLY A:U IN GOOD RESPONDER CBA MICE

Pretreatment *		Mean Log$_2$ Titer ± S.E. After Challenge †			Thyroiditis	
Day −10	Day −3	Day 0 Challenge †	Day 0 ‡	Day 14	Mean Index ± S.E.	No. Positive/Total
MTg 200 μg	MTg 200 μg	MTg in CFA	< 1.0	12.0 ± 0.7	1.8 ± 0.2	7/7
MTg 200 μg	MTg 200 μg	MTg in CFA	2.3 § ± 0.5	2.3 § ± 0.5	0.0 ‖	0/7
Poly A:U 300 μg	Poly A:U 300 μg	MTg in CFA	4.9 § ± 0.3	10.0 ± 0.5	1.3 ± 0.2	6/7
MTg 200 μg	Poly A:U 300 μg	MTg in CFA	4.0 § ± 0.2	5.3 ± 0.5	0.4 ± 0.2 ‖	3/7
Poly A:U 300 μg	Poly A:U 300 μg	MTg in CFA	< 1.0	11.4 ± 0.5	2.4 ± 0.2	7/7
MTg 200 μg Poly A:U 300 μg	Poly A:U 300 μg	—	4.9 § ± 0.3	5.9 ± 0.6	0.3 ± 0.1 ‖	3/7

* Poly A:U was given i.v. 3 h after MTg.
† 60 μg MTg in CFA into the hind footpads.
‡ Serum samples obtained immediately before challenge.
§ Mercaptoethanol-sensitive.
‖ p ≤ 0.001 when compared to control group without MTg pretreatment.

Effect of TSH and TRH on Induction of Tolerance

To determine if an endogenously raised MTg level could influence the susceptibility of good responder mice to induction of autoimmunity, either TSH or TRH was administered to CBA mice. TSH is of bovine origin and thus could be immunogenic for mice. TRH, on the other hand, is a synthetic tripeptide and acts on the pituitary to release endogeneous TSH; its use permits a comparison of the effects of exogenous and endogenous TSH. TABLE 6 shows that, when three doses of TSH or TRH were given on days 0, 7, and 14, no autoantibodies to MTg were found for three weeks; the data obtained on different days are pooled for presentation. After challenge with MTg plus LPS on days 28, 35, and 49, antibody responses on days 56 and 63 were lower in the TSH- and TRH-treated mice than in the control mice. Whereas all mice that had not received hormonal treatment produced IgG antibodies, only 33% and 60% of the animals receiving TSH and TRH, respectively, produced IgG antibodies. In contrast, 100% of the animals in all groups produced IgM antibodies. We also injected 20 µg LPS into two other groups 24 h after each hormone dose to determine if LPS could act as an adjuvant to any MTg released endogenously as a result of hormonal treatment. The inclusion of LPS led to very low transient titers (2.3) of IgM antibody during hormonal administration. After challenge, suppression of IgG formation was even more pronounced in mice that had received LPS in addition to TSH or TRH.

In another series of experiments, we injected TSH or TRH daily for 14 d. As shown in TABLE 7, autoantibodies to MTg were not observed in the hormone-treated groups during the first three weeks. After injection of an immunogenic regimen of MTg and LPS, significantly lower antibody titers were observed in the hormone-treated groups. Thyroid pathology was present in only 17% or less of the animals. We also injected LPS on days 1, 8, and 15 to determine if suppression due to TSH or TRH could be circumvented. Again, suppression was greatest in LPS-treated mice on the basis of antibody titers. Thyroid pathology was reduced to the same extent as in TSH- or TRH-treated mice without LPS. To ascertain the specificity of suppression, 100 µg ovalbumin was given on days 21 and 39. All animals responded with the expected antibody titers to ovalbumin, with the exception of one group of mice treated with TRH and LPS. In all other experiments, however, mice treated with TRH and LPS yielded anti-ovalbumin titers equivalent to the TRH-treated or -untreated mice.

Because of the bovine source of TSH, the animals might form antibodies to bovine proteins and render the TSH inactive. Accordingly, sera obtained on days 14 and 21 in several experiments were tested for antibodies to the TSH preparations used. No significant amounts of hemagglutinins were detected in any of the sera tested.

DISCUSSION

The above findings show that the injection of two doses of soluble MTg at certain intervals induced tolerance to a subsequent immunizing regimen as expressed by markedly reduced antibody titer, greatly diminished *in vitro* lymphocyte proliferative response, and low incidence of thyroid lesions. Studies of the requirements for tolerization indicate that the effective regimen is two doses at concentrations between 20 and 200 µg (TABLE 3), with an optimal

TABLE 6

INDUCTION OF TOLERANCE IN GOOD RESPONDER CBA MICE BY PRETREATMENT WITH WEEKLY INJECTIONS OF TSH OR TRH

Treatment (Dose) TSH, TRH Days 0,7,14 LPS Days 1,8,15	Mean Log$_2$ Titer ± S.E.				IgG Ab Positive Day 63 (%)
	Preimmunization *	Postimmunization †			
		Day 42	Day 56	Day 63	
TSH (0.25 U)	<1.0	2.0 ‡ ± 0.5	4.3 ‡ ± 0.5	6.3 ± 1.1	33
TSH (0.25 U) + LPS (20 µg)	2.3 ‡ ± 0.2	2.2 ‡ ± 0.6	3.7 ‡ ± 0.8	4.0 ± 0.9	17
TRH (1 µg)	<1.0	3.4 ‡ ± 0.7	6.0 ± 1.1	8.4 ± 2.2	60
TRH (1 µg) + LPS (20 µg)	2.0 ‡ ± 0.6	3.5 ‡ ± 0.3	3.6 ‡ ± 0.3	4.3 ± 0.4	25
None	<1.0	5.5 ‡ ± 0.3	10.8 ± 0.5	11.0 ± 1.3	100

* Assayed on days 7, 14, and 21 and averaged.
† Immunized i.v. with 20 µg each of MTg and LPS on days 28, 35, and 49.
‡ Mercaptoethanol-sensitive.

TABLE 7

INDUCTION OF TOLERANCE IN GOOD RESPONDER CBA MICE BY PRETREATMENT WITH DAILY INJECTIONS OF TSH OR TRH

Treatment (Dose) TSH or TRH Days 0–13 LPS Days 1,8,15	Mean Log_2 Anti-MTg Titer ± S.E.			IgG Ab Positive Day 45 (%)	Thyroiditis Positive Day 45 (%)	Mean Log_2 Anti-Ovalbumin Titer ± S.E. Day 45
	Pre-immunization *	Postimmunization †				
		Day 35	Day 45			
TSH (0.25 U)	<1.0	2.8 ± 2.1	7.7 ± 1.4	67	0	9.3 ± 0.7
TSH (0.25 U) +LPS (20 µg)	1.5‡ ± 0.4	<1.0	5.2‡ ± 0.2	0	17	7.4 ± 0.9
TRH (1 µg)	<1.0	2.5 ± 1.6	7.8 ± 0.4	83	17	9.8 ± 0.9
TRH (1 µg) +LPS (20 µg)	1.9‡ ± 0.4	<1.0	5.0‡ ± 0.3	0	0	5.0 ± 2.0
None	<1.0	10.4 ± 0.6	13.8 ± 0.4	100	67	7.5 ± 0.4

* Assayed on days 7, 14, and 20 and averaged.
† Immunized i.v. with 20 µg each of MTg and LPS on days 21 and 28, and i.p. with 100 µg ovalbumin on days 21 and 39.
‡ Mercaptoethanol-sensitive.

interval of more than 1 d between the second injection of MTg and challenge (FIGURE 1). Tolerance is specific for MTg since it cannot be induced with liver extract; lymph node cells from tolerant mice proliferated in response, not to MTg, but to PPD, an antigen of CFA used in the challenge (TABLE 3). Tolerance persisted for at least 28 d; mice challenged 28 d after the tolerizing regimen still showed markedly suppressed antibody levels and reduced thyroid infiltration (FIGURE 1).

Soluble MTg apparently activates MTg-reactive Ts, since spleen cells from tolerant mice can transfer the suppression to normal syngeneic recipients challenged on the same day of transfer. This transfer is abrogated by cytotoxic anti-Thy 1 serum. We have previously reported that thymocytes from tolerant mice also transferred suppression, whereas thymocytes and spleen cells from normal mice had no effect.[5] We have considered two alternative explanations for the transfer of tolerance. One is that carry-over tolerogen by the donor cells induced tolerance in recipient mice. This possibility can be ruled out by the lack of suppression following the transfer of serum from tolerant mice as well as the fact that the time interval (1–3 h) between tolerogen introduction and challenge is inadequate to effect tolerance. A second alternative is that membrane-bound MTg on the transferred cells actively induced tolerance.[18] This appears unlikely, since anti-Thy 1–treated cells and adherent cells (data not shown) that could contain membrane-bound MTg were ineffective in transferring tolerance.

That poly A:U interferes with tolerance induction by MTg (TABLE 5) is further support for the involvement of Ts. Poly A:U prevents the formation of Ts to tolerogenic BGG in mice when given at a critical interval after the tolerogen; no transfer of suppression can be demonstrated.[19, 20] In the present studies, this critical interval of 3 h between MTg and poly A:U was employed. Moreover, when poly A:U was given with the second dose of MTg on day −3 rather than on both days −10 and −3, it was not very effective in preventing tolerance induction. This observation suggests that Ts had been activated by the first dose of MTg on day −10.

Efforts to prevent autoimmune disease by injecting soluble autoantigen have generally been unsuccessful. Tolerance induced by the use of retinal extract prevented autoimmune uveoretinitis in the guinea pig,[21] but no tolerance was observed after the injection of soluble thyroglobulin into the same species.[22] The injection of soluble myelin basic protein into the rat induced only a transient tolerance to experimental allergic encephalomyelitis that cannot be transferred.[23] Tolerance in the last two models required the use of antigen in incomplete Freund's adjuvant[22, 23] or membrane-bound thyroglobulin.[18] Since soluble MTg–induced tolerance, which is mediated by Ts, and thyroglobulin levels can be raised endogenously with the aid of specific hormones,[7, 10, 11] we administered TSH or TRH into genetically susceptible mice to determine if MTg levels would influence self tolerance or autoimmunity.

In two series of experiments, TSH and TRH were given either in 3 or 14 doses over a 14 d period. Despite the increase of circulating thyroglobulin levels,[7, 10, 11] treatment with hormones did not generate spontaneous production of MTg antibody at any time during the 21 d monitoring period. After challenge with MTg and LPS, both dosages of TSH and of TRH suppressed the formation of MTg antibodies (TABLES 6 and 7). While IgM levels in the hormone-treated mice were generally lower than in control mice, many did not make the switch to IgG formation, suggesting that the helper T cell (Th) function was inoperative. Not only was IgG formation suppressed, but also the incidence of thyroid lesions was much lower in the hormone-treated groups (TABLE 7). The suppression was not due to possible changes in metabolism brought on by thyroid stimulation, which may affect the immune response in general, since the animals made equivalent amounts of antibody to ovalbumin.

The mechanisms by which certain regimens of TSH and TRH prevent auto-immunity remain to be determined. Both TSH and TRH administrations induce an increase in circulatory thyroglobulin and thyroxine (T_4).[10, 11, 24] We have a preliminary indication that MTg as well as T_4 levels increase at the beginning of hormone administration by either repeated injections or steady infusion *via* an osmotic pump placed in the peritoneal cavity (M. Lewis and Y. M. Kong, unpublished). One possibility is that endogenously released MTg attains suffi-cient levels to activate Ts, as observed with two doses of injected MTg. Both exogenous (bovine) TSH and endogenous (mouse) TSH increased by TRH treatment had similar effects in inducing specific suppression of the response to MTg. In all these experiments, TRH was less effective than TSH in reducing antibody titers. This difference may be related to the feedback regulation of high levels of T_4 on TSH release by the pituitary during TRH treatment.[25] On the other hand, the continued injection of TSH could bypass the feedback inhibition, resulting in a greater effect on the thyroid than TRH administration. A sensitive assay for serum MTg levels would aid this study, and is being developed in our laboratory.

Interestingly, when LPS was given during the period of hormonal treatment, suppression of antibody formation was greater than in mice given hormones alone. The incidence of thyroiditis was similarly reduced. This observation suggests that suppression was not circumvented by the adjuvant action of LPS on MTg released endogenously. Since LPS can induce suppression when given at certain intervals with other T-dependent antigens,[26] it must be given at a critical time interval in relationship to serum MTg levels. This critical interval may influence whether self tolerance is strengthened or autoimmunity is initi-ated. Another possibility for the lack of adjuvant effect of LPS might be the inactivation of LPS at the time of challenge by antibodies produced during the first LPS exposure. To exclude this possibility, LPS from two different bacterial species was used in other experiments for initial treatment with hormones (*E. coli*) and for challenge (*S. enteriditis*). No differences in results were observed. The nonspecific suppression induced by LPS may act synergistically with the specific suppression resulting from hormonal treatment.

The present finding that soluble MTg in two doses at specified time intervals induced Ts, coupled with our previous observation that soluble MTg in 16 repeated doses activates Th,[8] led us to formulate the concept of clonal balance. This concept states that the ratio of self-reactive Ts to Th, rather than the clonal deletion of Th, maintains normal self tolerance.[5] The natural role of Ts in preventing autoimmune disease has been shown by Kojima *et al.*[27] and Penhale *et al.*[28] by means of early thymectomy and irradiation. Cantor and Gershon have also reported the spontaneous development of autoantibodies in mice repopulated with Lyt 1 cells,[29] presumably because Ts of the Lyt 2,3 lineage had been removed. These manipulations are nonspecific, in that differ-ent Ts clones are destroyed so that antibodies to thyroglobulin are not the only autoantibodies found.[29-31] By using hormones acting on the thyroid, we are in a position to determine specifically if clonal balance can be influenced by MTg levels raised endogenously. The use of thyroid-regulating hormones would, at the same time, provide a true self antigen, released in the natural way and not subjected to possible denaturation during extraction. The suppression obtained after TSH and TRH treatment supports our working hypothesis that circulatory levels of MTg and its manner of presentation influence the homeostatic balance between self tolerance and autoimmunity.

SUMMARY

Immunological tolerance was induced in a mouse model of autoimmune thyroiditis by using soluble mouse thyroglobulin. Good responder (H-2^k) strains, C3H and CBA, were given 200 μg MTg i.v. 10 and 3 d before challenge with an immunizing regimen of 20 μg each of MTg and LPS i.v. on days 0 and 7 or of 60 μg MTg in CFA into the hind footpads on day 0. The animals were monitored for up to 28 d. Tolerance was expressed by markedly reduced antibody titers, greatly diminished in vitro lymphocyte proliferative response to MTg, and low incidence of thyroid lesions. Similarly treated poor responder (H-2^d) Balb/c mice also showed reduced antibody levels; thyroid infiltration was not present. Tolerance in good responder mice persisted for at least 28 d and was specific. Spleen cells from MTg-pretreated mice suppressed the induction of autoimmune thyroiditis in normal syngeneic recipients. The suppressor cells were not adherent to plastic and were susceptible to cytotoxicity by anti-Thy 1 serum and complement, indicating the mediation of tolerance by suppressor T cells. Poly A:U, which interferes with the induction of Ts by tolerogen, prevented induction by soluble MTg.

We next studied the effect of endogenously raised MTg on tolerance induction. In two series of experiments, thyroid-regulating hormones, TSH and TRH, were given either on days 0, 7, and 17 or daily for 14 d. Treatment with hormones did not generate spontaneous production of MTg antibody. After challenge with MTg and LPS, only 33–60% and 60–83% of the animals receiving TSH and TRH, respectively, formed IgG antibodies, showing that the remaining mice did not have functional helper T cells. Thyroid pathology was observed in only 17% or less of the groups of animals. LPS administered on days 1, 8, and 15 produced even greater suppression in antibody formation than did hormonal treatment alone, and thyroid infiltration remained low. In all experiments, the animals responded normally to another antigen, ovalbumin.

The present findings that soluble MTg in two doses at specified time intervals induces antigen-specific Ts, coupled with our previous observation that soluble MTg in 16 repeated doses activates Th, led us to formulate the concept of clonal balance. This concept states that the ratio of self-reactive Ts to Th, rather than clonal deletion of Th, maintains normal self tolerance. The suppression obtained after TSH and TRH treatment supports our working hypothesis that circulatory levels of MTg and its manner of presentation influence the homeostatic balance between self tolerance and autoimmunity.

ACKNOWLEDGMENTS

The skillful assistance of Julia Gnadt, Shou-Jou Piston, and Margaret Clark is much appreciated. I. Okayasu was on leave from the Department of Pathology, School of Medicine, Tokyo Medical and Dental University, Japan.

REFERENCES

1. VLADUTIU, A. O. & N. R. ROSE. 1971. Science **174:** 1137–39.
2. VLADUTIU, A. O. & N. R. ROSE. 1975. Cell. Immunol. **17:** 106–13.
3. ESQUIVEL, P. S., N. R. ROSE & Y. M. KONG. 1977. J. Exp. Med. **145:** 1250–63.
4. ESQUIVEL, P. S., Y. M. KONG & N. R. Rose. 1978. Cell. Immunol. **37:** 14–19.
5. ROSE, N. R., Y. M. KONG, I. OKAYASU, A. A. GIRALDO, K. BEISEL & R. S. SUNDICK. 1981. Immunol. Rev. **55:** 299–314.
6. DANIEL, P. M., O. E. PRATT, I. M. ROITT & G. TORRIGIANI. 1967. Immunology **12:** 489–504.
7. VAN HERLE, A. J., G. VASSART & J. E. DUMONT. 1979. N. Engl. J. Med. **301:** 307–14.
8. ELREHEWY, M., Y. M. KONG, A. A. GIRALDO & N. R. ROSE. 1981. Eur. J. Immunol. **11:** 146–51.
9. OKAYASU, I., Y. M. KONG, N. R. ROSE & C. S. DAVID. 1980. Fed. Proc. Fed. Am. Soc. Exp. Biol. **39:** 667.
10. ULLER, R. P., A. J. VAN HERLE & I. J. CHOPRA. 1973. J. Clin. Endocrinol. Metab. **37:** 741–45.
11. VAN HERLE, A. J., R. P. ULLER, N. L. MATTHEWS & J. BROWN. 1973. J. Clin. Invest. **52:** 1320–27.
12. KONG, Y. M., C. S. DAVID, A. A. GIRALDO, M. ELREHEWY & N. R. ROSE. J. Immunol. **123:** 15–18.
13. OKAYASU, I., Y. M. KONG, C. S. DAVID & N. R. ROSE. 1981. Cell. Immunol. **61:** 32–39.
14. KONG, Y. M. & S. L. CAPANNA. 1974. Cell. Immunol. **11:** 488–92.
15. POSTON, N. R. 1974. J. Immunol. Methods **5:** 91–95.
16. ROSE, N. R., F. J. TWAROG & A. J. CROWLE. 1971. J. Immunol. **106:** 698–704.
17. SIEGEL, S. 1956. Nonparametric Statistics: 1–213. McGraw-Hill. New York.
18. BRALEY-MULLEN, H., J. G. TOMPSON, G. C. SHARP & M. KYRIAKAS. 1980. Cell. Immunol. **51:** 408–13.
19. CAPANNA, S. L. & Y. M. KONG. 1974. Immunology **27:** 647–53.
20. FESSIA, S. L. & Y. M. KONG. 1977. Scand. J. Immunol. **6:** 1209–16.
21. DE KOZAK, Y., J. P. FAURE, H. ARDY, M. USUI & B. THILLAYE. 1978. Ann. Immunol. (Paris) **129C:** 73–88.
22. BRALEY-MULLEN, H., G. C. SHARP, M. KYRIAKOS, N. HAYES, C. DUNN, P. JEPSEN & R. D. SANDERS. 1978. Cell. Immunol. **39:** 289–96.
23. SWIERKOSZ, J. E. & R. H. SWANBORG. 1977. J. Immunol. **119:** 1501–06.
24. CHOPRA, I. J. & D. H. SOLOMON. 1973. Endocrinology **92:** 1731–35.
25. SNYDER, P. J. & R. D. UTIGER. 1972. J. Clin. Invest. **51:** 2077–84.
26. HAAS, G., A. G. JOHNSON & A. NOWOTNY. 1978. J. Exp. Med. **148:** 1081–86.
27. KOJIMA, A., Y. TANAKA-KOJIMA, T. SAKAHURA & Y. NISHIZUKA. 1976. Lab. Invest. **34:** 550–57.
28. PENHALE, W. J., A. FARMER & W. J. IRVINE. 1975. Clin. Exp. Immunol. **21:** 362–75.
29. CANTOR, H. & R. K. GERSHON. 1979. Fed. Proc. Fed. Am. Soc. Exp. Biol. **38:** 2058–64.
30. KOJIMA, A., O. TAGUCHI & Y. NISHIZUKA. 1982. *In* Proc. 3d Int. Workshop on Nude Mice. N. D. Reed, Ed. Gustar Fisher. New York. In press.
31. AHMED, S. A. & W. J. PENHALE. 1982. Experientia. **37:** 1341–43.

DISCUSSION OF THE PAPER

D. R. GREEN (*Yale University, New Haven, Conn.*): Two points: Lila McVay-Boudreau demonstrated that removal of the Lyt 2 positive cells from a normal animal—B mice that were reconstituted with only Lyt 1 cells—had a spontaneous increase in their anti-thyroglobulin levels. Not as high as that seen in NZB mice but nevertheless significant. Replacing Lyt 2 positive cells from a normal animal with no deliberate immunization of any sort caused a drop in those levels.

My second point is a question hailing back to Dr. Weigle's work. I think it would be very interesting to see if, in your animals that have been suppressed or tolerized to thyroglobulin, that form of tolerance can be broken in the way Dr. Weigle has reported several times. Will rabbit thyroglobulin or maybe even your outbred mouse thyroglobulin induce a breaking of tolerance such that, even in the face of the suppression, autoimmunity can result? Have you tried that?

KONG: No. It's a good comment. As I mentioned earlier, our emphasis is on unmodified autoantigen. But I would expect from Dr. Weigle's experience that there would be some production of autoantibodies to bovine or goat thyroglobulin if one were to use it.

W. O. WEIGLE (*Scripps Clinic and Research Foundation, La Jolla, Calif.*): I think that the type of mechanism Dr. Kong is dealing with involves suppressor T cells. I think that the only thing you could do by injecting crossreacting antigens is bypass the suppressor mechanism, and it wouldn't be the same as activating nonspecific T cells and turning on competent B cells, as our model showed.

GREEN: Autoimmunity may be induced by overcoming suppression, a mechanism different from those proposed by others. It isn't that we have different groups of T cells, some of which are clonally deleted, some of which are not, and that we somehow can get to those that have not been clonally deleted. We're now bypassing a suppressor cell that should be capable of suppressing any response to the autoimmunogen, thyroglobulin; in fact, you've really boosted the suppressor cells. You've really got them going by your tolerance procedure. And yet, by sneaking in with a crossreactive antigen, one can pick out helper cells, which somehow these suppressor cells can't get at. Now, it might be due to the absence of suppressor determinants on the crossreactive antigens. Alternatively, there may be other mechanisms of bypassing suppression, and that's part of my point: we should be aware of the possible ways of escaping from suppression, as well as inducing it.

KONG: With the antibody production, one could probably bypass the suppressor T cells using a crossreactive antigen. But there's no guarantee that the thyroid will still be infiltrated, because our data show that the antibody level does not correlate with thyroid infiltration.

E. DIENER (*University of Alberta, Edmonton, Alta.*): You pointed out at the beginning that you have nanogram amounts of thyroglobulin in the serum of a mouse. That's not a sufficient argument to conclude that it's not a secluded antigen because you simply don't have enough of the antigen there to be immunogenic. Would you think, in view of this, that it would be an advantage to try and use neonatal animals?

KONG: Yes, we have considered doing it. [Note added in proof: It should be re-emphasized that measurable amounts of circulatory thyroglobulin would preclude its classification as a sequestered antigen. Evidence is available that the thyroid functions well in mice by day 18 of gestation (BEAMER, W. G. & L. A. CRESSWELL. 1982. Anat. Rec. **202:** 387–93), making neonatal treatment too late.]

S. D. MILLER (*University of Colorado Medical Center, Denver, Col.*): I noticed on your slide that you only show the thyroiditis index when you transfer the unresponsiveness. What effect does that transfer have on the antibody response in the recipients and on the proliferative response that you showed us in the donors that were simply tolerized?

KONG: The antibody response was greatly suppressed also. We're doing lymphocyte proliferation right now.

WEIGLE: I'd like to get your opinion on why, when you give the hormones—you apparently get release of the thyroglobulin in the circulation—you always get suppression and never see immunity? Now, if the reason that you never see immunity is that you're putting out a suppressive amount of the thyroglobulin, then you should be able to cut back on these hormones to the point that you actually immunize these animals by giving them less. Unless you can do this, I think you would have to consider that the antigen you're injecting into these animals may be altered, and this is one of the reasons why you're getting an immune response to it.

A second question: You also show a good correlation between the proliferative T cell response, which I assume is Lyt 1, a helper T cell. If it is, why do you see such a good correlation between this response in thyroiditis and why don't you see a good correlation with the antibody response and thyroiditis?

KONG: First, let me address the hormonal levels. We're currently cutting back on dosage to see if we could induce autoimmunity, because one reason we gave the LPS was to get an adjuvant effect to see whether we could induce autoimmunity in some animals and suppression in others. The fact that we don't get suppression in all animals gave us hope that we could—by varying hormonal levels, timing of adjuvant, and so on—someday show how autoimmunity may be derived. So we have a lot more experiments to do.

Now, we're puzzled, ourselves, as to why we show a good correlation between proliferation and autoimmune disease, because we couldn't show proliferation or lesions in poor responder animals. This is in spite of the fact that they show high antibody levels. One explanation that might be offered is the degree of stimulation. We only give one injection into the footpad with CFA. Alternatively, the proliferative response may reflect T cell subsets amplifying or becoming effector/cytotoxic T cells. It is evident that genetic factors play a great role.

IMMUNOLOGICAL UNRESPONSIVENESS
IN PRIMED B LYMPHOCYTES *

D. Elliot Parks,† Patricia A. Nelson,‡ Sharyn M. Walker,§
and William O. Weigle

Department of Immunopathology
Scripps Clinic and Research Foundation
La Jolla, California 92037

Exposure to antigen can result in either immunological responsiveness or immunological unresponsiveness. The establishment of unresponsiveness in lymphoid cells can be accomplished by a variety of experimental procedures and can be maintained by any of a number of mechanisms.[1, 2] The nature and extent of the unresponsive state is dependent on the form and route of antigen administration as well as the immune status and maturity of the susceptible lymphoid cells. Immature neonatal cells are more readily tolerized than are functionally more mature adult B cells.[3-14] However, unresponsiveness has been induced in adult B cells under the appropriate *in vitro* culture conditions.[5, 7, 11, 14-17]

The ability to induce unresponsiveness in individuals primed by previous exposure to antigen would be of limited advantage and has rarely been accomplished.[18-22] The factors responsible for the difficulty in inducing unresponsiveness in primed, as compared to unprimed, lymphoid cells may reflect the maturity of these cells or interference by circulating antibody or activated helper T cells (Th). Nevertheless, the induction of unresponsiveness in primed B cells has been demonstrated both *in vivo*[23] and *in vitro*[15-17, 24] in a variety of antigenic systems. The mechanisms by which primed B cells can be rendered unresponsive during subsequent antigenic exposure have not been systematically addressed. This paper investigates the induction of immunological unresponsiveness in B cells previously primed by a soluble protein antigen—human gamma globulin (HGG) or the hapten trinitrophenyl (TNP). Unresponsiveness is established *in vivo* with the heterologous gamma globulin, HGG, or *in vitro* with TNP conjugated to turkey gamma globulin (TGG). The kinetics of tolerance induction, the role of suppressor cells, and the surface isotype of the B cells rendered unresponsive are among the parameters assessed in this article.

* This is publication no. 2588 from the Department of Immunopathology, Scripps Clinic and Research Foundation, La Jolla, California. This research was supported, in part, by grants from the United States Public Health Service, nos. AI07007 and AG01629, the American Cancer Society, no. IM-42K, and the Biomedical Research Support Program, no. RRO-5514.

† Recipient of Junior Faculty Research Award JFRA-8 from the American Cancer Society.

‡ Recipient of a National Science Foundation Graduate Fellowship. This work is submitted in partial fulfillment of the requirements for the Ph.D. degree from the Department of Biology, University of California, San Diego, supported, in part, by a grant from the United States Public Health Service, no. CA09174.

§ Recipient of Junior Faculty Research Award JFRA-19 from the American Cancer Society.

210

The establishment of tolerance to HGG in A/J mice has been extensively characterized both as to the lymphoid cells rendered unresponsive [25] and the doses of antigen required to tolerize T and B lymphocytes.[26, 27] The induction of unresponsiveness was attempted in adult A/J mice after priming with 100 μg of immunogenic, heat-aggregated HGG (AHGG).[23] As illustrated in FIGURE 1, unresponsiveness could be induced in primed animals by the injection of 2.5 mg monomeric deaggregated HGG (DHGG)[27] if the mice were rested 76 d or more after priming. Although this dose of tolerogen will induce a completely unresponsive state when injected into unprimed mice,[25-27] injection of tolerogen 10 d following priming with AHGG resulted in the death of the primed mice by anaphylaxis. These results indicate that unresponsiveness can be induced in primed mice, but only if attempted after the level of circulating antibody has diminished.

The duration of unresponsiveness established in the spleens of previously primed mice was compared with that of unprimed tolerized mice. Unresponsive-

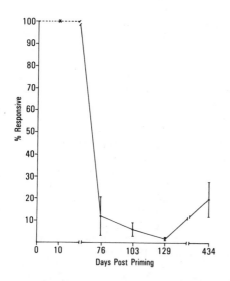

FIGURE 1. Induction of unresponsiveness following priming.

ness is established within 3 d in both Th and B cells of unprimed mice tolerized with 2.5 mg DHGG. Splenic B cells remain unresponsive for at least 45 d following tolerization and Th remain unresponsive for at least three months.[27] In contrast, when the same dose of DHGG is injected into mice primed 81 d after priming with AHGG, they are unresponsive for a considerably shorter period of time, as illustrated in FIGURE 2. Although the response of spleen cells from primed mice is depressed as early as 7 d after the injection of tolerogenic DHGG and remains depressed for at least three more weeks, complete responsiveness is observed five weeks after DHGG. These results indicate that both Th and B cells in primed mice recover responsiveness much more rapidly than do the lymphocyte subsets in unprimed tolerized mice. Furthermore, if tested at least five weeks after tolerization, primed tolerized cells demonstrate a response enhanced in comparison to that of primed cells not exposed to DHGG.

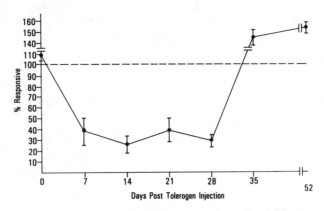

FIGURE 2. Duration of unresponsiveness in primed mice.

The intrinsic ability to induce unresponsiveness in primed spleen cells was investigated by removing those cells from the influence of the primed host. Two to six weeks after priming with AHGG, 60×10^6 spleen cells were injected into lethally irradiated normal recipients, which were then injected with 2.5 mg tolerogen (DHGG) and subsequently challenged with 400 μg immunogenic AHGG. The results of this experiment are shown in TABLE 1, which demonstrates that adoptively transferred normal spleen cells can be rendered unresponsive, whereas transferred primed spleen cells could not be when recipients were tested by challenge 3 d after the injection of tolerogen. However, if antigenic challenge was delayed until 10 d after the transfer and attempted tolerization, unresponsiveness could be established in primed spleen cells (TABLE 2). The possibility that the induction of unresponsiveness in primed spleen cells required a longer period of exposure to tolerogen than did induction in normal cells was explored by delaying antigenic challenge of irradiated recipients until 3, 6, 10, or 14 d after reconstitution with primed spleen cells and exposure to tolerogenic DHGG. As shown in FIGURE 3, these experiments demonstrated that unresponsiveness was established in primed and transferred spleen cells but that the unresponsiveness was transient (present only at day 6 to 10 after DHGG treatment). If antigenic challenge was delayed until 14 d after transfer and treatment, primed cells had recovered responsiveness and were hyperreactive, suggesting that antigen-specific B cells were not functionally deleted by exposure to DHGG but had been unresponsive to challenge on days 6 and 10 due either to receptor blockade or to the presence of suppressor cells.

TABLE 1

DIFFERENTIAL SUSCEPTIBILITY TO TOLERIZATION IN TRANSFERRED NORMAL AND PRIMED SPLEEN CELLS

Spleen Cells	DHGG	PFC per 10^6 Cells	Unresponsive (%)
Normal	—	300	
Normal	+	40	87
Primed	—	440	
Primed	+	810	0

TABLE 2

INDUCTION OF UNRESPONSIVENESS IN PRIMED SPLEEN CELLS
AFTER ADOPTIVE TRANSFER

Interval Between DHGG and Challenge	DHGG	PFC per 10^6 Cells	Unresponsive (%)
3	—	1720	
3	+	1450 N.S.	16
10	—	550	
10	+	80 $p < 0.05$	85

In order to assess their ability to induce unresponsiveness in primed B cells, splenic T cells were removed from primed spleen cell populations. Normal and primed spleen cells were treated with rabbit anti-thymocyte serum (ATS) plus C' immediately before adoptive transfer into normal irradiated recipients. As described for the transfer of unseparated primed spleen cells, 2.5 mg DHGG was injected 2 to 4 h after reconstitution with isolated splenic B cells.[23] 30×10^6 primed thymocytes were injected as a source of Th[28] at the time of antigenic challenge, 3 to 14 d after transfer and DHGG treatment. Unresponsiveness could be established in both normal and primed B cells if these cells were transferred and tolerized in the absence of T cells (TABLE 3). When challenged 14 d after exposure to tolerogen, transferred isolated primed B cells remained 95% unresponsive (TABLE 3), whereas unfractionated primed spleen cells were several times more responsive than primed cells not exposed to DHGG (FIGURE 3).

In order to determine the kinetic profile of the unresponsiveness induced in primed B cells following transfer and tolerization, the recipients were challenged 3, 6, 10, or 14 d after reconstitution with Th and antigen. As illustrated in FIGURE 4, unresponsiveness in transferred primed B cells is established within 3 d of the injection of DHGG and remains for at least two weeks after tolerization. The kinetics of unresponsiveness in primed B cells (FIGURE 4) contrast sharply with the kinetics of transient unresponsiveness induced in unfractionated primed spleen cells (FIGURE 3), but are very similar to the kinetics of unresponsiveness in untreated B cells tolerized in normal animals.[27]

The dose requirements for the induction of unresponsiveness in transferred, primed B cells was also investigated. Following ATS treatment and transfer

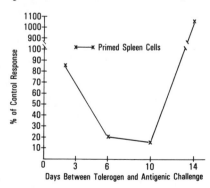

FIGURE 3. Kinetics of unresponsiveness in primed spleen cells after tolerogen.

TABLE 3

INDUCTION OF UNRESPONSIVENESS IN ISOLATED B CELLS AFTER ADOPTIVE TRANSFER

B Cells	DHGG	PFC per 10^6 Cells	Unresponsive (%)
Normal	—	70	
Normal	+	< 1 $p < 0.05$	99
Primed	—	390	
Primed	+	20 $p < 0.05$	95

into normal irradiated recipients, 30×10^6 primed B cells were exposed to increasing doses of DHGG from 100 µg to 2.5 mg. As depicted in FIGURE 5, unresponsiveness was not established in primed B cells following the injection of 100 µg tolerogen. However, a dose of 500 µg DHGG induced significant unresponsiveness and doses of 1 mg or more induced complete unresponsiveness. These data were obtained from recipients challenged 6 d after reconstitution and tolerization. The dose of tolerogen required to induce unresponsiveness in transferred primed B cells (FIGURE 5) is only slightly higher than the dose of DHGG previously reported to be necessary for the tolerization of unprimed B cells in the spleens of normal mice.[27] A possible involvement of antigen-specific suppressor cells in the establishment of unresponsiveness in primed lymphoid cells was investigated using recently developed in vitro techniques.[29] In this assay, 7.5×10^6 spleen cells from primed mice or from irradiated recipients reconstituted with primed cells were assayed for their ability to suppress 7.5×10^6 HGG-specific target cells. When putative effector cells were cocultured for 6 d with responsive target cells (FIGURE 6), suppressor cells could be detected in all primed spleen cell sources regardless of treatment. During the 6 d coculture, suppressor cells were generated from primed spleen cells, from the spleens of irradiated mice reconstituted with primed cells, and from the spleens of reconstituted mice that were also treated with DHGG.

The cells present in primed spleen cell populations responsible for the suppression detected in vitro appear to be T cells. Treatment of transferred or untransferred primed spleen cells with ATS plus C′ before coculture with HGG-specific target cells completely abolishes the ability to generate suppressor cell activity (FIGURE 7). These data indicate that the precursors and/or inducers of suppressor T cells (Ts) detected by this in vitro assay are present in all primed cell populations investigated.

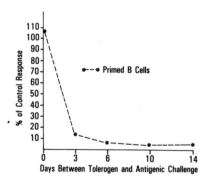

FIGURE 4. Kinetics of unresponsiveness in primed B cells after tolerogen.

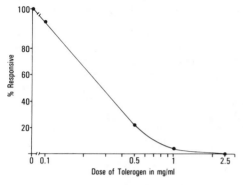

FIGURE 5. Dose requirements for unresponsiveness in primed B cells.

The ability to generate Ts *in vitro* from transferred primed spleen cells was compared with the ability to induce unresponsiveness in identical cells. Normal irradiated recipients were reconstituted with primed spleen cells and half of these recipients were injected with 2.5 mg DHGG. 2, 6, 10, or 14 d after transfer, spleen cells were removed from these recipients and cocultured for 6 d with responsive target cells. As illustrated in FIGURE 8, transferred primed spleen cells were equally capable of generating Ts at any of the times tested after transfer with or without tolerogen treatment. The level of suppression generated was equivalent to that detected in normal mice tolerized with DHGG and previously demonstrated to possess Ts both *in vivo* [30] and *in vitro*.[29] When compared with the kinetics of unresponsiveness induced in transferred primed spleen cells (FIGURE 3), the generation of Ts suppressing HGG-specific B cells

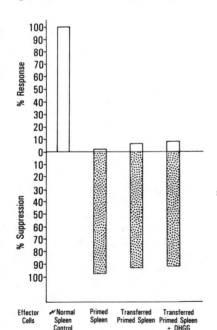

FIGURE 6. Suppressor cells in primed spleen cell populations.

in vitro demonstrates no correlation with the transient unresponsiveness induced in primed spleen cells.

Confirmation that *in vitro* induction of Ts in primed spleen cell populations does not correlate with the establishment of unresponsiveness in these primed cells is provided by the data presented in TABLE 4. Whereas primed spleen cells transferred into irradiated recipients respond to antigen challenge unless treated with DHGG, Ts can be generated from these transferred primed spleen cells *in vitro* regardless of their exposure or lack of exposure to DHGG in the reconstituted recipient. Therefore, the ability to induce mature effector Ts from inducer and/or precursor Ts in primed spleen cell populations appears to be unrelated to the induction of unresponsiveness in primed B cells with HGG.

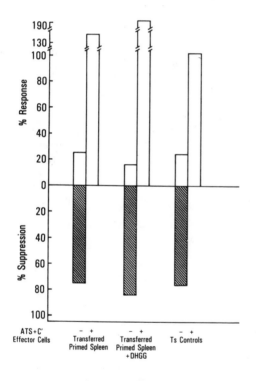

FIGURE 7. Anti-thymocyte serum sensitivity of suppression.

The presence of mature effector Ts in unresponsive primed spleen cell populations was also investigated. In order to circumvent the induction of Ts during *in vitro* culture, primed spleen cells were added to ongoing target cell cultures before or after transfer into irradiated recipients and exposure to DHGG. The primed cell population containing putative effector Ts were added for the last 2 d of 6 d cultures. FIGURE 9 illustrates the comparison between the results of the 6 d coculture to detect the *in vitro* generation of Ts and the 2 d coculture to detect the presence of mature effector Ts. Effector Ts cannot be detected in any of the three primed spleen sources regardless of transfer or exposure to tolerogen. However, as previously demonstrated in FIGURE 6, Ts can be generated from all primed cell populations after 6 d of culture *in vitro*. It can be concluded from these data that, whereas inducer and/or precursor Ts

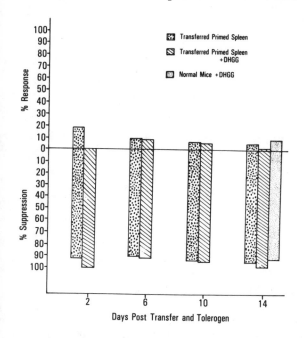

FIGURE 8. Kinetics of suppression *versus* time after transfer.

are present in primed spleen cells, the induction or presence of Ts is not responsible for the unresponsiveness that can be induced in primed B cells to HGG.

Helper T cells may, however, play a role in the prevention of tolerance induction in primed spleen cells. As illustrated in FIGURES 3 and 4, unresponsiveness is more readily induced and persists for a longer period in isolated B cells than in unfractionated spleen cells. Primed thymocytes or primed splenic T cells [23] were injected into recipients reconstituted with primed B cells during attempted

TABLE 4

In Vivo RESPONSIVENESS *Versus in Vitro* SUPPRESSION

In Vivo			
Donor Cells	DHGG	PFC per 10^6 Cells	Response (%)
Primed spleen	−	2490	100
Primed spleen	+	10	<1
In Vitro			
Primed Targets	Effector Cells	PFC per Culture	Response (%)
+	Normal spleen	3180	100
+	Transferred primed spleen	330	10
+	Transferred primed spleen + DHGG	290	9

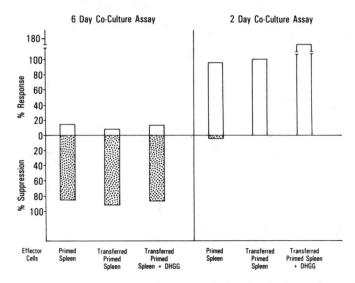

FIGURE 9. Induction of suppressor cells in primed spleen cells.

tolerization with DHGG. As demonstrated in FIGURE 10, coadministration of of either source of primed Th with tolerogen interfered with the induction of unresponsiveness in primed B cells. Therefore, the difficulty in establishing unresponsiveness in primed spleen cells may be attributed to the presence of primed Th present in this cell population, not to an intrinsic inability to tolerize primed B cells.

Although primed Th can interfere with the induction of tolerance in primed B cells, they cannot rescue these B cells once tolerance has been established. The results of the addition of excess primed Th to transferred primed spleen cells 6, 7, or 9 d following tolerization are presented in TABLE 5. Whereas

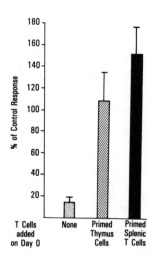

FIGURE 10. Interference with tolerance induction in primed B cells by primed T cells.

TABLE 5

STABILITY OF UNRESPONSIVENESS INDUCED IN TRANSFERRED
PRIMED SPLEEN CELLS

Donor Cells	DHGG	Addition of Helper Cells	Time of Challenge		
			6 d	7 d	9 d
Primed spleen	—	—	395 *	414	263
Primed spleen	+	—	20(5%) †	6(1%)	3(1%)
Primed spleen	+	+	18(5%)	2(1%)	7(3%)

* PFC per 10^6 cells.
† Percentage of responsiveness.

unresponsiveness was established by the injection of DHGG into irradiated recipients reconstituted with primed spleen cells, the addition of primed Th had no effect on this unresponsiveness.

Investigations of the susceptibility to tolerance induction of primed B cells and the mechanisms responsible for that unresponsive state were also performed in an *in vitro* culture system using hapten-primed B cells as the target for tolerance induction.[17] In this system, spleen cells previously primed and boosted *in vivo* with TNP-keyhole limpet hemocyanin (TNP-KLH) were cultured *in vitro* for 20 h at 37° C in the presence of the antigen TNP on a noncrossreactive carrier, TGG (FIGURE 11). This initial culture allows the interaction of B cells with tolerogen (TNP-TGG) in the absence of possible interference by primed Th. Following the initial culture, cells are extensively washed and cultured for another 4 d in the presence of 5 ng ml⁻¹ of antigenic TNP-KLH. This induces unresponsiveness in hapten-specific B cells only if these primed cells are exposed to tolerogen during the first 20 h of culture. Suppressor cells do not appear to be responsible for this unresponsive state, as indicated by the lack of suppression obtained when responsive and unresponsive cells are cocultured (FIGURE 11).

A lack of Ts in this hapten-specific unresponsive state in primed B cells is confirmed by experiments using anti-Lyt 2 antiserum. TABLE 6 illustrates the effects of the removal of T cells bearing Lyt 2⁺ surface phenotype from tolerized cells immediately before the 4 d assay culture. Neither the response to antigenic challenge with TNP-KLH nor the unresponsiveness in hapten-specific B cells induced by TNP-TGG is altered by the absence of Lyt 2⁺ Ts. As previouly demonstrated with HGG-specific B cells, the induction of unresponsiveness in primed B cells by heterologous gamma globulins is not dependent upon the presence of Ts.

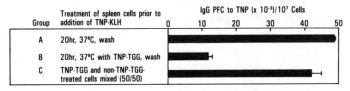

FIGURE 11. *In vitro* tolerization of TNP-specific B cells by preincubation with TNP-TGG.

TABLE 6

INDUCTION OF UNRESPONSIVENESS IN TNP-TGG WITH AND WITHOUT LYT 2+
SUPPRESSOR T CELLS

Treatment	TNP-TGG	PFC per 10^7 Cells	Suppression (%)
None	—	118 610	—
None	+	14 820	88
Anti-Lyt 2.2 + C	—	119 404	—
Anti-Lyt 2.2 + C	+	16 000	87

Because several laboratories have demonstrated that the appearance of IgD+ surface phenotype may reflect the maturation of B cells and the acquisition of increased resistance to tolerance induction,[31-33] the isotype of the primed and boosted TNP-specific B cells responding *in vitro* was assessed. Cells bearing IgM, IgD, or IgG$_1$ on their surface were removed by adherence to erythrocytes coated with heavy chain–specific antisera or by interference with function *in vitro* through the addition of specific antisera during culture.[17] As depicted in FIGURE 12, only depletion of IgG+ cells or blockade with anti-IgG serum had any inhibitory effect on the response to TNP-KLH *in vitro*. Depletion or inhibition of IgM+ or IgG+ B cells only enhanced the response of hapten-primed spleen cells. Therefore, it may be concluded that the surface phenotype of the primed and boosted B cells susceptible to tolerization *in vitro* was IgG+, IgM-, IgD-. These results are in agreement with reports that mature memory B cells are predominantly IgD-.[34, 35]

In conclusion, the establishment of immunological unresponsiveness in mice that have previously mounted an immune response to antigen exposure and presently possess memory T and/or B cells specific for the antigen is difficult. However, this resistance to tolerance induction does not reflect an intrinsic property of primed B cells. Primed B cells are not refractory to the induction of unresponsiveness mediated by previously encountered antigen. Nevertheless, the addition of primed helper T cells can interfere with the induction of unresponsiveness in primed B cells. Resistance to tolerance induction in primed cell populations may therefore be maintained by the presence of primed helper

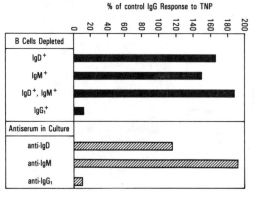

FIGURE 12. Surface isotype of primed B cells susceptible to *in vitro* tolerance induction.

T cells.[36] Suppressor T cells do not appear to be responsible for the unresponsive state induced in primed B cells. Evidence for both receptor blockade and functional deletion have been presented. Finally, the primed cells rendered unresponsive *in vitro* may represent mature memory cells bearing IgG⁺ surface phenotype but lacking membrane-bound IgD.

ACKNOWLEDGMENTS

The authors wish to thank Janet Kuhns for secretarial expertise in the preparation of this manuscript.

REFERENCES

1. WEIGLE, W. O. 1980. Adv. Immunol. **31:** 159–273.
2. PARKS, D. E. 1981. Clin. Immunol. Allergy **1:** 3–16.
3. WEIGLE, W. O. 1973. Adv. Immunol. **16:** 61–122.
4. METCALF, E. S. & N. R. KLINMAN. 1976. J. Exp. Med. **143:** 1327–40.
5. CAMBIER, J. C., J. R. KETTMAN, E. S. VITETTA & J. W. UHR. 1976. J. Exp. Med. **144:** 293–97.
6. ELSON, C. J. 1977. Eur. J. Immunol. **7:** 6–10.
7. CAMBIER, J. C., E. S. VITETTA, J. W. UHR & J. R. KETTMAN. 1977. J. Exp. Med. **145:** 778–83.
8. SEWCZUK, M. R. & G. W. SISKIND. 1977. J. Exp. Med. **145:** 1590–601.
9. METCALF, E. S. & N. R. KLINMAN. 1977. J. Immunol. **118:** 2111–16.
10. VENKATARAMAN, M. & D. W. SCOTT. 1977. J. Immunol. **119:** 1879–81.
11. NOSSAL, G. J. V. & B. L. PIKE. 1978. J. Exp. Med. **148:** 1161–70.
12. KETTMAN, J. R., J. C. CAMBIER, J. W. UHR, F. LIGLER & E. S. VITETTA. 1979. Immunol. Rev. **43:** 69–95.
13. METCALF, E. S., A. F. SCHRATER & N. R. KLINMAN. 1979. Immunol. Rev. **43:** 143–83.
14. PIKE, B. L., F. L. BATTYE & G. J. V. NOSSAL. 1981. J. Immunol. **126:** 89–94.
15. BYERS, V. S. & E. E. SERCARZ. 1968. J. Exp. Med. **128:** 715–28.
16. KATZ, D. H., T. HAMAOKA & B. BENACERRAF. 1974. J. Exp. Med. **139:** 1464–72.
17. WALKER, S. M. & W. O. WEIGLE. 1981. J. Exp. Med. **153:** 6563–64.
18. DORNER, M. M. & J. W. UHR. 1964. J. Exp. Med. **120:** 435–47.
19. DRESSER, D. W. 1965. Immunology **9:** 261–73.
20. SISKIND, G. W. & J. G. HOWARD. 1966. J. Exp. Med. **124:** 417–29.
21. VON FELTON, A. & W. O. WEIGLE. 1975. Cell. Immunol. **18:** 31–40.
22. SANFILIPPO, F. & D. W. SCOTT. 1977. Eur. J. Immunol. **7:** 283–287.
23. NELSON-RAMPY, P. A., D. E. PARKS & W. O. WEIGLE. 1981. J. Immunol. **127:** 1415–19.
24. WALKER, S. M., P. A. NELSON, D. E. PARKS & W. O. WEIGLE. 1981. *In* B Lymphocytes in the Immune Response: Functional, Developmental, and Interactive Properties. N. R. Klinman, D. E. Mosier, I. Scher, and E. S. Vitetta, Eds.: 267–74. Elsevier/North-Holland. New York.
25. CHILLER, J. M., G. S. HABICHT & W. O. WEIGLE. 1971. Science **171:** 813–15.
26. CHILLER, J. M. & W. O. WEIGLE. 1972. Contemp. Top. Immunobiol. **1:** 119–42.
27. PARKS, D. E. & W. O. WEIGLE. 1980. Clin. Exp. Immunol. **39:** 257–62.
28. PARKS, D. E., S. M. WALKER & W. O. WEIGLE. J. Immunol. **126:** 938–42.
29. PARKS, D. E., B. G. DUNBAR & W. O. WEIGLE. Submitted for publication.
30. PARKS, D. E., M. V. DOYLE & W. O. WEIGLE. 1978. J. Exp. Med. **148:** 625–38.

31. VITETTA, E. S., J. C. CAMBIER, F. S. LIGLER, J. R. KETTMAN & J. W. UHR. 1977. J. Exp. Med. **146:** 1804–8.
32. CAMBIER, J. C., E. S. VITETTA, J. R. KETTMAN, G. M. WETZEL & J. W. UHR. 1977. J. Exp. Med. **146:** 107–17.
33. SCOTT, D. W., J. E. LAYTON & G. J. V. NOSSAL. 1977. J. Exp. Med. **146:** 1473–83.
34. BLACK, S. J., W. VAN DER LOO, M. R. LAKES & L. A. HERZENBERG. J. Exp. Med. **147:** 984–96.
35. BLACK, S. J., T. TOKUHISA, L. A. HERZENBERG & L. A. HERZENBERG. 1980. Eur. J. Immunol. **10:** 846–51.
36. CHEN, S. & J. CERNY. 1980. J. Immunol. **125:** 1950–76.

DISCUSSION OF THE PAPER

E. DIENER (*University of Alberta, Edmonton, Alta*): Dr. Weigle, I always have a problem when you talk about long-lasting B cell tolerance. You claim that you have central tolerance in the absence of suppressors, but we know that it takes about seven days for immunocompetent B cells to mature. Even if one can't functionally demonstrate the presence of suppressors, wouldn't you still have to say that there has to be a suppressive mechanism active that prevents this recruitment from occurring when the antigen has disappeared?

WEIGLE: We have never made any claim for any long-term tolerance in B cells. As you recall, tolerance disappears very rapidly in B cells.

DIENER: I thought you said at the beginning that your B cell tolerance model can be extended over several weeks.

WEIGLE: If you give 2.5 mg of the DHGG, B cell tolerance lasts approximately 50 d and then starts to wane. The half-life of HGG in these animals is approximately eight days. Tolerance correlates very well with the presence of antigen. I think that the B cell tolerance is very short and disappears very rapidly after the antigen disappears.

D. R. GREEN (*Yale University, New Haven, Conn.*): I'd like to point out a similarity between what you're describing and some work we did, although, of course, it may not be the same mechanism. If T cells are the object of suppression and inactivation similar to this inactivation of the B cells, then hyperimmunized cells are capable of blocking the induction of suppression in T cells. In our system, we've characterized the T cell that's capable of blocking the induction of unresponsiveness and found it to be a Lyt 1+, Lyt 2-, I-J+ contrasuppressor cell. Have you results on phenotyping of that cell in your system?

WEIGLE: We have not used anti-I-J serum.

G. J. THORBECKE (*New York University Medical School, New York, N.Y.*): Have you tried to transfer the cells that were incubated with TNP–turkey gamma globulin into irradiated recipients to see if the unresponsiveness detected *in vitro* could also be detected *in vivo*? We have done similar experiments with B cells primed to TNP-KLH that are incubated with various TNP conjugates *in vitro*. In transfer situations, we find that things like TNP–gamma globulins do not really affect responsiveness, whereas TNP polysaccharide conjugates did. It seemed to be receptor blockade. *In vitro,* however, a very short incubation with TNP–gamma globulin did negatively influence their responsiveness. So there was a big difference in that respect.

WEIGLE: We haven't done those experiments, but certainly we're thinking about them. We have done some preliminary experiments with animals that had been immunized with TNP-KLH, then injected with TNP-turkey gamma-globulin, and, later, reinjected with TNP-KLH. In the preliminary experiments we could markedly suppress the response *in vivo.*

Y. BOREL (*Harvard Medical School, Boston, Mass.*): All the data we have seen so far has been in animals. I think that, if we believe that tolerance is something important, we should eventually apply these data to man, with the hope of influencing immunity in man by the induction of specific tolerance to antigens that are relevant to immune disease. In a first attempt to do that, we have examined whether we can induce tolerance in human peripheral blood lymphocytes *in vitro.* The work was done in Dr. Schlossman's laboratory by Dr. Morimoto, who has developed a model to detect hapten-specific antibody *in vitro* in the supernatant of cultured normal human peripheral blood lymphocytes.

In this experiment, hapten-specific tolerance was induced in human peripheral blood lymphocytes *in vitro.* It is specific for the hapten because another irrelevant hapten, such as penicilloyl on human gamma globulin, fails to induce tolerance to DNP. This demonstrates that it is not the carrier that is doing the work, but rather the hapten-carrier conjugate. In humans, isologous gamma globulin is the most important carrier. The only significant suppression was obtained when DNP was on human gamma globulin, not when it was on another species of gamma globulin, such as bovine or fowl gamma globulin or even a non-self human antigen, such as human serum albumin. So this confirms that we can induce hapten-specific tolerance in man. It also confirms the role of isologous gamma globulin as the relevant carrier to induce it.

Now, in concluding, I want to make a few comments and a few generalizations in an attempt to provoke some questions or comments from the audience. I think that we can fairly say that, at this meeting, we have seen two models that are very effective in inducing unresponsiveness. One is linking determinants to self cells, and the other is using soluble protein antigen or linking determinants to soluble carriers, such as isologous gamma globulin. I think that it's fair to say that the mechanism of unresponsiveness induced by determinants linked to cells is fairly complicated and may involve a network of suppressor cells. In contrast, the mechanism of unresponsiveness induced by soluble antigen does not appear to be dependent on suppressor cells, as we have just seen in Dr. Weigle's talk. So we certainly have a true mechanism of tolerance. What is this mechanism? Several mechanisms have been proposed. I think that there are a number of possibilities: clonal abortion, clonal deletion, receptor blockade, or permanent deletion of a receptor. We don't really know if any of these mechanisms are operating for natural antigens *in vivo.*

I think one can say that antigen is necessary to induce unresponsiveness. Not only to induce it, but probably to maintain it. I don't think it has been demonstrated whether the cell in which unresponsiveness is induced is aborted or deleted. Personally, I believe that the cell is always there, that the cell that is truly unresponsive is always present in the host, and that what maintains unresponsiveness is the antigen. When the antigen disappears, unresponsiveness disappears. What we're probably doing when we induce tolerance is just presenting this antigen to a receptor in such a manner that it can stay on the surface of the cell. Tolerance is then accomplished by some mechanism—initially by a receptor blockade mechanism, and then by a mechanism that we don't understand.

WEIGLE: I would like to say that the opinion of one of the chairmen of this session does not reflect the views of both chairmen.

C. A. WATERS (*University of Alberta, Edmonton, Alta.*): Dr. Weigle, you seem to be proposing that you have T cell deletion and no antigen present after one year in these normal A/J mice. How do you reconcile those two facts?

WEIGLE: I don't know how much antigen is present after one year in these mice. Apparently there is some. It takes extremely small doses of antigen to make T cells tolerant. I think that, once T cells are deleted, if that's what happens, they stay deleted until they recover by some sort of somatic mutation, or whatever makes these cells come back.

WATERS: But presumably you have to deal with the continual regeneration of cells.

WEIGLE: That's right, but it takes time for these cells to regenerate.

A. NISONOFF (*Brandeis University, Waltham, Mass.*): Dr. Weigle, in what particulars do the two chairmen disagree?

WEIGLE: I personally believe that the cells tolerized during neonatal life are deleted when the repertoire is being generated. This depletion is antigen-driven. Perhaps the somatic mutation that occurs at this time is also antigen-driven. My suggestion would be that, in immature B cells of neonatal animals, there is much more somatic mutation going on than in mature B cells of adult animals. This somatic mutation allows these cells to mutate away from the specificity of the antigen, so they're not really clonally deleted. I would call it clonal conversion.

D. W. SCOTT (*Duke University Medical Center, Durham, N.C.*): First of all, Dr. Borel, I want to thank you for saving me the task of summarizing the meeting, although the summary I may give tomorrow may be slightly different. I also want to point out that, in an *in vitro* system, Brigitte Groui in Pierre Galanand's lab has essentially done the same sort of experiment, except that she used hapten-modified lymphocytes. So the modified-self tolerance system has been adapted in a human *in vitro* model and shows similar characteristics, although it's far behind the system, as yet.

H. N. CLAMAN (*University of Colorado Medical School, Denver, Col.*): Dr. Weigle, how do you reconcile your ideas about clonal deletion with the very beautiful data presented today by Yi-chi Kong, by which I was fairly well convinced that reactive clones were present in adult animals?

WEIGLE: We don't get the same data as Dr. Kong.

CLAMAN: But you're not doing precisely the same experiments.

WEIGLE: We don't get significant proliferating T cells in animals that have been immunized with mouse thyroglobulin in complete Freund's adjuvant, although we can see it in animals that are immunized with bovine thyroglobulin or human thyroglobulin. With thyroglobulin, one just can't get tolerance if the antigen isn't there. If thyroglobulin isn't present in sufficient concentrations to keep the T cells and B cells tolerant, then these cells are not going to be tolerant. What I think is happening with Dr. Kong's system is that the T cells are tolerant because the level of antigen is present in sufficient quantities to make the T cells "tolerant," but not completely tolerant. Then one presses "leaky" tolerane by giving complete Freund's adjuvant or, perhaps, by giving very small amounts in repeated injections. One can then coax a limited number of these T cells to be activated. But I'm sure there are some antigens, for example, myelin basic protein, or, better yet, the acetylcholine receptor, that are present in a mouse in amounts not great enough to make either the T or the B cells tolerant. So there is no deletion of any clones. One has competent T cells and competent B cells, and if one injects the acetylcholine into these animals, they get a good antibody response and disease. I don't understand how that's difficult to deal with. You don't get deletions of cells if you don't have antigen there in sufficient concentrations to delete them.

CLAMAN: But then you're making rather subtle distinctions in quantitation.

WEIGLE: Right.

CLAMAN: So we're going to have a spectrum in which we have self-antigens that are not generally available, sequestered antigens, if you will. We're going to have self-antigens available in low concentrations and we're going to have self-antigens available in high concentrations, like serum albumin. Therefore, the question of clonal deletion, suppressor cells, modulation, and coaxing of reactive clones may depend, among other things, upon the availability of antigen to those cells. I have no ax to grind either way—I'm just trying to clarify my thoughts.

WEIGLE: I think the induction of tolerance depends on several things. First, I assume that there is a clonal deletion of some sort. Second, I assume that there is a difference in the amount of antigen required to make T cells and B cells tolerant. I also assume that the duration and degree of tolerance that one gets depends on the concentration of that antigen in the microenvironment of the participating cells.

BOREL: I think, as Sir Peter Medawar said, that it's very difficult to design an experiment that will distinguish between the absence of a reactive cell and the presence of a nonreactive cell. I think that all discussion of clonal deletion is extraordinarily difficult because there is no way to prove or disprove it.

H. F. HAVAS (*Temple University School of Medicine, Philadelphia, Penn.*): I have a little difficulty reconciling deletion with the maturing of the immune response that we and others have shown. If they're all gone, how can they mature?

WEIGLE: I don't believe they're all gone. You may have antigen at a low enough level that it won't trigger or tolerize cells that may be there. I think some balance between antigen levels and responsive cells prevents an antibody response. Certainly we know that there is a lot of low-level autoimmunity. We're probably making antibodies to something in the body all the time without getting any clinical symptoms. It's very transient, and we recover. These cells are not completely inhibited or completely deleted. They're just deleted to the level that we don't get in trouble.

E. S. GOLUB (*Purdue University, West Lafayette, Ind.*): Dr. Weigle, picking up on that last point and following the final statement of Dr. Naor's presentation, Cudkowicz has made the argument that NK cells serve the function in nature of homeostatic regulators. As you know from the preprint I sent you and which I'm sure you read, I'm making the argument that this could be the primary function of the immune response. I think this has been kind of rippling through the meeting—that over the last several years, the subleties of immune reactions have been growing. The grossest reactions are antibody formation, killing reactions. But now, subtle interactions of suppression, of proliferation, of regulation—it's as if we've been flirting around with the tip of the iceberg. If all MHC restriction and anti- and autoidiotype data are looked at in this context, couldn't we pick up your last statement that the body is always responding in some way to itself, perhaps to regulate itself, and that what we're talking about in tolerance is a regulatory mechanism for eliminating those destructive clones? Even though you're not making anti-eyeball and so you don't have clinical symptoms, you're always responding to something of self. So there can be functional deletion of destructive clones, and suppressing mechanisms and a variety of other mechanisms can be postulated. But to talk about the absence of clones—there is an accumulating amount of data that makes that difficult to defend, I think.

WEIGLE: I'm not quite brave enough to push my argument that far. But I'm glad you were.

GOLUB: I had a good teacher.

WEIGLE: One of the things that people don't consider when they're talking about tolerance induction *in vivo* is the *in vivo* behavior of the antigen. If you inject antigens, like keyhole hemocyanin, into an animal, it's going to be gone very quickly, in that it's broken down very rapidly and doesn't equilibrate between the intra- and extravascular fluid spaces, and thus never gets to all the potential antibody reactive cells. The same thing is true if one injects sheep red blood cells. With SRBC, one would not expect to get an unresponsiveness that results in the deletion of any cell. Sheep red blood cells have to be injected continuously; when one stops, an antibody response ensues. Any unresponsiveness that we have with these types of antigens is usually due to suppressor cell activity. And what people don't take into consideration, when they put TNP on things like HGG or BSA, is that these antigens are not handled the same way as the native serum proteins. The latter equilibrate between intra- and extravascular fluid spaces, they persist with a given half-life, and they do come in contact with all the potential antibody reactive cells. The former are usually rapidly eliminated.

B. N. WAKSMAN (*National MS Society, New York, N.Y.*): Well, since you're engaged in discussing philosophy, I thought I'd ask whether there is any evidence that you know of on the following question. We normally talk about suppressor T cells that suppress the reactions of either T cell populations or B cell populations that are present in the system. In other words, they suppress the response of existing cells. What I didn't hear discussed at any time is the possibility that there may be a class of T cell–mediated suppression that carries out the function of deleting clones, whether that deletion be real deletion or some sort of functional deletion in the sense that Yves Borel was talking about.

GREEN: We recently presented evidence—actually, it's now gotten a lot tighter—that coculturing a helper T cell with a suppressor T cell or a suppressor

T cell factor will specifically remove the ability of that helper cell to present help to a B cell even after you remove the suppressor cell. We removed the suppressors after 48 h with anti-Lyt 2, and then showed that the remaining cells are capable of making low responses to antigens such as horse red blood cells or burro red blood cells. The sheep red blood cell response, however, is completely removed. We've done that experiment by using a double Marbrook chamber, showing that this inactivation of helper T cells will actually proceed across a nucleopore membrane. Those suppressor cells can be removed very effectively by simply removing the chamber containing the suppressor cells and those helper cells have no activity for sheep red blood cells *in vitro*.

WEIGLE: In order to look at the role of the suppressor cells in maintaining tolerance to self, it is important to look to see if one can tolerize suppressor cells. You can't do this very easily with the antigens that actually induce suppressor cells, but you certainly can do this with antigens that don't. Elliot Parks has looked at this with HGG, and he certainly can induce an unresponsive state in suppressor cells with almost the same level of DHGG that it takes to induce unresponsiveness in helper T cells.

Y. M. KONG (*Wayne State University School of Medicine, Detroit, Mich.*): One reason that we do favor the concept of clonal balance is that it's hard to reconcile the fact of clonal deletion. This way, you don't have to postulate that T cell suppressor cells are no longer there; it's just that they're in small numbers or that T helper cells are not there and that they can delete it or that they are held in check by suppressor cells. Besides, our data show that we can selectively activate helper cells or suppressor T cells, and have shown that we could remove suppressor cells by thymectomy and irradiation, and then spontaneously get autoimmune disease. Thyroiditis was seen due to the fact that there were no longer any suppressor cells holding the autoreactive T cells in check. So I think that's further evidence for a balance of some sort. Of course, we don't know how the T suppressor cells hold the autoreactive T cells in check.

I do want to thank Dr. Claman and Dr. Weigle for helping me interpret the data of my presentation. I would like to suggest that the difference that Dr. Weigle and I have shown on the T cell proliferation assay is just a technical difficulty. It's very difficult to show really good proliferation with thyroglobulin, which is a weak antigen. We find that we have to keep the background counts very low. We don't use fetal calf serum, for example. We use mouse serum. Furthermore, we use genetically susceptible high-responder animals in order to show the proliferation.

WEIGLE: I think that's a good point. One of the things you have to consider when you mention that mouse thyroglobulin is a weak antigen in the mouse is that bovine and human thyroglobulins are good antigens in a mouse. This suggests that there is at least a partial state of tolerance to the autologous thyroglobulin.

THE INDUCTION OF TOLERANCE
TO ALLERGENIC CHEMICALS *

Merrill W. Chase

Laboratory of Immunology and Hypersensitivity
The Rockefeller University
New York, New York 10021

INTRODUCTION: HISTORY

In 1943, an unexpected finding was observed during studies on the induction of contact dermatitis to picryl chloride in guinea pigs. Sensitization was accomplished then by 10 to 12 daily intradermal (i.d.) injections, each of 0.25 μg picryl chloride (2,4,6-trinitrochlorobenzene, TNCB). After a suitable rest period, the animals were subjected to contact tests by spreading 0.03 ml olive oil containing 1% TNCB gently over an area about 20 mm in diameter on the close-clipped skin and recording the development of a delayed-type dermatitis. Along with this testing, three normal guinea pigs of the same weight and sex would be added to reveal any irritation that could result from the clipping procedure, the olive oil used as solvent, and general handling, as a standard for judging the responsiveness of the experimental group. After such a testing, in which no reaction was observed on these "toxicity controls," it happened that these three animals were added to the next experimental group to be sensitized. As expected, all animals became sensitized except these former "toxicity controls." This solid evidence of tolerance, induced by placing 1% of the chemical in olive oil on the skin, opened a new chapter for study. This original observation, however, could not be duplicated usefully (we return to this subject below), and sixteen other types of treatments were then explored to secure tolerance. Again unexpectedly, guinea pigs that had been fed daily with gelatin capsules containing ground 2,4-dinitrochlorobenzene (DNCB) mixed with lactose proved to be unresponsive to sensitization with DNCB. Later, direct feedings of TNCB or DNCB dissolved to 1% in triglyceride oil [1] were made with a variety of chemical allergens. Not only could guinea pigs of suitable genetic constitution [2, 3] be sensitized regularly to provide a standard against which the degree of tolerance could be assessed, but it was found that tolerance established by feeding did not recede with later attempts at sensitization with the same allergenic chemical.

There had been a prior observation of tolerance to a chemical allergen, neosalvarsan, although we were not aware of the observation. In 1928, Wilhelm Frei had been able to sensitize human volunteers by a single injection of neosalvarsan i.d.,[4] but not men who had received prior intravenous injections as treatment for syphilis, and this observation was confirmed shortly.[5] Frei had

* This research was supported by a grant from the National Institute of Allergy and Infectious Diseases, no. AI–01258, and by a postdoctoral fellowship (GF–4487) to my former colleague Dr. Jack R. Battisto. Also, thanks are due to Dr. Roy E. Ritts, C. Dean Dukes, and Stephen O. Atherton, who participated in portions of this work, and to Thelma H. Carter.

also succeeded in sensitizing guinea pigs by the same single-injection procedure.[6] Sulzberger, then working in the same laboratory in Breslau, extended Frei's work by attempting to block sensitization of guinea pigs by an intravenous injection of 6 mg neosalvarsan (one-third the lethal dose) one day after making an i.d. sensitizing injection of the chemical. At the intradermal test made four weeks later, the six guinea pigs that had received the i.v. dose were unresponsive, like Frei's treated syphilitic men, and the "positive control" group exhibited significant degrees of hypersensitivity.[7, 8] Unfortunately, this single experiment stood alone, for Sulzberger, returning to America, found that guinea pigs in New York City would not develop a hypersensitivity to neosalvarsan by a single i.d. injection of the chemical (see Reference 9). The insusceptibility to allergic conversion was attributed variously to diet and a necessary critical concentration of ascorbic acid in the diet; genetic factors may also have played a role. The basic problem was put aside, and no other trial of allergenic chemicals was attempted. An effect of diet, with a suggestion that a vitamin C–poor diet may be favorable for sensitization with neosalvarsan (neoarsphenamine), was confirmed much later, and differences in the sensitizing capacity of different batches were noted.[10, 11]

In 1961, we turned to a serious investigation of the Frei-Sulzberger phenomenon.[9] We could effect satisfactory sensitization to neosalvarsan by making five i.d. injections at weekly intervals instead of one injection, or by a single injection of "Old Salvarsan" (Ehrlich's 606). With this information, we employed our own routine for studying tolerance instead of the Sulzberger procedure. In one experiment, a single i.v. injection of 6 mg neosalvarsan was made; the animals were rested for six weeks and then sensitized by five weekly i.d. injections of the same chemical, with inclusion of new guinea pigs as positive controls. The Sulzberger observation was finally and neatly confirmed. We then used Old Salvarsan, which sensitizes by a single intradermal injection. This was neutralized, mixed with guinea pig serum, and injected i.v. at 6 mg per guinea pig. Six weeks later these animals and controls were injected i.d. with Old Salvarsan. At the final skin test, 5 out of 12 were found to have become tolerant and 2 out of 12 partially tolerant. Accordingly, there is one underlying principle for establishing tolerance to allergenic chemicals and it is appropriate to refer to a "Frei-Sulzberger-Chase" phenomenon. Frey et al. confirmed our successful repetition of the Frei-Sulzberger experiment with neoarsphenamine,[12] adopting the Chase routine of making the intravenous injection several weeks before attempting sensitization.

The experimental induction of tolerance to picryl chloride by feeding shortly revealed that the unresponsiveness was not limited to deviating delayed-type hypersensitivity, but that the unresponsiveness extended to depression of the antibody-forming apparatus (see Reference 13). This subject and studies by others are discussed below. The interference with the capacity to make antigen-specific immunoglobulin pertains to self-coupling of the allergens, yet even if antibody does arise it does not vitiate the persisting tolerance to development of contact sensitivity.

MATERIALS AND METHODS

Animals and Feeding

Albino guinea pigs of the Moen-Chase strain [2, 3] were used, highly selected for susceptibility for sensitization with haptens. Feedings were commenced at about three months of age. Animals were restrained by being wrapped in a large square of muslin, then held with mouth upwards. A tapered triangle of brass wire was inserted behind the canine teeth to hold the lips apart. Feedings were made from a 1 ml glass pipet with fire-polished tip, clean on the outside and passed below the molar teeth. One or two preliminary feedings were made with 0.2 ml olive oil or corn oil, then feedings with oil containing 1% TNCB or DNCB were commenced. Two patterns were used: (1) five or six daily feedings in one week, repeated twice with one week of rest between courses; (2) three successive feedings per week on each of three weeks. Later, Dr. Roy E. Ritts introduced feeding by a stomach tube made of 125 mm of the terminal end of Pharmaseal's K-30 infants' feeding tubing, size 8 French, attached to an all-glass 5 ml syringe through a size C polyethylene tubing adaptor (Clay-Adams, Inc., New York, N.Y.).[14] The tubing was passed through the bore of a 3 cm length of 7 mm i.d. glass tubing; this was lowered into the mouth after the feeding and served to prevent spatter as the K9 tubing was withdrawn. The animals were caged by threes and separated if the animals were not compatible. Only animals with uninjured skin were accepted for active sensitization.

Sensitization and Testing

Recrystallized picryl chloride (TNCB) was prepared using absolute alcohol: benzene (2:1) and dinitrochlorobenzene (DNCB) was recrystallized from absolute ethyl alcohol. Solutions for sensitizing, intradermal injections, routines (0.1 ml alcoholic saline = 0.25 µg), and methods of testing have been described.[15] After using simple intradermal injections to sensitize, final tests were made with 1% TNCB or DNCB in olive oil, according to the sensitizing chemical. Degrees of sensitivity as read at 24 h were rated on this scale: ++++, pink, slightly thickened; +++, pink but either somewhat pale or slightly macular; ++, pale pink; +, faint pink, even; ±, faint pink but not confluent; ±, many small faint pink spots; tr, or strong trace, few faint pink spots; tr., trace; f.tr., faint trace; prac. 0, practically zero; 0, negative. Intergrade readings, e.g., +++±, were made as appropriate.

A special method for sensitizing, used to secure extraordinarily high contactant sensitivity, is the "combination method." An initial but low-grade sensitivity is established by intramuscularly injecting picrylated (TNP-) "ghosts," or stromata of guinea pig erythrocytes, in aqueous suspension within a type of complete Freund's adjuvant (CFA). Thereafter, a series of contact tests are made with the simple chemical in triglyceride oil; this causes a stepwise increase in the degree of hypersensitivity, even up to 1:400 of 1% TNCB[15, 16] (see table 2 of Reference 16). The readings scale is expanded, since the final tests, even with dilute solutions of hapten, can give intense reactions.[15]

Preparation of Hapten-Protein Conjugates

Soluble conjugates were prepared by several methods; an early method[15] is applicable, and necessary, for coupling water-reactive haptens such as o-chlorobenzoyl chloride, citraconic anhydride, and the like; it has been used with TNCB and dinitrofluorobenzene (DNFB) also. Later refinements with TNCB, DNFB, and trinitrobenzene sulfonic acid (TNBS) used control of temperature and pH through a Radiometer pH meter TTT-1C and stepwise addition of the reacting hapten in absolute alcohol.

The preparation of conjugates with guinea pig erythrocyte stromata followed procedures previously described.[15, 17] Such products were held at 4° C in saline with 0.25% phenol.

Anaphylaxis and Passive Cutaneous Anaphylaxis

Systemic anaphylaxis was tested by direct injection of soluble antigens into the jugular vein, the small opening in the neck skin being sutured by one or two ties. Passive cutaneous anaphylaxis was carried out to detect and partially quantitate the amount of IgG_1 antibody produced by the guinea pigs.[18, 19]

Adoptive Transfers of White Cells

Cells of paraffin oil–induced exudates at 48 h, lymph nodes, and spleens were prepared and injected intravenously into recipient guinea pigs as described.[14, 18, 20]

RESULTS

Establishment of Tolerance towards Contact Sensitization

While the most solid tolerance encountered was induced by long-term feeding of capsules containing lactose and DNCB, ensuring passage of the capsules past the molar teeth was time-consuming. We found it sufficient, albeit not best, to force the jaws apart and have the guinea pigs swallow 0.3 ml triglyceride oil containing 1% of the allergen, avoiding contact of allergen with the lips. Typical results with this simple technique are shown in FIGURE 1, the guinea pigs having been raised from parental stock that had been selected for high susceptibility with DNCB.[2, 3] The controls responded to the sensitizing procedure with great regularity; the pre-fed animals are seen to be displaced decidedly towards the right. About 18% were negative or essentially negative, while 43% showed only low degrees of reactivity, such as ±, +, or +±. The displacement was sufficient to permit the use of 7–10 fed animals in exploring different facets of unresponsiveness. TABLE 1 presents details of one experiment carried out with 11 pre-fed and 11 normal animals.[21]

A comparison of the effectiveness of routes of application in securing unresponsiveness is shown in TABLE 2.[13] Experiment A was conducted by Stephen O. Atherton: three animals, perhaps five, show meaningful degrees of tolerance by simple application of hapten in olive oil to the skin. (Probably my own first success with this method was due to a fortuitous use of genetically suitable animals among the outbred guinea pigs, or to a different timing, see FIGURE 2c.) In experiment B, feedings produced the usual pattern of tolerance among 14 animals, while intrajugular injection yielded 15 to 20 guinea pigs showing a measure of tolerance; only 4 (14%) fall within categories +++ to ++++ versus 59% for the "positive control" group. Animals exhibiting decided tolerance after i.v. injection are just as tolerant as those receiving

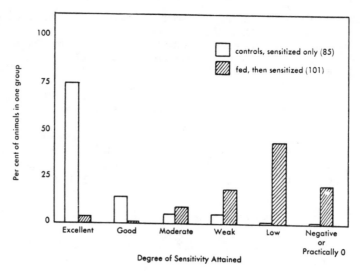

FIGURE 1. Inhibition of drug allergy caused by prior feeding of the inciting agent (2,4-dinitrochlorobenzene). (Combined table.) Each feeding was 0.3 ml olive oil containing 3 mg of the allergen; 15–18 feedings were made. After a rest period, contact tests with 0.03 ml olive oil containing 1% DNCB were applied by spreading the oil evenly over an area of 25 mm diameter. Readings were recorded at 24 h. (From Reference 13, by permission of Harper and Row.)

feedings, but, obviously, animals prepared by i.v. injection must be sensitized to determine their status, whereas a group prepared by feeding can be put into an experiment without prior testing, e.g., adoptive transfer, and so on, provided that a subset of the fed group can be shown to be unresponsive when challenged with the experimental and normal controls.

Characteristics of the Unresponsiveness to Dermal Sensitization

The degree of tolerance secured by our feedings of TNCB or DNCB is profound but not absolute, yet partial or low-level tolerance is stable and remains at the same level despite further i.d. courses of sensitizing injections.

The persistence of unresponsiveness is demonstrated in TABLE 3, in which the sensitizing procedure, following the feedings of 31 animals at the same time, was applied only after rest periods staggered between 73 and 298 days.[13] Each test group was accompanied by normal, aging animals as positive controls. Further pursuit of the duration of unresponsiveness by this procedure would not be rewarding, since guinea pigs aged one year or more do not sensitize to contact reactivity as well as younger stock, and a degree of false unresponsiveness enters into the tabulation.

The specificity of the induced tolerance is illustrated in TABLE 4. Tolerance is limited to the chemical that has been fed.[13] (It had been determined in a prior experiment that concurrent use of a second allergen does not appreciably distort the observed degree of tolerance even though both allergens couple to self carriers.)

Constraints on Antibody Synthesis by Tolerizing with Haptens

A majority of guinea pigs sensitized to TNCB by a series of i.d. injections (0.25 μg each) will produce some amount of detectable anti-TNP antibody of IgG_1 class, the antibody that is responsible for anaphylaxis in this animal. It was therefore surprising that animals fed TNCB gave little evidence of anaphylaxis after the sensitizing course, whether tested with picrylated (TNP) proteins of guinea pig serum or with TNP-casein (TABLE 5). In a more revealing experiment, fed animals were injected i.p. with 5 mg TNP–guinea pig serum on five occasions, rested for four weeks, and tested for anaphylaxis with TNP-casein as a hapten-specific antigen: there were only traces of anaphylactic reactivity; in contrast, all controls died. The resistance to antibody synthesis pertains only to stimulation by hapten coupling with self and by preformed hapten–guinea pig

TABLE 1

UNRESPONSIVENESS TO SENSITIZATION SECURED BY PRIOR FEEDING
OF 2,4-DINITROCHLOROBENZENE *

	Contact Tests		
Treatment	1%	0.33%	0.1%
Feeding of DNCB	+±	tr.	0
	(+±)	(tr.)	(tr.)
	(±)	0	0
	(±)	0	0
	±	tr.	f.tr.
	(tr)	tr.	0
	tr.	f.tr.	0
	(f.tr.)	0	0
	(f.tr.)	0	0
	f.tr.	0?	0
	0?	0	0
None	(+++++)	(+++++)	(+)
	+++++	++++	(±)
	+++++	+++±	(±)
	+++++	+++	±
	+++++	(+++±)	tr.
	++++	+++	(±)
	+++++	++	±
	++++	(++)	±
	+++±	++	tr.
	+++	±	0

* Male guinea pigs (375 to 450 g) were fed 3 mg DNCB in 0.3 ml olive oil on days 1 to 6, 15 to 20, and 29 to 34. Intradermal sensitizing injections of 2.5 μg DNCB were made on days 50, 51, 53, 55, 57, 59, and 61. Contact tests of single drops of differing concentrations of DNCB in olive oil, placed on day 78, were read at 24 and 48 h. The highest reaction is recorded (within parentheses for 48 h readings). Animals were also tested with the oil vehicle, without reaction. Four normal animals were tested in the same way, also without reaction.

NOTE: The reading scale is described in Materials and Methods. (Adapted from Reference 22, by permission of Academic Press.)

TABLE 2

ESTABLISHMENT OF UNRESPONSIVENESS BY ADMINISTERING PICRYL CHLORIDE

	Experiment A		Experiment B		
Rating	Controls	Percutaneous (contact)	Controls	Intravenous	Feeding
0				5	4
Prac. 0				1	2
f. tr.				1	1
tr.				3	
tr		3	4	5	4
±, ∓		2	1	4	3
+	1			2	
+±		2	1	2	
++			1	2	
+++	1		2	2	
++++	2	2	4	1	
++++±	2		1	1	
+++++	2		3		

NOTE: The numbers of animals falling into each category of contactant sensitivity under Ratings in two experiments are indicated; the "positive" controls were not pretreated before experimental sensitization, along with the pretreated animals, with picryl chloride. Categories are described in Materials and Methods. (Adapted from Reference 13, table 1, with permission.)

conjugates (TABLE 5).[13] If TNP-coupled bovine gamma globulin was used as a non-self carrier, the animals developed anti-TNP precipitins as much as normal animals (TABLE 6) and they succumbed anaphylactically to i.v. injection of TNP-casein. Both IgG_2 and IgG_1 antibodies seem to have been formed. Yet, even with this activated antibody-forming apparatus, they did not respond to contact testing with TNCB.[16]

Unresponsiveness was also demonstrated by feeding picric acid to the guinea

TABLE 3

PERSISTENCE OF UNRESPONSIVENESS (FEEDINGS OF PICRYL CHLORIDE)

Rest Period (d)	Contact Test 1%
73	0, 0, 0, 0, 0, 0, 0, ±
94	0, 0, 0, f. tr.
275	0, 0, 0, 0, 0, 0, 0, ∓, +±, +++±
298	0, 0, 0, 0, 0, tr, ±, ±, +

NOTE: After standard courses of feedings with picryl chloride, no further treatment was given. At the intervals stated, fed animals, along with paired normal animals of equal age, were subjected to 14 or 15 intradermal injections, one per day, then rested for two or three weeks. Contact tests were applied, and a satisfactory degree of contact reactivity was shown in all control groups. Only contact tests in the previously fed animals are shown above. (Adapted from Reference 13, by permission of Harper and Row.)

pigs, for which a special sensitizing method is required, called the "split-adjuvant" technique.[14]

With more reactive allergens—citraconic anhydride, o-chlorobenzoyl chloride, and phthalic anhydride—self-coupling after i.d. injection did produce a low level of circulating antibody and weak contact-type reactivity, but very much less than in the positive control groups. The experience with citraconic

TABLE 4

SPECIFICITY OF UNRESPONSIVENESS: DOUBLE SENSITIZATIONS

	Contact Tests			
	DNCB	o-ClBCl		Olive
Group	1%	10%	2%	Oil
Not fed	+ + + + + +	+ + + + + +	+ + +	prac. 0
	+ + + + ±	+ + + + ±	+ +	0
	+ + +	+ + + + + ±	+ +	0
	+ + + ±	+ + + + +	+ +	0
	+ + + + ±	+ + + + + + ±	+ + + + + ±	0
Fed DNCB	+ +	+ + + + + + ±	+ + + ±	prac. 0
	+ ±	+ + + + + + ±	+ + ±	tr
	±	+ + + + + + ±	+ + +	tr.
	tr.	+ +	tr	0
	±	+ + + + + + ±	+ + + +	prac. 0
	tr.	+ + + + + ±	+ + + ±	prac. 0
Fed o-ClBCl	+ + + + ±	+ +	±	tr
	+ ±	+	±	0
	+ + + +	+	±	prac. 0
	+ + + + +	+ ±	tr	0
	+ + + + +	+ ±	±	0
	+ + + + + ±	+ + + + +	+ + + + +	±
Toxicity controls	0	prac. 0	0	0
	f.tr.	tr	prac. 0	prac. 0
	0	prac. 0	0	0

NOTE: To ensure sensitization to two chemical allergens (top row), it was necessary to alternate the injections, one on every other day, until six injections of DNCB and five injections of ortho-chlorobenzoyl chloride (o-ClBCl) had been given. DNCB was injected in 0.1 ml alcoholic saline i.d. to deliver 0.25 μg, o-ClBCl in 0.05 ml olive oil to deliver 10 μg. Of the doubly sensitized animals, one group had previously been fed with DNCB, another group with o-ClBCl, and the others not fed. All were tested at one time, and readings at 24 h are recorded. (Adapted from Reference 13, by permission of Harper and Row.)

anhydride will be described in some detail. This chemical, α-methyl maleyl anhydride, reacts immediately with water to yield citraconic acid. A total of 18 or 30 feedings were given, each 0.3 ml corn oil containing 1% anhydride. Two animals fed 30 times were then shown to have developed no IgG_1 antibody, since they were not anaphylactically sensitive to citraconyl–guinea pig serum proteins. The remaining 16 fed animals plus 11 normal animals were subjected

TABLE 5

INHIBITION OF ANAPHYLACTIC SENSITIZATION BY PRIOR FEEDINGS
OF PICRYL CHLORIDE

Antigen i.v. Conjugate	Dose (mg)	Animals Fed Picryl Chloride	Control Animals
	Part A:	Sensitized by intradermal injections of picryl chloride	
Picryl-GPS	10	0, 0?, tr?, tr., tr.	
	6	Slight	
	5		D_3*
	2		D_4, +++, +, ∓
	Part B:	Sensitized with picrylated guinea pig serum	
Picryl Casein	30	+±, 0, 0, 0, 0	
	20	D_4, tr., 0, 0	D_{32}, tr.
	15		D_5
	10	0, 0?, 0?, 0?	D_5, D_6, +, +
	5		D_6, D_{15}, ++++$_{240}$, +++

* Subscripts represent the time in minutes. Nonfatal anaphylactic symptoms are rated + to +++. D = death; tr. = trace; 0 = negative; 0? indicates slight chewing; GPS = guinea pig serum.

NOTE: In Part A, 16 feedings of 3 mg picryl chloride were made over a period of 30 d. After 26 d, 12 injections of 2.5 µg picryl chloride were made (0.1 ml volumes) intradermally into all animals over 22 d. After a resting period of 19 d, contact tests were made, and 10 d later the above tests were carried out.

In Part B, 15 feedings of 3 mg picryl chloride or of the vehicle (corn oil) were made over a period of 31 d. After a further 45 d, 5 mg picrylated guinea pig serum was injected intraperitoneally on five occasions during a period of two weeks. Testing for the anaphylactic state, as shown, was made one month later. (Adapted from Reference 13, by permission of Harper and Row.)

to sensitization after a resting period of 32 d, five i.d. injections with 50 µg of the anhydride in 0.05 ml corn oil being given over three weeks. On day 9, after the third i.d. injection, the control animals exhibited 14 to 19 mm reactions at 24 h, with livid and scabby centers. The fed animals showed a mild but positive skin reaction. Following the fifth i.d. injection, the controls gave pronounced "mixed" reactions, both cellular sensitivity and Arthus-type antibody-mediated reactions; only four of the pre-fed animals exhibited such large reactions. Because the circulating antibody masked the cell-mediated reactivity, we performed superficial scratch tests using a sewing needle drawn across a droplet of 25% anhydride in dioxane. The fed animals gave no significant reaction at 24 h, unlike the positive controls, which had pronounced reactions of equal width on both ventral and dorsal sides of the scratch on the midline of a flank.

The experience with feeding phthalic anhydride was similar and is summarized in TABLE 7. Also, the feeding of another water-labile allergen, o-chlorobenzoyl chloride, led to the same result, a mild production of antibody and only slight contactant reaction, as opposed to the pronounced reactivity of the controls.

With the application of a special method of sensitizing, the combination method described in Materials and Methods, even animals fed with TNCB could be rendered contact-sensitive to a degree: they responded in contact testing to 0.3% TNCB in corn oil, whereas the controls responded to concentrations 50 to 100 times smaller.[16] Such an outcome reinforces the concept of low-level partial tolerance, not the "wiping out" of reactive clones.

Other Studies with Pre-Fed Guinea Pigs

Serum of pre-fed animals, not subjected to sensitization, contained no blocking antibody, and passively administered (i.v.) guinea pig IgG_1 anti-TNP antibody showed no accelerated decay in the circulation, which event would signal the existence of hapten-protein complexes *in vivo*.[18] Nor were any such depots apparent in the subsequent experiments of Dr. Roy E. Ritts, who fed 1-^{14}C-picryl chloride and examined sections by autoradiography.[13] Transfer of the cells of unresponsive animals to normal outbred recipients did not impose any evident degree of tolerance.[18]

When tolerant guinea pigs were used as recipients of cells from outbred TNCB-sensitized donors (cells of paraffin oil–induced peritoneal exudates taken at 48 h, or spleens, or lymph nodes), they reacted normally in acceptance of contact reactivity, but their inherent tolerance remained. Normal animals undergo a boosting effect from skin tests made immediately after cellular transfer and develop a moderate degree of active sensitization, but the tolerant recipients reverted to the unresponsive state as soon as the donated cells were rejected.[21, 22] Polak, using allogeneic recipients in such a transfer and noting some persistence of the sensitivity, concluded that the donated cells "terminated the state of immunological tolerance!"[23]

Attempts were made to overcome the tolerant state to TNCB by transferring the cells of normal animals before undertaking active sensitization. All such

TABLE 6

PRODUCTION OF PICRYL-SPECIFIC ANTIBODY BY PICRYL CHLORIDE–FED GUINEA PIGS WITHOUT INCITEMENT OF PICRYL-SPECIFIC DELAYED HYPERSENSITIVITY

Group	Initial Treatment	Method of Attempted Sensitization *	Contact Sensitivity to 1% PCl	Immunization Attempted †	Anti-picryl Precipitins Detected †	Method of Attempted Sensitization *	Contact Sensitivity to PCl ⅓%	1%
A ‡	PCl-fed	i.d.	0/4	PBGG+alumina	3/4	—	—	0/4
B	PCl-fed	—	—	PBGG+alumina	7/7	i.d.	1/7	1/7
C	None	—	—	PBGG+alumina	6/7	i.d.	5/7	5/7
D	None	—	—	—	—	i.d.	5/7	6/7

* A shortened series of four daily injections of 2.5 μg picryl chloride, made intradermally (i.d.), was given.

† The precipitin test, conducted with picrylated chicken serum albumin, measured picryl-specific antibody.

‡ Animals of this group were fed on various abbreviated schedules: one received a 2% solution four times in one week, others were fed a 1% solution, one on four occasions in two weeks, and the remainder on nine occasions in three weeks.

NOTE: Adapted from Reference 16, by permission of the Journal of Experimental Medicine.

238 Annals New York Academy of Sciences

attempts failed. In order to secure a lasting "adoptive" transfer, members of Sewell Wright's family 13 guinea pigs were used. Since our breeding program had led us to establish inbred sublines of family 13, we used closely related animals as donors and recipients, such as parents, uncles, sibs, and children within the same subline. Family 13 cells were transferred i.v. either directly or after mild x-irradiation of the recipients; also, cells were taken from animals presensitized to o-chlorobenzoyl chloride and providing clones capable of transferring contactant hypersensitivity, tuberculin hypersensitivity, and a continuing synthesis of IgG$_1$-specific anti-o-chlorobenzoyl-conjugate antibody. Such procedures did not convert TNCB-tolerant family 13 guinea pigs into animals that could be sensitized with TNCB, although the "signal" clones continued to synthesize antibody for several months and maintained the contact sensitivity and tuberculin sensitivity (unpublished experiments).

TABLE 7

ESTABLISHMENT OF TOLERANCE TO CONTACT DERMATITIS
BY ADMINISTERING PHTHALIC ANHYDRIDE

Ratings	Test with 7.5% Phthalyl Chloride		Test with 5% Phthalyl Chloride	
	Pre-Fed	Controls	Pre-Fed	Controls
Prac. 0			1	
f. tr.			1	
tr	1		3	
±, +	2		1	1
+	1		1	
++, ++	2		1	2
++, +++	2	1		
++++		1		
+++++		2		5
++++++		3		

NOTE: Guinea pigs were fed 0.4 ml corn oil containing 2.4 mg phthalic anhydride in 30 feedings over 34 d, then rested for 22 d. Two tested and shown not to be anaphylactically sensitive to phthalyl–guinea pig serum proteins. The remaining eight animals and eight normals were sensitized by 5 i.d. injections of 0.05 ml corn oil with 100 μg phthalic anhydride. While both groups produced anti-phthalyl antibodies, the amount produced by the pre-fed animals was only in a low concentration. The reactions of two animals are pictured in figure 2 of Reference 13.

A Role of Tolerance in Active Sensitizations

The above-mentioned experiments have been concerned with establishing substantial degrees of unresponsiveness to chemical allergens. Unanticipated information pointing to a regular role of low-level unresponsiveness came to light when Dr. Egon Macher injected very small amounts of radiolabeled TNCB (0.25 μg, 1 nmol) or DNCB (5 μg, or 25 nmol) i.d. into an ear to trace the temporal development of sensitivity in relation to timed excisions of the injected ear.[24, 25] It is sufficient to state that the event of sensitization could be linked with the very small proportion of these doses that became bound locally in the ear tissue. The amount of hapten that passed directly into the blood vessels of the ear was measured, and the equivalent amount was injected i.v. into normal animals. These, along with new animals, were then sensitized.[25] Evidence was obtained for a measure of tolerance in these animals. Deliberate applications were then made of small doses of the haptens by various routes (FIGURE 2). In FIGURE 2bB, i.v. injection of a subsensitizing amount of cold DNCB was given. Similarly, subsensitizing doses of TNCB (FIGURE 2aA) or DNCB (FIGURE 2bA) were given intradermally. Further, single contact applications of 0.02 ml olive oil with 1% cold TNCB were made on 27 animals (FIGURE 2c). In all these procedures, 50 to 60% of the animals were rated $+$ or less after the deliberate sensitizing course and final contact test; the remainder were somewhat displaced in the ratings scale from the positive controls, but they showed substantial contactant sensitivity. From these and other—unpublished—experiments, we are sure that every active sensitization with simple chemical haptens is a result of two opposing forces, namely, sensitization and a measure of tolerance.

Other Experiments Prior to the Concept of Suppressor Cells

These experiments employed feedings of 27 mg in three weeks, or 45–54 mg over five weeks, yet it seemed that the tolerance was being established by low-dose retention. Radiolabeled TNCB, studied by Dr. Ritts, was rapidly excreted in urine, bile, and feces, chiefly as picric acid. Mistakenly, and stubbornly, we persisted in the idea that long-term tolerance must rest upon retained hapten fixed to tissue, but such a depot was sought in vain. Passively administered specific antibody had a normal clearance time,[18] autoradiographic studies of tissue sections exposed for many months were negative—apart from a trace in one thymus—and tissue sections examined with fluorescent rabbit anti-picryl antibody were not stained (Dukes and Chase, unpublished).

That low-dose tolerance indeed was sufficient was shown in 1966 by Battisto and Miller, who injected 12.5 to 50 μg TNCB directly into the mesenteric vein (or the jugular vein) on two occasions: 19 out of 44 (43%) were unresponsive.[26] In a further step, Battisto and Bloom made a single i.v. injection of TNP-guinea pig "membranes" (picrylated spleen cells living or heated, erythrocyte stromata, erythrocytes) and secured unresponsiveness in 43 out of 54 (79%) of the treated animals.[27] This was not the first trial: in 1941, the writer had injected citraconyl–guinea pig stromata into guinea pigs i.p. and had secured some cases of tolerance, but the method was not promising if the goal was to induce tolerance regularly. Yet, despite the variability of the method, Battisto and Bloom properly pointed out that animals that responded to hapten-coupled particulates demonstrated that the tolerizing antigen need "not reach all potentially immunocompetent cells." [28] But few workers were then ready to muse on precursors and cell types with special functions. Still, the concept of tolerance struck home, and other studies were undertaken, strikingly by Leskowitz with arsanilic acid conjugated to acetylated tyrosine.[29, 30]

Particularly in the sixties, excellent studies of experimental sensitization were made with guinea pigs. The phenomenon of tolerance was confirmed and new facts came to the fore. Such studies were made in this country by Salvin and his colleagues Smith and Coe,[31-33] in England by Turk *et al.* and Asherson,

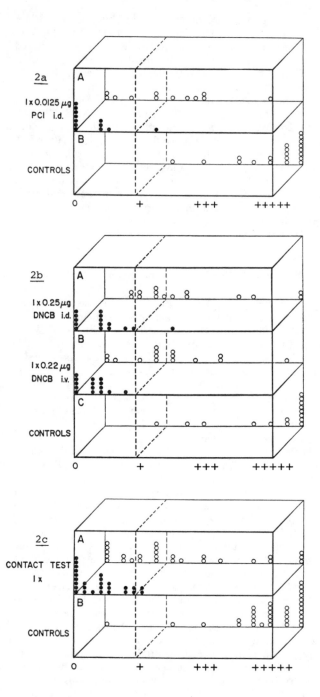

in Switzerland by J. A. Frey *et al.*, a team that Polak joined in 1968; he is building on these observations with great originality.[34] We shall mention several facets of studies from these sources, but we shall not consider the recent studies with isologous and congenic mice, which appear elsewhere in this volume.

A variety of experiments was undertaken to seek possible factors in the induction of tolerance. Tolerance was not changed by initial splenectomy (Ritts and Chase, unpublished) or thymectomy.[35] And young germ-free guinea pigs, with their underdeveloped lymphatic apparatus, could be tolerized.[36] Results suggesting circulating cells as active components came later: tolerized mothers gave birth to normal offspring [37] (seen also in early experiments by Chase), unless unresponsiveness was induced in late pregnancy.[37] Further, parabiosis between tolerized and normal autologous partners rendered the normal partner tolerant within 10 days.[38]

The reports of tolerance led several dermatologists to turn to man without prior study of their procedures on animals. White and Baer made 23 applications of highly dilute DNCB on the skin of one forearm; [39] Grolnick had his volunteers swallow tincture of krameria before meals for many weeks.[40] Neither procedure was effective. Later, from 1964–1971, Lowney made an orderly approach, first with *para*-nitrosodimethyl aniline (NDMA) on guinea pigs and later with DNCB in man.[41-44] These studies showed that an infusion into the bowel of a guinea pig with 0.2 to 2.0 mg NDMA would result in low or depressed sensitization scores. In human subjects (FIGURE 3), DNCB in acetone was applied to the buccal surface of alternate cheeks; the subjects breathed rapidly to evaporate the acetone and deposit the allergen. Later, these volunteers and 37 normal individuals were given a sensitizing course. By this procedure, only 21% of the new volunteers failed to become sensitive (FIGURE 3, bottom panel); the pretreated individuals (FIGURE 3, upper panels) were unresponsive to the extent of 55–58%.[44]

Pomeranz undertook to establish unresponsiveness by giving a single feeding (60 mg) of TNCB to starved guinea pigs.[46-48] The first feedings, made with rapidly absorbable solvents, led to a high level of antibody, although tolerance to contact was secured. (This is a prime example of "split tolerance." [49]) When olive oil was the solvent, rapid absorption did not occur and the animals were both contact-negative and antibody-negative. With this single dose, a minimum of 9 d, optimally 18 d, was needed for tolerance to develop, in agreement with other studies by de Weck, Frey, *et al.*[50-52]

A possible insight into the mechanism of this type of split tolerance comes from Cantor and Dumont.[53] Dogs that were fed DNCB and then injected with the chemical subcutaneously produced no anti-DNP antibody, unlike dogs given a complete portacaval transportation before feeding. The authors suggested that the antigenic complexes that form are normally removed by Kupffer cells in the liver sinusoids and so suppress antibody formation.

FIGURE 2. Partial tolerogenic effects of small doses of simple haptens. In all panels, the near plane (animals represented by filled circles) shows the distribution of sensitivities at the first contact test made with one droplet of 1% hapten in olive oil; readings below the dashed plane ($+$) are judged insignificant. The far plane (animals represented by open circles) shows the distribution of these same animals' sensitivities and those of newly introduced controls (bottom panels) after active sensitization with ten daily injections of 2.5 µg of either picryl chloride (PC1, or TNCB) or DNCB. The significance of these tests is given in the text. (From Reference 25, by permission of the Journal of Experimental Medicine.)

A new and basic concept in understanding the mechanism of tolerance—and perhaps sustained partial tolerance—was introduced by Gershon et al.; that is, the existence of suppressor cells.[54] The outreach of this concept would finally explain early reports on the role of cyclophosphamide in inducing types of unresponsiveness [55, 56] as well as later experiments.[57, 58] These facts are presented in more detail by Dr. Polak (this volume).

DISCUSSION

Our early experiments were reviewed, showing that guinea pigs pretreated with simple allergenic chemicals would be unresponsive, or "tolerant," in subse-

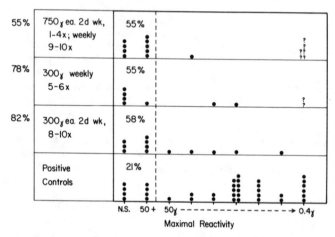

FIGURE 3. Topical sensitization following application of DNCB to buccal mucosa of human volunteers. Acetone solutions of DNCB were applied in the patterns shown at the left, viz., the top row indicates that treatments were given, first, at two-week intervals and then continued at weekly intervals for nine or ten weeks. The sensitizing procedure consisted of applications of 150 μg DNCB in acetone on four sites 2.5 cm in diameter once a week for eight weeks or until sensitivity was noted. The baseline is divided by a dashed line. To the left, individuals were either not sensitive (N.S.) or required more than 50 μg to evidence any reactivity. To the right, the degree of sensitivity is recorded as the smallest dose to which the patients responded. (Adapted from Reference 44, by permission.)

quent attempts to sensitize them with the same chemical (FIGURE 1 and TABLES 1, 4, and 7). Once induced by pre-feeding, tolerance is retained for more than 298 days (TABLE 3), and it is specific for the chemical fed (TABLE 4 and Reference 32).

Although specific unresponsiveness was first encountered following percutaneous application, the most efficient routine was found to be feeding guinea pigs gelatin capsules containing allergen or introducing small amounts of olive oil containing 1% of the chemical past the molar teeth. The efficiency of tolerization by this method was adequate to allow us to assume that tolerance was attained in experiments where sensitizing contacts with the chemical were to be avoided, but confirmed always by attempts to sensitize a subset of the same fed group of animals. Intravenous injections and percutaneous applications were compared with feeding (TABLE 2)—65% and 55%, respectively, were rendered tolerant, and not less so than by feeding, but the successfully tolerized animals had to be discovered by sensitization procedures. In later experiments,[25] single intradermal injections of subsensitizing doses rendered 46–50% of the animals tolerant, while single contact tests with picryl chloride or single intravenous doses of DNCB tolerized 53–55% of the guinea pigs (FIGURE 2).

Similar degrees of successful tolerization were secured by Battisto and Miller by injecting small amounts of TNCB directly into the mesenteric vein on two occasions (43%),[26] and by Battisto and Bloom by intravenous injection of TNP-coupled guinea pig "membranes" (79%).[22] The importance of these successes lies in the demonstration that (1) tolerance is indeed attained as a "low-dose" response, and (2) tolerance can be attained, even if irregularly, by methods in which the tolerizing antigen "need not reach all potentially immunocompetent cells." A further example is cited from the work of Lowney,[44] who treated human volunteers with DNCB on the buccal mucosal surfaces (FIGURE 3). Successful tolerization was encountered in about 35% of his subjects.

Only selected modes of establishing haptenated self will induce significant degrees of unresponsiveness. In work done using groups of mice, the tolerizing efficacy of the adopted route of application is often not established. Instead, the prevalent term is relative "suppression," a statistical average of the responses among groups of mice that will include tolerant, partially tolerant, barely tolerant, and not tolerant individuals.

Evidence is also presented that tolerization that occurs after feedings by self coupling results in a significant disturbance in the formation of anti-hapten immunoglobulin (TABLE 5), but that there is no such "block" if immunization of tolerized animals is conducted with haptenated foreign protein (TABLE 6). In experiments with water-labile sensitizers used for pre-feeding, there is found, in addition to a rather solid degree of contactant-type unresponsiveness, a small but not insignificant synthesis of antibody to haptenated self (TABLE 7).

An explanation for continued long-term tolerance was first thought to be retention of a hapten-protein depot, but searches failed to support the idea. In 1972, Gershon et al. suggested the presence of a class of suppressor cells, which could far outnumber the effector cells.[54] Actual experiments, mostly with the use of cyclophosphamide, have reinforced this concept,[23, 24, 55-58] which is presented in experiments with guinea pigs by Dr. Polak (this volume).

It is shown that immunological tolerance does, indeed, extend to cell-mediated hypersensitivity, even if an extensive review of 1975, broadly titled *Immunological Tolerance*, chose to ignore this aspect of tolerance.[59]

SUMMARY

The first recognition of tolerance and partial tolerance to attempted sensitization with simple allergenic chemicals is described. A proper designation would be the Frei-Sulzberger-Chase phenomenon. Coupling with self occurs in these experiments; there is not only resistance to developing contactant-type sensitivity but also to synthesis of immunoglobulins toward hapten-self complexes. The onset of tolerance is initiated by small doses of haptens.

Various facets of these investigations speak strongly against a concept of clonal deletion as an explanation. The concept of the relative numbers of suppressor and effector cells also argues against clonal deletion. Evidence exists that tolerance can be transferred to syngeneic animals by cells during parabiosis (Polak, this volume).

Contact sensitivity can be imposed on a tolerized guinea pig through a transfer of cells from outbred sensitized donors, but the tolerance remains after the transferred cells have been rejected.

Tolerance could not be overcome in inbred guinea pigs by infusing normal or functionally "labeled" cell populations from close relatives before attempting sensitization, a fact that supports the existence of overwhelmingly large numbers of suppressor cells.

Various routes of application have been explored to find a way to establish the tolerant state. The most successful are (1) feeding of small doses and (2) two intravenous injections of massive doses of DNP- or TNP-benzene sulfonates. Several other methods will effect tolerance in about half the animals, but experimental sensitization is the only method that will locate the tolerized animals.

REFERENCES

1. CHASE, M. W. 1946. Inhibition of experimental drug allergy by prior feeding of the sensitizing agent. Proc. Soc. Exp. Biol. Med. **61:** 257–59.
2. CHASE, M. W. 1941. Inheritance in guinea pigs of the susceptibility to skin sensitization with simple chemical compounds. J. Exp. Med. **73:** 711–26.
3. CHASE, M. W. 1953. The inheritance of susceptibility to drug allergy in guinea pigs. Trans. N.Y. Acad. Sci. Ser. 2 **15:** 78–82.
4. FREI, W. 1928. Ueber willkürliche Sensibilisierung gegen chemisch definierte Substanzen. I. Mitteilung: Untersuchungen mit Neosalvarsan am Menschen. Klin. Wochenschr. **7:** 539–42.
5. KAPLUN, B. J. & J. M. MOREINIS. 1930. Versuch der experimentellen Sensibilisierung gegen Salvarsan, bei Menschen und Tieren. Acta Derm. Venereol. **11:** 295–304.
6. FREI, W. 1928. Ueber willkürliche Sensibilisierung gegen chemisch definierte Substanzen. II. Mitteilung: Untersuchungen mit Neosalvarsan am Tier. (Salvarsanexantheme beim Tier.) Klin. Wochenschr. **7:** 1026–31.
7. SULZBERGER, M. B. 1929. Zur Frage der experimentellen Salvarsan Ueberempfindlichkeit. Klin. Wochenschr. **8:** 253–54.
8. SULZBERGER, M. B. 1929. Hypersensitiveness to neoarsphenamine in guinea pigs: Experiments in prevention and desensitization. Arch. Dermatol. Syphilis **20:** 669–97.
9. CHASE, M. W. 1963. Tolerance towards chemical allergens. *In* La Tolérance Acquise et la Tolérance Naturelle à l'Egard de Substances Antigéniques Définies. Colloques Internationaux du Centre National de la Recherche Scientifique, No. 116: 139–58.
10. FREY, J. R., A. L. DE WECK & H. GELEICK. 1966. Sensitization, immunological tolerance and desensitization of guinea pigs to neoarsphenamine. I. Sensitization to NEO. Overall results and experiments on the skin sensitizing techniques. Int. Arch. Allergy Appl. Immunol. **30:** 288–312.
11. FREY, J. R., A. L. DE WECK & H. GELEICK. 1966. Sensitization, immunological tolerance and desensitization of guinea pigs to neoarsphenamine. II. Influence of various factors on sensitization to NEO. Int. Arch. Allergy Appl. Immunol. **30:** 385–404.
12. FREY, J. R., A. L. DE WECK & H. GELEICK. 1966. Sensitization, immunological

tolerance and desensitization of guinea pigs to neoarsphenamine. III. Immunological tolerance to NEO. Int. Arch. Allergy Appl. Immunol. **30:** 428–45.

13. CHASE, M. W., J. R. BATTISTO & R. E. RITTS. 1963. The Acquisition of Immunologic Tolerance *via* Simple Allergenic Chemicals. *In* Conceptual Advances in Immunology and Oncology, 16th Ann. Symp. Fundamental Cancer Research, 1962 at Univ. Texas M.D. Anderson Hosp. & Tumor Inst., Houston, Texas: 395–416. Harper and Row. New York.

14. CHASE, M. W. & H. C. MAGUIRE, JR. 1973. Studies on the sensitization of animals with simple chemical compounds. XIV. Further studies on sensitization of guinea pigs with picric acid. Int. Arch. Allergy Appl. Immunol. **45:** 513–42.

15. CHASE, M. W. 1954. Experimental sensitization with particular reference to picryl chloride. Int. Arch. Allergy Appl. Immunol. **5:** 163–91.

16. BATTISTO, J. B. & M. W. CHASE. 1965. Induced unresponsiveness to simple allergenic chemicals. II. Independence of delayed-type hypersensitivity and formation of circulating antibody. J. Exp. Med. **121:** 591–606.

17. LANDSTEINER, K. & M. W. CHASE. 1941. Studies on the sensitization of animals with simple chemical compounds. IX. Skin sensitization induced by injections of conjugates. J. Exp. Med. **73:** 431–38.

18. BATTISTO, J. R. & M. W. CHASE. 1963. Immunological unresponsiveness to sensitization with simple chemical compounds. A search for antibody-absorbing depots of allergen. J. Exp. Med. **118:** 1021–35.

19. CHASE, M. W. 1976. Semiquantitative passive cutaneous anaphylaxis. *In* Methods in Immunology and Immunochemistry, Vol. 5. C. A. Williams and M. W. Chase, Eds.: 22–26. Academic Press. New York.

20. BLOOM, B. R. & M. W. CHASE. 1967. Transfer of delayed-type hypersensitivity: A critical review and experimental study in the guinea pig. Prog. Allergy **10:** 151–255.

21. CHASE, M. W. 1959. Models for hypersensitivity studies. *In* Cellular and Humoral Aspects of the Hypersensitive States. H. S. Lawrence, Ed.: 251–78. Hoeber-Harper. New York.

22. CHASE, M. W. 1967. Hypersensitivity to simple chemicals. The Harvey Lectures, Series **61:** 169–203. Academic Press. New York.

23. POLAK, L. 1977. Immunological Aspects of Contact Sensitivity. *In* Advances in Modern Toxicology, Vol. 4: Dermatotoxicology and Pharmacology. F. N. Marzulli & H. I. Maibach, Eds.: 225–88. Hemisphere. Washington, D.C.

24. MACHER, E. & M. W. CHASE. 1969. Studies on the sensitization of animals with simple chemical compounds. XI. The fate of labeled picryl chloride and dinitrochlorobenzene after sensitizing injections. J. Exp. Med. **129:** 81–102.

25. MACHER, E. & M. W. CHASE. 1969. Studies on the sensitization of animals with simple chemical compounds. XII. The influence of excision of allergenic depots on onset of delayed hypersensitivity and tolerance. J. Exp. Med **129:** 103–21.

26. BATTISTO, J. R. & J. MILLER. 1962. Immunologic unresponsiveness produced in adult guinea pigs by parenteral introduction of minute quantities of hapten or protein. Proc. Soc. Exp. Biol. Med. **111:** 111–15.

27. BATTISTO, J. R. & B. R. BLOOM. 1966. Mechanism of immunologic unresponsiveness: A new approach. Fed. Proc. Fed. Am. Soc. Exp. Biol. **25:** 152–59.

28. BATTISTO, J. R. & B. R. BLOOM. 1966. Dual immunological unresponsiveness induced by cell membrane coupled hapten or antigen. Nature (London) **212:** 156–57.

29. LESKOWITZ, S. 1967. Production of hapten-specific unresponsiveness in adult guinea-pigs by prior injection of monovalent conjugates. Immunology **13:** 9–17.

30. COLLOTTI, C. & S. LESKOWITZ. 1968. Immunogens and non-immunogens in the induction of tolerance. Nature (London) 222: 97–99.
31. SMITH, R. F. 1961. Immunological tolerance of non-living antigens. Adv. Immunol. 1: 67–129.
32. COE, J. E. & S. B. SALVIN. 1963. The specificity of allergic reactions. VI. Unresponsiveness to simple chemicals. J. Exp. Med. 117: 401–23.
33. SALVIN, S. B. & R. F. SMITH. 1964. The specificity of allergic reactions. VII. Immunologic unresponsiveness, delayed hypersensitivity, and circulating antibodies to proteins and hapten-protein conjugates J. Exp. Med. 119: 851–68.
34. POLAK, L. 1980. Immunological aspects of contact sensitivity: An experimental study. Monogr. Allergy 15: 1–170.
35. FOLLETT, D. A., J. R. BATTISTO & B. R. BLOOM. 1966. Tolerance to defined chemical hapten produced in adult guinea pigs after thymectomy. Immunology 11: 73–76.
36. FRIEDLAENDER, M. H., H. BAER & P. R. B. MCMASTER. 1972. Contact sensitivity and immunologic tolerance in germ-free guinea pigs. Proc. Soc. Exp. Biol. Med. 141: 522–26.
37. POLAK, L. & C. RINCK. 1979. Induction of tolerance to DNCB-contact sensitivity in guinea pig fetuses. In Function and Structure of the Immune System. W. Müller-Ruchholtz and H. K. Müller-Hermelink, Eds.: 313–17. Plenum. New York.
38. POLAK, L. 1975. The transfer of tolerance to DNCB-contact sensitivity in guinea pigs by parabiosis J. Immunol. 114: 988–91.
39. WHITE, W. A. & R. L. BAER. 1950. Failure to prevent experimental eczematous sensitization; observations on "spontaneous" flare-up phenomenon. J. Allergy 21: 344–48.
40. GROLNICK, M. 1951. Studies in contact dermatitis. VIII. The effect of feeding antigen on the subsequent development of skin sensitization. J. Allergy 22: 170–74.
41. LOWNEY, E. D. 1965. Immunologic unresponsiveness appearing after topical application of contact sensitizers in the guinea pig. J. Immunol. 95: 397–403.
42. LOWNEY, E. D. 1968. Attenuation of contact sensitization in man. J. Invest. Dermatol. 50: 244–49.
43. LOWNEY, E. D. 1968. Immunologic unresponsiveness to a contact sensitizer in man. J. Invest. Dermatol. 51: 411–19.
44. LOWNEY, E. D. 1971. Tolerance of dinitrochlorobenzene, a contact sensitizer, in man. J. Allergy Clin. Immunol. 48: 28–35.
45. POMERANZ, J. R. & P. S. NORMAN. 1966. Concomitant anaphylactic sensitization and contact unresponsiveness following the infusion or feeding of picryl chloride to guinea pigs. J. Exp. Med. 124: 69–80.
46. POMERANZ, J. R. 1969. Induction of tolerance by a single feeding of picryl chloride. Clin. Res. 17: 277.
47. POMERANZ, J. R. 1970 Immunologic unresponsiveness following a single feeding of picryl chloride. J. Immunol. 104: 1486–90.
48. POMERANZ, J. R. 1971. Studies on the evolution of immunologic unresponsiveness following hapten feeding. J. Invest. Dermatol. 56: 451–45.
49. BRENT, L. & H. COURTENOY. 1962. On the induction of split tolerance. In Mechanisms of Immunological Tolerance. M. Hašek, A. Lengerová & M. Voytišková, Eds.: 113–21 Czechoslovak Academy of Sciences. Prague. Academic Press. New York.
50. DE WECK, A. L. & J. R. FREY. 1966. Immunotolerance to simple chemicals. Monogr. Allergy 1: 1–142.
51. FREY, J. R., A. L. DEWECK, H. GELEICK & L. POLAK. 1971. Immunological tolerance in contact hypersensitivity to DNCB. Dose and time dependence. Cellular kinetics. Immunology 21: 483–87.

52. FREY, J. R., A. L. DE WECK, H. GELEICK & L. POLAK. 1972. The induction of immunological tolerance during the primary response. Int. Arch. Allergy Appl. Immunol. **42:** 278–99.
53. CANTOR, H. M. & A. E. DUMONT. 1967. Hepatic suppression of sensitization to antigen absorbed into the portal system. Nature (London) **215:** 744–45.
54. GERSHON, R. K., P. COHEN, R. HENCIN & S. A. LIEBHAGER. 1972. Suppressor T cells. J. Immunol. **108:** 586–90.
55. MAGUIRE, H. C., JR. & H. I. MAIBACH. 1961. Specific immune tolerance to anaphylactic sensitization (egg albumin) induced in the guinea pig by cyclophosphamide. J. Allergy **32:** 406–8.
56. MAGUIRE, H. C., JR., H. I. MAIBACH & L. W. MINISCE, JR. 1961. Inhibition of guinea pig anaphylactic sensitization with cyclophosphamide. J. Invest. Dermatol. **36:** 235–36.
57. PARKER, D., J. L. TURK & R. J. SCHEPER. 1975. Central and peripheral action of suppressor cells in contact sensitivity in the guinea-pig. Immunology **30:** 593–97.
58. SOMMER, G., D. PARKER & J. L. TURK. 1975. Epicutaneous induction of hyporeactivity to contact sensitization. Demonstration of suppressor cells induced by contact with 2,4-dinitrothiocyanate benzene. Immunology **29:** 517–25.
59. HOWARD, J. G. & N. A. MITCHISON. 1975. Immunological tolerance. Prog. Allergy **18:** 97–204.

ORAL TOLERANCE

Martin F. Kagnoff

Department of Medicine
University of California, San Diego
La Jolla, California 92093

INTRODUCTION

Food, bacterial, viral, parasitic, and chemical antigens encountered in the gastrointestinal tract present a major antigenic challenge to the host and are important in the development and function of the host immune system. A great deal has been learned over the past several years about the character and regulation of immune responses initiated by enteric antigen exposure. Studies from many different laboratories have increased our understanding of the gastrointestinal immune system, its function in normal host-environment interactions, and its role in the pathogenesis of certain intestinal and systemic diseases.[1, 2] My laboratory has had a particular interest in the intestinal immune response and in host-environment interactions that are mediated by the gastrointestinal immune system. As described below, diminished or absent systemic immune responsiveness to an antigen after exposure to that antigen by the enteric route appears to be an important facet of the host's interaction with many different antigens in the gastrointestinal tract. This phenomenon has been termed "oral tolerance."

ORAL TOLERANCE

Antigen encountered by the gastrointestinal route can stimulate an intestinal mucosal IgA antibody response, often in the absence of a measurable systemic immune response.[3, 4] This local IgA antibody is thought to prevent the absorption of antigenic material from the intestinal tract and to mediate local protective immunity to viruses and bacteria. In addition, as shown initially by Wells using proteins[5] and by Chase using dinitrochlorobenzene,[6] the ability to stimulate an immune response in sites outside the intestine may be decreased if the animal has previously been exposed to the same antigen by the enteric route. Considering the ability of varying quantities of antigenic material to be absorbed across the normal or inflamed intestine, it seems logical that mechanisms resulting in decreased systemic immune responses to such antigens might be highly advantageous to the host, particularly since absorbed antigenic material could initiate potentially harmful allergic responses or crossreact with self components and result in the induction of autoimmune reactions.[7]

Several investigators, including ourselves, have studied the factors responsible for decreased immune responses observed during systemic challenge with an antigen originally encountered by the gastrointestinal route.[8-30] These studies have made use of a variety of different antigens and test systems. Different types of immune responses have been assessed (*e.g.*, antibody-forming cells, circulating antibody, passive cutaneous anaphylaxis, delayed-type hypersensi-

0077-8923/82/0392-0248 $1.75/0 © 1982, NYAS

tivity (DTH), cytotoxic allograft reactions, and T cell proliferative responses). In the various studies, decreased systemic immune responses after antigen feeding have been reported to result from mechanisms involving antibody (possibly including anti-idiotypic antibody), antigen-antibody complexes, soluble factors, and suppressor T cells. Despite marked differences in experimental design (feeding protocols, antigen and species of animal used, and type of response measured), a common feature of all studies has been the fact that the decreased immune responses after antigen feeding are, to a remarkable degree, antigen specific. This paper summarizes our studies on the development of systemic immune unresponsiveness after antigen feeding.

SUPPRESSION OF HUMORAL ANTIBODY RESPONSES TO ERYTHROCYTE ANTIGENS

The ability of enterically administered antigens to alter humoral- and cell-mediated immune responses in extraintestinal sites in mice has been studied using heterologous erythrocytes. As shown in FIGURE 1, profound suppression of the splenic anti-SRBC (sheep red blood cell) response was seen when SRBC-fed mice were subsequently challenged parenterally with that antigen. The IgM response in mice that had continuously ingested SRBC for more than three weeks was diminished by approximately 75 to 90% compared with that seen in controls. In contrast, IgA and IgG responses initially increased greater than 2.5-fold after erythrocyte feeding; but, with continuous ingestion of SRBC for eight weeks or more, they too were significantly diminished. Suppression of the anti-SRBC response in SRBC-fed mice persisted for more than four months after the feeding was stopped.

The reduction in the IgM response was not due to a lack of IgM B cell precursors for SRBC.[17] Instead, active suppression appeared to be responsible for the diminished IgM response. Adoptive transfer studies failed to show that T suppressor cells were responsible.[17] Rather, suppression appeared to be due to a soluble factor in the serum of mice fed the antigen. Suppression could be transferred to normal mice by the injection of serum from SRBC-fed mice (TABLE 1). The suppressor factor also suppressed the induction of IgM anti-SRBC responses in normal spleen cell cultures (TABLE 1). Both in vivo and in vitro suppression was highly antigen specific (TABLE 1). Although the serum factor suppressed the induction of IgM anti-SRBC responses, it did not block the expression of previously established splenic IgM anti-SRBC responses in vivo or in vitro.[17] As characterized in culture, suppression mediated by the factor was not H-2 restricted.[17] The suppressor factor was shown to have a molecular weight of approximately 150 000 (FIGURE 2), was heat stable (60° C, 30 min), and contained immunoglobulin determinants (FIGURE 3), but lacked detectable erythrocyte determinants.[17, 26] IgA and IgG in vitro secondary anti-SRBC responses were not inhibited by the serum factor, but were inhibited by hyperimmune mouse anti-SRBC serum (TABLE 2). Thus, the sensitivity of IgM responses to suppression by the serum factor may be higher than that of IgG or IgA responses. Alternatively, separate suppressor factors or suppressor mechanisms may exist for IgM compared with IgA and IgG responses.

Adsorption with SRBC of the sera from SRBC-fed mice totally removed suppressor activity from approximately one-third of the samples examined. Of the remaining samples, one-third retained all suppressor activity after adsorption and one-third retained 50–70% of their suppressor activity. In parallel experiments, adsorption of sera with SRBC consistently removed all suppressor

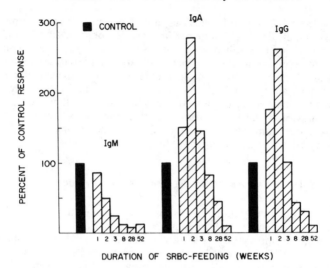

FIGURE 1. Suppression of splenic IgM, IgA, and IgG anti-SRBC responses after i.p. SRBC challenge of SRBC-fed and control mice. BDF_1 mice that had ingested approximately 2×10^9 SRBC per day for 1–52 weeks (hatched bars) and control littermate mice (solid bars) were immunized i.p. with 2×10^8 SRBC. Maximum IgM, IgA, and IgG plaque-forming cell (PFC) responses in SRBC-fed mice are expressed as a percentage of the maximum control response, which was taken at 100%. Control IgM, IgA, and IgG responses were 89 900, 48 600, and 136 900 anti-SRBC PFC per spleen, respectively. IgM anti-sera responses were greatest on day 5 in both fed and control mice, whereas IgA and IgG anti-SRBC responses were greatest on day 9 in control mice and on day 5 in mice fed SRBC for more than eight weeks.

activity from hyperimmune mouse and rabbit anti-SRBC serum with anti-SRBC titers several thousand times greater than those in the sera from SRBC-fed mice.

Several explanations are possible for the variations in the removal of suppressor activity from the serum of SRBC-fed mice after SRBC adsorption.[26] In two-thirds of the sera, SRBC adsorption removed all or part of the suppressor activity and suppression appeared to be mediated, partially or completely, by anti-SRBC antibody. However, SRBC adsorption might not remove suppressor activity mediated by anti-SRBC antibody if such antibody had a low binding affinity for SRBC or was directed against determinants sparsely represented on the SRBC membrane. Alternatively, the erythrocyte determinants presented to the immune system after intestinal digestion of SRBC may induce an antibody response not normally produced after challenge with intact SRBC. Such antibody, although not adsorbed by intact SRBC, might nonetheless suppress an antibody response to SRBC. Further, the variable removal of suppressor activity by SRBC adsorption could be due to the fact that some of the sera contained several types of suppressor factors. SRBC adsorption would not be predicted to remove suppressor activity mediated by either immune complexes or anti-idiotypic antibody. As for immune complexes, the size of the suppressor factor and the failure to remove the suppressor factor by anti-SRBC immuno-adsorbants argue against such complexes playing a major role in the serum-mediated suppression. We have no data for or against the possibility that anti-idiotypic antibody in some sera may be involved in the suppressor mechanism. Finally, we have demonstrated a serum factor in mice injected with a soluble SRBC lysate that is indistinguishable by several criteria from the serum suppressor factor found in SRBC-fed mice.[26] Those studies suggest that exposure to antigen by the enteric route is not required for the production of serum suppressor factors similar or identical to those produced after SRBC feeding.

In other studies, suppression of anti-SRBC responses has been attributed to different serum factors or to soluble factors derived from lymphoid cells of SRBC-fed animals.[9, 28] André et al. described a serum suppressor factor in SRBC-fed mice thought to be an immune complex containing IgA antibody.[9] Unlike ours, their serum factor suppressed the expression of already established IgM anti-SRBC plaque-forming cell (PFC) responses. Moreover, IgM, as well as IgA and IgG, responses were reportedly decreased in mice fed four daily doses of SRBC before intraperitoneal (i.p.) challenge with SRBC.[9] The identical feeding protocol[9] in our laboratory resulted in increased IgA and IgG responses after i.p. SRBC challenge,[17] suggesting that feeding had resulted in priming rather than a decrease in immune responsiveness. Recently, Mattingly and his coworkers have reported the appearance of suppressor cells for SRBC in rats fed with that antigen[18] and have shown that spleen cells from erythrocyte-fed mice can produce two different factors in vitro that have a marked influence on the induction of the in vitro anti-SRBC response.[28] These factors have a molecular weight of 30–40×10^3 and 60–75×10^3 daltons. It was not shown whether or not the factors contained immunoglobulin determinants, and larger molecular weight material in the void volume was reportedly discarded during the purification procedure on Sephadex G-100.[28]

TABLE 1

ABILITY OF SERUM FROM SRBC-FED MICE TO SUPPRESS THE PRODUCTION
OF SPLENIC IgM ANTI-SRBC RESPONSES in Vivo AND in Vitro

Source of Serum Injected or Added to Culture	IgM Anti-SRBC Response after SRBC Challenge	IgM Anti-HRBC Response after HRBC Challenge
In vivo *	PFC per spleen ± S.E.	
None	93 280±10 740	42 470±6940
Normal mouse serum	89 156±8042	Not tested
SRBC-fed mouse serum	8250±1110	40 840±3210
In vitro †	PFC per 10^6 cultured cells ± S.E.	
Normal mouse serum	1306±120	1073±94
SRBC-fed mouse serum ‡	38±14	1133±111

* For in vivo experiments, normal BDF₁ mice were injected with 0.5 ml serum i.p. as indicated and, 8 h later, challenged with either 2×10^8 SRBC or 2×10^8 HRBC i.p. Splenic anti-RBC responses were assayed five days later.

† For in vitro experiments, 1 μl of pooled normal BDF₁ mouse serum or pooled serum from SRBC-fed BDF₁ mice was added to normal spleen cell cultures at the initiation of culture. Cultures were stimulated with 6×10^5 SRBC or HRBC as indicated and assayed four days later.

‡ Cultures stimulated with both SRBC and HRBC showed 90% suppression of the anti-SRBC response, but no significant suppression of the anti-HRBC response, (not shown).

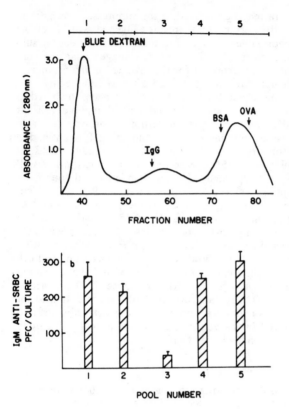

FIGURE 2. Suppressor activity in serum from SRBC-fed BDF₁ mice fractionated on Sephadex G-200. (a) Elution profile of serum from SRBC-fed mice. Individual fractions were placed into five major pools, as depicted. Column markers are depicted by arrows. (b) IgM anti-SRBC responses in cultures of normal BDF₁ spleen cells. Ten μl from pools 1 to 5 of Sephadex G-200–passed serum from SRBC-fed mice were added to cultures containing 10^6 spleen cells. Cultures were then stimulated with SRBC. Values are expressed as the mean $\pm$ SEM of six replicate cultures. Suppressor activity was found predominantly in pool 3.

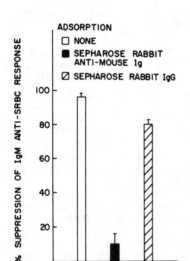

FIGURE 3. Removal of suppressor activity from SRBC-fed mouse serum by Sepharose-coupled anti-mouse immunoglobulin. Sera from SRBC-fed mice that were not adsorbed, or had been adsorbed with Sepharose-coupled rabbit anti-mouse immunoglobulin (Ig) or, as a control, Sepharose-coupled rabbit IgG, were added to cultures containing 10^6 normal BDF₁ spleen cells. Cultures were stimulated with 6×10^5 SRBC and assayed for IgM anti-SRBC responses four days later. As shown, approximately 90% of the suppressor activity was removed from SRBC-fed mouse serum by adsorption with anti-mouse immunoglobulin, but not by adsorption with normal rabbit IgG.

SUPPRESSION OF DELAYED-TYPE HYPERSENSITIVITY REACTIONS TO ERYTHROCYTE ANTIGENS

Feeding mice erythrocyte antigens also resulted in decreased systemic immune responses to the erythrocyte used for feeding as assessed by DTH. Mice fed sheep or horse erythrocytes for two or more weeks could not produce significant DTH reactions to such erythrocytes. Suppression of DTH was specific for the fed antigen, and persisted in part for more than six months after

TABLE 2

EFFECT OF SERUM FROM SRBC-FED MICE AND HYPERIMMUNE MOUSE ANTI-SRBC SERUM ON SPLENIC ANTI-SRBC SECONDARY RESPONSES IN CULTURE *

Source of Serum Added to Culture	Quantity of Serum Added (μl)	IgA and IgG Anti-SRBC PFC per 10^6 Cultured Cells †	
		IgG	IgA
Experiment 1			
Serum, SRBC-fed mice ‡	100	4395	3120
Normal mouse serum	100	4420	3845
No serum	—	3290	3440
Experiment 2			
Mouse anti-SRBC serum ‡§	100	580	0
Normal mouse serum		11 350	11 680
Mouse anti-SRBC serum	10	2475	1030
Normal mouse serum		12 400	14 380
Mouse anti-SRBC serum	1	3990	2640
Normal mouse serum		10 900	10 100
Mouse anti-SRBC serum	0.1	5430	4960
Normal mouse serum		12 280	12 175
No serum	—	12 250	11 350

* Cultures containing 5×10^6 spleen cells from multiply SRBC-primed BDF$_1$ mice were stimulated with 6×10^5 SRBC and assayed five days later.

† Arithmetic mean of triplicate cultures.

‡ These sera suppressed the induction of primary IgM anti-SRBC responses by more than 90% in parallel control cultures containing spleen cells from unprimed mice.

§ The hemagglutination titer of mouse anti-SRBC serum was 1:20 000. The final hemagglutination titer of anti-SRBC sera in culture ranged from 1:4000 to 1:4. Hyperimmune mouse anti-SRBC serum at these concentrations, or diluted as much as 20- or 100-fold beyond a detectable hemagglutination titer, inhibited primary IgM anti-SRBC culture responses by more than 90%.

erythrocyte feeding was stopped (TABLES 3 and 4).[16] Diminished DTH responses were shown to be due to suppressor cells, and not due to antibody.[16] As shown in TABLE 5, adoptive transfer of spleen cells from erythrocyte-fed mice to normal mice inhibited the induction of DTH in the normal mice. Although suppressor cells inhibited the induction phase, or afferent limb of sensitization for DTH, they did not inhibit elicitation of the DTH response in mice with established DTH immunity.[16] Thus, spleen cells sensitized for DTH

TABLE 3

SPECIFICITY OF DIMINISHED DTH REACTIONS IN ERYTHROCYTE-FED MICE *

	DTH Reaction to	
Antigen Fed	SRBC	HRBC
None	65.5±3.3	46.1±4.8
SRBC	2.1±1.3	34.0±0.9
HRBC	58.0±5.1	1.0±0.4

* Mice fed SRBC or horse erythrocytes (HRBC) for four weeks before the study were sensitized with 2.5×10^5 SRBC or HRBC i.v. and footpad challenged with 1.2×10^8 SRBC or HRBC four days later. DTH reactions are expressed as the percentage increase in footpad thickness ± s.e. 24 h after footpad challenge.

could transfer positive DTH reactions equally well to erythrocyte-fed and normal control mice, indicating that suppression was not due to effector blockade.[16]

Although DTH to SRBC was diminished in mice fed SRBC for more than two weeks, examination of the spleens of such mice revealed cells sensitized for DTH as well as suppressor cells. The former were readily demonstrated by footpad swelling after spleen cells were transferred from erythrocyte-fed mice into the footpads of normal mice, followed by local SRBC challenge.[16] In addition, priming for DTH rather than suppression of DTH was seen in the first week after SRBC feeding. Thus, DTH reactions to SRBC were produced by direct SRBC footpad challenge in mice fed SRBC for six to eight days, but not in mice fed SRBC for more than two weeks. Many parallels appear to exist between the suppression of DTH after erythrocyte feeding and the suppression of DTH after ovalbumin feeding.[24]

TABLE 4

DTH REACTIONS AFTER CESSATION OF SRBC FEEDING

	% Increase Footpad Thickness (DTH) ± s.e.		Suppression of DTH in Fed Mice † (%)
Time after SRBC Feeding Discontinued *	Controls	Mice Previously Fed SRBC	
24 h	73±1.1	6.5±1.1	91
2 wk	61±9.7	7.3±3.7	88
6 wk	69±5.1	43±5.0	38
13 wk	59±4.2	25±6.9	58
6 mo	59±5.7	37±4.0	37

* Mice were fed SRBC for four weeks. DTH reactions were studied 24 h to six months after SRBC feeding was discontinued.

† DTH reactions in mice previously fed SRBC compared to DTH reactions in control littermates studied in parallel. DTH reactions were significantly diminished ($p < 0.05$) in previously fed mice at all times examined between 24 h and six months after SRBC feeding was discontinued.

SUPPRESSION OF HUMORAL ANTIBODY RESPONSES TO PROTEIN ANTIGENS

The decreased systemic immune response to soluble proteins after protein feeding has been examined extensively,[11, 13, 14, 19-25] using proteins such as ovalbumin, keyhole limpet hemocyanin, and human gamma globulin. Investigations have demonstrated a decrease in IgG antibody responses, passive cutaneous anaphylaxis, and T cell proliferative responses. In these systems, decreased responses appear to be mediated, at least in part, by suppressor T cells [19-21, 23] that may arise initially in Peyer's patches.[19] Studies using hapten-protein conjugates have demonstrated functional B cells after antigen feeding and suggested that T helper cells may be the target of suppression.[21]

TABLE 5

SPLEEN CELLS FROM SRBC-FED MICE CAN INHIBIT THE INDUCTION
OF DTH REACTIONS IN NORMAL MICE

Source of Spleen Cells *	Number of Spleen Cells Transferred	Increase in Footpad thickness (DTH) ± S.E. (%)
None		44 ± 3.4
SRBC-fed mice	2×10^8	25 ± 2.9 †
Normal mice	2×10^8	65 ± 4.0
SRBC-fed mice	1×10^8	19 ± 1.7 †
Normal mice	1×10^8	48 ± 7.4
SRBC-fed mice	5×10^7	18 ± 3.0 †
Normal mice	5×10^7	N.T. ‡
SRBC-fed mice	1×10^7	23 ± 4.2 †
Normal mice	1×10^7	49 ± 3.2

* Spleen cells from SRBC-fed or normal mice were transferred into normal recipient mice. One hour later, recipients were challenged with 2.5×10^5 SRBC i.v. After four days, mice were footpad challenged with SRBC.
† Values significantly different from mice receiving spleen cells from normal mice or no spleen cells ($p < 0.05$).
‡ N.T., not tested in this experiment. In two different experiments, transfer of 5×10^7 normal spleen cells to control mice did not inhibit the production of DTH.

We have found markedly diminished splenic PFC responses to fowl gamma globulin (FGG) in C57BL/6 mice fed FGG and parenterally challenged with FGG 7–10 d later (TABLE 6). Two or more 20 mg intragastric doses of FGG were consistently required to suppress the IgA and IgG anti-FGG response to i.p. FGG challenge. In mice challenged i.p. with FGG 7–10 d after a single 20 mg FGG feeding, priming rather than suppression of the IgA and IgG anti-FGG response was noted. As with SRBC feeding, serum from FGG-fed mice could transfer suppression to normal mice (TABLE 7).

Spleens from multiply FGG-fed mice yielded normal anti-FGG responses when transferred into lethally irradiated syngeneic recipients. In these experiments, the IgG and IgA anti-FGG response peaked earlier (day 8) when cells from FGG-fed mice, rather than cells from littermate control mice (day 12)

TABLE 6

SUPPRESSION OF ANTI-FGG RESPONSE IN FGG-FED MICE
CHALLENGED PARENTERALLY WITH FGG *

Antigen Feeding	Anti-FGG PFC per Spleen †‡		
	IgM (day 5)	IgG (day 9)	IgA (day 9)
None	2250	56 500	23 600
FGG	170	3575	3180

* C57B1/6 mice fed 20 mg FGG intragastrically for three consecutive days were injected ten days later with 250 μg FGG in alum-pertussis i.p. Splenic anti-FGG responses were assayed five and nine days later.

† IgG and IgA anti-FGG responses were greatest on day 9. IgM anti-FGG responses were greatest on day 5.

‡ Compared to controls, mice fed 20 mg FGG for one day only and later challenged with FGG i.p. demonstrated markedly increased IgG and IgA anti-FGG responses, which were greatest on day 5 (not shown). In contrast, IgM anti-FGG responses were diminished 50 to 75% compared to controls in mice challenged i.p. with FGG seven to ten days after one FGG feeding (not shown).

were transferred. Thus, although decreased responses are seen after FGG feeding, priming also seems to have occurred.

Our data using FGG are similar to the results seen in the SRBC feeding model. However, they contrast with the data reported after ovalbumin feeding. Thus, transfer of suppression from fed to normal mice with serum has not been reported after ovalbumin feeding,[22] unresponsiveness to ovalbumin persisted when spleen cells from fed mice were adoptively transferred to irradiated syngeneic recipients,[20] and systemic antibody responses decreased strikingly after a single 20 mg dose of ovalbumin.[14, 19, 20, 21-23] Our studies suggest that, in addition to T cell suppressor cells, serum factors (e.g., antibody or antigen-antibody complexes) may be important in oral tolerance after protein feeding.

TABLE 7

SERUM FROM FGG-FED MICE SUPPRESSES ANTI-FGG RESPONSES
IN NORMAL MICE *

Serum Transferred	Anti-FGG Response in FGG-Injected Mice (PFC per spleen)		
	IgM	IgG	IgA
None	4500	299 200	159 900
Serum from FGG-fed mice, 0.5 ml †	330	34 500	17 100

* Normal C57B1/6 mice were injected with 0.5 ml serum from FGG-fed mice and challenged 8 h later with 250 μg FGG in alum-pertussis i.p. Splenic anti-FGG responses were assayed nine days later.

† Serum from mice that had been fed 20 mg FGG daily for three days and were bled seven days later.

SUPPRESSION OF HUMORAL ANTIBODY RESPONSES TO POLYSACCHARIDE ANTIGENS

Mice fed the bacterial capsular polysaccharide dextran B1355 [31, 32] had a markedly diminished antibody response to α1,3 determinants on dextran when they were challenged i.p. with that antigen (TABLE 8). These results with a thymus-independent antigen differ from those reported by others.[21] Thus, lipopolysaccharide, polyvinyl pyrolidone, and dinitrophenyl-ficoll did not suppress antibody responses when mice fed these antigens were subsequently challenged parenterally with the same antigens.[21] The differences in these results may be a function of the differences in experimental protocols, particularly in feeding protocols, rather than differences in the effects of the different antigens. Lipopolysaccharide, polyvinyl pyrolidone, and dinitrophenyl-ficoll were fed as single doses of 20 mg or as 20 mg divided over 3 d.[21] Dextran was fed daily for at least 6 d (10 mg per dose) before suppression was noted.

TABLE 8

SUPPRESSION OF THE ANTI-α1,3 DEXTRAN B1355 RESPONSE
IN DEXTRAN-FED MICE CHALLENGED PARENTERALLY WITH DEXTRAN *

Mice	Anti-α1,3 Dextran B1355 Response (PFC per 10^6 spleen cells)		
	IgM	IgA	
Control	3127 ± 385	3673 ± 87	
		$p < 0.001$	$p < 0.01$
Dextran-fed	778 ± 185	204 ± 62	

* Control Balb/c mice and Balb/c mice fed dextran B1355 (10 mg d^{-1}) for eight days were challenged with 100 μg dextran B1355 i.p. seven days after feeding was stopped. Splenic anti-α1,3 dextran responses were assayed five days later. The results are expressed as the arithmetic mean ±S.E.

FAILURE TO SUPPRESS CYTOTOXIC ALLOGRAFT REACTIONS

Priming rather than suppression was seen after mice were fed with cells having different H-2 or non-H-2 gene-coded cell surface alloantigens. Thus, feeding such tumor or spleen cells increased, rather than decreased, precursor cytotoxic T cell populations responding to those antigens in the spleen (FIGURE 4).[15] In addition, mice fed such cells did not have prolonged survival of skin grafts transplanted from donor mice having the same H-2 or non-H-2 gene-coded alloantigenic differences as the cells used for feeding.

DISCUSSION

Enteric exposure to erythrocyte, protein, reactive chemical, and bacterial antigens can decrease the magnitude of a systemic immune response to the same antigen subsequently given by the parenteral route, a phenomenon known as oral tolerance. Feeding such antigens has been variously reported to decrease

IgM, IgG, and IgE serum antibody responses, splenic plaque-forming cell responses, delayed-type hypersensitivity reactions, and *in vitro* T cell proliferative responses.[8-30] Many antigens encountered in the gastrointestinal tract may be absorbed to varying degrees, either intact or as fragments, across the intestine. Processes that result in decreased systemic immune responses to such antigenic material would seem advantageous, in some instances, to the host. This is particularly the case since otherwise harmless nonpathogenic antigens absorbed from the intestine might stimulate systemic allergic reactions or crossreact with self components and lead to autoimmune responses.[7] Although decreased systemic immune responses to food antigens and certain bacterial components and chemicals may be biologically beneficial, systemic unresponsiveness to pathogenic bacteria and viruses that invade the host from the gut often would not be in the host's best interest. Such antigens should activate pathways that result in the production of appropriate protective systemic immune responses.

Our antigen-feeding experiments consistently found evidence for initial priming as well as for subsequent suppression of immune responses in extra-

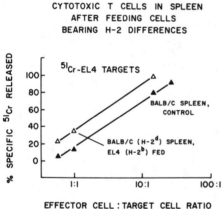

CYTOTOXIC T CELLS IN SPLEEN
AFTER FEEDING CELLS
BEARING H-2 DIFFERENCES

FIGURE 4. Expansion of precursor cytotoxic T lymphocytes in spleen after feeding mice cells having alloantigenic differences coded for by the H-2 major histocompatability complex. Spleen cells from control Balb/c (H-2^d) mice (▲—▲) or Balb/c mice fed 10^7 EL4 (H-2^b) cells three times weekly for one month (△—△) were stimulated in culture for five days with irradiated C57BL/6 (H-2^b) spleen cells. Cytotoxicity was determined using ^{51}Cr-EL4 target cells. Spleens from EL4-fed mice contained approximately 2–3-fold more cytotoxic T lymphocytes against ^{51}Cr-EL4 than spleens from control mice. In additional controls, cytotoxicity was demonstrated to be T cell mediated and specific for H-2^b.

intestinal sites when both were carefully sought. Whether decreased systemic immune responses or priming for the induction of greater systemic immune responses is seen after enteric antigen exposure appears to depend on several factors. Among these factors are the nature of the antigen (*e.g.,* soluble proteins, particulate antigens, cell surface alloantigens, and replicating viruses and microorganisms), the dose, duration, and frequency of antigen exposure, the host's prior enteric and parenteral antigen exposure, the species, strain, and age of the animal used for study, the gastrointestinal microflora (*i.e.,* germ-free or conventional), the type of immune response being evaluated (*i.e.,* antibody or DTH), the time interval between antigen exposure and parenteral stimulation of the systemic immune response, and, possibly, the lymphoid site at which the antigen is first encountered (*e.g.,* some replicating pathogens may invade through the gut mucosa while other antigens are first encountered after uptake into Peyer's patches).

Four of the factors cited above warrant further comment. First, the intestinal microflora seem important to the production of oral tolerance after antigen feeding. SRBC fed to germ-free, but not conventional, mice stimulated a systemic anti-SRBC antibody response.[33] In addition, antibody responses to SRBC i.p. were produced in C3H/HeJ lipopolysaccharide (LPS) nonresponder mice that had been previously fed SRBC, whereas significant responses were not produced by SRBC i.p. in SRBC-fed LPS responder C3H/HeN mice.[34] These findings were interpreted to suggest that LPS derived from gram-negative intestinal bacteria are important in oral tolerance, perhaps by activating suppressor T cells in Peyer's patches.[34] Second, the host's past antigenic exposure is important when considering oral tolerance. We and others have been unable thus far to consistently suppress, and have often increased, serum antibody and splenic PFC responses by antigen feeding of mice previously primed parenterally by the same antigen.[21, 23, 35] However, with increased knowledge of the mechanisms and pathways involved in the production of oral tolerance, it may be possible to develop feeding protocols for producing suppression of immune responses in already primed mice. Such studies are particularly important when considering the prevention and treatment of allergic reactions. Third, species differences may be important. Decreased delayed contact-type hypersensitivity reactions and decreased serum antibody responses to parenteral challenge have been reported in humans after mucosal exposure to reactive chemicals or protein antigens.[36, 37] However, we and others have noted that rabbits fed bovine serum albumin[38, 39] or erythrocyte antigens (Kagnoff, unpublished observations) produced increased rather than decreased serum antibody responses when challenged with such antigens parenterally. Whether this is related to fundamental differences between the species or to other factors such as experimental design has not been established. Finally, the age at which antigen feeding is initiated is important. Thus, young children, but not adults, fed milk proteins often develop serum antibodies to such antigens[40] and newborn mice do not develop oral tolerance after ovalbumin feeding.[41]

Peyer's patches are a major sampling site for gut antigens[42] and are crucial in the initiation and generation of the mucosal IgA response.[43, 44] After enteric antigen challenge with a variety of antigens (e.g., heterologous erythrocytes and proteins), lymphocyte populations in Peyer's patches appear to be primed.[42, 45] As illustrated in FIGURE 5, activated lymphocytes are thought to migrate from Peyer's patches to the mesenteric lymph nodes (MLN).[1] Gut antigens may also enter the intestinal lymphatics directly and activate MLN cells, after which MLN cells enter the thoracic duct lymph and then the systemic circulation.[1] A population of the B cells that originated in the Peyer's patches and MLN return to the lamina propria of the intestinal mucosa, where, after stimulation with antigen, they produce IgA that is secreted into the intestinal lumen.[1, 43] Such IgA binds antigen in the intestinal tract and diminishes its further absorption. Other MLN B cells migrate to various parts of the mucosal immune system (e.g., mammary gland, female genital tract, and bronchus-associated lymphoid tissue) and produce IgA in those sites.[1, 44] T cells populating the lamina propria and intraepithelial regions of the intestinal mucosa also appear to derive from Peyer's patches and MLN, following similar migratory pathways.[46]

As shown in FIGURE 5, other lymphocytes activated by enteric antigen in Peyer's patches and perhaps in MLN (e.g., suppressor T lymphocytes) may selectively migrate to extraintestinal lymphoid tissue such as the spleen and suppress immune responses in those sites.[10, 18, 19, 29] Such suppression is revealed as oral tolerance if antigen-fed mice are challenged parenterally with the same antigen used for feeding. It is not clear to what extent helper T cells and primed B cells from Peyer's patches and MLN also migrate to extra-intestinal lymphoid tissue and play a role in the initial priming and induction of immune responses seen after antigen feeding. Also, as shown in FIGURE 5, antigens (and perhaps antigen-antibody complexes) may gain access to the

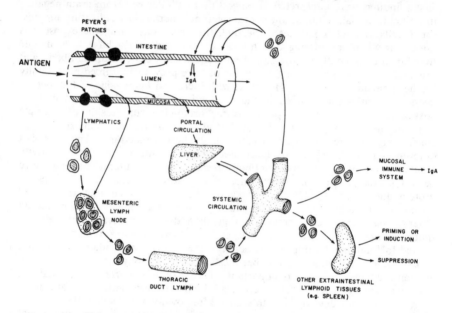

FIGURE 5. Pathways resulting in oral tolerance. Antigens in the intestine can activate B and T lymphocytes in Peyer's patches. After exiting Peyer's patches, such lymphocytes migrate *via* the lymphatics to the mesenteric lymph nodes (MLN). Antigens from the gut may also enter the intestinal lymphatics directly and activate populations of MLN cells. Cells from MLN subsequently enter the thoracic duct lymph and then the systemic circulation. Some of the B cells selectively migrate to the lamina propria of the intestinal mucosa, where, after stimulation with antigen, they produce IgA, which is secreted into the intestinal lumen. Such IgA binds and prevents further antigen absorption. Other B cells from MLN migrate to different parts of the mucosal immune system (*e.g.*, mammary gland, female genital tract, and bronchus-associated lymphoid tissue) and produce IgA. Still other lymphocytes activated by enteric antigen in Peyer's patches and perhaps in MLN (*e.g.*, suppressor T lymphocytes) may selectively migrate to extraintestinal lymphoid tissue *e.g.*, spleen), and ultimately suppress the production of systemic immune responses. Antigen from the intestine (or antigen-antibody complexes) that gains access to the systemic circulation *via* the portal circulation and liver may also stimulate lymphocyte populations in extraintestinal sites and activate mechanisms that result in suppression (or priming or induction) of system immune responses.

portal circulation and, after passage through the liver, enter the systemic circulation and stimulate lymphocyte populations in the extraintestinal lymphoid tissues. Such interactions may result either in suppression or in priming and induction of systemic immune responses in extraintestinal sites. By virtue of its interposition between the portal and systemic circulation, and of its receipt of blood from both, the liver has a role in oral tolerance [47] and in the host's interaction with intestinal antigens. Thus, absorbed antigen from the intestine and antigen-antibody complexes can be removed from the portal or systemic circulation by the hepatic reticuloendothelial system (*i.e.,* Kupffer cells). In addition, circulating IgA-antigen complexes that are postulated to play a role in oral tolerance [9] and to be deposited in the skin or kidneys in certain diseases,[49] can be removed from the serum and then secreted into bile, which subsequently enters the intestine.[49, 50]

It is clear that antigen in the intestine can activate a dual process that involves the production of an IgA mucosal antibody response and a diminished systemic immune response to the same antigen.[25, 29] The former mechanism appears to decrease antigen absorption while the latter prevents the host from developing undesirable immune reactions in extraintestinal tissues to otherwise harmless antigenic material that crosses the intestinal mucosa. The clinical relevance of such biological mechanisms is perhaps best illustrated in individuals with a selective IgA deficiency.[2] Finally, oral tolerance has been reported to be mediated by mechanisms variously involving T cells, B cells, soluble factors that may be derived from T cells, antibody (possibly anti-idiotypic antibody), and antigen-antibody complexes. Although such mechanisms appear to be activated by antigen interacting with gut-associated lymphoid tissue in sites such as the Peyer's patches and MLN, or by antigen (or antigen-antibody complexes) directly inducing suppressor mechanisms in extraintestinal lymphoid tissues, the relative contribution of each to the production and maintenance of oral tolerance is unknown.

Several key tasks lie ahead. For example, the mechanisms responsible for initiating and maintaining suppression or enhancement of systemic immune responses to different types of antigens encountered in the gastrointestinal tract need further study. How the site of the immune encounter with antigen in the gastrointestinal tract and invasive microorganisms and normal intestinal microflora influence subsequent systemic immune responses also needs to be determined. With such information, it may be possible to develop effective strategies for manipulating systemic and intestinal immune responses in a highly specific manner by enteric antigen challenge with well-defined antigenic stimuli. Hopefully, more effective oral immunization programs will evolve from a thorough understanding of the mucosal immune system and its interactions with the systemic immune system.

ACKNOWLEDGMENTS

I am grateful to Mr. Raleigh Austin, whose technical expertise has been extremely valuable to these studies over the past several years. I also wish to thank the National Institute of Arthritis, Metabolism, and Digestive Diseases (National Institutes of Health), and the National Foundation for Ileitis and Colitis for their generous financial support of our investigations. Finally, I wish to thank Ms. Debby Glazer for typing this manuscript.

REFERENCES

1. KAGNOFF, M. F. 1981. Immunology of the digestive system. *In* Physiology of the Gastrointestinal Tract. J. Christensen, G. Jacobson, S. Schultz, and M. Grossman, Eds.: 1337–59. Raven Press. New York.

2. KAGNOFF, M. F. 1982. Immunology and diseases of the gastrointestinal tract. *In* Gastrointestinal Disease, 3rd Ed. M. H. Sleisenger and J. S. Fordtran, Eds. W. B. Saunders. Philadelphia. In press.
3. DAVIES, A. 1922. An investigation into the serological properties of dysentery stools. Lancet **203:** 1009–12.
4. OGRA, P. L. & D. T. KARZON. 1969. Poliovirus antibody response in serum and nasal secretions following intranasal inoculation with inactivated poliovaccine. J. Immunol. **102:** 15–23.
5. WELLS, H. G. 1911. Studies on the chemistry of anaphylaxis. III. Experiments with isolated proteins, especially those of the hen's egg. J. Infect. Dis. **9:** 147–71.
6. CHASE, M. W. 1946. Inhibition of experimental drug allergy by prior feeding of the sensitizing agent. Proc. Soc. Exp. Biol. Med. **61:** 257–59.
7. KAGNOFF, M. F. 1974. Induction and paralysis: A conceptual framework from which to examine the intestinal immune system. Gastroenterology **66:** 1240–56.
8. THOMAS, H. C. & D. M. V. PARROTT. 1974. The induction of tolerance to a soluble protein antigen by oral administration. Immunology **27:** 631–39.
9. ANDRÉ, C., J. F. HEREMANS, J. P. VAERMAN & C. L. CAMBIASO. 1975. A mechanism for the induction of immunological tolerance by antigen feeding: Antigen-antibody complexes. J. Exp. Med. **142:** 1509–19.
10. ASHERSON, G. L., M. ZEMBALA, M. A. C. C. PERERA, B. MAYHEW & W. R. THOMAS. 1977. Production of immunity and unresponsiveness in the mouse by feeding contact sensitizing agents and the role of suppressor cells in the Peyer's patches, mesenteric lymph nodes and other lymphoid tissues. Cell. Immunol. **33:** 145–55.
11. BAZIN, H. & B. PLATTEAU. 1977. Oral feeding of ovalbumin can make rats tolerant to an intraperitoneal injection of dinitrophenylated ovalbumin and *Bordetella pertussis* vaccine. Biochem. Soc. Trans. **5:** 1571–73.
12. DAVID, M. F. 1977. Prevention of homocytotropic antibody formation and anaphylactic sensitization by prefeeding antigen. J. Allergy Clin. Immunol. **60:** 180–87.
13. HANSON, D. G., N. M. VAZ, L. C. S. MAIA, M. M. HORNBROOK, J. M. LYNCH & C. A. ROY. 1977. Inhibition of specific immune responses by feeding protein antigens. Int. Arch. Allergy Appl. Immunol. **55:** 526–32.
14. VAZ, N. M., L. C. S. MAIA, D. G. HANSON & J. M. LYNCH. 1977. Inhibition of homocytotropic antibody responses in adult inbred mice by previous feeding of the specific antigen. J. Allergy Clin. Immunol. **60:** 110–15.
15. KAGNOFF, M. F. 1978. Effects of antigen-feeding on intestinal and systemic immune responses. I. Priming of precursor cytotoxic T cells by antigen feeding. J. Immunol. **120:** 395–99.
16. KAGNOFF, M. F. 1978. Effects of antigen-feeding on intestinal and systemic immune responses. II. Suppression of delayed-type hypersensitivity reactions. J. Immunol. **120:** 1509–13.
17. KAGNOFF, M. F. 1978. Effects of antigen-feeding on intestinal and systemic immune responses. III. Antigen-specific serum-mediated suppression of humoral antibody responses after antigen feeding. Cell. Immunol. **40:** 186–203.
18. MATTINGLY, J. A. & B. H. WAKSMAN. 1978. Immunologic suppression after oral administration of antigen. I. Specific suppressor cells formed in rat Peyer's patches after oral administration of sheep erythrocytes and their systemic migration. J. Immunol. **121:** 1878–83.
19. NGAN, J. & L. S. KIND. 1978. Suppressor T cells for IgE and IgG in Peyer's patches of mice made tolerant by the oral administration of ovalbumin. J. Immunol. **120:** 861–65.
20. RICHMAN, L. K., J. M. CHILLER, W. R. BROWN, D. G. HANSON & N. M. VAZ.

1978. Enterically induced immunologic tolerance. I. Induction of suppressor T lymphocytes by intragastric administration of soluble proteins. J. Immunol. **121:** 2429–34.

21. CHILLER, J. M., R. G. TITUS & H. M. ETLINGER. 1979. Cellular dissection of tolerant states induced by the oral route or in neonatal animals. *In* Immunologic Tolerance and Macrophage Function. P. Baram, J. R. Battisto & C. W. Pierce, Eds.: 195–221. Elsevier/North Holland. Amsterdam.

22. HANSON, D. G., N. M. VAZ, L. C. S. MAIA & J. M. LYNCH. 1979. Inhibition of specific immune responses by feeding protein antigens. III. Evidence against maintenance of tolerance to ovalbumin by orally induced antibodies. J. Immunol. **123:** 2337–43.

23. HANSON, D. G., N. M. VAZ, L. A. RAWLINGS & J. M. LYNCH. 1979. Inhibition of specific immune responses by feeding protein antigens. II. Effects of prior passive and active immunization. J. Immunol. **122:** 2261–66.

24. MILLER, S. D. & D. G. HANSON. 1979. Inhibition of specific immune responses by feeding protein antigens. IV. Evidence for tolerance and specific active suppression of cell-mediated immune responses to ovalbumin. J. Immunol. **123:** 2344–50.

25. SWARBRICK, E. T., C. R. STOKES & J. F. SOOTHILL. 1979. Absorption of antigens after oral immunization and simultaneous induction of specific systemic tolerance. Gut **20:** 121–25.

26. KAGNOFF, M. F. 1980. Effects of antigen-feeding on intestinal and systemic immune responses. IV. Similarity between the suppressor factor in mice after erythrocyte-lysate injection and erythrocyte feeding. Gastroenterology **79:** 54–61.

27. MATTINGLY, J. A. & B. H. WAKSMAN. 1980. Immunologic suppression after oral administration of antigen. II. Antigen-specific helper and suppressor factors produced by spleen cells of rats fed sheep erythrocytes. J. Immunol. **125:** 1044–47.

28. MATTINGLY, J. A., J. M. KAPLAN & C. A. JANEWAY, JR. 1980. Two distinct antigen-specific suppressor factors induced by the oral administration of antigen. J. Exp. Med. **152:** 545–54.

29. CHALLACOMBE, S. J. & T. B. TOMASI, JR. 1980. Systemic tolerance and secretory immunity after oral immunization. J. Exp. Med. **152:** 1459–72.

30. PERERA, M. A. C. C. & G. L. ASHERSON. 1981. Effect of adult thymectomy on the contact sensitivity skin reaction and the unresponsiveness caused by feeding contact sensitizing agents. Immunology **43:** 613–18.

31. KAGNOFF, M. F. 1979. IgA anti-dextran B1355 responses. J. Immunol. **122:** 866–70.

32. TREFTS, P. E., D. RIVIER & M. F. KAGNOFF. 1981. T cell–dependent IgA anti-polysaccharide response in vitro. Nature (London) **292:** 163–65.

33. HEREMANS, J. F. & H. BAZIN. 1971. Antibodies induced by local antigenic stimulation of mucosal surfaces. Ann. N.Y. Acad. Sci. **190:** 268–75.

34. MCGHEE, J. R., S. M. MICHALEK, H. KIYONO, J. L. BABB, M. P. CLARK & L. M. MOSTELLER. 1981. Endotoxin and IgA responses. *In* Recent Advances in Mucosal Immunity. In press.

35. KAGNOFF, M. F. Immunological unresponsiveness after enteric antigen administration. *In* Recent Advances in Mucosal Immunity. In press.

36. LOWNEY, E. D. 1968. Immunologic unresponsiveness to a contact sensitizer in man. J. Dermatol. **51:** 411–17.

37. KORENBLAT, P. E., R. M. ROTHBERG, P. MINDEN & R. S. FARR. 1968. Immune responses of human adults after oral and parenteral exposure to bovine serum albumin. J. Allergy **41:** 226–35.

38. ROTHBERG, R. M., S. C. KRAFT & R. S. FARR. 1967. Similarities between rabbit antibodies produced following ingestion of bovine serum albumin and following parenteral immunization. J. Immunol. **98:** 386–95.

39. ROTHBERG, R. M., S. C. KRAFT & S. M. MICHALEK. 1973. Systemic immunity after local antigenic stimulation of the lymphoid tissue of the gastrointestinal tract. J. Immunol. **111:** 1906–13.
40. ROTHBERG, R. M. & R. S. FARR. 1965. Anti-bovine serum albumin and anti-alpha lactalbumin in the serum of children and adults. Pediatrics **35:** 571–88.
41. HANSON, D. G. 1981. Ontogeny of orally induced tolerance to soluble proteins in mice. I. Priming and tolerance in newborns. J. Immunol. **127:** 1518–24.
42. KAGNOFF, M. F. 1977. Functional characteristics of Peyer's patch lymphoid cells. IV. Effect of antigen feeding on the frequency of antigen-specific B cells. J. Immunol. **118:** 992–97.
43. CEBRA, J., J. R. KAMAT, P. J. GEARHART, S. M. ROBERTSON & J. TSENG. 1977. The secretory IgA system of the gut. Ciba Found. Symp. **46:** 5–28.
44. McDERMOTT, M. R. & J. BIENENSTOCK. 1979. Evidence for a common mucosal immunologic system. I. Migration of B immunoblasts into intestinal, respiratory, and genital tissues. J. Immunol. **122:** 1892–98.
45. KAGNOFF, M. F. 1975. Functional characteristics of Peyer's patch cells. III. Carrier priming of T cells by antigen feeding. J. Exp. Med. **142:** 1425–35.
46. GUY-GRAND, D., C. GRISCELLI & P. VASSALLI. 1978. The mouse gut T lymphocyte, a novel type of T cell. Nature, origin and traffic in mice in normal and graft-versus-host conditions. J. Exp. Med. **148:** 1661–67.
47. CANTOR, H. M. & A. E. DUMONT. 1967. Hepatic suppression of sensitization to antigen absorbed into the portal system. Nature (London) **215:** 744–45.
48. ANDRÉ, C., F. C. BERTHOUX, F. ANDRÉ, J. GILLON, C. GENIN & A. C. SABATIER. 1980. Prevalence of IgA2 deposits in IgA nephropathies. A clue to their pathogenesis. N. Engl. J. Med. **303:** 1343–46.
49. PEPPARD, J., E. ORLANS, A. W. R. PAYNE & E. ANDREW. 1981. The elimination of circulating complexes containing polymeric IgA by excretion in the bile. Immunology **42:** 83–89.
50. RUSSELL, M. W., T. A. BROWN & J. MESTECKY. 1981. Role of serum IgA hepatobiliary transport of circulating antigen. J. Exp. Med. **153:** 968–76.

DISCUSSION OF THE PAPER

J. W. STREILEIN (*University of Texas Health Science Center, Dallas, Tx.*): I have two questions. One: Can you tell us about the technique by which you feed the antigen that would lead you to suspect that Peyer's patches are the first sites at which antigen recognition could take place in the gut?

KAGNOFF: A number of studies, both from our laboratory and from others' point out that Peyer's patches are key to the initiation of a subsequent mucosal immune response.

STREILEIN: In terms of an IgA response?

KAGNOFF: Yes. Also, there's evidence for priming T cell populations such as helper T cells, suppressor T cells, and cytotoxic T cells after feeding antigen. For example, investigators have taken cells from Peyer's patches after short periods of feeding, done adoptive transfers, and shown that there are suppressor cells present that subsequently appear in mesenteric nodes and later in spleen. I don't think we know definitively that Peyer's patches are the first sites of antigenic contact. I would predict they would be for certain types of antigens.

STREILEIN: What would you expect would be the first site for sheep red blood cells?

KAGNOFF: Sheep red blood cells and other particulate antigens may enter Peyer's patches first since they would not normally cross the mucosa at other sites to any significant extent.

STREILEIN: My second question is related to that. You used, in the one example, EL4 cells to try to induce tolerance to histocompatibility antigens. Those cells, of course, are very good at getting across surfaces and migrating. Have you ever tried to induce tolerance to antigens by using immobile cells?

KAGNOFF: We've used both spleen cells and tumor cells, and find the same sorts of results.

STREILEIN: Epidermal cells?

KAGNOFF: No.

CONSEQUENCES OF PRENATAL EXPOSURE
TO MATERNAL ALLOANTIGENS *

Frank L. Adler and Louise T. Adler

*Division of Immunology
St. Jude Children's Research Hospital
Memphis, Tennessee 38101*

INTRODUCTION

Increased susceptibility to the induction of specific immunological unresponsiveness has often, but not invariably, been associated with immaturity of the immune system. Thus, fetal and neonatal animals are thought to be most readily tolerized, especially to transplantation antigens, and it has been suggested that tolerance for self is generated during this critical period. In more recent work, it has been shown that B lymphocytes from the immature animal are more readily tolerized than those from mature donors [1, 2] and that suppression through T cells is highly active in the very young. [3]

In apparent contrast to these findings are reports of active immune responses by fetuses against various antigens in response to infection or injection [4] and observations of "spontaneous" antibody responses to noninherited maternal allotypic immunoglobulin antigens. Such responses have been described in humans, [5-7] pigs, [8] mice, [9] and rabbits. [10, 11] While long-lasting antibody formation has been emphasized in some of these studies, [5-8, 10, 11] others have stressed that the immune response is preceded by specific unresponsiveness. [9]

We have called attention to the apparent coexistence of persisting but low-level antibody formation and a similarly persistent state of decreased responsiveness to the allotypic antigen, *i.e.*, a lasting state of partial tolerance. [10] This report describes further studies on rabbits in which both the route and the time of exposure to foreign allotypic determinants were varied in order to examine the significance of these variables. We also present preliminary findings relevant to the induction of partial tolerance based on *in vitro* studies with spleen cells from adult rabbits.

RESULTS

Elimination of Immunoglobulin Passively Acquired by Various Routes

In our previous studies, we had examined the progeny of heterozygous dams nursed by their natural mothers until they were eight weeks old. In such young rabbits, maternal immunoglobulin (Ig) of the noninherited allotype disappeared from their sera (<10 μg ml^{-1}) when they were 8–10 weeks old. [10] More recently, we have examined young rabbits born to chimeric dams whose sera contained about 10–30% Ig of the allotype made by donor cells. [12] The young

* This research was supported by grants from the National Institutes of Health, nos. CA 23709, AI 13159, and CA 21765 (CORE), and by ALSAC.

266

acquired prope tionally less of such maternal Ig than Ig corresponding to the dam's genotype, and it disappeared sooner, to be followed by demonstrable antibody formation in many of the offspring.

In order to obtain some insight into the respective roles of Ig acquisition across the placenta and of maternal Ig obtained through nursing, a number of litters were fostered at birth to dams of an allotype foreign to them. In such animals, while the peak concentration of Ig carrying the fostering dam's allotype was 300–600 μg ml^{-1} serum in the first bleeding taken at three weeks of age, less than 10 μg ml^{-1} was found at ages 8–10 weeks. Nursing activity of the young declines sharply after six weeks and it is not clear to what extent diminished intake of milk, decreasing Ig concentration in the milk, and declining absorption from the gut contributed to the depletion of maternal Ig.

Immune responses to Ig of a foreign allotype acquired solely through postnatal feeding occurred regularly. In a typical experiment, nine young from two litters, all of allotype b^9b^9, were fostered to three dams of allotype b^4b^4. Antibody for the b4 allotype was demonstrable in six rabbits, with the onset of its formation between days 88 and 177. The three nonresponders were from one litter: two were nursed by one foster dam and one by another. In a second experiment, a group of nine b^4b^5 newborns were nursed by b^9b^9 females. All eliminated Ig of the b9 allotype between days 42 and 56; antibody against b9 Ig became detectable in eight rabbits between days 56 and 88 and could be demonstrated in the ninth rabbit on day 210. There was no evidence for an acceleration in the clearance of b9 Ig just before its total elimination.

The question of immune elimination of Ig carrying a foreign allotype acquired from the natural or the foster mother appeared to be of particular interest because of its implications for the regulation of gene expression in the Ig system by network controls in general and in the "latent allotype" problem in particular.[13] We therefore examined three rabbits that had been exposed to foreign allotypes *in utero* and through nursing. When they were 6–8 months old, they were injected i.v. with Ig carrying the allotype markers to which they had been exposed and also, for control purposes, with Ig of an irrelevant allotype. The results shown in TABLE 1 reveal no difference in the rates of elimination of the Ig carrying relevant and of the Ig carrying irrelevant allotypic markers. Both Ig types, after initial equilibration, were eliminated with an apparent half-life of about seven days. It appears, therefore, that pre- or neonatal priming and the ensuing low-level antibody responses do not contribute to a significant acceleration in the elimination of a challenge dose, a result consistent with our finding that these rabbits show little evidence of effective priming for specific immune responses,[10] which will be documented further below.

Responses of Perinatally Primed Rabbits to Parenteral Immunization

Our earlier findings showed a long-lasting but low-level antibody response to allotypic determinants but an absence of demonstrable memory in animals that had been exposed to large doses of the antigen neonatally. This study was then extended through the use of antigenic challenges with the appropriate Ig in Freund's adjuvant. Two intramuscular injections of 5 mg each were given, the first in complete, the second in incomplete adjuvant. This procedure elicits antibody, albeit in widely varying amounts, in all normal controls.

The results obtained in two groups of rabbits, all 6–8 months old and of the b^4b^5 allotype, are shown in FIGURE 1. Responses are shown as peak titers after the first and after the second injection. One of the groups, consisting of 14 rabbits, had been nursed on b^9b^9 foster dams, while the second group of 11 rabbits had been nursed on their own b^4b^4 or b^5b^5 mothers. All were injected with b9 Ig. There was clearly no difference in the responses of the two groups, even though most of the animals in the first group had made or were making low levels of anti-b9 at the time of the injections. It should be noted that one rabbit in the experimental group remained unresponsive.

Additional data on responses to challenge injections using the procedure just described may be seen in TABLES 2 and 3. Shown there are the responses

TABLE 1

PERINATAL EXPOSURE TO FOREIGN ALLOTYPE WITH OR WITHOUT
SUBSEQUENT ANTIBODY FORMATION DOES NOT RESULT IN IMMUNE ELIMINATION

Rabbit	Allotype	Exposed to	Injected with	Ig	Day 0.01	1	5	7	9	14
206	a^3a^3/b^5b^5	b4, b6	b9, b4, b6	b5	7680 *	7680	15 360	15 360		
				b9	538	269	134	67	67	50
				b4	538	269	134	67	67	34
				b6	538	269	67	67	67	34
204	a^3a^3/b^4b^5	b6	b9, b6	b5	3840	3840	3840	3840		
				b9	538	268	134	134	67	67
				b6	269	134	67	67	67	34
198	a^1a^3/b^4b^4	b5, b6	a2, b5, b6	b4	7680	3840	7680	7680		
				a2	202	67	50	50	34	17
				b5	538	269	134	134	134	67
				b6	269	134	134	67	67	34

* μg per ml serum.

NOTES: These rabbits were born to chimeric females with high serum levels of donor-type Ig carrying allotypic markers as noted in the "Exposed to" column.

Weighing 2.2–3.3 kg at the time of injection, they received weight-adjusted amounts of appropriately pooled normal sera containing equal amounts of Ig of each of the specificities listed in the column "Injected with."

For control purposes, rabbits 204 and 206 received Ig b9 and rabbit 198 Ig a2. For additional control purposes, one of the markers on the recipient's own Ig was titrated (b5 for rabbits 204 and 206, b4 for rabbit 198).

of control rabbits and of rabbits exposed to foreign allotypic determinants *in utero,* orally, or by intraperitoneal injection during the first week of life, or by a combination of two or more of these procedures. It will be noted that complete or nearly complete unresponsiveness to the challenges was observed in seven rabbits that had been exposed to the allotypic determinant both *in utero* and through nursing (rabbits 113, 114, T399, T486, T490, TABLE 2, and rabbits 118, 119, TABLE 3). Three of these animals had also been injected with serum containing the appropriate allotype shortly after birth. When the neonatal exposure to foreign allotype was by means of such injections alone, or was obtained through nursing alone, neither overt tolerance nor a significantly enhanced response to either of the challenge injections resulted. This point is

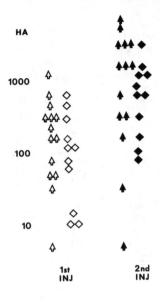

FIGURE 1. Anti-b9 responses of b^4b^5 rabbits in response to two injections of Igb9.
▲ Rabbits nursed on b^9b^9 dams
◆ Control rabbits

illustrated in more detail in FIGURE 2, which depicts the responses to b9 Ig in three rabbits that had been nursed on b^9b^9 dams and in three control animals. While the responses of the three pre-exposed rabbits might have been slightly greater than those of the three controls, reference to the data in FIGURE 1 will illustrate the lack of significance of these apparent differences.

The data just presented extend the descriptive phase of the consequences of fetal or neonatal exposures, under physiological conditions, to large amounts

TABLE 2

ANTI-b4 RESPONSES AFTER CHALLENGE WITH IG b4
IN RABBITS EXPOSED TO b4 PERINATALLY

			Weeks post challenge		
Rabbit	Allotype	Exposure	3	4	5
113	a^3a^3/b^5b^5	i.u., p.o.	<4	<4	<4
114	a^2a^3/b^5b^6		<4	<4	<4
T399			32	32	16
T486	a^3a^3/b^5b^6	i.u., p.o., i.p.	<4	<4	<4
T490			<4		
T464			3200	1600	1600
T466	a^1a^3/b^9b^9	p.o.	1600	1600	3200
T465			1600	1600	3200
T513	a^2a^2/b^9b^9	p.o.	100	100	100
T531	a^3a^3/b^9b^9		800	400	400

NOTES: i.u.: *in utero*; p.o.: *per os* (nursing); i.p.: i.p. injection of serum.
Antibody titers of control rabbits ranged from 100–25 600; the median ≅ 3200.

TABLE 3

ANTI-b5 RESPONSES AFTER CHALLENGE WITH IG b5
IN RABBITS EXPOSED TO b5 PERINATALLY AND IN CONTROLS

Rabbit	Allotype	Exposure	Weeks post challenge		
			3	4	5
120	a^1a^3/b^6b^6	i.u., p.o.	128	128	256
118	a^1a^3/b^6b^6		64	32	32
119	a^3a^3/b^6b^6		<4	<4	<4
T333	a^2a^3/b^4b^6		1600	1600	1600
T358	a^1a^3/b^4b^4	i.p.	800	400	400
T359	a^2a^3/b^4b^6		400	400	400
111	a^2a^2/b^4b^6		400	400	400
115	a^2a^3/b^4b^6	—	800	1600	1600
110	a^1a^3/b^4b^6		400	400	400
120	a^1a^3/b^6b^6		100	100	200

NOTES: As per TABLE 2.

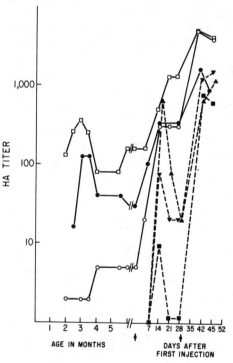

FIGURE 2. Antibody against Ig b9 produced by b^4b^5 rabbits. Six rabbits at six months of age were injected twice with Ig b9 in adjuvant (arrows). Solid lines depict the responses of rabbits nursed by b^9b^9 dams; broken lines depict the responses of controls.

of weak allogeneic antigens. The overt immunity observed in the majority of the animals was not accompanied by increased responsiveness to injections of the antigen. Some of the rabbits were totally unresponsive, while others reacted like control animals. These findings suggest that partial tolerance, probably mediated by an active suppression mechanism, is initiated and coexists with immunity in an equilibrium state that allows for some variation in individual animals. It remains for future investigations to perform the appropriate cell separations required for the demonstration and identification of suppressor cells *in vitro,* or by transfer to histocompatible recipients.

An in Vitro *Model for the Simultaneous Induction of Active Immunity and Tolerance*

In view of the palpable need for a model that allows more rapid progress, and also because the findings just presented raised questions regarding the significance both of age at the time of first exposure and of the allogeneic nature of the antigens, we turned to an *in vitro* model already well established in our

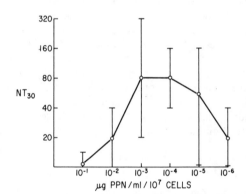

FIGURE 3. *In vitro* responses to varying amounts of S-T2 antigen. Spleen cells were pulsed for 2 h at 37° C with the amounts of solubilized phage antigen (μg protein N per ml per 10^7 cells) shown and cultures were incubated 4–5 d. The responses were measured as NT^{30} (the highest dilution of culture fluid mediating more than 30% neutralization).

laboratory in which antibody formation and specific unresponsiveness are readily induced.

The model is the primary IgM antibody response of rabbit spleen cells to solubilized antigens of bacteriophage T2. This system has been characterized as one that is independent of demonstrable requirements for help by either T cells or macrophages. However, it is sensitive to suppression by antigen-specific T suppressor cells. Both antibody formation and suppression are inducible by the treatment of spleen cells with antigen during a 2 h pulse, and the induction of tolerance requires 100–1000 times the amount of antigen optimal for the initiation of antibody formation.[14, 15] A typical dose response curve for this system is shown in FIGURE 3, which defines the optimal immunogenic dose as 10^{-3}–10^{-4} μg of antigen N per ml per 10^7 cells, and the tolerogenic dose as 10^{-1}–10^{-2} μg N. The curve is drawn through the mean response values and the brackets indicate the total range encountered in the responses of all the spleens tested.

We wished to test the hypothesis that the apparently tolerogenic amounts of antigen also stimulate antigen-specific B cells but that antibody formation remains unexpressed because of the simultaneous induction of T suppression. This idea was tested in two ways. Assuming that the frequency of precursors of specific B and Ts cells was not likely to be the same, we diluted tolerized spleen cells in a suspension of autologous thymocytes, using these cells as filler, and assayed the resulting cultures for antibody formation in the usual manner.

Shown in TABLE 4 are the results of one such experiment. It is evident that only minimal antibody formation occurred when 1.2×10^6 tolerized spleen cells were cultured. However, 3×10^5 or 6×10^5 such cells made optimal amounts of antibody, comparable to that produced by similar numbers of spleen cells that had been treated with the immunogenic dose of antigen. Little or no antibody was formed by 7×10^4 or 1.5×10^5 cells, whether they had been treated with one or the other antigen dose. We believe that these data suggest that precursors of antibody-producing B cells outnumber precursors of antigen-specific Ts cells in the spleens of adult normal rabbits. More elaborate experiments of the type just described will permit quantitation of these two cell populations.

A second approach involved the removal of T cells from the spleen cell suspension, either before or after pulse treatment with antigen in the tolerogenic concentration. Data from two such experiments are shown in TABLE 5. In both experiments, depletion of T cells was achieved by removing those cells which formed rosettes with autologous papainized erythrocytes,[16] leaving a population in which about 85% of the cells were Ig+. It will be noted that the amount of antigen that was tolerogenic for the unfractionated cells was immunogenic for the T cell–depleted population. There is also a suggestion that the T-depleted cultures responded somewhat better to antigen doses in the immunogenic range (FIGURE 3), an observation in accord with the notion that some degree of suppression may be induced even by the immunogenic doses.

TABLE 4

DILUTION OF TOLERIZED CELLS REVEALS IMMUNIZATION

Spleen Cells	A			B		
	1	2	3	1	2	3
1.2×10^6	10	10	20	160	80	160
6×10^5	160	80	40	80	80	40
3×10^5	80–160	80	40	20–40	80	20–40
1.5×10^5	10–20	5	5	10	10	20–40
7×10^4	<5	<5	<5	<5	<5	<5
None	<5	<5	<5	<5	<5	<5

NOTES: Spleen cells were diluted with autologous thymocytes so that the final cell concentration in each culture was 1.2×10^6 cells per 0.25 ml.

Group A: Spleen cells were pulsed for 2 h with 10^{-1} μg S-T2 N per 10^7 cells ("tolerogenic dose").

Group B: Spleen cells were pulsed for 2 h with 10^{-3} μg S-T2 N per 10^7 cells ("immunogenic dose").

For each experimental point, triplicate cultures were assayed.

Data are expressed as NT 30.[14]

TABLE 5

T CELL DEPLETION CONVERTS TOLEROGENIC INTO IMMUNOGENIC STIMULI

S-T2 (μg per ml per 10^7 cells)	Experiment 1		Experiment 2	
	Total Spleen Cells	Splenic B Cells	Total Spleen Cells	Splenic B Cells
10^{-1}	20	320	<5–5	160
10^{-2}	320	640	20–40	160
10^{-3}	320	640	40	160
10^{-4}	320	320	20	80
10^{-5}	80	40	10	10
10^{-6}	<5	5	<5	NT

NOTE: T cell depletion was achieved by removing cells that form rosettes with papainized autologous red cells. The remaining cells were 85% Ig$^+$.

DISCUSSION

The data presented here and in a previous paper[10] suggest to us that the spontaneous response of rabbits to maternal allotypic Ig determinants is one of balanced immunity and specific unresponsiveness, in which persistent antibody formation at low levels is a measure of the former and ineffective responses to parenteral challenge are an indication of the latter. Data presented here show that the degree of tolerance varies widely, since some rabbits fail to respond to challenge injections completely while others produce antibody that does not, however, exceed that produced by unprimed controls. These findings in the rabbit model would appear to reconcile those made in humans and swine,[5–8] which emphasized the lasting antibody responses, with those made in mice,[9] which stressed the establishment of tolerance prior to immunity. It should be noted, however, that tolerance in mice was deduced from their failure to respond to challenge at a time when antigen acquired *in utero* or through nursing was still present and in the light of the proposition that tolerance persists only in the presence of critical amounts of antigen.

Our data show that maternal Ig is generally completely absent from sera at three months of age and that antibody formation is usually demonstrable two to four weeks later. We have not observed any significant acceleration in the rate of antigen elimination during the final phase; thus, the time of onset of antibody formation is not likely to be much earlier than that indicated by the titration results, which detect free antibody in concentrations greater than 0.01 μg ml^{-1} serum. Also of interest is the observation that immune elimination of a challenge dose of Ig given to such animals as adults could not be demonstrated, a result consistent with persistence of tolerance but in striking contrast to the rapid elimination of Ig carrying a latent allotypic marker in rabbits that had intermittently produced such Ig but had no measurable antibody of the appropriate specificity.[13]

Our earlier data pertaining to the frequency and magnitude of spontaneous responses to maternal allotypic determinants[10] have been analyzed by Hagen *et al.* together with their own data and have led them to propose that the immune response is under polygenic control.[11] While this may well be correct, it is our belief that, in measuring antibody responses, we determine the net result of the balance between overt immunity and tolerance. The concept of such partial tolerance has been invoked in transplantation studies by Hasek and Chutna, who have discussed its possible role in the regulation of immune responses in general.[17] Among a number of reports on partial tolerance induction in adult animals, that of Weitzman et al. draws attention to the simultaneous induction of a plaque-forming B cell immune response and of Ts after the injection of supraoptimal doses of sheep erythrocytes,[18] a finding similar to our observation in the in vitro model. Papers by Richman et al.[19] and Araneo et al.[20] are also of particular interest, in that they present evidence for the simultaneous induction of isotype- and antigen-specific T suppressor and helper cells and for localized antibody responses in putatively nonresponding mice. Our in vitro model, for which we report preliminary evidence here, demonstrates, we believe, the induction of a covert immunity analogous to that seen by others in the in vivo studies just cited.

While the in vitro model is admittedly remote from our in vivo studies on responses to the perinatal exposure to maternal alloantigens, it illustrates that the induction of partial tolerance is not restricted to the prenatal or neonatal period, as already demonstrated in work by others.[18-20] It also shows that it is not restricted to allotypic determinants of Ig molecules in the rabbit, a point that seems worthy of consideration, since isologous Ig has been acclaimed as a particularly effective tolerogenic carrier for attached haptens in the mouse[21] and could function in a similar manner with respect to an endogenous determinant.

An interesting aspect of the response to maternal allotype markers is its long duration in the absence of demonstrable antigen. While colonization of the young with a few maternal B cells is one possible source of continuing antigenic stimulation, temporary bursts of latent allotype production might also be a possibility. We see as one likely mechanism a sequence of events in which exposure to the maternal allotype during the perinatal period results in the induction of suppression, possibly through Ts cells, and antibody production by B cells. The antiallotypic antibody response of the rabbit is preponderantly one of molecules sharing common idiotypes (References 23–25 and D. Metzger, personal communication), and autoantibody formation against the common idiotype in rabbits making anti-maternal allotype antibody has recently been demonstrated (L. S. Rodkey, personal communication). Such anti-idiotypic antibody could serve as a surrogate for the maternal allotype in stimulating a lasting antibody response.[26] Assuming that the recognition site of the putative Ts cells bears the common idiotype, one could visualize extended stimulation of these cells as well. Ongoing studies in our laboratory are aimed at the elucidation of these problems.

ACKNOWLEDGMENTS

We gratefully acknowledge the technical assistance of Ms. Carol Smith and Ms. Sabrina Walker and the secretarial help of Ms. Chris Winston.

REFERENCES

1. METCALF, E. S. & N. R. KLINMAN. 1976. J. Exp. Med. **143**: 1327.
2. NOSSAL, G. J. V. & B. L. PIKE. 1978. J. Exp. Med. **148**: 1161.
3. ARGYRIS, B. F. 1978. Cell. Immunol. **36**: 354.
4. SILVERSTEIN, A .M. 1964. Science **144**: 1423.
5. STEINBERG, A. G. & J. A. WILSON. 1963. Science **140**: 303.
6. WILSON, J. A. & A. G. STEINBERG. 1965. Transfusion (Philadelphia) **5**: 516.
7. SPEISER, P. 1966. Ann. Pediatr. (Paris) **207**: 20.
8. RASMUSEN, B. A. 1965. Science **148**: 1742.
9. WARNER, N. L. & L. A. HERZENBERG. 1970. J. Exp. Med. **132**: 440.
10. ADLER, F. L. & R. J. NOELLE. 1975. J. Immunol. **115**: 620.
11. HAGEN, K. L., L. E. YOUNG, R. G. TISSOT & C. COHEN. 1978. Immunogenetics **6**: 355.
12. ADLER, L. T., F. L. ADLER, C. COHEN & R. G. TISSOT. 1981. J. Exp. Med. **154**: 1085.
13. YARMUSH, M. L., J. A. SOGN, P. D. KERN & T. J. KINDT. 1981. J. Exp. Med. **153**: 196.
14. SCHAEFER, A. E., L. T. ADLER & M. FISHMAN. 1975. J. Immunol. **114**: 1281.
15. ADLER, F. L., M. NAKAO, L. T. ADLER & M. FISHMAN. 1981. Proc. 19th Int. Symp. on Biological Models, Brno, Czechoslovakia. *In* Cellular and Molecular Mechanisms of Immunological Tolerance. T. Hraba and M. Hasek, Eds.: 313. Marcel Dekker. New York.
16. NAKO, M., F. L. ADLER, L. T. ADLER & M. FISHMAN. 1981. Cell. Immunol. **58**: 448.
17. HASEK, M. & J. CHUTNA. 1979. Immunol. Rev. **46**: 3.
18. WEITZMAN, S., F. W. SHEN & H. CANTOR. 1976. J. Immunol. **117**: 2209.
19. RICHMAN, L. K., A. S. GRAEFF, R. YARCHOAN & W. STROBER. 1981. J. Immunol. **126**: 2079.
20. ARANEO, B. A., R. L. YOWELL & E. E. SERCARZ. 1979. J. Immunol. **123**: 961.
21. BOREL, Y. 1976. Transplant. Rev. **31**: 3.
22. URBAIN, J., C. COLLIGNON, J. D. FRANSSEN, M. MAREME, O. LEO, G. URBAIN-VANSANTEN, P. V.D.WALLE, M. WIKLER & C. WUILMART. 1979. Ann. Immunol. (Paris) **130C**: 281.
23. ROLAND, J. & P.-A. CAZENAVE. 1979. C. R. Acad. Sci. Ser. D **288**: 571.
24. GILMAN-SACHS, A., S. DRAY & W. J. HORNG. 1980. J. Immunol. **125**: 96.
25. ROLAND, J. & P.-A. CAZENAVE. 1981. Eur. J. Immunol. **11**: 469.
26. EICHMANN, K. & K. RAJEWSKI. 1975. Eur. J. Immunol. **5**: 661.

DISCUSSION OF THE PAPER

J. CHILLER (*Scripps Clinical Research Foundation, La Jolla, Calif.*): With respect to the reconstitution of the suppression by the addition of T cells, how specific is that phenomenon? Will normal T cells do the same thing?

F. L. ADLER: No, these are highly antigen specific. When T cells from a spleen stimulated with an entirely unrelated phage are used, they do not impose unresponsiveness on these cells. So it's antigen specific.

ACTIVE CLONAL DELETION
IN NEONATAL *H-2* TOLERANCE *

J. Wayne Streilein, Rebecca S. Gruchalla, Peter Wood, and
Phoebe Strome

Departments of Cell Biology and Internal Medicine
The University of Texas Health Science Center at Dallas
Dallas, Texas 75235

INTRODUCTION

Transplantation tolerance induced by the inoculation of allogeneic hemato-poietic cells into neonatal mice was first achieved approximately thirty years ago.[1,2] With this singular achievement, experimental verification was claimed for the clonal selection hypothesis as formulated by F. M. Burnet.[3] Over the next several decades, a conceptual paradigm concerning the mechanism of self/non-self discrimination came to dominate immunological thinking. While numerous other models of immunological tolerance and specific unresponsive-ness have emerged subsequently, the discipline continues to return to the classical model as the standard by which contemporary ideas are judged. At present, numerous laboratories around the world are engaged in a renaissance of experi-mentation with neonatal transplantation tolerance and an exciting new set of observations has emerged.[4] We have joined this pursuit, but have restricted the scope of our approaches to immunogenetic considerations. That is, by employ-ing a wide assortment of genetically defined *H-2* recombinant and congenic mouse strains, we have explored the immunogenetic basis of tolerance produced by administering semiallogeneic spleen and bone marrow cells intravenously to neonatal recipients. By selecting strain combinations disparate at one or more regions of the *H-2* complex, we hoped to compare and contrast the type and degree of tolerance thus achieved. Our initial experiments confirmed the validity of this approach by revealing the following important findings.

(1) While transplantation tolerance can be induced in neonatal mice to any and all alloantigens encoded by *H-2* genes, not all determinants are equally tolerogenic. Class II major histocompatibility (MHC) antigens (Ia) induce specific tolerance with great facility; class I determinants do so with considerably more difficulty.[5]

(2) Class II antigens have the further property of improving the tolerogenic potential of class I antigens if the tolerance-conferring inoculum expresses dis-parities of both types of determinants. Genetic mapping of this effect has been localized to the *I-J/E* subregions of *H-2*, a portion of this chromosomal segment that has been suspected in other systems of governing immune suppression.[6]

(3) Long-term *H-2*-tolerant adult mice are capable of rejecting, in a seemingly inappropriate fashion, third party skin allografts expressing a unique array of *H-2* determinants subsumed by the aggregate genetic information of the host and the donor of the tolerance-conferring inoculum. These results hint at the possibility that *I* region molecules on the graft restrict and direct

* This research was supported, in part, by grants from the United States Public Health Service, nos. AI–10678 and CA–09082.

0077–8923/82/0392–0276 $1.75/0 © 1982, NYAS

the activities of alloreactive cells putatively present, but suppressed, in tolerant mice.[7] Support for this idea has been generated by other investigators.[8]

Although this collection of data can be used to mount an argument in favor of the hypothesis that neonatal transplantation tolerance results from an active process rather than from passive clonal deletion, the evidence is largely circum-stantial. The studies to be described in this article were designed to seek out, identify, and exploit differences between the tolerant states induced by class I and class II MHC alloantigens.

It is worth noting, at the outset, that these studies were initiated without any preconceived notions concerning the nature of the tolerance-conferring event. In a stable adult *H-2* tolerant mouse it is impossible to know *a priori* whether the phenotype of tolerance represents (1) a passively procured state achieved at a single time in early lymphocyte ontogeny, (2) an active process in which tolerance is being continually induced as a central event, or (3) an active process that suppresses the alloreactivities of mature antigen-reactive lymphocytes in the periphery. We were prepared to accept any or all of these mechanisms as important in achieving the clinical state of *H-2* tolerance.

On the Homogeneity of Tolerant Phenotype in Neonatal Transplantation Tolerance

H-2 tolerance has been studied in numerous murine strain combinations representing various types of disparity. While all combinations were *H-2* congenic, and therefore genetically identical at all non-*H-2* loci, four different types of disparity were employed: entire *H-2* segment, class I alone (*K* or *D*), class II alone, and partial *I* region plus *D*.

We have established certain criteria for the designation of animals as *H-2* tolerant: tolerant animals must accept skin grafts bearing the tolerated allo-antigens in impeccable condition for more than 60 d, but they should reject third party (*H-2*) skin grafts in typical first set fashion; lymphoid cells harvested from tolerant animals must fail to respond specifically in mixed lymphocyte reactions (MLR), in cell-mediated lympholysis (CML) assays, and in local graft *versus* host reactions (GVHR).[9, 10] Using these criteria, we have documented several other parameters by which animals designated as tolerant are also homogeneous, even though the types of H-2 tolerogens differ (TABLE 1). (1) Thymocytes from adult tolerant animals fail to respond to the tolerated antigens *in vitro*, and lymph node and spleen cells from tolerant animals, even when activated polyclonally with concanavalin A (con A), fail specifically to kill target cells bearing the tolerated determinants.[10] Since thymocytes from normal adult mice possess alloreactivity in mixed lymphocyte reactions, we presume that cells capable of recognizing tolerated antigens have been phenotypically deleted from the thymus glands of *H-2*-tolerant mice. Moreover, the failure to activate polyclonally cytotoxic cells specific for the tolerated antigens indicates that these precursor cells must not be present among spleen and lymph node cells of tolerant mice. This is an important finding, in that the use of a polyclonal mitogen sidesteps the need for inducer cells, which have been implicated as targets of specific T suppressor cells, in the cell-mediated cytotoxicity (CMC) assay. These data do not address the question of whether T inducer cells specific for the tolerated antigens exist in tolerant mice. However, a strong case exists for the conclusion that cytotoxic cells and their precursors do not.

(2) Dr. Peter Wood in our laboratory has made a systematic study of the ontogeny of *H-2* tolerance during the first three weeks of life. He has assayed MLR and CML responses among thymocytes and splenocytes from animals that received semiallogeneic cells intravenously at birth.[11] Initially, it was confirmed that thymocytes from normal neonatal mice already possess MLR and CML toward H-2 antigens and that their spleens acquire this reactivity as early as the first three or four days of life, finally reaching adult levels after 14–21 d. When animals inoculated with semiallogeneic cells were examined, alloreactivity to H-2 antigens expressed on the inoculated cells was rapidly quenched within the neonatal thymus: MLR and CML fell to background levels within 4–5 d and never developed within spleens, even though these animals displayed normal reactivity to third party H-2 antigens. These findings are interesting on at least two counts. First, the tolerant state, as revealed by these *in vitro* tests, develops with surprising speed. By seven days of age, lymphoid cells from tolerant mice fail to react to donor-type alloantigens in a highly specific manner. Second,

TABLE 1

CHARACTERISTICS OF NEONATALLY INDUCED H-2 TOLERANCE

Accepts skin grafts bearing tolerated antigens indefinitely; rejects third party skin grafts in first-set fashion.

Fails to respond to tolerated antigens in mixed lymphocyte reactions, cell-mediated cytotoxicity, and local graft *versus* host reactions; responds normally to third party alloantigens in these assays.

Thymocytes and polyclonally activated peripheral lymphocytes from adult tolerant mice fail specifically to respond to tolerated antigens *in vitro*.

Specific alloreactivity is rapidly depleted from neonatal thymus glands after inoculation of semiallogeneic cells.

Specific alloreactivity to tolerated antigens never develops in spleens of neonatally injected mice.

Suppressor cells, active in MLR, CML, and GVHR assays, are not present in lymphoid cell suspensions prepared from adult tolerant mice.

Chimerism in spleen, lymph nodes, and bone marrow ranges from 0.5 to 4.0%; chimeric cells are rarely found in thymuses.

H-2 tolerance can be established in the face of already extant alloreactivity directed at the putative tolerogens: Although thymus cells of uninjected neonatal mice already possess alloreactivity, this reactivity is lost from the thymus over the several days after inoculation and does not appear in the spleen at any time thereafter. These data strongly suggest that an active process interferes with the expression of alloreactivity that has already formed within the thymus gland of newborn mice. Comparable ontogenetic studies of specific alloreactivity have been conducted in strain combinations representing various types of H-2 incompatibility, and the pattern is similar for all. Disparities of class II share with entire *H-2* disparities a rapid quenching of specific alloreactivity in thymus glands of injected neonates who never acquire detectable specific alloreactivity in their spleens.

(3) R. S. Gruchalla has extensively examined lymph node and spleen cells from *H-2* tolerant mice for their capacity to suppress normal alloreactive cells

in three different assays: mixed lymphocyte reaction, cell-mediated cytotoxicity, and local graft *versus* host reactions. In no instance was it possible to demonstrate that the addition of tolerant cells interfered with (suppressed) the alloreactivity of admixed normal cells. At least for tolerant animals of the type produced and studied in this laboratory, conventional assays for suppressor cell activity have been of no value in dissecting the tolerant phenotype.[10]

(4) Chimerism, of a rather low order, is regularly established in all animals who become *H-2* tolerant. By employing fluorescein isothiocyanate (FITC)-labeled semiallogeneic cells at the time of neonatal inoculation, labeled cells of donor origin have been found in spleen, liver, and bone marrow. Only very rarely are similarly labeled cells detected by fluorescent microscopy among thymocytes of mice inoculated at birth. In stable adult tolerant mice, descendants of the original donor inoculum have been identified in spleen, lymph nodes, and bone marrow using fluorescence microscopy with the aid of alloantigen-specific monoclonal antibodies. The degree of chimerism varies, but is always a small percentage, ranging from 0.2 to 4.0% of the number of cells within each of these lymphoid compartments. The degree of detectable chimerism within the thymus is exceedingly small, usually comprising less than 0.1% of cells; in many instances, no chimeric cells could be detected. In the case of mice rendered tolerant of Ia antigens alone, the actual degree of chimerism is likely to be higher than these figures suggest. Only a portion of the cellular descendants of the original semiallogeneic cells will express class II MHC determinants during any stage of differentiation. Thus, Ia-tolerant mice may contain a higher degree of chimerism than the data indicate. Assuming that the proportion of spleen cells that are Ia+ will be the same for descendants of the tolerance-conferring inoculum as for normal cell populations, then as many as 8–10% of spleen cells in Ia-tolerant mice may actually be descended from the original donor cells. In any event, the degree of chimerism in Ia-tolerant mice is of approximately the same order of magnitude as that for other types of *H-2* tolerance.

Thus, irrespective of the type of H-2 antigen used for tolerance induction, all adult tolerant mice possess a uniform phenotype by the criteria just described. Yet we were convinced that more than one mechanism was operative in our tolerant animals. In an effort to identify these putative mechanisms, we designed several experimental approaches toward unmasking them. First, we tested the tolerance-conferring efficacy of semiallogeneic cells when admixed with equal numbers of immunocompetent lymph node and spleen cells from adult mice syngeneic with neonatal recipients of the inoculum. Second, we attempted to abolish the tolerant state in adult mice by administering cellular suspensions prepared from syngeneic lymph node spleen and bone marrow. Third, we attempted to transfer the tolerant state to untreated syngeneic recipients with spleen and lymph node cells and with bone marrow cells from tolerant mice. The results, which successfully reveal that more than one mechanism operates in the induction and maintenance of the tolerant state, follow.

INDUCTION OF TOLERANCE WITH MIXTURES
OF ADULT SYNGENEIC AND SEMIALLOGENEIC LYMPHOHEMATOPOIETIC CELLS

The amazing rapidity with which *H-2* tolerance becomes established in neonatal mice led us to consider the possibility that an active process was being exerted against already formed immunocompetent alloreactive cells. Specifically, we had found that neonatal thymocytes, which had already acquired alloreactivity to *H-2* alloantigens, lost this reactivity within four or five days of the inoculation of semiallogeneic cells. The cells in question are thought to be ontogenetically mature and poised to disseminate from thymus to peripheral lymph structures. Yet, after the injection of semiallogeneic cells, these cells were depleted from the thymus and failed to take up residence in peripheral lymphoid organs, suggesting that they had been deleted or suppressed. As a means of testing this possibility, we constructed mixtures of lymphohematopoietic cells from adult semiallogeneic donors and from donors syngeneic with the neonatal mice to be injected. It was reasoned that the latter population, which is known to contain mature alloreactive lymphocytes specific for the tolerogens on the semiallogeneic cells, should be susceptible to specific quenching of alloreactivity in the injected neonatal recipient similar to that hypothesized to occur within the recipient's own thymus gland. While this line of experiments has not been completed, preliminary results are revealing and are presented in TABLE 2. When the disparity was limited to class II alloantigens, tolerance was established even though mature alloreactive cells were present in the tolerance-conferring inoculum. By contrast, B10.S mice, injected at birth with a mixture of semiallogeneic (B10.S × 9R)F$_1$ hematopoietic cells and B10.S spleen cells, failed to develop tolerance. Since B10.S neonates injected at birth with (B10.S × 9R)F$_1$ cells are easily tolerized, this failure is a significant one. These results indicate that the induction of tolerance to different *H-2* alloantigens proceeds differently and involves at least partially nonoverlapping cell types. At least for the specific genetic relationships used, mature lymphocytes capable of recognizing Ia alloantigens can be inhibited from responding to these antigens in the neonatal environment, whereas similarly mature lymphocytes reactive with D region antigens are impervious to this effect. Presumably, these latter cells mount an effective attack against the admixed semiallogeneic cells and prevent the establishment of stable chimerism. Studies to document this interpretation are in progress.

ABOLITION OF TOLERANCE IN ADULT MICE WITH SYNGENEIC LYMPHOHEMATOPOIETIC CELLS

Adult tolerant mice with long-standing (>60 d) skin grafts bearing the tolerated antigens received intravenously either 100×10^6 lymph node and spleen cells or a similar number of bone marrow cells harvested from syngeneic donors. During the next 45 d, the resident grafts were examined for evidence of rejection. In animals whose tolerated grafts were healthy at 45 d, a second skin graft, syngeneic with the first, was placed orthotopically. The survival patterns of these grafts were then examined over the following 30 d. The results of these experiments, conducted chiefly by R. S. Gruchalla, are presented in TABLE 3. The various types of immunogenetic disparity are presented separately. Three groups performed similarly: class I alone, entire H-2, and partial class II plus class I. The majority of these recipients of syngeneic lymph node and spleen cells rejected their long-standing skin allografts, evidence that the tolerant state had been abolished; moreover, virtually all the remaining animals strongly rejected second skin grafts of the same genotype. Thus, immunocompetent syngeneic lymphoid cells are able to fully abolish the tolerant state

TABLE 2

TOLERANCE-CONFERRING POTENTIAL OF SEMIALLOGENEIC HEMATOPOIETIC CELLS ALONE
AND WHEN ADMIXED WITH SYNGENEIC IMMUNOCOMPETENT CELLS

Neonatal Recipients	Inoculum	N	Percentage Tolerant
B10.S	(B10.S × 9R)F₁	27	96
B10.S	B10.S + (B10.S × 9R)F₁	15	0
B10.AQR	(B10.AQR × 6R)F₁	29	90
B10.AQR	B10.AQR + (B10.AQR × 6R)F₁	18	50

in mice tolerant of entire *H-2* and single class I antigens. However, no similar success was observed in mice tolerant only of Ia alloantigens. A small minority of *I* region–tolerant mice that received immunocompetent syngeneic cells rejected their long-standing tolerated grafts, and less than 50% of the remainder rejected the second test graft. Thus, in a majority of Ia-tolerant mice, the tolerant state appeared to be so firmly entrenched that the administration of large numbers of mature alloreactive syngeneic cells failed to abolish it. These results strongly suggest that an active process exists within Ia-tolerant mice that is capable of deleting or suppressing the reactivities of mature alloreactive lymphoid cells.

As a further confirmation of this notion, lymphoid cells harvested from spleen and lymph nodes of Ia-tolerant mice whose tolerance had not been abolished by the administration of syngeneic lymphoid cells responded *in vitro* in mixed lymphocyte reactions to the tolerated antigens. Nonetheless, these animals retained their test allografts in impeccable condition.

It was of considerable interest to examine the fate of tolerance when adult mice received inoculations of syngeneic bone marrow cells (see TABLE 3). If simple clonal deletion was the mechanism of *H-2* tolerance induction, achieved as a single irrevocable effect during neonatal life, then supplying an adult

TABLE 3

ABOLITION OF H-2 TOLERANCE WITH SYNGENEIC CELLS

Disparity	Inoculum *	N	Tolerance Abolished †
Class I	LN + SPL	25	96
	Bone marrow	24	20
	None	52	19
Class II	LN + SPL	19	43
	None	38	20
Entire H-2	LN + SPL	15	100
Partial II plus I	LN + SPL	12	100
	None	37	37

* 100 × 10⁶ syngeneic cells injected intravenously into adult tolerant mice.
† Tolerance was considered to be abolished if the first or second test skin graft was rejected within 45 or 30 d, respectively.

tolerant mouse with stem cell progenitors of specific alloreactive cells should suffice to reconstitute the alloreactivity of these mice. When class I tolerant mice were inoculated with 100×10^6 syngeneic bone marrow cells, their long-standing grafts remained unperturbed throughout the 45 d observation period. Moreover, application of a second test graft, syngeneic with the tolerated graft, resulted in the indefinite survival of both grafts. At face value, this result implies that an active process directed at deleting alloantigen-specific lymphoid cell precursors, but not their mature descendants, operates in stable tolerant mice of this type.

ADOPTIVE TRANSFER OF THE H-2 TOLERANT STATE

While the two previous experimental paradigms examined the ability of the tolerant state to modify the alloreactivity of normal mature lymphoid cells in the developing or established tolerant environment, the next procedure was designed to examine the reactivities of tolerant lymphoid cells placed in an immunocompetent, but naive environment. Adoptive transfer of *H-2* tolerance was attempted by two different protocols devised to examine the possibility that suppressor cells mediate tolerance at induction and at effectuation of the alloimmune response. In the first, recipient mice, syngeneic with the tolerant donor, received 250 rad gamma irradiation 24 h before an intravenous injection of 100×10^6 lymph node and spleen cells from *H-2*-tolerant donors. Three days later, recipients were grafted orthotopically with skin bearing the tolerated antigens. In the second protocol, 100×10^6 lymphoid cells from tolerant donors were injected intravenously into syngeneic recipients that had been grafted orthotopically with skin of the tolerated haplotype four days previously. The survival patterns of these test grafts were compared with those of grafts placed on control mice that received normal syngeneic lymphoid cells. The results of these experiments are shown in TABLES 4 and 5. When the first protocol was used, successful adoptive transfer of tolerance was achieved when the tolerated antigens were derived exclusively from the *I* region of *H-2*. More limited success was observed when the tolerogens were derived from partial class II plus single class I disparities. However, tolerance to isolated class I antigens and to the entire *H-2* segment could not be transferred by this method. When the second protocol was employed, successful transfer was achieved with all four different types of immunogenetic disparity, but as many experiments failed as succeeded. To date we have been unable to control the capriciousness of results with the second protocol, and have elected to delay further analysis. However, the results of experiments with the first protocol are consistent with those from the previously described experiments and corroborate the hypothesis that tolerance of Ia alloantigens is maintained by an active process that differs from the mechanisms operative in tolerance of class I alloantigens.

In an effort to identify the cellular basis for successful transfer of Ia tolerance, negative selection experiments were conducted in which lymphoid cell suspensions prepared from Ia-tolerant donors were treated with either (1) an anti–T cell reagent or (2) an alloantiserum directed at the relevant Ia antigens, before inoculation into untreated syngeneic recipients. These experimental results are displayed in TABLE 6. Deletion of T cells from spleen and lymph node suspensions of tolerant mice failed to prevent transfer of the tolerant state. Moreover, deletion of Ia+ cells from the adoptive transfer inoculum also failed

TABLE 4

ADOPTIVE TRANSFER OF H-2 TOLERANCE: FIRST PROTOCOL

Type of Disparity	Number of Experiments	Number of Recipients	Incidence of Successful Transfer Experiments	
			N	(%)
Class I	9	60	0	0
Class II	3	24	3	100
Entire H-2	5	31	0	0
I-J through D	3	22	2	67

NOTES: First protocol: (1) day 0: irradiate normal adult recipients with 300 rad, (2) day 1: inoculate 100×10^6 lymph node and spleen cells from tolerant donor intravenously into irradiated syngeneic recipients, (3) day 4: graft recipients with skin bearing tolerated antigens, and (4) observe for evidence of rejection.

Successful transfer: the median survival time of test grafts on recipients of putative tolerant lymphoid cells was significantly greater than that of test grafts on recipients of normal syngeneic lymphoid cells.

to prevent recipient mice from accepting Ia-disparate skin allografts for prolonged, and sometimes indefinite, periods. From a wide assortment of mechanisms that could account for Ia tolerance in this system, these experiments appear to rule out several important possibilities. Deletion of T cells had no effect; therefore, we conclude that suppressor T cells, whether of host or semiallogeneic origin, do not participate in the aspect of *H-2* tolerance revealed by adoptive transfer. Depletion of Ia-bearing cells was similarly without effect; thus, Ia-bearing cells in the transfer inoculum play no role or are not required to reestablish the tolerant state under the conditions of these experiments. However, this realization does not rule out a participatory role for semiallogeneic cells in *H-2* tolerance; only a minority of the cellular descendants of the original tolerance-conferring inoculum would be expected to bear Ia determinants, and then only during certain stages of their developmental life. The possibility

TABLE 5

ADOPTIVE TRANSFER OF H-2 TOLERANCE: SECOND PROTOCOL

Type of Disparity	Number of Experiments	Number of Recipients	Incidence of Successful Transfer Experiments	
			N	(%)
Class I	4	29	2	50
Class II	2	7	2	100
Entire H-2	2	12	2	100
I-J through D	1	6	1	100

NOTES: Second protocol: (1) day 0: graft normal adult recipients with skin bearing tolerated antigens, (2) day 4: inoculate 100×10^6 lymph node and spleen cells from tolerant donor intravenously into syngeneic recipients bearing test allografts, and (3) observe for evidence of rejection.

Successful transfer is described in TABLE 4.

exists, therefore, that non-Ia-bearing cells of original donor origin might still prove to be critical in the maintenance of tolerance. In addition, several other possibilities are consistent with these results and are discussed below.

In fairness, it should be pointed out that our arguments concerning an active process in Ia tolerance are based upon a major assumption: that the Ia-tolerant state is antigen specific. It is impossible to test this possibility directly, since appropriate *H-2* recombinant mouse strains have not yet been developed. If it should turn out that the tolerance in question lacks antigen specificity, then nonspecific suppressor mechanisms, unrelated to T cells or Ia-bearing semi-allogeneic cells, could account for the active process. We do know that Ia-tolerant mice reject skin grafts bearing third party class I alloantigens that are not expressed on cells in the tolerance-conferring inoculum. If their tolerance is a nonspecific one, then it extends only to class II determinants—an unlikely possibility.

Multiple Mechanisms Operate to Produce H-2 Transplantation Tolerance

From our earliest experimental results, we have been convinced of the likelihood that simple passive clonal deletion could never completely explain *H-2* transplantation tolerance. On the basis of the several studies just described, we feel confident in stating that active processes contribute to the tolerance phenotype. A summary of the data bearing on this important point is presented in Table 7 in such a manner that tolerance induced by class I MHC antigens can be compared with tolerance induced by class II determinants. Although the analysis is not yet complete, at this stage it seems reasonable to place tolerance to isolated Ia alloantigens in a separate category, perhaps as a subset of phenomena associated with neonatal *H-2* tolerance. Justification for this categorization rests on the following points. (1) Tolerance to this class of

TABLE 6

ADOPTIVE TRANSFER OF H-2 TOLERANCE BY FIRST PROTOCOL: DEPLETION OF SELECTED CELL TYPES FROM DONOR INOCULUM

Donor of Cells for Transfer	Antiserum Pretreatment	Number of Recipients	Median Survival Time of Test Skin Allografts (d)
Experiment 1			
B10.AQR tol 6R	anti-Thy 1.2 + C	8	45
B10.AQR tol 6R	MOPC-104E + C	7	>50
None	—	7	14.7
Experiment 2			
B10.AQR tol 6R	Anti-Ia^q + C	7	28.5
B10.AQR tol 6R	Normal mouse serum	7	21.0
None	—	6	13.2

TABLE 7

EVIDENCE CONCERNING ACTIVE MECHANISMS IN TOLERANCE DIRECTED
AT *H-2* ALLOANTIGENS

Parameter	Type of H-2 Disparity	
	Class I	Class II
Very effective as neonatal tolerogen	No	Yes
Alloreactivity rapidly quenched in neonatal thymus	Yes	Yes
Mixtures of immunocompetent syngeneic lymphoid cells and semiallogeneic cells induce neonatal tolerance	No	Yes
Tolerance can be abolished with syngeneic immunocompetent lymphocytes	Yes	No
Tolerance can be abolished with syngeneic hematopoietic cells	No	No
Tolerance can be transferred adoptively with lymph node and spleen cells		
First Protocol	No	Yes
Second Protocol	Yes	Yes

antigens, unlike class I antigens, is achieved readily after neonatal inoculation of semiallogeneic cells. (2) Ia tolerance can be enforced upon immunocompetent lymphoid cells already possessing the relevant alloreactivity. Supporting evidence includes (a) rapid loss of alloreactivity among immunocompetent thymocytes of injected neonates, (b) successful induction of tolerance by semiallogeneic cells mixed with immunocompetent cells at the time of neonatal injection, (c) failure of immunocompetent lymphoid cells to abolish the adult tolerant state, and (d) successful adoptive transfer of Ia tolerance to naive recipients. (3) Healthy skin grafts persist both on recipients of adoptive transfer and on tolerant recipients of immunocompetent lymphoid cells despite the fact that specific alloreactive cells can be identified by MLR in their spleens and lymph nodes. Simple suppression systems, of the type revealed in MLR, CMC, and GVHR assays, are apparently not involved; moreover, host T cells are not responsible for adoptive transfer, nor are the cells bearing the tolerated Ia antigens at the time of adoptive transfer. This concentration of baffling requirements and restrictions is not easily accommodated in a simple hypothesis. Nonetheless, placing special emphasis on the fact that Ia tolerance can be enforced upon mature peripheral lymphoid cells, we would suggest that a suppression system, perhaps mediated by antigen- or idjotype-specific B cells and their antibody products, could be operating. We have no direct data to support this notion, although a formidable array of negative data are consistent with it. Since the hypothesis lends itself readily to testing, its validity can be determined.

But what of neonatally induced tolerance to class I and entire H-2 disparities? A peripheral mechanism similar to that invoked for Ia antigen tolerance apparently does not operate for other types of *H-2* tolerance. In the latter case, evidence in favor of active mechanisms is scantier and the phenotype of clonal deletion is much more pervasive. The prompt abolition of class I and entire *H-2* tolerance by the systemic administration of syngeneic immunocompetent lymphoid cells and the failure to adoptively transfer the tolerant state of immunocompetent recipients (by the first protocol) indicate that this type of tolerance can not be impressed upon mature antigen-reactive cells in the periphery; if an active process operates, these data imply that the process operates on less mature cells with the aid of peanut agglutinin (PNA). We have investigated mature (PNA⁻) and immature (PNA⁺) thymocytes in the adult tolerant state. PNA⁺ thymocytes are thought to represent immature cells that bear antigen-specific receptors on their surface but have not yet differentiated into fully functional T cells. When these cells are placed in mixed lymphocyte cultures with allogeneic stimulator cells, they fail to respond; however, if T cell growth factor (interleukin-2) is added to the culture medium, a proliferative response ensues. By employing this assay, it has been determined that the thymus glands of adult *H-2* tolerant mice lack PNA⁺ cells capable of responding to the tolerated antigens, although PNA⁺ cells that react to third party alloantigens do exist. Thus, the phenotype of clonal deletion extends to the earliest identifiable thymocytes and raises the possibility that the deletion process may even take place prethymically. Our finding that exceedingly few (if any) FITC-labeled semiallogeneic cells ever appear in the thymus glands of neonatal recipient mice is consistent with a prethymic site of deletion, since it is difficult to envision how so few cells could be so strategically located within the thymus that they achieve deletion. This does not represent proof, however; merely circumstantial evidence.

The finding that syngeneic adult bone marrow cells were unable to abolish tolerance in stable class I tolerant mice is also consistent with an active process maintaining the tolerant state and focuses attention on the hematopoietic marrow as a possible site. Direct experimental verification of this possibility represents a formidable challenge. We have accumulated a disappointing list of negative experiments that have attempted to test the idea that tolerance is actively induced within the hematopoietic marrow by the presence of semiallogeneic cells: (1) H-2 tolerance can not be transferred adoptively to untolerized adult mice with bone marrow cells harvested from tolerant donors; (2) tolerance can not be induced in adult mice by the intravenous inoculation of mixtures of syngeneic normal lymphoid cells and semiallogeneic bone marrow cells; (3) tolerance can not be achieved in adult mice by the intravenous inoculation of semiallogeneic bone marrow cells depleted of Ia antigen–positive cells by treatment with specific alloantiserum and complement. Preliminary attempts to isolate thymic precursors from bone marrow suspensions, force their differentiation *in vitro* in the presence of thymosin, and then test their alloreactivity in the presence of interleukin-2 have failed. This approach would be an attractive way to determine whether, in tolerant animals, antigen-specific thymic precursors exist in the bone marrow even though they can not be identified in the thymus. An alternative approach would be to devise an experimental protocol in which bone marrow cells from a tolerant animal (from which semiallogeneic cells had been depleted) could be placed in an inert recipient in which the tempo of the emergence of tolerogen-specific antigen-reactive cells could be studied. In a sense, this experimental approach has been successfully employed by Dorsch and Roser in a rat transplantation tolerance model.[12] The idea is also related to a set of experiments conducted by Scott to evaluate T cell unresponsiveness to nontransplantation antigens.[13]

Lest the focus on bone marrow as the site of tolerance induction and maintenance dominate our thinking, we recognize that other tissue sites could as easily be involved. Since the early days in which chimerical analysis of neo-natally induced tolerance was conducted by chromosomal counting methods and with cytotoxic alloantisera, it has been stated that the level of chimerism in mice made *H-2* tolerant with semiallogeneic cells is exceedingly low—usually below the level of resolution of the assays. Now that monoclonal antibodies specific for *H-2* alloantigens are available, accurate detection and quantification of chimerism is possible. In our laboratory, descendants of semiallogeneic cells used to induce tolerance can regularly be found in lymphoid tissues of adult tolerant mice; the frequency ranges from 0.2–4.0%. While this number seems quite small, it represents, in the aggregate, a sizable pool of antigen-bearing cells. Since chimerism is essential to the maintenance of *H-2* tolerance, it is relevant to consider the proportion of chimeric cells within tolerant animals. Two observations indicate the extent to which chimeric cells infiltrate tissues where immune responses are induced and expressed. Forman and Streilein have reported that when *H-2* tolerant mice are primed *in vivo* to minor H antigens, their splenic cells can be converted *in vitro* into cytotoxic T cells that are restricted by the class I antigens of the host as well as by those of the chimeric cells.[14]

This observation indicates that chimeric cells are present in relevant lymph organs to permit recognition of minor H antigens in the context of "tolerated" class I determinants. In addition, we have recently confirmed Steinmuller's observation that skin grafts prepared from *H-2* tolerant mice, when placed orthotopically on syngeneic recipients, induce alloimmunity to the tolerated antigens; this is revealed by the fact that these recipients reject, in second-set fashion, skin bearing the putative tolerogens.[15] While Steinmuller was unable to document the degree of chimerism in his animals, we know that lympho-hematopoietic chimerism in our animals may approach 4%. Epidermal Langerhans cells are an important alloantigenic cell within skin grafts. Recognizing that Langerhans cells are derived from bone marrow precursors,[16] we presume that the skin of tolerant mice would be comprised of comparable proportions of host and chimeric Langerhans cells. The epidermis of murine skin contains approximately 700–800 Langerhans cells per mm^2.[17] Thus, each skin graft (175 mm^2) used in these studies contained as many as 5000 semiallogeneic Langerhans cells. A similar number of spleen cells has been shown to be sufficient to immunize mice to *H-2* alloantigens.[18] Considering the size of the cutaneous surface in a mouse, the number of donor-descended Langerhans cells is almost staggering and represents an enormous reservoir of tolerated antigen.

These points are made merely to emphasize the magnitude of the expression of semiallogeneic antigens in adult H-2 tolerant mice whose level of chimerism is usually stated to be quite low. On the contrary, chimeric cell antigens are expressed throughout all the tissues of tolerant animals, and not only within bone marrow and organized lymphoid tissues. Thus, there are virtually un-limited anatomical possibilities for confrontations between emerging antigen-reactive cells and tolerated antigens. Identifying the relevant site or sites is another formidable challenge.

SUMMARY

Based on our studies to date, as well as the results of others, we are of the opinion that the phenomenon of neonatally induced *H-2* tolerance (in which the phenotypes of *in vivo* and *in vitro* alloreactivities are homogenous) does not result from a single process. Our evidence identifies (1) a peripheral process that can prevent mature alloreactive lymphocytes from responding to class II alloantigens, (2) a central mechanism that functionally deletes tolerogen-specific lymphocyte precursors, perhaps even before they reach the thymus, and (3) a genetic mechanism that endows Ia antigens with the capacity to promote tolerance induction of class I alloantigens in neonatal mice. We believe, but have no direct proof, that neonatally induced *H-2* tolerance is achieved through an interlocking network of fail-safe mechanisms in which "forbidden" allo-reactive clones, from the moment they acquire the capacity to recognize toler-ated antigens, are confronted by sequential barriers to their functional matura-tion and to their ultimate participation in alloimmune responses. Conceptually, it is reasonable to identify the following as likely participants in the erection of these barriers: (1) alloantigen-bearing chimeric cells, (2) alloantigen-specific T suppressor cells and B cells (responsible for enhancing antibodies), (3) idiotypically oriented host T suppressors, as well as alloantigen-receptor oriented T cells of chimeric origin. But, practically, the data that verify the role of any of these participants are embarrassingly shallow. If neonatal *H-2* tolerance can be imagined as a hologram, one gets the feeling that squinting through the currently available data might reveal only the barest outlines of its form.

ACKNOWLEDGMENTS

The numerous contributions to this work at many levels by Dr. R. E. Billingham are deeply appreciated. We wish to thank Mr. John Peeler for expert technical assistance and Ms. Helen Patterson for careful preparation of the manuscript.

REFERENCES

1. BILLINGHAM, R. E., L. BRENT & P. MEDAWAR. 1953. Actively acquired tolerance of foreign cells. Nature (London) **172:** 603–6.
2. BILLINGHAM, R. E., L. BRENT & P. B. MEDAWAR. 1956. Quantitative studies on tissue transplantation immunity. III. Actively acquired tolerance. Proc. R. Soc. London Ser. B **239:** 357–415.
3. BURNET, F. M. 1959. The Clonal Selection Theory of Acquired Immunity. Cambridge University Press. Cambridge.
4. MÖLLER, G., Ed. 1979. Transplantation Tolerance. Immunol. Rev. **46:** 3–146.S.
5. STREILEIN, J. W. & J. KLEIN. 1977. Neonatal tolerance to *K* and *D* region alloantigens of *H-2* complex. J. Immunol. **119:** 2147–50.
6. STREILEIN, J. W. & J. KLEIN. 1980. Neonatal tolerance of H-2 alloantigens. I. *I* region modulation of tolerogenic potential of K and D antigens. Proc. R. Soc. London Ser. B **207:** 461–74.
7. STREILEIN, J. W. 1980. Neonatal tolerance of H-2 alloantigens. II. *I* region dependence of tolerance expressed to K and D antigens. Proc. R. Soc. London Ser. B **207:** 475–86.
8. CZITROM, A. A., G. H. SUNSHINE & N. A. MITCHISON. 1980. Suppression of the proliferative response to *H-2D* by *I-J* subregion products. Immuno-genetics **11:** 97–102.
9. STREILEIN, J. W. & R. S. GRUCHALLA. 1981. Analysis of neonatally induced

tolerance of H-2 alloantigens. I. Adoptive transfer indicates that tolerance of class I and class II antigens is maintained by distinct mechanisms. Immunogenetics **12:** 161–74.

10. GRUCHALLA, R. S. & J. W. STREILEIN. 1982. Analysis of neonatally induced tolerance of H-2 alloantigens. II. Failure to detect alloantigen-specific T lymphocyte precursors and suppressors. Immunogenetics. **15:** 111–27.
11. WOOD, P. J. & J. W. STREILEIN. 1982. Ontogeny of acquired immunological tolerance to H-2 alloantigens. Eur. J. Immunol. **12:** 188–94.
12. ROSER, B. & S. DORSCH. 1979. The cellular basis of transplantation tolerance in the rat. Immunol. Rev. **46:** 55–86.
13. COHN, M. L. & D. W. SCOTT. 1979. Functional differentiation of T cell precursors. 1. Parameters of carrier-specific tolerance in murine helper T cell precursors. J. Immunol. **123:** 2083–87.
14. FORMAN, J. & J. W. STREILEIN. 1979. T cells recognize minor histocompatibility antigens on *H-2* allogeneic cells. J. Exp. Med. **150:** 1001–7.
15. STEINMULLER, D. 1967. Immunization with skin isografts taken from tolerant mice. Science **158:** 127–29.
16. KATZ, S. I., K. TAMAKI & D. H. SACHS. 1979. Epidermal Langerhans cells are derived from cells originating in bone marrow. Nature (London) **282:** 324–26.
17. BERGSTRESSER, P. R., C. FLETCHER & J. W. STREILEIN. 1980. Surface densities of Langerhans cells in relation to rodent epidermal sites with special immunologic properties. J. Invest. Dermatol. **74:** 77–80.
18. BILLINGHAM, R. E. & L. BRENT. 1959. Quantitative studies on tissue transplantation immunity. IV. Induction of tolerance in newborn mice and studies on the phenomenon of runt disease. Philos. Trans. R. Soc. London Ser. **242:** 439–77.

DISCUSSION OF THE PAPER

D. R. GREEN (*Yale University, New Haven, Conn.*): The cell that transfers tolerance doesn't appear to be a T cell in this system. How about the cells that block the induction of tolerance in the neonate or help break tolerance?

STREILEIN: We have not looked at them.

A. M. MARCHAND (*Santurce, Puerto Rico*): Do you have any data as to the risk of cancer in these animals—the incidence of cancers?

STREILEIN: We have not made any effort to collect that kind of data in a systematic way. The animals actually have a noticeable incidence of lymphoid neoplasms. The ones that we've identified so far all seem to be of the T cell variety, and some of them even have interesting reactivities with the alloantigens in question.

J. CHILLER (*Scripps Clinic and Research Foundation, La Jolla, Calif.*): The inability to induce tolerance in the class I system is where you cotransfer normal and immunocompetent donor cells, is that right?

STREILEIN: That's right.

CHILLER: How do you explain that phenomenon? First, what are these cells immunocompetent to?

STREILEIN: In these experiments, I took the spleen and lymph node cells out of an adult B10.S mouse and mixed them with a (B10.S × 9R)F$_1$ cell population and injected that mixture into a neonate. Now I presume, but have no direct evidence, that the B10.S adult cells are immunocompetent in that environment and are able, somehow, in their reaction against the 9R alloantigens, to prevent the successful establishment of chimerism. If that is what is happening, it does not appear to take place with class II antigens.

CHILLER: Will the phenomenon no longer hold if you take cells from a tolerant adult animal and do the same transfer—in other words, if you eliminate that alloreactive population?

STREILEIN: We have not done that experiment precisely, but the ability to transfer tolerance with bone marrow and spleen cells from tolerant animals to untolerized animals, such as neonates, has been shown before.

QUESTION: Can you transfer tolerance with thymic or bone marrow populations from your tolerant animals?

STREILEIN: I cannot answer with regard to the thymus. We have been unable to transfer tolerance with bone marrow from tolerant animals.

QUESTION: Have you any indication that, if you inject bone marrow cells into syngeneic animals, they will differentiate and you will have T cell differentiation? Or do they not compete with the local bone marrow cells?

STREILEIN: In which experiment?

QUESTION: The one in which you inject syngeneic bone marrow cells into tolerant animals. I don't think there's a chance that bone marrow will be accepted in a normal nonirradiated animal even if it is syngeneic.

STREILEIN: I agree. That's not a very strong experiment. I couldn't think of how else to do that. We have no evidence that the marrow was, in fact, engrafted.

B. HALL (*R.P.A. Hospital, Camperdown, N.S.W., Australia*): The experiments you did with adoptive transfer were negative selection experiments, in that you depleted T cells or depleted Ia-bearing cells. Have you ever done the positive selection experiment and determined if pure populations of T cells or pure populations of Ia-positive cells will adoptively transfer tolerance?

STREILEIN: No, we've not tried to purify T cells from the tolerant animals and get them to work. We are unable to establish tolerance in adult animals after irradiation by giving them F$_1$ Ia-bearing cells. But that's not exactly the experiment you're suggesting. No, we've not done that.

HALL: Ia-bearing cells from normal animals?

STREILEIN: From normal animals.

HALL: Do you think there are two mechanisms operating? Perhaps, after you delete the suppressor T cell, the Ia residual population cell operates; then, when you do the experiment the other way around, the other mechanism operates.

STREILEIN: I'm not sure whether there're two mechanisms or whether there's a single mechanism that requires two participants, both of which need to be present in order for it to work. I can't answer that.

T CELL SIGNALS IN TOLERANCE *

Henry N. Claman

Departments of Medicine and of Microbiology and Immunology
University of Colorado Health Sciences Center
Denver, Colorado 80262

INTRODUCTION

My purpose is to discuss signals that turn T cells on and off. I will do this primarily by using data from the model of dinitrofluorobenzene (DNFB) contact sensitivity and tolerance. I shall try to bring together some experimental observations and integrate them into our knowledge of cellular immunology. As our knowledge has grown over the past few years, we have come to recognize that regulatory mechanisms controlling T cell responses are complex—in fact, even more complex than the basic T cell mechanisms themselves.

I will discuss separately the following two subjects: first, the results of presenting DNP to unprimed or naive T cells. If the signal is "on," we call it induction, sensitization, or priming. If the signal is "off," we call it tolerance.[1] Second, the results of presenting DNP to primed systems. If the result is "on," we call it boosting or anamnesis. If the signal is "off," we call it desensitization. I make a distinction between naive systems and primed systems because the phenomenology is different. Whether the differences are qualitative or merely quantitative remains to be seen.

SIGNALS FOR T_{DH} IN AN UNPRIMED SYSTEM

On Signals for Unprimed T Cells

In contact sensitization to DNP, the phenomenology tells us that DNP must be closely associated with self components and that sensitization occurs best when DNP is on Ia-bearing cells, *e.g.*, Langerhans cells in the skin. That is, the sensitizing antigen is DNP-self. The sensitizing antigen stimulates at least three antigen-specific cells (TABLE 1). (1) The delayed hypersensitivity T cell (T_{DH} presumably from a T_{DH} precursor, pT_{DH}), which is id+, Ia-, Lyt 1+, and functionally able to transfer the sensitized state to naive syngeneic recipients in a classic Landsteiner-Chase passive transfer experiment. This cell does not appear to proliferate *in vitro* when restimulated. (2) The T proliferative cell (T_{prlf}, which may be a helper cell), which is id+, Ia+, and proliferates *in vitro* when restimulated with antigen. (3) The Ts-auxiliary cell (Ts-aux), which is id+, I-J+, and functionally interacts with efferent suppressor T cells and with anti-id.

The stimulation of pT_{DH} occurs by associative recognition of DNP-self and another signal (perhaps contributed by the T proliferative or helper cell);

* This research was supported, in part, by a grant from the United States Public Health Service, no. AI–12685.

0077-8923/82/0392-0291 $1.75/0 © 1982, NYAS

TABLE 1

CELLS INDUCED BY SENSITIZATION TO DNFB
(ALL IDIOTYPE POSITIVE)

TDH	Ia⁻
	Passively transfers contact sensitivity.
Tprlf	Ia⁺
	Proliferates *in vitro*. A helper?
Ts-aux	I-J⁺
	Delivers a negative signal to TDH in suppression.

thus, there are two signals involved in contact sensitization. I call DNP-self signal 1 and the other signal, as yet unidentified, signal 2. It is likely that signal 2 is a nonspecific interleukin-type stimulus. This is diagrammed in FIGURE 1. (We know there are two signals because we will see later that presentation of signal 1 only may not turn the system "on" and, indeed, may turn it "off"—see below.)

It seems that the two signals do not have to be presented together for priming to occur. This is exemplified by experiments in which DNP-self (signal 1) is given i.v. This is actually an "off" signal; but, when concanavalin A (con A) is given soon after, the combination results in sensitization.[2] (Con A by itself seems to do nothing in this system.) Thus, con A serves as signal 2, which, when added to signal 1, results in priming (FIGURE 2). Similarly, sensitization results when dinitrobenzene sulfonic acid (DNBSO₃) is signal 1 and amphotericin B is signal 2.[3] Cohn calls this an abnormal form of induction that may be related to autoimmunity.[4] The original example was by Dresser, who was the first to discuss immunity and tolerance in terms of two signals *versus* one signal. In his experiments, bovine gamma globulin (BGG) was the tolerogen (signal 1) and Freund's adjuvant was signal 2. The two signals could be given separately to get immunity.[5]

Off Signals for Unprimed T Cells

In contact sensitivity, tolerance may be produced by presenting the antigen (or congers of it) by special routes. This includes the intravenous route [6] and, as first shown by Merrill Chase for dinitrochlorobenzene, the oral route.[7] Even topical DNFB can produce tolerance if it is presented on skin poor in antigen-presenting Langerhans cells.[8] With DNFB, tolerance can occur after intravenous presentation of DNFB, DNBSO₃, dinitrophenylated red blood cells (DNP-RBC), and DNP-lymphocytes, but not with DNP-lysine or DNP-mouse gamma globulin (DNP-MGG).[9] We showed that, among the different cell types asso-

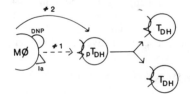

FIGURE 1. Ordinarily, signals 1 and 2 are closely linked.

ciated with DNFB, the most efficient tolerance was produced by cells bearing the most Ia antigens.[10] This makes it likely that the tolerogenic signal (1) is, in fact, DNP associated with Ia, which is what is believed to be signal 1 for induction of sensitivity. (Many experiments have shown that, in this model, tolerogenic signals also turn on T suppressors (Ts). Since the inducers of Ts appear to be sensitive to cyclophosphamide (Cy) and tolerance can be produced by signal 1 after Cy treatment,[11] I believe that these tolerogens can provide "off" signals directly to pT_{DH}.) It should be clear that, in order to preserve the tolerogenic function of signal 1, it must be processed by methods that evade the endogenous production of signal two, which would convert the tolerogen into an immunogen. An example is TNP-lymphoid cells, which are tolerogenic if given intravenously but immunogenic if given subcutaneously.[12] Somehow, "host processing" by the subcutaneous route adds signal 2 to the tolerogen and results in sensitization. Nevertheless, the i.v. route is not always tolerogenic (just as the epicutaneous route does not always sensitize). Certain Ia^+ cells, such as Langerhans epidermal cells, coupled with hapten will sensitize if given intravenously.[13] Thus, both the form and the route of the antigen determine the outcome.

DNP-lysine given i.v. does not tolerize, and so does not appear to be recognized by pT_{DH} as any type of signal.[14] Again, this agrees with the concept that signal 1 is DNP associated with Ia. As DNP-lysine is not chemically

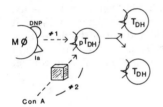

FIGURE 2. Signals 1 and 2 can be delivered separately (non-associatively).

reactive; it is not able to join a membrane to make signal 1. DNP-MGG is an interesting case; it is a potent B cell tolerogen [15] but does not tolerize in contact sensitivity to DNFB.[16] Thus, "off" signals for B cells may be different from "off" signals for T cells. Actually, as B cells recognize free antigen, one would not expect a requirement for self to constitute a tolerizing signal 1 for B cells.

REGULATION OF THE PRIMED T_{DH} SYSTEM

On Signals—Anamnestic Responses

T cell memory exists in contact sensitivity; resensitization with booster epicutaneous doses of DNFB will give increased contact responses. Thus, primed T_{DH} may be reactivated by both signals, 1 and 2, given by topical DNFB. Little work has been done to measure booster responses in Tprlf or Ts-aux. The system is complicated, however, since repeated applications of contact sensitizer also raise anti-hapten antibodies.[17, 18]

Off Signals—Desensitization

This is a much more interesting question, and can be restated as, What signals are necessary either to turn off primed T_{DH} or to prevent their reactivation? The answers are complex and interesting.

Anti-Idiotypic Antibody

Anti-idiotypic antibody (anti-id) can negatively regulate established contact sensitivity responses. Normally occurring anti-id arises during contact sensitivity to DNFB and down regulates it in the animal.[19] An anti-id antiserum that behaves like the normally occurring anti-id has been raised by repeatedly immunizing mice with syngeneic cells rich in T_{DH}. Thus, the anti-id appears to be induced by T_{DH} and can down regulate T_{DH} either in the animal itself or by inhibiting the classical Landsteiner-Chase passive transfer of contact sensitivity.[20] As it is an antibody and shows no MHC restriction in its action,[19] one might predict that it would act directly on the idiotype of T cells reactive to DNP (presumably DNP-self). This is a form of nonassociative recognition and could be thought of as a kind of signal 1 (although that is usually considered to be antigen and not anti-id). The surprising finding is that, although this anti-id appears to be raised by T_{DH} and although T_{DH}-rich populations bind to and adsorb anti-id, its action is through another id+ cell, namely Ts-aux. Anti-id activates Ts-aux, which then delivers some negative signal to T_{DH}. It seems paradoxical that, although T_{DH} induces anti-id and anti-id binds to T_{DH}, anti-id has as yet no discernible action directly on T_{DH}. In summary, anti-id can serve as a negatively regulating signal that acts indirectly on T_{DH} in contact sensitivity.

Desensitization by Antigen (Signal 1)

Desensitization in vivo. Negative regulation by suppressive mechanisms, often including anti-idiotypes (as above), are so pervasive in immunology that one wonders about simpler mechanisms in which antigens are used to desensitize. Desensitization of DTH has been accomplished on occasion.[21, 22] In experimental contact sensitivity, the results are not dramatic. DeWeck showed that, in guinea pigs, DNP-lysine did not desensitize and $DNBSO_3$ did so only transiently.[23] We also showed that injection of large amounts of $DNBSO_3$ induced a temporary state of unresponsiveness that lasted only 2–3 d. It was accompanied by and correlated with proliferation of some unidentified cells in the mouse.[24] Thus, $DNBSO_3$, which appears to be a tolerogenic signal 1 in naive animals, is not effective in the desensitization of primed animals. It also seems to induce active processes such as cell proliferation, which would not be characteristic of "pure" signal 1 substances. These phenomena also raise the question of whether the signals for pT_{DH} in naive animals are different from the signals for mature or induced T_{DH} in primed animals.

Desensitization or Blocking Induced by Antigen in Vitro. The above experiments show that it is difficult to use antigen alone to desensitize animals with contact sensitivity *in vivo*. If it could be done, it might be done *via* indirect mechanisms, such as provocation of anti-hapten or anti-id antibodies, or directly *via* the often discussed but rarely proven mechanism of "receptor blockade." Recently, John Moorhead has done experiments that bear on this question.[25] He has blocked the passive transfer of contact sensitivity by a brief incubation of DNFB-primed cells with small amounts of DNP-lysine. Such DNP-lysine-treated cells fail to transfer contact sensitivity. The inhibition is antigen-specific and apparently does not involve suppressor cells, since populations depleted of Lyt 2[+] cells are also blocked. However, the blockade is weak, in that it is readily reversed by incubating the blocked cells in media free of DNP-lysine. These data are of interest for several reasons. First, the inhibition occurs *via* the same receptor that binds anti-id antibody. Second, it implies that the primed T cells can recognize free antigen and thus makes it likely either that the T cell has two receptors, or that it has one that, perhaps in part, recognizes DNP. Third, it suggests that receptor blockade, independent of indirect influences from suppressor cells, can directly down regulate T_{DH}.

In terms of signal theory, I would interpret these data as follows. First, DNP-lysine can act as signal 1 (although weakly) and directly down regulate primed T_{DH} by occupying the idiotype. Second, this appears to be a weak interaction that is readily reversible *in vitro*. This probably explains why DNP-lysine is a poor desensitizer *in vivo*—it is undoubtedly very difficult to get a high enough tolerogen concentration *in vivo* for such a weak antigen-idiotype interaction. Third, the reversible nature of the interaction between receptor and antigen (signal 1) indicates that such an interaction, although leading to cell inactivation, is only temporary and does not deliver a long-lasting negative signal ("turn off") to the T_{DH}.

The role of anti-antigen antibody (blocking antibody) in desensitization is outside the scope of this presentation but may well be another possible mechanism.

QUESTIONS RAISED BY THESE DATA

Many questions are raised and I shall discuss only a few.

How Different Are Signals for Unprimed and Primed Systems?

(1) DNP-lysine does not affect either one *in vivo*. It weakly blocks primed T_{DH} *in vitro* but does not stimulate Tprlf.[14] It has not been tested on pT_{DH}. (2) $DNBSO_3$ acts as signal 1 on unprimed cells and also triggers suppressive mechanisms. Its desensitizing action on primed systems is temporary and one wonders why it doesn't appear to turn on suppressive mechanisms in primed systems and lead to more effective down regulation.

What Happens When Idiotypes Are Occupied?

Perhaps the interaction between T_{DH} and DNP-lysine is weak because this cell usually sees DNP-self. In this case, DNP-lysine is a sort of signal ½; perhaps better desensitization would occur if the T_{DH} met with a whole signal 1, *e.g.*, DNP-Ia membrane. How is the interaction of idiotype with DNP-lysine different from the interaction with anti-idiotype? DNP-lysine seems to block T_{DH} but anti-id has no discernible effect. In terms of Ts-aux, however, anti-id activates the cell to down regulate T_{DH} while DNP-lysine appears to have no effect. If Ts have a higher avidity for antigen [26] and recognize antigen in nonassociative ways, why doesn't DNP-lysine activate Ts-aux, leading to efficient down regulation of T_{DH}? Perhaps activation of Ts-aux requires crosslinking of id; this could be accomplished by anti-id but not by monovalent DNP-lysine. In view of the postulated "partial" recognition of id by DNP-lysine, it is possible that crosslinking of id would not occur even by polyvalent DNP-protein.

What Is the Role of Antigen in Desensitization?

From what has gone before, it would seem to be a weak agent when it works directly on id+ cells. Antigen seems to be more effective when it works through suppressor mechanisms or when it is linked to something like antigen-induced clone proliferation followed by cytotoxic drugs.

SUMMARY

In contact sensitivity (and other forms of T cell sensitivities), T cell activation and priming of the system requires at least two signals. Signal 1 includes specific antigen and signal 2 is a nonspecific stimulus. Ordinarily, the signals are invoked in an associative manner, but they can be delivered separately. The physicochemical nature of the antigen and the manner of host processing are critical to the delivery of signal 2.

Tolerance in unprimed systems is induced by the presentation of signal 1 (antigen) in forms and by routes that do not activate signal 2. This seems to invoke suppressor mechanisms and to directly inactivate T_{DH} cells.

In primed systems where contact sensitivity is present, signals 1 and 2 boost the response.

In primed systems, "off signals" (desensitization) may be provided by some anti-id antibodies, which act by stimulating suppressor mechanisms that finally work to down regulate T_{DH}. Antigen alone (signal 1) also appears to be capable of directly down regulating T_{DH}, but so far it has not proved a powerful tool in desensitizing primed T cells.

REFERENCES

1. CLAMAN, H. N. 1979. T-cell tolerance—one signal? Cell. Immunol. **48:** 201–7.
2. CLEVELAND, R. P. & H. N. CLAMAN. 1980. T cell signals: Tolerance to DNFB is converted to sensitization by a separate nonspecific second signal. J. Immunol. **124:** 474–80.
3. SHIRLEY, S. F. & J. R. LITTLE. 1979. Immunopotentiating effects of amphotericin B. I. Enhanced contact sensitivity in mice. J. Immunol. **123:** 2878–82.
4. COHN, M. 1981. Conversations with Niels Kaj Jerne on immune regulation: Associative versus network regulation. Cell. Immunol. **61:** 425–36.
5. DRESSER, D. W. 1962. Specific inhibition of antibody production. II. Paralysis induced in adult mice by small quantities of protein antigen. Immunology **5:** 378.

6. CLAMAN, H. N., S. D. MILLER, M. S. SY & J. W. MOORHEAD. 1980. Suppressive mechanisms involving sensitization and tolerance in contact allergy. Immunol. Rev. **50:** 105–32.

7. CHASE, M. W. 1946. Inhibition of experimental drug allergy by prior feeding of the sensitizing agent. Proc. Soc. Exp. Biol. Med. **61:** 257–59.

8. TOEWS, G. B., P. R. BERGSTRESSER & J. W. STREILEIN. 1980. Epidermal Langerhans cell density determines whether contact hypersensitivity or unresponsiveness follows skin painting with DNFB. J. Immunol. **124:** 445.

9. CLAMAN, H. N., S. D. MILLER, P. J. CONLON & J. W. MOORHEAD. 1980. Control of experimental contact sensitivity. Adv. Immunol. **30:** 121–57.

10. CONLON, P. J., J. W. MOORHEAD & H. N. CLAMAN. 1979. Efficient induction of immediate tolerance to contact sensitivity by hapten-modified spleen cells requires Ia+ cells compatible with recipient. Nature (London) **278:** 257–59.

11. MILLER, S. D., M. S. SY & H. N. CLAMAN. 1977. The induction of hapten-specific T cell tolerance using hapten-modified lymphoid membranes. II. Relative roles of suppressor T cells and clone inhibition in the tolerant state. Eur. J. Immunol. **7:** 165–70.

12. GREENE, M. I., M. SUGIMOTO & B. BENACERRAF. 1978. Mechanisms of regulation of cell-mediated immune responses. I. Effect of the route of immunization with TNP-coupled syngeneic cells on the induction and suppression of contact sensitivity to picryl chloride. J. Immunol. **120:** 1604–11.

13. PTAK, W., D. ROZYCKA, P. W. ASKENASE & R. K. GERSHON. 1980. Role of antigen-presenting cells in the development and persistence of contact hypersensitivity. J. Exp. Med. **151:** 362–75.

14. CLAMAN, H. N. & S. D. MILLER. 1976. Requirements for induction of T cell tolerance to DNFB: Efficiency of membrane-associated DNFB. J. Immunol. **117:** 480–85.

15. GOLAN, D. T. & Y. BOREL. 1971. Nonantigenicity and immunologic tolerance: The role of the carrier in the induction of tolerance to the hapten. J. Exp. Med. **134:** 1046.

16. CLAMAN, H. N., S. D. MILLER & J. W. MOORHEAD. 1977. Tolerance: Two pathways of negative immunoregulation in contact sensitivity to DNFB. Cold Spring Harbor Symp. Quant. Biol. **41:** 105–11.

17. TAYLOR, R. B. & G. M. IVERSON. 1971. Hapten competition and the nature of cell-cooperation in the antibody response. Proc. R. Soc. London Ser. B **176:** 393.

18. TAKAHASHI, C., S. NISHIKAWA, Y. KATSURA & T. IZUMI. 1977. Anti-DNP antibody response after the topical application of DNFB in mice. J. Immunol. **33:** 589.

19. SY, M. S., J. W. MOORHEAD & H. N. CLAMAN. 1979. Regulation of cell mediated immunity by antibodies: Possible role of anti-receptor antibodies in the regulation of contact sensitivity to DNFB in mice. J. Immunol. **123:** 2593–98.

20. MOORHEAD, J. W. 1982. Antigen receptors on murine T lymphocytes in contact sensitivity. III. Mechanism of negative feedback regulation by auto-anti-idiotypic antibody. J. Exp. Med. **155:** 820–30.

21. LESKOWITZ, S. & V. E. JONES. 1965. Immunochemical study of antigenic specificity in delayed hypersensitivity. III. Suppression of hapten-specific delayed hypersensitivity by conjugates of varying size. J. Immunol. **95:** 331.

22. KANTOR, F. S. 1968. Delayed hypersensitivity. I. Effect of in vitro exposure of cells to antigen upon leukocytic transfer of delayed hypersensitivity. J. Exp. Med. **127:** 251.

23. DEWECK, A. L. & J. R. FREY. 1966. Immunotolerance to simple chemicals. Monogr. Allergy. **1.**

24. PHANUPHAK, P., J. W. MOORHEAD & H. N. CLAMAN. 1975. Tolerance and

contact sensitivity to DNFB in mice. IV. Desensitization as a manifestation of increased proliferation of sensitized cells. J. Immunol. **114:** 1147.
25. MOORHEAD, J. W. 1982. Antigen receptors on murine T lymphocytes in contact sensitivity. I. Functional inhibition of effector T cells by monovalent DNP: Implication for a two-receptor model. J. Exp. Med. **154:** 1811–26.
26. OKUMURA, K., T. TAKEMORI, T. TOKUHISA & T. TADA. 1977. Specific enrichment of the suppressor T cell bearing I-J determinants. J. Exp. Med. **146:** 1234–45.

DISCUSSION OF THE PAPER

A. H. SEHON (*University of Manitoba, Winnipeg, Man.*): You mentioned, with regard to desensitization *in vitro*, that the DNP-lysine is not effective. What about a polyvinyl form of DNP, such as coupled to proteins or any other carrier?

CLAMAN: Well, Dr. Sehon was kind enough to give me some DNP-polyvinyl alcohol, which is sitting on my desk in Denver, and the experiments haven't been done. Certainly they're worth doing.

SEHON: But in this case, I would think that, even without polyvinyl, coupling DNP to protein *in vitro* through crosslinking may—

CLAMAN: Are you talking about *in vitro* experiments?

SEHON: Yes.

CLAMAN: Well, DNP-lysine will desensitize the cells *in vitro* to the extent that they block the paths of transfer. And DNP-BSA will do the same. It's *in vivo* that DNP-lysine seems to do nothing. That may be just a technical problem.

SEHON: But you said weak.

CLAMAN: It's weak because the bond between the DNP-lysine is easily reversed by incubating the blocked cells in medium free of DNP-lysine. Is Dr. Moorhead here? You've blocked cells with DNP-BSA. What's the bond between the T_{DH} cell and DNP-BSA?

J. W. MOORHEAD (*University of Colorado Medical School, Denver, Col.*): It appears to be somewhat stronger, but it's weak, as well.

J. CHILLER (*Scripps Clinic and Research Foundation, La Jolla, Calif.*): It's only fitting that the last question of today's meeting be asked by Dr. Chase.

M. W. CHASE (*Rockefeller University, New York, N.Y.*): I want to make three observations. First, if we put picryl chloride on a normal guinea pig's skin, and let's say we get 15 to 30% unresponsive, where are the missing Langerhan's cells? Then, I want to mention an experiment of Dr. Polak's of some time ago. After a single injection of dinitrobenzene sulfonate when the cells are transiently suppressed, he divides them into two portions and treats one half with trypsin. He puts the untreated cells back into an isologous animal and finds that the animal has no sensitivity. But animals receiving cells treated with trypsin show positive skin reactivity. This could possibly indicate that there are surface receptors that have been occupied for a time.

The final observation I want to make is that I think that the injection of dinitrobenzene sulfonate for securing transient-type sensitivity is very much over-rated. Our speaker, I believe, thinks that also. But if we have supersensitive guinea pigs, that is, those sensitive to a 1:450 dilution of a 1% solution of hapten, and we put stronger concentrations of hapten on the skin and we retest them within the next week, they're completely nonreactive. So a discharge can occur with relatively little material put upon the skin. And you don't have to use 500 mg per kg intravenously to get the same effect. Now, these are things that have to be put into the total pattern, I would suggest. Otherwise, I think that what we have heard today is very edifying.

CLAMAN: That's the nicest thing he's ever said to me.

CHILLER: We'd better stop, then.

SUPPRESSOR T CELL CIRCUITS

Baruj Benacerraf, Mark I. Greene, Man-Sun Sy, and
Martin E. Dorf

Department of Pathology
Harvard Medical School
Boston, Massachusetts 02115

INTRODUCTION

Over the last few years, several laboratories have intensively studied specific suppression by antigen-specific T cells. This has revealed the existence of unsuspected complexity in the manner in which the immune response is negatively regulated by T cells. The salient findings are that (1) The specific suppression phenomena involve the interactions of several sets of T cells with defined properties and characteristic surface markers.[1] (2) These T cells each produce specific factors that can be shown to mediate their precise regulatory function.[2] (3) Their specificity is either for the antigen or for the immunoglobulin idiotypes that determine certain aspects of their interactions. (4) Certain of the suppressor T cells (Ts) in these circuits bear determinants coded for by the I-J subregion of the murine H-2 complex, which also appears to restrict the interactions at certain critical steps in the pathway, in a way similar to the restrictions imposed by the I-A and I-E subregions on helper T cell (Th) interactions.[1] (5) Accordingly, suppressor T cell interactions in the circuit can be shown to be governed by both V_H genes and major histocompatibility complex (MHC) genes at appropriate steps.

Based primarily on the results obtained in our laboratories, where the regulation of several models by suppressor T cells has been investigated, we have recently proposed that T cell suppression in all murine systems proceeds by a common major pathway involving the sequential interactions of three T cell subsets with distinct properties, which we have termed Ts_1, Ts_2, and Ts_3.[1] We have also proposed that this overall scheme may be used to integrate the data obtained in systems developed in other laboratories.

We now propose to review the criteria that we have used to distinguish and identify the distinct cells in the pathway. We shall also describe the latest data from our laboratories on the analysis of T cell suppressor circuits, their cells, and their specific products. We shall then discuss the problems we have encountered and are now facing in integrating the complex data in a generalizable scheme to determine to what extent one needs to postulate variants unique to certain systems. Finally, we shall try to address some of the major unresolved fundamental issues, such as the significance of the observed I-J restrictions at the molecular level and the possible role of antigen presentation by accessory cells in the T cell suppressor pathway. TABLE 1 describes the criteria used to analyze the systems under investigation. The major distinguishing points considered were: (1) the binding specificity of the relevant cell or factor and, in particular, whether its receptor is idiotypic (antigen specific) or anti-idiotypic, (2) the membrane phenotype and drug sensitivity of the factor producer and the acceptor cell, (3) the involvement of genetic restrictions (H-2 or V_H) in

300

0077–8923/82/0392–0300 $1.75/0 © 1982, NYAS

the interactions at the level of the cells or the factors, and (4) the mode of suppression, *i.e.*, early acting, or afferent, *versus* late acting, or efferent. Only efferent suppressors are effective on immune cells.

SUPPRESSION OF DELAYED-TYPE HYPERSENSITIVITY RESPONSES TO ABA OR NP

We chose to study the suppression of delayed-type hypersensitivity (DTH) responses in haptenic systems that, in selected mouse strains, are characterized by the presence of predominant crossreactive idiotypes on specific anti-hapten antibody, such as the azobenzene arsonate (ABA) system in mice with the Igh^e-linked CRI [3] or the 4-hydroxy-3-nitrophenyl acetyl (NP) system in mice with the Igh^b NP^b idiotype.[4]

The studies of ABA-specific suppression were carried out by a group headed by Mark Greene and involving Man-Sun Sy, Al Nisonoff, and Ronald Germain, while the studies on NP-specific suppression were performed in Martin Dorf's laboratory. It is remarkable that, except for some details unique to each system, essentially identical results were obtained independently by both laboratories and identical conclusions were reached.

TABLE 1

ANALYSIS OF SUPPRESSOR T CELLS AND FACTORS

1. Binding specificity: (a) Antigen
   (b) Anti-idiotypic
2. Lyt phenotype and drug sensitivity of T suppressor factor producer and acceptor cells
3. Genetic restrictions on cell-cell interactions or factor-cell interactions
4. Afferent or efferent suppressor function

PROPERTIES OF Ts_1 AND TsF_1

The intravenous injection of haptenated syngeneic spleen cells in both systems triggers cyclophosphamide (Cy)-sensitive pre-Ts cells that mature into antigen-binding Ts_1 cells. These Ts_1 cells in the ABA system have been shown to express the Lyt $1^+,2^-$ phenotype. Ts_1 cells are idiotype-positive in both systems and function as afferent and not efferent suppressors.[5-8] ABA- and NP-specific Ts_1 cells have been successfully hybridized with the lymphoma BW 5147 and stable hybridoma lines have been produced with the characteristic properties of the hapten-specific Ts_1 factors.[9, 10] Such hybrid lines bear the respective idiotypic determinants and produce suppressor factors (TsF_1) that are idiotypic, antigen-binding, and bear I-J coded determinants in their culture supernatant.

TsF_1 products in both ABA and NP systems function by stimulating non-immune Cy-resistant T cells to become Ts_2, which, in these two systems, are anti-idiotypic rather than antigen specific.[7, 11] This has been verified with TsF_1 obtained from both immune spleen cell populations and Ts_1 hybridoma cell lines.[12] In the latter case, it could be verified that, in these two systems, hybridoma-derived ABA and NP TsF_1 factors stimulate Ts_2 cells in the absence of antigen, in contrast to what was observed in the GAT system;[13] an interesting point, considering that the Ts_2 induced in the GAT system appear to be antigen specific rather than anti-idiotypic.[14]

Another important property of Ts_1 cells and their factors, TsF_1, is their ability to function without genetic restrictions. Thus, both ABA and NP TsF_1 factors can stimulate Ts_2 cells across V_H and MHC differences.[7, 15]

PROPERTIES OF Ts_2 AND TsF_2

The finding that T cell suppressor factor can induce the appearance of another population of Ts was originally made by Waltenbaugh while working with GT-specific TsF in our laboratories.[16] Tada soon reached the similar conclusion that keyhole limpet hemocyanin (KLH) TsF stimulates the generation of suppressor T cells.[17] Our analysis of the suppressor pathway in the ABA and NP systems showed that the role of TsF_1 is, indeed, the stimulation of a new population of suppressor cells, Ts_2.[7, 11]

Ts_2 differ radically from Ts_1 in their properties and function. In the ABA and NP systems, Ts_2 cells are anti-idiotypic and can be shown to bind to idiotype-coated plates; they bear Lyt 2^+ determinants and, as shown in the NP system, I-J coded specificities; and they function as efferent suppressors, i.e., they are able to suppress DTH reactions and plaque-forming cell (PFC) responses in an already immune animal. Another very important difference between Ts_1 and Ts_2 concerns the genetic restrictions that govern their interactions with their targets. Ts_2 are restricted both by V_H genes and by the I-J subregion of the MHC in expressing their suppressive activity.[18, 19]

T cell hybridomas with the properties of Ts_2 have been produced in the NP system. Such Ts_2 hybridomas have all the properties of the Ts_2 parent.[19] Ts_2 factors function by producing a soluble factor, TsF_2, which, in these two systems, is anti-idiotypic and also bears I-J subregion–coded determinants. TsF_2 suppress in the efferent mode and display MHC and V_H restrictions in their ability to mediate suppression.

PROPERTIES OF Ts_3 AND TsF_3

The efferent property of Ts_2 led us to think that these cells might be the final effectors. However, this proved not to be the case. Earlier work by Sy et al. in the DNP system had revealed the need for an additional cell, which they called the auxiliary cell, in the final effector pathway.[20] Such a cell, which, for internal consistency, we termed Ts_3, was soon identified in both the ABA and the NP systems.[21, 22]

The discovery of Ts_3 was stimulated by the observation that the injection of Ts_2 or TsF_2 did not result in suppression of an immune animal if the recipient mouse had been treated with low doses of Cy shortly after immunization. It was clear, therefore, that a highly Cy-sensitive cell was the target of TsF_2 in the suppressor circuit. It was also shown that the Ts_3 subset is always induced as part of the conventional immunization that stimulates DTH sensitivity, i.e., immunization with adjuvant or percutaneous sensitization. Antigen-activated Ts_3 cells are inactive until they are appropriately triggered by Ts_2 or TsF_2.

We then undertook to document the properties of this new set of cells in the suppressor circuit in both the ABA and the NP systems. Ts_3 cells in these systems are antigen specific and presumably MHC restricted. They express the Lyt 2 phenotype and bear, as verified in the NP system, I-J coded determinants. Ts_3 cells produce an antigen-specific TsF_3 that mediates efferent suppression in these systems. The suppressive activity of Ts_3 and TsF_3 in the NP system can be demonstrated in Cy-treated recipients and, as in the case of TsF_2, is restricted by both V_H and MHC (I-J) genes.

Ts_3 hybridomas have been obtained in the NP system.[23] The properties of these cells and their products are currently being investigated.

In some systems, the specific activation of Ts_3 cells results in suppression that is, to some extent, nonspecific. Thus, in the ABA system, we have been able to devise conditions whereby the activation of ABA-specific Ts_3 results in the suppression of mice differing at the Igh-1 locus, and even in suppression of a DTH reaction of a different specificity.[21]

COMPARISONS WITH OTHER SYSTEMS

In TABLE 2, we present the properties and interactions of the cells and factors of the suppressor circuit responsible for the suppression of DTH responses in systems characterized by a predominant idiotype, *i.e.,* the ABA and NP systems. We will now discuss the extent to which the model we propose can apply, with appropriate modifications, to other well-investigated suppressor systems.

Ts_1 IN OTHER SYSTEMS

Ts_1 can be considered to function as an inducer of the suppressor circuit. It bears the unique Lyt $1^+,2^-,$I-J$^+$ phenotype. A similar Ts_1 inducer has been identified by Eardley, Cantor, Gershon, and associates in the suppression of antibody responses to sheep red blood cells (SRBC) [24, 25] and is activated concomitantly with immunization. Many of its features are similar to those of the model developed for ABA and NP suppression. The Ts_1 in this system is also Lyt 1^+ and produces a TsF that activates unprimed Lyt $1^+,2^+$ cells. As in our systems, this interaction initiates V_H restrictions.

Ts_1 factors with similar properties have not yet been identified in Tada's KLH system [17] or in the suppression of contact sensitivity to DNP or TNP studied by Clamon, Miller, and Moorhead.[26] However, one may argue that Ts_1 are very early cells and that Tada's system was studied fairly late in immunization, after the Ts_1 stage. Similarly, the system studied by Claman and associates employs DNP conjugates, which are strong antigens and are capable of direct stimulation of Ts_2 cells. The Ts_1 cell was not specifically looked for, and might have been induced but gone undetected.

Ts_2 IN OTHER SYSTEMS

As mentioned earlier, there are several reported instances of the induction of a second-order suppressor T cell by a factor extracted or secreted by an

TABLE 2

PROPERTIES OF SUPPRESSOR T CELLS AND FACTORS

Property	Cells			Factors		
	Ts_1	Ts_2	Ts_3	TsF_1	TsF_2	TsF_3
H-2I determinants	I-J	I-J	I-J	I-J	I-J	I-J
Lyt determinants	$1^+, 2^-$	$(1^+), 2^+$	2^+	—	—	—
Igh determinants	Igh-V	?	Igh-V	Igh-V	?	Igh-V
Specificity	antiantigen	anti-idiotype	antiantigen	antiantigen	anti-idiotype	antiantigen
Phase of action	induction	effector	effector	induction	effector	effector
Genetic restriction	—	H-2 + Igh	—	none	I-J + Igh	I-J + Igh
Cellular target	—	—	—	pre-Ts_2	Ts_3	?
Activity in cyclophosphamide-treated recipients	?	no	yes	?	no	yes

NOTE: Ts_1 and Ts_3 are induced by antigen, presumably in the context of MHC products, whereas Ts_2 are induced by TsF_1. The determinants on TsF_1 impart genetic restrictions.

earlier suppressor. Such Ts$_2$ have been demonstrated in the GT and GAT systems, the KLH system,[17] and the SRBC system,[24, 25] as well as in our systems, and has been documented in the suppression of both humoral and cellular immunity. The generation of Ts$_2$ by TsF$_1$ may be, therefore, considered well accepted.

Some important differences remain in the Ts$_2$ described; the major one concerns the specificity of these cells. In the ABA and NP systems, Ts$_2$ cells are anti-idiotypic, whereas, in all other systems discussed above, including the GAT system, they are antigen specific. It may be that the anti-idiotypic nature of the ABA and NP Ts$_2$ cells and factors is due to the presence of predominant CRI in these systems. In other systems, such as the GAT system, the activation of Ts$_2$ may, therefore, require an antigen signal as well as TsF$_1$ dependence; this can be accomplished by antigen bridging.

Ts$_3$ in Other Systems

A Ts$_3$-type cell was originally described by Sy *et al.* as essential for suppression of contact sensitivity.[20] Such a cell is also found in the terminal effector phase of antibody suppression in the SRBC system of Eardley *et al.*[24, 25] and the product of such a cell was reported to mediate nonspecific suppression.[27] It is reasonable to conclude that the existence of Ts$_3$-like cells in many systems is based on solid evidence from several laboratories and can now be accepted.

Unresolved Issues

Several major issues remain unresolved.

(1) What are the signals that trigger Ts$_1$ and Ts$_3$?

(2) What is the significance of the MHC restriction in the T cell circuit, and what is the relationship between the role of I-J as restriction specificity for the T cell circuit and the presence of I-J-coded determinants on suppressor factors?

(3) What is the real importance of idiotype-anti-idiotype interactions in the regulation of suppressor T cell interactions, and what is the significance of V$_H$ restrictions in the T cell suppressor circuit? Is it only related to the anti-idiotype specificity of the Ts$_2$ or does it reflect the role of immunoglobulin specificities as restriction elements in cell interactions like the MHC, as proposed by Gershon?

A major concern is the mode of stimulation of Ts$_1$ and Ts$_3$. Do these cells require presentation of antigen by appropriate accessory cells? It is highly probable that the requirements for the stimulation of Ts$_1$ and Ts$_3$ differ considerably, based on the fact that Ts$_3$ is MHC restricted while Ts$_1$ is not. How is the I-J restriction brought about? Does it depend on antigen presentation by I-J-bearing accessory cells? All these points are amenable to experimental solutions within a relatively short time.

Another set of important questions relates to the role of idiotype and anti-idiotype in triggering various cells in the T cell suppressor network. For instance, studies on the ABA system in our laboratory have shown that afferent suppressor idiotype-bearing Ts$_1$ cells are stimulated when anti-idiotype is administered intravenously,[28] while the administration of idiotype-conjugated spleen cells stimulates anti-idiotype Ts_2-like cells with the activity of efferent suppressors.[29] Thus, efferent Ts_2 suppressors can be induced by either TsF_1 or idiotype administered on spleen cells. This raises the issue of whether the two inductions are analogous and whether idiotype-conjugated spleen cells behave like a conventional antigen when conjugated to spleen cells and stimulate an anti-idiotypic Ts_1 afferent cell that goes undetected, while, together with idiotype, this Ts_1 cell in turn stimulates the Ts_2 anti-idiotype efferent cell that we have detected in our experiments. If this is indeed the case, the situation would be analogous to the sequence of events in the GAT and the KLH systems, where both Ts_1 and Ts_2 share the same specificity and also require the immunizing antigen to ensure specific interaction. This possibility can also be explored experimentally by searching deliberately for an early anti-idiotype Lyt 1^+ inducer Ts_1 in animals injected with idiotype-conjugated spleen cells.

REFERENCES

1. GERMAIN, R. N. & B. BENACERRAF. 1981. A single major pathway of T lymphocyte interactions. Scand. J. Immunol. **13**: 1–10.
2. GERMAIN, R. N. & B. BENACERRAF. 1980. Helper and suppressor T cell factors. Springer Sem. Immunopathology **3**: 93–128.
3. NISONOFF, A., S.-T. JU & F. L. OWEN. 1977. Studies of structure and immunosuppression of a cross-reactive idiotype in strain A mice. Immunol. Rev. **34**: 89–118.
4. IMANISHI, T. & O. MAKELA. 1974. Inheritance on antibody specificity. I. Anti-(4-hydroxy-3-nitrophenyl)acetyl of the mouse primary response. J. Exp. Med. **140**: 1498–510.
5. WEINBERGER, J. Z., R. N. GERMAIN, S.-T. JU, M. I. GREENE, B. BENACERRAF & M. E. DORF. 1979. Hapten-specific T-cell responses to 4-hydroxy-3-nitrophenyl acetyl. II. Demonstration of idiotypic determinants on suppressor T cells. J. Exp. Med. **150**: 761–76.
6. GREENE, M. I. & B. BENACERRAF. 1980. Studies on hapten specific T cell immunity and suppression. Immunol. Rev. **50**: 163–86.
7. SY, M. S., M. H. DIETZ, R. N. GERMAIN, B. BENACERRAF & M. I. GREENE. 1980. Antigen and receptor driven regulatory mechanisms. IV. Idiotype bearing I-J$^+$ suppressor T cell factor (TsF) induced second order suppressor T cells (Ts-2) which express anti-idiotypic receptors. J. Exp. Med. **151**: 1183–95.
8. DIETZ, M. H., M. S. SY, M. I. GREENE, A. NISONOFF, B. BENACERRAF & R. N. GERMAIN. 1980. Antigen and receptor driven regulatory mechanisms. VI. Demonstration of cross-reactive idiotypic determinants of azobenzenearsonate specific antigen binding suppressor cells producing soluble suppressor factor(s). J. Immunol. **125**: 2374–79.
9. OKUDA, K., M. MINAMI, S.-T. JU & M. E. DORF. 1981. Functional association of idiotypic and I-J determinants on the antigen receptor of suppressor T cells. Proc. Nat. Acad. Sci. USA **78**: 4557–61.
10. WHITAKER, R. B., J. T. NEPOM, M. S. SY, M. TAKAOKI, C. F. GRAMM, I. FOX, R. N. GERMAIN, M. J. NELLES, M. I. GREENE & B. BENACERRAF. 1981. Suppressor factor from a T cell hybrid inhibits delayed type hypersensitivity to azobenzenearsonate (ABA). Proc. Nat. Acad. Sci. USA. **78**: 6441.
11. WEINBERGER, J. Z., R. N. GERMAIN, B. BENACERRAF & M. E. DORF. 1980. Hapten specific T-cell response to 4-hydroxy-3-nitrophenyl acetyl. V. Role of idiotypes in the suppressor pathway. J. Exp. Med. **152**: 161–69.
12. TAKAOKI, M., M. S. SY, B. WHITAKER, J. NEPOM, R. FINBERG, R. N. GERMAIN, A. NISONOFF, B. BENACERRAF & M. I. GREENE. 1982. Biological activity

of an idiotype bearing suppressor T cell factor produced by a long term T cell hybridoma. J. Immunol. **128:** 49.

13. GERMAIN, R. N., J. THEZE, J. A. KAPP & B. BENACERRAF. 1978. Antigen-specific T-cell mediated suppression. I. Induction of L-glutamic acid[60]-L-alanine[30]-L-tyrosine[10] specific suppressor T cells in vitro require both antigen specific T-cell suppressor factor and antigen. J. Exp. Med. **147:** 123–36.

14. KAPP, J. A. Personal communication.

15. OKUDA, K., M. MINAMI, D. H. SHERR & M. E. DORF. 1981. Hapten specific T-cell responses to 4-hydroxy-3-nitrophenyl acetyl. XI. Pseudogenetic restrictions of hybridoma suppressor factors. J. Exp. Med. **154:** 468–79.

16. WALTENBAUGH, C., J. THEZE, J. A. KAPP & B. BENACERRAF. 1977. Immuno-suppressive factor specific for L-glutamic acid[50]-L-tyrosine[50] (GT). III. Generation of suppressor T cells by a suppressive extract derived from GT primed lymphoid cells. J. Exp. Med. **146:** 970–85.

17. TADA, T. & K. OKUMURA. 1980. The role of antigen specific T cell factors in the immune response. Adv. Immunol. **28:** 1–87.

18. DIETZ, M. H., M.-S. SY, B. BENACERRAF, A. NISONOFF, M. I. GREENE & R. N. GERMAIN. 1981. Antigen- and receptor-driven regulatory mechanisms. VII. H-2 restricted anti-idiotypic suppressor factor from efferent suppressor T cells. J. Exp. Med. **153:** 450–63.

19. MINAMI, M., K. OKUDA, S. FURUSAWA, B. BENACERRAF & M. E. DORF. 1981. Analysis of T cell hybridoma. I. Characterization of H-2 and Igh restricted monoclonal suppressor factors. J. Exp. Med. **154:** 1390.

20. SY, M. S., S. D. MILLER, J. W. MOORHEAD & H. N. CLAMAN. 1979. Active suppression of 1-fluoro-2,4-dinitrobenzene-immune T cells. Requirement for an auxiliary T cell induced by antigen. J. Exp. Med. **149:** 1197–207.

21. SY, M. S., A. NISONOFF, R. N. GERMAIN, B. BENACERRAF & M. I. GREENE. 1981. Antigen and receptor driven regulatory mechanisms. VIII. Suppression of idiotype negative ABA specific T cells results from the interaction of an anti-idiotypic Ts-2 with a CRI[+] ABA primed T cell target. J. Exp. Med. **153:** 1415–25.

22. SUNDAY, M. E., B. BENACERRAF & M. E. DORF. 1981. Hapten specific T cell responses to 4-hydroxy-3-nitrophenyl acetyl. VIII. Suppressor cell pathways in cutaneous sensitivity responses. J. Exp. Med. **153:** 811–22.

23. OKUDA, K., M. MINAMI, S. FURUSAWA & M. E. DORF. 1981. Analysis of T cell hybridomas. II. Comparisons among three distinct types of monoclonal suppressor factors. J. Exp. Med. **154:** 1838.

24. EARDLEY, D. D., J. HUGENBERGER, L. MCVAY-BOUDREAU, F. W. SHER, R. K. GERSHON, & H. CANTOR. 1979. Immunoregulatory circuits among T cell sets: effect of mode of immunization on determining which Ly T cell will be activated. J. Immunol. **122:** 1663–65.

25. EARDLEY, D. D., F. W. SHER, H. CANTOR & R. K. GERSHON. 1979. Genetic control of immunoregulatory circuits: Genes linked to the Ig locus govern communication between regulatory T-cell sets. J. Exp. Med. **150:** 44–59.

26. CLAMAN, H. N., S. D. MILLER, M. S. SY & J. W. MOORHEAD. 1980. Suppressive mechanisms involving sensitization and tolerance in contact allergy. Immunol. Rev. **50:** 105–32.

27. FRESNO, M., L. MCVAY-BOUDREAU, G. NABEL & H. CANTOR. 1981. Antigen-specific T lymphocyte clones. I. Purification and biological characterization of an antigen-specific suppressive protein synthesized by clone T cells. J. Exp. Med. **153:** 1260–74.

28. SY, M. S., B. A. BACH, Y. DOHI, A. NISONOFF, B. BENACERRAF & M. I. GREENE. 1979. Antigen and receptor driven regulatory mechanisms. I. Induction of suppressor T cells with anti-idiotypic antibodies. J. Exp. Med. **150:** 1216–28.

29. SY, M. S., B. A. BACH, A. R. BROWN, A. NISONOFF, B. BENACERRAF & M. I.
GREENE. 1979. Antigen and receptor driven regulatory mechanisms. II.
Induction of suppressor T cells with idiotype coupled syngeneic spleen cells.
J. Exp. Med. **150:** 1229–40.

DISCUSSION OF THE PAPER

J. CHILLER (*Scripps Clinic and Research Foundation, La Jolla, Calif.*):
Can you tell us about the relative constitutive nature or the inducibility of the
hybridomas? Can the Ts_2 producer be induced with Ts_1, or with the idiotype
or anti-idiotype, respectively, *et cetera*?

BENACERRAF: These experiments are in progress.

H. N. CLAMAN (*University of Colorado Health Sciences Center, Denver,
Col.*): Can you tell us a little about TsF_3 and the hybridoma that makes it?
How does it exert its antigen-nonspecific effect? Does it bind to antigen? What
does it bind to?

BENACERRAF: The nonspecificity, as far as we could see, was only found
in the ABA system, not in the NP system. We only have these hybridomas in
the NP system. This hybridoma, as well as its product, is specific in its action as
well as in its specificity. It only suppresses the idiotype response of that particular specificity.

J. R. BATTISTO (*Cleveland Clinic Foundation, Cleveland, Oh.*): Do any of
the inhibitory factors interact at all with any of the helper factors, the interleukins?

BENACERRAF: I don't know.

ACTIVATIONAL SIGNALS FOR
IMMUNE EFFECTOR AND SUPPRESSOR T CELLS
REACTIVE WITH HAPTENIC DETERMINANTS

Akira Tominaga, Jonathan S. Bromberg, Muneo Takaoki,
Sophie Lefort, John Noseworthy, Baruj Benacerraf, and
Mark I. Greene

Department of Pathology
Harvard Medical School
Boston, Massachusetts 02115

The immune response to haptens linked to cell surface proteins has been studied in many different experimental systems and laboratories.[1-5] Our own interest in the nature of the immune response to haptens has focused on what discrete characteristics of the ligand-host relationship determine whether suppressor or effector T cells are activated. Over the last several years we have analyzed the haptens trinitophenyl (TNP) and azobenzene arsonate (ABA).

ROUTE OF ADMINISTRATION

In the TNP system it was observed, in agreement with the studies of Battisto and Bloom [1] and Miller and Claman,[2] that the intravenous administration of syngeneic splenocytes, coupled under conditions of 10 mM TNBS, led to unresponsiveness in the recipient and the induction of hapten-specific suppressor T cells for contact sensitivity. Other routes of administration were analyzed for their ability to induce immunity or suppression. Both intravenous (i.v.) and intraperitoneal (i.p.) administration of hapten-coupled cells led to unresponsiveness, while subcutaneous (s.c.) administration of the same cells primed a variety of effector T cell subsets. These include hapten-specific T cells mediating contact sensitivity (Tcs), delayed type hypersensitivity (T_{DH}), proliferation (Tp), and helper cells (Th) active in augmenting T cell–mediated cytotoxicity (Tc). Radiolabeled hapten-coupled cells clearly revealed that i.v. administration resulted in the accumulation of cells in the spleen, while s.c. administration resulted in labeled cells being concentrated in the draining lymph nodes. Thus, a single major determinant of whether immune effector or suppressor T cells are activated is related to the differential effect of central *versus* peripheral ligand exposure.[5]

ROLE OF ANTIGEN-PRESENTING CELLS *in Vivo*

Other studies in the TNP system revealed another major determinant of the choice between the activation of effector and the activation of suppressor T cells is the *in vivo* function of antigen-presenting cells (APC). Exposure of mice to ultraviolet radiation (270–300 nm, 1.2 J M^{-2} s^{-1}, 30 min a day for five consecutive days), followed by subcutaneously priming with either normal hapten-coupled splenocytes or hapten-coupled splenocytes obtained from uv-

0077–8923/82/0392–0309 $1.75/0 © 1982, NYAS

treated donors, resulted in distinctly different response patterns.[6] Ultraviolet-treated mice were effectively primed by normal hapten-coupled splenocytes, but were not primed at all if splenocytes were obtained from uv-treated donors. Normal mice were also effectively primed by hapten-coupled uv-treated splenocytes. These studies suggested that the exposure of mice to uv irradiation resulted in the systemic loss of cells capable of presenting antigen. In addition, uv-treated mice inoculated with uv-treated hapten-coupled APC developed a population of hapten-specific suppressor T cells capable, upon adoptive transfer, of inhibiting the generation of T cell immunity in mice.

ACTIVATION SIGNALS OF APC

To determine whether APC mediate other signals or functions independent of linking antigen with I region–determined molecules, we evaluated the ability of certain hormones (interleukins) to complement the functional capacity of uv-inactivated APC in the generation of effector T cells.[7] Ultraviolet-treated hapten-coupled APC, while incapable of activating Te in a uv-treated recipient, can stimulate T cells if the uv-treated recipient is given pure interleukin-1 (IL-1) intravenously. Therefore, another type of signal necessary to activate Te is IL-1 related activity in conjunction with ligand on the appropriate APC cell surface.

SIGNALS ASSOCIATED WITH I REGION MOLECULES

To more precisely analyze hapten presentation by specialized APC *in vivo*, we evaluated the ability of anti-I-A region antibodies to abrogate hapten presentation by APC.[8] Animals immunized with hapten-coupled APC subcutaneously that simultaneously received anti-I-A antibody intravenously were unable to generate effector T cells. Instead, specific Ts were induced. Appropriate use of parental and F_1 cells and antisera against each parental specificity showed that the antibodies were directed against the hapten-coupled APC. Therefore, the I-A molecule seems critical to the activation of effector T cells, but not decisive in triggering the APC required to trigger Ts. Moreover, recent studies by Sprent have extended this notion by showing that anti-I-A antibody administered *in vivo* could effectively abrogate helper cell activation.[9] More recently, the efficacy of monoclonal anti-I-A antibodies in abrogating T cell proliferative responses *in vitro* has also been shown to be due, in part, to the triggering of suppression.[10] Bromberg *et al.* have approached the monoclonal anti-I-A effect *in vivo* in a novel way.[11] By coupling hapten to the monoclonal antibody, it was possible to show that ABA-coupled anti-I-A antibody administered *in vivo* could lead to hapten-specific unresponsiveness. Thus, activational signals associated with I-A molecules can be manipulated to lead to unresponsiveness.

ACTIVATION OF EFFECTOR CELLS

To document the activation requirements of effector cells, we have begun to analyze the special role of antigen-presenting cells *in vivo* and *in vitro*. As discussed above, uv irradiation sensitivity clearly identifies one of the physical characteristics of cells relevant to immunity. More recently, we have subjected adherent cells to density gradient separation, as originally described by Steinman *et al.*,[12] and have also characterized the cell surface markers, using a panel of monoclonal antibodies. By density separation, the APC cells relevant to activation of T effector cells are contained within the low density fraction. High density cells are ineffective in triggering hapten-specific effector cells. Moreover, the relevant low density APC were I-A⁺ and sensitive to a very brief exposure (20 s) of uv irradiation ($1.2-1.4$ J m^{-2} s^{-1} at 20 cm), yet resistant to 1500 rads of x-ray irradiation. Activational requirements for T effector cells are associated with a subset of adherent cells with the following characteristics: low density, 1500 rad resistant, uv sensitive, and I-A⁺.

ACTIVATION OF Te CELLS BY DISTINCT TYPES OF I REGION MOLECULES

In order to evaluate the relative contribution of the H-2 to the control of the Te cells, we analyzed the ability of a panel of inbred strains to respond to immunization with hapten-coupled syngeneic APC. Of all strains studied, Balb/c mice responded best to immunization by this means. A/J responded least well. Moreover, (Balb/c $\times$ A/J)F$_1$ mice responded with an intermediate value to both parental types. We next evaluated the effect of varying the hapten density of a panel of syngeneic or allogeneic cells on presenting hapten to either Balb/c, C3H, or C57B1/6 recipients. We observed that lightly derivatized cells were very weakly immunogenic, whereas heavily haptenated cells were efficient immunogens. Moreover, we observed that B6 cells activate Te in Balb/c recipients over a range of hapten densities. Comparing the hapten-presenting abilities of cells from other species, we clearly observed that, whereas sheep, chicken, guinea pig, and rabbit cells coupled with hapten could not activate Te, rat cells similarly coupled could trigger Te to a moderate degree. This led us to consider the fact that B6 mice and Balb/c share the Ia-8 determinant, which might explain the observed ability of the B6-hapten-coupled cells to trigger Balb/c mice. Thus, it is likely that T cells respond to more common determinants of the major histocompatibility complex (MHC), such as public antigens plus nominal antigens. The ability of certain rat cells to be moderately immunogenic implies that these putative shared public specificities have been conserved in certain species through evolution and that the receptor for these determinants has similarly been retained.

THE CELL SURFACE CHARACTERISTICS OF LIGAND-INDUCED Ts

The ability to activate subsets of suppressor T cells by these regimens prompted our evaluation of the cell surface characteristics of such cells. We were unable to fully define the fine characteristics of suppressor cells using TNP and so turned to the azobenzene arsonate (ABA) hapten. Nisonoff and colleagues showed that the ABA hapten, when coupled to protein carriers, evoked a relatively homogeneous antibody response in certain strains of mice. It was possible to show that 20–70% of the anti-ABA antibodies in A strain mice carried a structural marker known as the crossreactive idiotype (CRI).[13] Rabbit antibodies (anti-idiotypes) to A/J anti-ABA antibodies were used to define this structural characteristic. Other strains of mice were evaluated and it was found that C.AL-20 mice (H-2^{d}Igh-1^d), which have the A1/N allotype on the Balb/c background, also made CRI-bearing anti-ABA antibodies. This latter study indicated a linkage of idiotype to allotype. Moreover, Nisonoff and colleagues established that certain aspects of CRI determinants were associated with the ligand-binding site of the antibody (*i.e.*, an interaction structure of the light and heavy chain variable regions), while other CRI structures were associated solely with the variable (V_H) region of the heavy chain. These subsets of CRI determinants are clearly a part of a larger set known as the CRI family (see TABLE 1).

We initiated the study of the ABA hapten to determine whether the extensive data on the structure of anti-ABA molecules might also be of use in the characterization of T cell ligand-binding structures.

Subcutaneous administration of ABA-coupled syngeneic spleen cells (SC) to A/J mice was able to readily induce ABA-specific T_{DH}.[5] These cells do not seem to bear CRI determinants on the cell surface. Intravenous administration of ABA-SC activated a population of ABA-specific suppressor T cells. Although the ABA-specific Ts could be induced in any strain of mice, A/J ABA-specific Ts, but not Balb/c Ts, could be lysed with rabbit anti-idiotype plus complement.

TABLE 1

IDIOTYPES IN THE ABA SYSTEM
CROSS-REACTIVE IDIOTYPE FAMILY

Idiotypes associated with the ligand binding site: example—on immunoglobulins (Ig)
Idiotypes associated with heavy and light chain interactions: example—on Ig
Idiotypes associated with nonbinding site–related areas: example—on Ig and T cell suppressor factors
Idiotypes associated with the V_H region only: example—T cell suppressor factors

Therefore, certain strains of mice that have been stimulated to develop ABA-specific Ts used similar, if not identical, V region genes to encode the ligand-binding receptors of both B and T cells.

To more precisely delineate the type of CRI used by suppressor T cells, we developed a series of mice that had appropriate V_H genes but inappropriate V_L genes. We observed that, whereas these mice were unable to make discernible CRI+ anti-ABA antibody, they could be stimulated to generate ABA-specific suppressor molecules that could be bound by anti-idiotype antibody. A detailed study of anti-idiotypic antibodies capable of binding suppressor factors from ABA-specific Ts_1 has revealed that anti-idiotypes to the nonbinding site V_H gene product react with the T cell molecules. Although such studies have been performed with the Ts induced by ligand, so-called first order, Ts_1, cells, similar experiments remain to be done with other suppressor subsets. At least two other Ts sets have been defined and will be discussed below: second order, Ts_2, cells and the Ts_3 subset.

THE ROLE OF HAPTEN DENSITY

The density of hapten plays a decisive role in the activation of suppressor cells. In the course of studying the genetic restrictions of Ts, we attempted to generate Ts with lightly haptenated cells (0.01 mM TNBS) and determine if such putative Ts would function in syngeneic or allogeneic transfers. Ts induced by sub-optimal doses of antigen had no apparent functional ability when transferred into a syngeneic recipient. However, lightly haptenated cells did stimulate a set of Ts precursors (pre-Ts), which, when transferred into an allogeneic recipient, was able to manifest suppression. The allogeneic effect induced by the transfer seems to act as an activational signal for the pre-Ts. Further detailed analyses of this phenomenon revealed that highly defined intra–I region (I-J) allogeneic effects directed against the pre-Ts were necessary and sufficient for its activation.[15, 16] Other allogeneic effects were completely ineffective. We explained the occurrence of this specific triggering of pre-Ts by virtue of allogeneic effect molecules generated during the allogeneic interactions. These anti-I-J molecules were capable of binding in a specific manner to I-J determinants present on the pre-Ts surface. After this second signal, pre-Ts either differentiated or expanded to participate in suppressor cell pathways.

An *in vitro*–derived I-J allogeneic effect factor (AEF), produced and tested in conjunction with T. L. Delovitch, Toronto, can replace the signaling provided by the allogeneic effect. Several components in the AEF were capable of activating pre-Ts and B cells. Similar types of molecules were reported by Delovitch to be made by allogeneic effects against the I-A region structures and to lead to activation of B cells.[17] Melchers and associates have shown that a molecule produced by a cloned Th line is similar to that described by Delovitch (by molecular weight and specificity) and can also activate certain B cells.[18] It can therefore be assumed that molecules created by the allogeneic effect, and other molecules derived from other cellular interactions, may be useful in transmitting the second signals necessary for either suppressor T cell or B cell activation. These signals appear to be highly specific and function *via* a defined interaction with I region molecules.

SIGNALING BY SUPPRESSOR FACTORS

The concept of the existence of suppressor cell pathways was first introduced by Tada and colleagues[19] and then expanded upon by Eardley and associates.[20, 21]

In the ABA system, we were able to demonstrate that suppressor cells activated by ligand produced a factor. Ligand-activated Ts (or first order Ts$_1$) elaborated an ABA-specific TsF$_1$ that bore crossreactive idiotypic structures as well as I-J subregion encoded elements.[22] To determine if ABA-induced Ts$_1$ participated in a suppressor pathway, an experiment similar to that described by Waltenbaugh and colleagues[23] was performed. CRI+, I-J+ TsF$_1$ was administered to untreated A/J mice. Splenocytes from these mice were removed and found to transfer suppression. Thus, another type of activation mechanism, independent of ligand and other signals such as the allogeneic effect, was shown to be triggering cells to become suppressive.

Cells induced by TsF$_1$ (so-called Ts$_2$, or second order cells) were anti-idiotypic. In further studies, we also found a third set of T cells (Ts$_3$), which are apparently triggered by anti-idiotypic Ts$_2$-released (TsF$_2$) molecules. Thus, suppressor molecules play a major and determining role in stimulating other subsets of cells in the suppressor pathway. The Ts$_3$ cell, once activated, can suppress reactions in a receptor- and antigen-nonspecific way.[24]

Triggering of Suppressor Cells by Other Interactions

In order to assess whether antibodies were capable of activating effector or suppressor T cells, two distinct approaches were followed. In the first instance, we evaluated whether anti-idiotypic antibody could activate Ts. We had observed that rabbit anti-idiotype, and even mouse monoclonal anti-idiotype (unpublished), could prime for Te activity when administered subcutaneously.[25] When given intravenously, anti-idiotypic antibody leads to the stimulation of an idiotype-bearing Ts. In this instance, the activational signals relate to the interaction of an idiotypic T suppressor cell with an anti-idiotypic antibody. Ligand itself does not appear to be necessary for the triggering of either the effector or the suppressor cell.

As a second approach, we evaluated whether or not an antibody to a specific receptor on lymphocyte cells might trigger T cells. The reovirus hemagglutinin binds to subsets of both B and T cells.[26] In terms of the T cell, reovirus binds predominantly to Lyt 23 cells (Howard Weiner and Rochelle Epstein, personal communication) and has been shown to activate suppressor T cells nonspecifi-

TABLE 2

Cell Type Activated	Manipulation of Host
Ts	i.v. route of administration of ligand-coupled cells
Te	s.c. route of administration of ligand-coupled cells
Ts	uv treatment of mice prior to s.c. route of administration of uv-treated ligand-coupled cells
Te	uv treatment of mice plus IL-1 administration
Ts	anti-I-A antibody administered *in vivo*
Te	anti-idiotype s.c.
Ts	anti-idiotype i.v.
?Ts	anti-reovirus receptor antibody

cally. We developed an antibody to this nonclonally expressed receptor and showed that it generates unresponsiveness in the same manner as virus. Thus, an interaction of antibody with an apparently nonclonal receptor on a subset of T cells causes them to be activated to manifest nonspecific suppression. It is of interest that this receptor also appears on a subset of human suppressor/cytotoxic cells. We can explain this kind of triggering as a result of some major but undefined function of this receptor on these cells. Clearly, this type of triggering is radically different from the signals associated with specific T cell factors or even from anti-idiotype interacting with clonally distributed idiotypic receptors. The precise mechanism underlying this is presently under study.

Conclusion

Of the mechanisms that determine the outcome of immunological perturbation of the mouse, we have considered several distinct stimuli (TABLE 2). At the basis of the decisive events that determine whether suppression or immunity is dominant is the route of administration of ligand and the effectiveness of the specialized APC necessary to trigger Te. If these two features are manipulated, then one can preferentially generate suppression or effective immunity. The I-A⁺ APC seem to determine if Te cells are triggered; if they are blocked by anti-I-A antibodies or rendered ineffective by uv response, then suppression occurs. These observations might suggest that another set of APC with different I region structures and different physical characteristics (uv resistance?) may be essential for activating suppressor cells. This issue is currently under study in our laboratory. A second major principle is that certain types of molecules, like allogeneic effect factor, can interact with H-2 encoded products and trigger subsets of suppressor cells to become active. Furthermore, signals from one subset of suppressor cells (Ts_1) to another (Ts_2) are clearly mediated through a characterized TsF molecule. Finally, we have assumed that special receptors, such as the hemagglutinin binding site, once bound by antibodies, can lead to activation of the cells. It is likely that, with time, common features of these activational mechanisms will be understood.

REFERENCES

1. BATTISTO, J. R. & B. R. BLOOM. 1966. Dual immunological unresponsiveness induced by cell membrane coupled hapten or antigen. Nature (London) **212:** 156–57.
2. MILLER, S. D. & H. N. CLAMAN. 1976. The induction of hapten specific T cell tolerance using hapten modified lymphoid cells. I. Characteristics of tolerance induction. J. Immunol. **117:** 1519–26.
3. OKUDA, J., M. MINAMI, D. H. SHERR & M. E. DORF. 1981. Hapten-specific T cell responses to 4-hydroxy-3-nitrophenyl acetyl. XI. Pseudogenetic restrictions of hybridoma suppressor factors. J. Exp. Med. **154:** 468–79.
4. PIERRES, A., J. S. BROMBERG, M. S. SY, B. BENACERRAF & M. I. GREENE. 1980. Mechanisms of regulation of the induction of genetically restricted suppressor cells. J. Immunol. **124:** 343–48.
5. BACH, B. A., L. SHERMAN, B. BENACERRAF & M. I. GREENE. 1978. Mechanisms of regulation of cell-mediated immunity. II. Induction and suppression of delayed-type hypersensitivity to azobenzenearsonate-coupled syngeneic cells. J. Immunol. **121:** 1460–68.
6. GREENE, M. I., M. S. SY, M. KRIPKE & B. BENACERRAF. 1979. Impairment of antigen presenting cell function by ultraviolet radiation. Proc. Nat. Acad. Sci. USA **76:** 6591–95.
7. LEFORT, S. *et al.* In preparation.
8. PERRY, L. L., M. E. DORF, B. A. BACH, B. BENACERRAF & M. I. GREENE. 1980. Mechanisms of regulation of cell mediated immunity. VIII. Anti-I-A allo-antisera interferes with induction and expression of T cell mediated immunity to cell bound antigen *in vivo.* Clin. Immunol. Immunopathol. **15:** 279–92.
9. SPRENT, J. 1980. Effects of blocking helper T cell induction *in vivo* with anti-Ia antibodies. Possible role of I-A/E hybrid molecules as restriction elements. J. Exp. Med. **152:** 996–1010.
10. SPRENT, J. E., E. A. LERNER, J. BROUCE & F. W. SYMINGTON. 1981. Inhibition of T cell activation *in vivo* with mixtures of monoclonal antibodies for I-A and I-A/E molecules. J. Exp. Med. **53:** 188–92.
11. BROMBERG, J. S., J. NEPOM, B. BENACERRAF & M. I. GREENE. Hapten coupled monoclonal anti-I-A antibodies provide a first signal for the induction of suppression. Submitted.
12. STEINMAN, R. M. & Z. A. COHN. 1974. Identification of a novel cell type in peripheral lymphoid organs or mice. II. Functional properties *in vitro.* J. Exp. Med. **139:** 380–97.

13. KUETTNER, M. G., A. L. WANG & A. NISONOFF. 1972. Quantitative investigations of idiotypic antibodies. VI. Idiotype specificity as a potential genetic marker for the variable regions of mouse immunoglobulin polypeptide chains. J. Exp. Med. 135: 579–95.

14. SY, M. S., A. BROWN, B. A. BACK, B. BENACERRAF, P. D. GOTTLIEB, A. NISONOFF & M. I. GREENE. 1981. Genetic and serological analysis of the expression of crossreactive idiotypic determinants on anti-p-azobenzenearsonate antibodies and p-azobenzenarsonate-specific suppressor T cell factors. Proc. Nat. Acad. Sci. USA 78: 1143–47.

15. BROMBERG, J. S., B. BENACERRAF & M. I. GREENE. 1981. Mechanisms of regulation of cell-mediated immunity. VII. Suppressor T cells induced by suboptimal doses of antigen plus an I-J specific allogeneic effect. J. Exp. Med. 153: 437–49.

16. BROMBERG, J. S., M. S. SY, B. BENACERRAF & M. I. GREENE. 1981. T cell–T cell interaction in the generation of first order idiotype bearing suppressor cells. Clin. Immunol. Immunopathol. In press.

17. DELOVITCH, T. L., J. WATSON, R. BATTISTELLA, J. F. HARRIS, J. SHAW & V. PAETKAU. 1981. In vitro analysis of allogeneic lymphocyte interaction V. Identification and characterization of two components of allogeneic effect factor, one of which displays H-2-restricted helper activity and the other, T cell-growth factor activity. J. Exp. Med. 153: 107–28.

18. ANDERSON, J. & F. MELCHERS. 1981. T cell-dependent activation of resting B cells: Requirement for both nonspecific unrestricted and antigen-specific IA-restricted soluble factors. Proc. Nat. Acad. Sci. USA 78: 2497–501.

19. TADA, T. & K. OKUMURA. 1980. The role of antigen specific T cell factors in the immune response. Adv. Immunol. 28: 1–87.

20. EARDLEY, D. D., J. KEMP, F.-W. SHEN, H. CANTOR & R. K. GERSHON. 1979. Immunoregulatory circuits along T cell sets: Effect of mode of immunization on determining which Lyl T cell sets will be activated. J. Immunol. 122: 1663–65.

21. EARDLEY, D. D., D. B. MURPHY, J. D. KEMP, F. W. SHEN, H. CANTOR & R. K. GERSHON. 1980. Ly-1 inducer and Ly-1.2 acceptor T cells in the feedback suppression circuit bear an I-J subregion controlled determinant. Immunogenetics 11: 549–57.

22. SY, M. S., M. H. DIETZ, R. N. GERMAIN, B. BENACERRAF & M. I. GREENE. 1980. Antigen and receptor-driven regulatory mechanisms. IV. Idiotype-bearing I-J$^+$ suppressor T cell factors induce second-order suppressor T cells which express anti-idiotypic receptors. J. Exp. Med. 151: 1183–95.

23. WALTENBAUGH, C., J. THEZE, J. A. KAPP & B. BENACERRAF. 1977. Immunosuppressive factor(s) specific for L-glutamic acid^{50}–L-tyrosine^{50} (GT). IV. Generation of suppressor T cells by a suppressive extract derived from GT primed lymphoid cells. J. Exp. Med. 146: 970–85.

24. SY, M. S., A. NISONOFF, R. N. GERMAIN, B. BENACERRAF & M. I. GREENE. 1981. Antigen- and receptor-driven regulatory mechanisms. VIII. Suppression of idiotype-negative. p-azobenzenearsonate-specific T cells results from the interaction of an anti-idiotypic second-order T suppressor cell with a cross-reactive-idiotype-positive, p-azobenzenearsonate-primed T cell target. J. Exp. Med. 153: 1415–25.

25. SY, M. S., A. R. BROWN, A. NISONOFF, B. BENACERRAF & M. I. GREENE. 1980. Antigen and receptor driven regulatory mechanisms. III. Induction of delayed type hypersensitivity to azobenzenearsonate with anti-cross-reactive idiotypic antibodies. J. Exp. Med. 151: 896–909.

26. NEPOM, J. T., H. L. WEINER, M. DICHTER, D. SPRIGGS, L. POWERS, B. FIELDS & M. I. GREENE. 1981. Identification of hemagglutinin specific idiotype associated with reovirus recognition shared by lymphoid and neuronal cells. J. Exp. Med. In press.

DISCUSSION OF THE PAPER

J. CHILLER (*Scripps Clinic and Research Foundation, La Jolla, Calif.*): Does the conversion of pre-Ts to Ts_1 *in vitro* require the presence of macrophages?

GREENE: Unfortunately, I can't answer that question because we use spleen populations that have been neither extensively purified for T cells nor deprived of macrophages. However, there is another set of experiments in which mice are subjected to a regimen that makes their total antigen-presenting cell population completely ineffective, and they are still capable of generating Ts_1 cells.

CHILLER: Do you have cells frozen as pre-Ts that can be converted to Ts at the hybridoma level with allogeneic factors?

GREENE: We have not done that.

HYPERIMMUNITY
AND THE DECISION TO BE INTOLERANT *

Douglas R. Green

Departments of Pathology and Biology
Yale University School of Medicine
New Haven, Connecticut 06510

Richard K. Gershon

Laboratory of Cellular Immunology
Howard Hughes Medical Institute
Yale University School of Medicine
New Haven, Connecticut 06510

INTRODUCTION

The Oulipo (derived from Ouvroir de Litterature Potentielle) is a French group of writers and mathematicians who revel in wordplay such as the devising of algorithms for the transformation of prose and poetry. These transformations often produce results that appear, at first, almost nonsensical, but, upon inspection, reveal surprising properties of language and literature.[1]

Taking our lead from the Oulipo, we have chosen to discuss, not tolerance, but its antipodal sibling on the immunological continuum—hyperimmunity. For, through understanding why and how a system can be frozen in an "on" state, we might gain insight into what sort of signals might, instead, have turned it off.

Recently, we described and characterized the elements of a regulatory T cell circuit, the contrasuppressor circuit, which is capable of producing just this sort of "on" state. In this discussion, we shall consider the evidence for this circuit in the generation and maintenance of the hyperimmune state. Then, using the logic of the Oulipo, we shall briefly examine the possibility that tolerance exists (in some forms) because of an absence of such activity.

THE PARADOX OF HYPERIMMUNITY

The ability to respond in a specific and accelerated fashion to a previously experienced antigen is a hallmark of the immune system, without which there would be no need for a generation of diversity. (A simple algorithm could then be devised, such as: Nonspecifically reject any material that does not fit an anti-self receptor. Note that such an algorithm also simplifies the principle of self tolerance but cannot explain acquired tolerance or memory.) Repeated antigenic challenge produces an elevated response, a state that can be described as "hyperimmunity."

It has been shown that serum from hyperimmune animals, which contains very high titers of antigen-specific antibody, will completely suppress the ability

* This research was supported by training grant no. AI–07019.

318

of a naive recipient (receiving as little as 2 μl of serum i.p.) to make a primary response to the antigen.[2] Recently, Iverson *et al.* demonstrated the presence of extraordinarily high concentrations of antigen-specific T cell–derived suppressor factor (up to 1 mg ml^{-1}) in such sera.[3]

Yet, immune responses proceed in these animals. That is the first part of the paradox.

This observation shows that the immune memory in these animals is not carried exclusively in the serum (as might be predicted by idiotypic network theory). Transfer of the cells into naive recipients transfers both immunity and resistance to the suppressive effects of the immune serum.[4] Tada *et al.*[5] and Eardley and Gershon,[6] however, have shown that secondary antibody responses cannot be transferred with immunized cells into untreated naive recipients. Transfer requires low-dose irradiation or cyclophosphamide (Cy) treatment of the recipient.[6, 7] This is the second part of the paradox. This observation tells us that the hyperimmune state differs qualitatively from the state produced by a single exposure to antigen. It does not tell us what this difference might be.

Contact sensitivity to picryl chloride can be transferred by the intravenous injection of immune splenocytes into naive recipients.[8] Recently, we have shown that this transfer requires two immune Lyt 1 T cells: an I-J$^-$ subset that carries the immunity and can transfer it to animals treated with a low dose (20 mg kg^{-1}) of Cy and an I-J$^+$ population that is required if the immunity is to be transferred to untreated recipients.[9]

The effector of the contrasuppressor circuit is an I-J$^+$ Lyt 1 T cell that has the ability to render helper T cells resistant to suppression.[10] The activity of such an immunoregulatory circuit in hyperimmune animals would help resolve the above paradox.

THE DOUBLE MARBROOK MODIFICATION OF THE INTERMEDIATE CULTURE SYSTEM

In order to study T cell–T cell interactions in the regulation of helper T cells (in the absence of B cells), we used an intermediate culture system.[11] Helper and regulatory T cells were mixed, cultured together for 24–48 h, and then separated by the use of antisera directed against cell surface markers present only on the regulatory cells. Using this system, we were able to demonstrate the following. (1) Helper T cells can be inactivated by suppressor T cells such that, when recovered, these helper cells have lost the ability to provide help to fresh cultures of B cells plus antigen.[11] (2) T suppressor inducer cells can also be inactivated by suppressor cells such that they subsequently fail to induce suppression when added to cultures of whole spleen and antigen.[11] (3) Contrasuppressor effector cells are capable of blocking the inactivation of helper cells by suppressor cells.[10] (4) Such "contrasuppressed" helpers are subsequently relatively resistant to additional suppressor cell signals.[10]

An improvement has recently been made on this intermediate culture system. Helper cells were placed in the lower chamber of a periscopic double Marbrook chamber, while other regulatory cells were placed in the upper chamber. Following a 48 h incubation, the helpers were readily recovered without fear of contamination by the other cells. These helpers were added to fresh B cells plus antigen and cultured for five days. The resulting PFC response represents a measure of the helper potential in the regulated helper T cell population (FIGURE 1).

HYPERIMMUNE SPLEEN CELLS AS A SOURCE OF CONTRASUPPRESSION

The experimental design is shown in FIGURE 1. Lyt 1 helper cells were placed in the lower chamber in all cases (with SRBC). The upper chamber could then hold the precultured suppressor cells and SRBC hyperimmune spleen cells† (passed over goat anti-mouse Ig plates to remove B cells). SRBC were added to control for potential effects of antigen carryover on the immune cells. The antigen was not required in this chamber for suppression to occur, however (unpublished observation).

Following a 48 h culture, the cells in the lower chamber were harvested and tested for helper activity by adding them to fresh B cells (anti-Thy 1–treated spleen cells) under conditions for *in vitro* SRBC responses. In addition, fresh suppressor cells were added at this point to test the helper cells for resistance to suppression. The results of this experiment are shown in FIGURE 2.

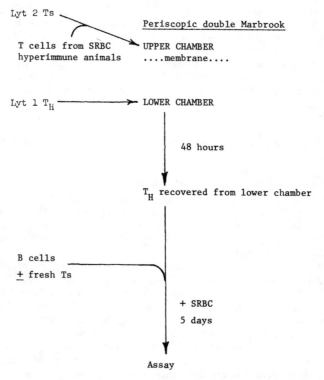

FIGURE 1. Double Marbrook modification of the intermediate culture system.

† Mice were given at least six weekly injections and had hemagglutination titers of 10 doubling dilutions or better.

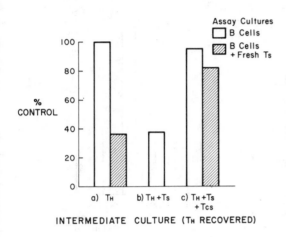

FIGURE 2. T cells from SRBC-primed animals (T_H) were cultured in the lower chamber of a periscopic double Marbook culture. Nonspecific suppressor T cells (Ts) were placed in the upper chamber, with or without T cells from SRBC hyperimmunized animals (T_{HI}). After 48 h, the T_H cells were retrieved from the lower chamber and added to B cells (anti-Thy 1 plus complement-treated spleen cells) under conditions for an *in vitro* SRBC response. Some cultures received fresh suppressor cells. The results are expressed as a percentage of the PFC response of controls (T + B cells). The control had approximately 900 PFC per culture.

As can be seen, helper cells treated in this way were capable of giving good help to B cells (group a).

Suppressor cells in the upper chamber were capable of inactivating these T helper cells, this effect persisting after retrieval (group b). Presence of hyperimmune spleen cells in the upper chamber, however, completely blocked this suppressor effect, leaving the helper cells in the lower chamber active (group c). The difference between groups a and c could be seen upon addition of fresh suppressors to the assay cultures. The normal helpers in group a were easily suppressed, while the "contrasuppressed" helpers in group c were rendered resistant to the suppressors. Thus, hyperimmune spleen cells contain a population that can produce effects identical to cultured neonatal contrasuppressors; that is, rendering helper T cells resistant to suppression.[10]

FIGURE 3 shows experiments that characterize the hyperimmune contrasuppressor population. When the plate passed, SRBC hyperimmune T cells were treated with either anti-Lyt 1 or anti-I-J plus complement, and the ability of these cells to block suppression (or render helper cells resistant to suppression) was removed. The evidence, then, for an I-J+ Lyt 1 contrasuppressor effector in the spleens of SRBC hyperimmune animals is supported functionally and by cell surface profile.

Unlike cultured neonatal contrasuppressors,[10] the hyperimmune contrasuppressors were generated by the action of antigen on the immune system. Yamauchi *et al.* demonstrated that Lyt 2 cells from antigen (SRBC)-primed animals produce an antigen-specific suppressor factor and a contrasuppressor inducer factor.[12] This TcsiF can be absorbed on sheep and on some, but not all, mammalian heterologous erythrocytes, suggesting some antigen specificity, but one broader than that of the suppressor factor. This TcsiF was found to act upon Lyt 1,2 transducers to produce contrasuppression. In this discussion,

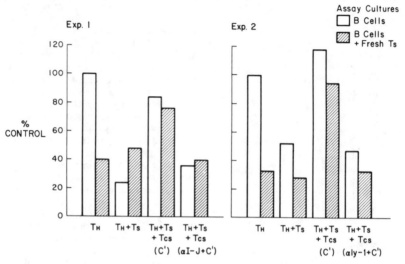

FIGURE 3. Conditions were as described in FIGURE 2, with the following modifications: (1) T_H were treated with anti-Lyt 2 plus complement before intermediate culture and (2) T_{HI} were treated with complement (C') or specific antisera plus complement (anti-Lyt 1.2 or anti-I-J^b) before intermediate culture. The control, for experiment 1, had approximately 1000 PFC per culture; that for experiment 2, approximately 1000 PFC per culture.

successive immunizations with the same antigen (SRBC) push the circuit into the effector (Lyt 1) mode *in vivo*.

ANTIGEN SPECIFICITY OF THE CONTRASUPPRESSOR EFFECTOR

While no antigen specificity was attributable to neonatal contrasuppressors (effective for SRBC, TNP, and oxazalone,[10, 13] as well as burro and horse red blood cells, data unpublished), the hyperimmune contrasuppressors might show some specificity. In FIGURE 4, an experiment to test this idea is shown.

The lower chamber in this experiment contained either burro red blood cell (BRBC)-primed or SRBC-primed Lyt 1 helper cells. The upper chamber contained the nonspecific precultured suppressors and SRBC hyperimmune spleen cells. While the appropriate antigen was added to the lower chamber (BRBC or SRBC), only SRBC were added to the upper chamber.

The results show that, whereas the suppressors were capable of inactivating both helper cell populations, only the SRBC-specific responses could be contrasuppressed by the addition of SRBC hyperimmune spleen cells. Once again, the contrasuppressor cells rendered the SRBC-specific helper cells resistant to subsequent suppressor cell signals. Thus, Lyt 1 contrasuppressor cells from SRBC hyperimmune mice showed a degree of antigen specificity, in that they had no effect upon the inactivation of BRBC-specific helper cells.

The Hyperimmune State

The demonstration of the existence of contrasuppressor effector cells with a degree of antigen specificity in the spleens of hyperimmune animals helps to explain how an immune response can proceed in these animals in the face of so much immunosuppressive material in their serum. Why, however, is there so much immunosuppressive material in the serum of these animals? The answer may involve the interaction of the suppressor and contrasuppressor circuits. We have previously demonstrated the action of suppressor T cells upon both helper T cells and the inducers of suppression.[11] This latter effect, the feedback of suppressor activity on inducers, suggests that large amounts of suppressor effector product should not be made, since the interaction of the inducer and effector is required for the production of suppressor activity (see Reference 14) and the inducer activity will have been abated by the effector itself. This feedback, however, could be blocked if the inducer cell, like the helper T cell, can serve as a target of contrasuppression as well as feedback suppression. If so, then, in the presence of the activity of both circuits, suppressor cells will continue to produce large amounts of suppressive material without feedback, for this suppressive material will have difficulty in inhibiting the contrasuppressed feedback inducer cells (or the contrasuppressed helper T cells). This seems to be the case in both hyperimmune and some autoimmune animals (MRL), *i.e.*, large amounts of systemic suppression that are ignored by responding cells.[15] This model explains why suppressor factors are best derived from immune rather than tolerant animals (which have inactivated their suppressor mechanism by feedback).

The action of contrasuppressors upon feedback inducer cells is implied by

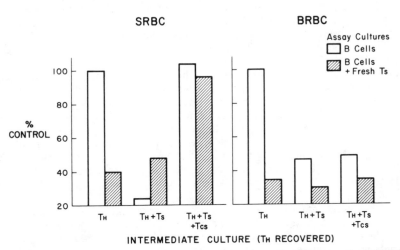

FIGURE 4. Conditions were as described in FIGURE 2. T_H cells were from SRBC- or BRBC-primed animals; all T_HI were from SRBC-hyperimmunized animals. Recovered T_H were cultured with B cells with the appropriate red blood cell (SRBC or BRBC). The assays were made against the appropriate red blood cell. The control for SRBC had approximately 1000 PFC per culture; that for BRBC had approximately 1600 PFC per culture.

the above argument but is rather difficult, in practice, to prove. Any attempt to contrasuppress the suppressor inducers simultaneously produces suppressor-resistant helper cells. These, in turn, mask any suppression that might be induced. Further improvements in the intermediate culture system are required before this model can be addressed experimentally.

THE TRANSITION TO HYPERIMMUNITY

Having characterized the hyperimmune state, in part, we are left with the question, How does multiple exposure to antigen produce such a state?

In recent years an attractive hypothesis has suggested that antigen-presenting cells direct antigen into one or more immunoregulatory circuits,[16, 17] presumably in response to both internal and external conditions. With regard to hyperimmunity, Haughton has demonstrated that immune peritoneal exudate (PE) macrophages incubated with naive T cells drive the T cells into a state such that these cells can block the suppressive effects of hyperimmune serum *in vivo*.[18]

Preliminary experiments from our lab indicate that incubation of naive T cells with plastic adherent peritoneal exudate cells (PEC) from hyperimmune animals for 24 h allows the generation of a cell capable of blocking suppressor cell activity *in vitro* (see FIGURE 5). Unimmunized PEC plus T cells and immunized PEC in the absence of T cells fail to produce this effect.

While it remains to be shown whether these T cells bear phenotypic characteristics of the contrasuppressor circuit, we may still speculate on the role of the antigen-presenting cell in hyperimmunity and contrasuppression. We shall take a slightly circuitous route to this end.

Macher and Chase showed that if an area that has been painted with a sensitizing reagent is removed a short time after painting, then tolerance to the antigen, rather than immunity, is generated.[19] Why, then, does the intact painted skin of sensitized animals shift this regulatory balance in favor of immunity?

There is good presumptive evidence that haptenated standard antigen-presenting cells induce both helper and suppressor systems. The question of which of these two systems will dominate the response depends, to a large extent, on the relative numbers of suppressor cells stimulated at the time of immunization. While tolerance is produced by intravenous injection of haptenated macrophages, immunity is often the result of subcutaneous administration.[20, 21] The latter route presumably bypasses the suppressor circuit, since lymph node–localizing T cells are depleted of suppressor cells compared to spleen-localizing T cells.[22] Another method of bypassing the suppressor circuit is to treat animals with low doses (20 mg kg^{-1}) of cyclophosphamide.[23] Haptenated macrophages injected i.v. into cyclophosphamide-pretreated mice produces significant immunity.[20]

It has been demonstrated that help and suppression in this system can be shifted in favor of immunity by the administration of contrasuppressors.[13] Thus, even in cases in which the suppressor circuit is not bypassed, active contrasuppression can allow dominant immunity.

One could therefore postulate that optimal modes of immunization, including intradermal injection of antigen and the use of adjuvants (or antigens with "inherent adjuvanticity"[24]), all lead to potent immunity because of local activation of cells in the contrasuppressor circuit.

Support for this idea comes from studies of Langerhans cells, the antigen-

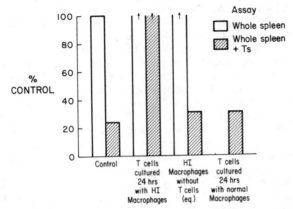

FIGURE 5. Plastic adherent cells from the peritoneal exudate of normal or hyperimmunized animals were cultured 24 h with naive T cells. These were added to spleen cells with or without suppressor cells (Ts) under conditions for an *in vitro* PFC response to SRBC. The control response (for spleen cells alone) was 5350 PFC per culture.

presenting cells of the skin. Unlike haptenated macrophages, intravenous injection of haptenated Langerhans cells leads to immunity without requiring any manipulation of the suppressor system.[20] Even in the presence of concomitant activation of suppressor cells by other haptenated cells, immunity induced by the Langerhans cells can be dominant. Thus, in the experiments of Macher and Chase discussed above,[19] signals from the haptenated epidermal Langerhans cells activated other cells that overcame the tolerogenic signals delivered by hapten that leaked through the skin and localized on other molecules in the spleen.

The splenic dendritic cell, another antigen-presenting cell, behaves like a Langerhans cell experimentally.[25] When antigen-coupled spleen cells containing both splenic macrophages (tolerogenic) and dendritic cells (immunogenic) are injected intravenously, suppressor cells—which can be demonstrated if a Lyt 1 cell that "neutralizes" suppression is removed[26]—are generated. This strongly supports the idea that immunity is a question of balance, often between suppression and contrasuppression, with the helper cell as the focus of attention.[27]

Thus, by switching antigen into the suppressor or contrasuppressor circuits, antigen-presenting cells have a major role in tipping this balance in favor of tolerance or immunity. As we have seen, the PEC of hyperimmune animals seem capable of inducing a positive contrasuppressor-inducing potential in cocultured naive T cells. It may be, then, that it is the antigen-presenting cells that predispose an actively challenged animals towards hyperimmunity.

TOLERANCE AND THE ABSENCE OF CONTRASUPPRESSION

Some years ago, it was postulated that the appearance of tolerance might be produced by a lack of contrasuppressive activity upon exposure to antigen.[28] We are now in a position to examine this prospect in more detail.

As we have shown, all immunogenic challenges may induce both suppression and contrasuppression. Suppose, for the sake of argument, that tolerogenic protocols not only fail to induce contrasuppression but can, in some cases, completely inactivate certain cells of this circuit. The tolerogenic stimulus then activates suppressor cells but deletes contrasuppression (we are prejudiciously ignoring other possible and relevant properties of tolerogens, such as paralysis). As we have previously shown, Lyt 2 suppressor T cells are capable of inactivating both helper T cells and the suppressor circuit itself. We should observe a transient period of suppression followed by a (self-imposed) loss of suppressor activity with no return of helper function.

Recall, however, that we have theoretically deleted the contrasuppressor circuit as well. Subsequently, then, re-exposure to immunogenic doses of antigen, which normally induces both suppression and contrasuppression, will, in our tolerized animal, only induce suppression.

Over time, contrasuppressor potential may slowly return, so that antigenic challenge will have the effect of inducing less and less suppressive effects. Eventually, so much contrasuppression will have returned that no suppression will be seen. At this point, tolerance will break.

When tolerance is induced in adult mice with dHGG, this is exactly what is observed.[29] A period of active suppression is soon followed by an absence of demonstrable suppression, although the animal remains unresponsive. Antigenic challenge subsequently induces suppressor cell activity, but this potential decreases with time. Eventually, no suppression can be observed upon challenge and, shortly thereafter, tolerance breaks.

We do not suggest that all forms of tolerance proceed as outlined (although William of Occam might), only that this is at least one of (perhaps several) strategies to unresponsiveness. We do suggest, however, that, to understand how the immune system turns on and off, it is necessary to study both positive and negative mechanisms of immunoregulation and how they interact. Thus, in considering a continuum of immune responsiveness, hyperimmunity may result from decreased suppression, increased contrasuppression, or both; tolerance may result from increased suppression, decreased contrasuppression, or both.[30]

With regard to stating the above thesis, undoubtedly the Oulipo (who are notoriously fond of anagrams) would have a preference:

Note: "Tolerance and no contrasuppression"
sounds a lot nicer to a person 'pon entrance.‡

REFERENCES

1. GARDNER, M. 1977. Mathematical games Sci. Am. **241:** 121.
2. HAUGHTON, G. & D. R. NASH. 1969. Specific immunosuppression by minute doses of passive antibody. Transplant. Proc. **1:** 616.
3. IVERSON, G. M., D. D. EARDLEY, C. A. JANEWAY & R. K. GERSHON. Isolation of circulating IgT with the use of anti-idiotype immunoabsorbants. Proc. Nat. Acad. Sci. USA. In press.
4. HAUGHTON, G. 1971. Specific immunosuppression by minute doses of passive antibody. III. Reversal of suppression by peritoneal exudate cells from immune animals. Cell. Immunol. **2:** 567.

‡ The second line is an anagram of the first.

5. TADA, T. & T. TAKEMORI. 1974. Selective role of thymus-derived lymphocytes in the antibody response. I. Differential suppressive effect of carrier-primed T cells on hapten-specific IgM and IgG antibody responses. J. Exp. Med. **140:** 239.
6. EARDLEY, D. D. & R. K. GERSHON. 1975. Feedback induction of suppressor T cell activity. J. Exp. Med. **142:** 524.
7. CELADA, F. 1966. Quantitative studies of the adoptive immunological memory in mice. I. An age dependent barrier to syngeneic transplantation. J. Exp. Med. **124:** 7.
8. ASHERSON, G. L. & W. PTAK. 1968. Contact and delayed hypersensitivity in the mouse. I. Active sensitization and passive transfer. Immunology **15:** 405.
9. IVERSON, G. M., W. PTAK, D. R. GREEN & R. K. GERSHON. The role of contrasuppression in the adoptive transfer of immunity. Submitted.
10. GREEN, D. R., D. D. EARDLEY, A. KIMURA, D. B. MURPHY, K. YAMAUCHI & R. K. GERSHON. 1981. Immunoregulatory circuits which modulate responsiveness to suppressor circuit. Eur. J. Immunol. **11:** 973.
11. GREEN, D. R., R. K. GERSHON & D. D. EARDLEY. 1981. Functional deletion of different Ly-1 cell inducer subset activities by Ly-2 suppressor T lymphocytes. Proc. Nat. Acad. Sci. USA. **78:** 3819.
12. YAMAUCHI, K., D. R. GREEN, D. D. EARDLEY, D. B. MURPHY & R. K. GERSHON. 1981. Immunoregulatory circuits that modulate responsiveness to suppressor cell signals: The failure of B10 mice to respond to suppressor factors can be overcome by quenching the contrasuppressor circuit. J. Exp. Med. **153:** 1547.
13. PTAK, W., D. R. GREEN, S. K. DURUM, A. KIMURA, D. B. MURPHY & R. K. GERSHON. 1981. Immunoregulatory circuits that modulate responsiveness to suppressor cell signals: Contrasuppressor cells can convert an *in vivo* tolerogenic signal into an immunogenic one. Eur. J. Immunol. **11:** 980.
14. GERSHON, R. K. 1980. Immunoregulation circa 1980: Some comments on the state of the art. J. Allergy Clin. Immunol. **66:** 18.
15. GERSHON, R. K., M. HOROWITZ, J. D. KEMP, D. B. MURPHY & D. MURPHY. 1978. The cellular site of immunoregulatory breakdown in the *lpr* mouse. *In* Genetic Control of Autoimmune Disease. N. R. Rose, R. E. Bigazzi, and N. L. Warner, Eds.: 223. Elsevier/North Holland. New York.
16. GERSHON, R. K., K. F. NAIDORF & W. PTAK. 1980. Information transfer between T cell sets: The macrophage is the message. *In* Macrophage Regulation of Immunity. E. R. Unanue and A. S. Rosenthal, Eds.: 431. Academic Press. New York.
17. MITCHISON, N. A. 1980. MHC molecules as guides for T lymphocyte parallel sets. *In* Strategies of Immune Regulation. E. E. Sercarz and A. J. Cunningham, Eds.: 121. Academic Press. New York.
18. HAUGHTON, G. 1974. Specific immunosuppression by minute doses of passive antibody. V. Participation of macrophages in reversal of suppression by peritoneal exudate cells from immune animals. Cell. Immunol. **13:** 230.
19. MACHER, E. & M. W. CHASE. 1969. Studies on the sensitization of animals with simple chemical compounds. XI. The influence of excision of allergenic depots on onset of delayed hypersensitivity and tolerance. J. Exp. Med. **129:** 81.
20. PTAK, W., D. ROZYCKA, P. W. ASKENASE, & R. K. GERSHON. 1980. Role of antigen-presenting cells in the development and persistence of contact hypersensitivity. J. Exp. Med. **151:** 362.
21. GREENE, M. I. & B. BENACERRAF. 1980. Studies on hapten specific T cell immunity and suppression. Immunol. Rev. **50:** 163.
22. GERSHON, R. K., E. M. LANCE & K. KONDO. 1974. Immuno-regulatory role of spleen localizing thymocytes. J. Immunol. **112:** 546.

23. COHEN, P. & R. K. GERSHON. 1975. The role of cortisone-sensitive thymocytes in DNA synthetic responses to antigen. Ann. N.Y. Acad. Sci. **249:** 451.
24. DRESSER, D. W. 1962. Specific inhibition of antibody production. II. Paralysis induced in adult mice by small quantities of protein antigen. Immunology **5:** 378.
25. BRITZ, J. S., P. W. ASKENASE, W. PTAK, R. M. STEINMAN & R. K. GERSHON. Specialized antigen-presenting cells: Splenic dendritic cells, and peritoneal exudate cells induced by mycobacteria activate effector T cells that are resistant to suppression. J. Exp. Med. In press.
26. BRALEY-MULLEN, H. 1980. Direct demonstration of splenic suppressor T cells in mice tolerant to type III pneumococcal polysaccharide: Two-step requirement for development of detectable suppressor cells. J. Immunol. **125:** 1849.
27. GREEN, D. R. & R. K. GERSHON. 1981. The immunological orchestra, circa 1981. *In* Immunoglobulin Idiotypes. C. A. Janeway, E. E. Sercarz, H. Wigzell, and C. F. Fox, Eds.: 893. Academic Press. New York.
28. GERSHON, R. K. 1974. Lack of activity of contra-suppressor T cells as a mechanism of tolerance. *In* Immunological Tolerance: Mechanisms and Potential Therapeutic Applications. D. H. Katz and B. Benacerraf, Eds.: 441. Academic Press. New York.
29. PARKS, D. E. 1981. Decreased ability to demonstrate suppressor T cell activity during tolerance. J. Supramol. Struct. **5:** 197.
30. GREEN, D. R. & D. D. EARDLEY. 1981. Modelling a continuum of immune responsiveness. *In* Immunoglobulin Idiotypes and Their Expression. C. A. Janeway, E. E. Sercarz, H. Wigzell, and C. F. Fox, Eds.: 673. Academic Press. New York.

DISCUSSION OF THE PAPER

H. N. CLAMAN (*University of Colorado Medical School, Denver, Col.*): Both the suppressor-inducer factor and the contrasuppressor cells are derived from mice hyperimmunized to sheep cells. Is the hyperimmunization necessary? I wish you'd also comment on the role of the factor or the contrasuppressor cell in either naive animals or animals just given an ordinary immunogenic regimen.

GERSHON: To produce the suppressor molecules, we took a protocol that had been developed by Okamura and Tada, in which they inject antigen on day zero. Two weeks later they inject antigen again. They then wait two weeks and put the cells in culture. I cannot comment on whether this is the exact protocol that's needed, but it works. Contrasuppressor cells can be found in naive animals. But they are controlled by another set of cells and, in order to see them, you have to get rid of that other set of cells. The optimal system for looking at this is in the B-10 mouse, because the B-10 mouse does not have an acceptor cell for the second order suppressor cells that control the contrasuppressor cells. So the B-10 mouse in this system, in Tada's system, and in the system developed by Janeway is a dominant contrasuppressor in these types of assays. You can treat their cells with anti-I-J and get perfectly good suppression.

CLAMAN: Then what is the necessity for hyperimmunizing the mice to get the contrasuppressor cells that you mentioned today?

GERSHON: Dr. Green, are you here? Can you answer that?

GREEN: I use hyperimmunization because, in order to get these sorts of effects, you need immunization. Hyperimmunization is by far the easiest way to demonstrate the effects. Haughton has shown that, by manipulating cells from immune animals, he can produce effects resembling these; that is, overcoming suppression *in vivo*. He found a requirement for only a single immunization. I did not find that I could do that, which was the reason for going after the hyperimmune animals as a source of contrasuppressors. But I don't know how many immunizations it takes.

CLAMAN: I'm not interested in precisely how many immunizations. I want to know if the animals that are treated to produce contrasuppressor cells also have other cells that produce suppressor-inducer factors at the same time.

GERSHON: Yes. Much more than normal. The higher the level of contrasuppression that you can assay, the higher the level of suppression. The two go up simultaneously. The most striking example is the MLR autoimmune mouse. If you take very small numbers of spleen cells from MRL mice and ask them to suppress the response of their congenic partners, they suppress it to zero. Their spleen cells will not suppress their own cells. But, after Dr. Green has treated their cells with an anti-contrasuppressor serum, they can suppress their own cells. These mice wind up with lymph nodes that are approximately 100 to 200 times normal size. So we think that that is an example of circuitous interruptus, where the contrasuppressor cell prevents the suppressor cell from acting and the suppressor cell just keeps making more and more material.

J. CHILLER (*Scripps Clinic and Research Foundation, La Jolla, Calif.*): What is the specificity of the contrasuppressor and its mode of action on its target cell? Is the target of contrasuppression the helper cell?

GERSHON: It is a target; not the target.

CHILLER: A target. Is there recognition of specificity?

GERSHON: No.

REGULATION OF THE MAJOR CROSSREACTIVE IDIOTYPE ASSOCIATED WITH ANTI-p-AZOPHENYLARSONATE ANTIBODIES OF A/J MICE

Mitchell J. Nelles,* Yoshitane Dohi †, and Alfred Nisonoff *

*Department of Biology
and
Rosenstiel Basic Medical Sciences Research Center
Brandeis University
Waltham, Massachusetts 02254

† Department of Immunology
Research Institute for Microbial Diseases
Osaka University
Osaka, Japan

INTRODUCTION

In this paper, we will review recent investigations of suppression of the humoral response mediated by intrastrain crossreactive idiotypic determinants present on anti-p-azophenylarsonate (anti-Ar) antibodies of A/J mice. These studies complement investigations of T cell responses carried out in the laboratories of M. I. Greene and B. Benacerraf, which are reviewed elsewhere in this volume. The work to be described deals with regulation of the major cross-reactive idiotype (CRI) induced by inoculation of syngeneic cells to which CRI+ antibodies are conjugated and with the existence of idiotype-suppressor factors with idiotypic or anti-idiotypic receptors. In addition, we will discuss regulation of the CRI mediated by idiotopes present on monoclonal CRI+ antibodies and by monoclonal antibodies directed to idiotopes associated with the major CRI.

Suppression of the CRI response with anti-idiotypic reagents became feasible after the existence of the intrastrain idiotypic crossreaction had been demonstrated.[1] Thus, in the system we have investigated, it was possible to attempt to suppress an A/J mouse with anti-CRI prepared against anti-Ar antibodies of another A/J mouse or of a pool.[2] Using this approach, it was found that inoculation of rabbit anti-CRI into adult recipients results in selective suppression of the major idiotypic component of the anti-Ar response.[2] There is little effect on the total anti-Ar production upon subsequent immunization with keyhole limpet hemocyanin (KLH)-Ar.[3] At about the same time, in vitro suppression of an idiotypic response to phosphorylcholine was demonstrated by Cosenza and Köhler;[4] this was subsequently extended to in vivo responses by Strayer et al.[5] A significant advance was made by Eichmann in 1974, when he demonstrated that suppression with anti-Id results in the induction of idiotype-suppressor T cells that can adoptively transfer the idiotype-suppressed state to untreated adult syngeneic recipient mice.[6] Again, the recipients were able to produce antibody (anti-streptococcal group A) upon subsequent immunization, but the antibodies lacked the major crossreactive idiotype characteristic of the A strain of mice.

330

0077–8923/82/0392–0330 $1.75/0 © 1982, NYAS

There is evidence that, once established, idiotype suppression may be maintained in part by the dominance of secondary B cells; *i.e.,* cells with receptors lacking the major idiotype may dominate the response because of their large numbers and because they are more easily triggered than any primary CRI[+] B cells that may have emerged from suppression. The potency of this mechanism was demonstrated by experiments in which mice of the CRI[-] Balb/c strain were immunized with KLH-Ar and their enriched B cells transferred into CRI[+] allotype-congenic C.AL-20 recipients.[7] The C.AL-20 mice failed to produce the major idiotype upon subsequent immunization. Quantitative experiments showed that this suppression was due to the B cells transferred and not to contaminating T cells. The importance of B cell dominance was subsequently extended to show temporary but marked suppression of an entire allotypic response using appropriate congenic strains of mice.[8]

RESULTS AND DISCUSSION

Regulation of the Idiotypic Component of the A/J Anti-Ar Humoral Response with Idiotype-Conjugated Thymocytes

Studies carried out in collaboration with Frances L. Owen demonstrated the existence of idiotype-suppressor T cells with anti-idiotypic receptors.[9, 10] It was found that such cells were present in high concentrations in the spleens of mice that had been immunologically suppressed by inoculation of rabbit anti-CRI antibody, hyperimmunized with KLH-Ar, and allowed to rest for 8–12 weeks. Both the immunization and rest period were essential for the development of large numbers of anti-idiotypic suppressor T cells. These cells were identified through their capacity to form rosettes with syngeneic erythrocytes coated with Fab fragments derived from CRI[+] anti-Ar antibodies. Idiotypic specificity of the interaction was demonstrated by the inhibition observed with CRI[+] anti-Ar antibodies, anti-CRI, or free hapten. In addition, the splenocytes failed to form rosettes with red blood cells coated with nonspecific Fab fragments. It was further demonstrated that the rosette-forming cells constituted most of the suppressor activity present in hyperimmunized suppressed mice. Depletion of the rosette-forming cells by centrifugation resulted in an almost complete loss of suppressor activity and the rosettes themselves were found to be much more inhibitory than the unfractionated splenic T cell population.

The existence of anti-idiotypic suppressor T cells raised the possibility that idiotype suppression could be induced without the use of anti-idiotypic antibodies or antigen. In this experiment, we attempted to stimulate the anti-idiotypic suppressor T cells by inoculation of CRI[+] antibody conjugated to syngeneic thymocytes. Rowley *et al.* had previously demonstrated the suppression of an antibody response to phosphorylcholine in Balb/c mice by preinoculation of idiotype-positive molecules.[11] Because the major idiotype comprises such a large fraction of the Balb/c response, it was not ascertained whether the suppression was idiotype or antigen specific; the formation of suppressor T cells was not investigated at that time. TABLE 1 shows the effects of two pre-inoculations of idiotype-conjugated thymocytes followed by immunization with KLH-Ar.[12] Details of the experimental protocol are contained in footnotes to the table. The concentrations of idiotype in unknown samples were estimated from their inhibitory capacity per unit weight of anti-Ar antibody in the standard radioimmune assay for CRI; this assay employs radiolabeled purified A/J anti-Ar antibody, slightly less than an equivalent amount of rabbit anti-CRI serum and excess goat anti-rabbit Fc. The data indicate that A/J mice that receive idiotype-conjugated thymocytes before immunization with KLH-Ar produce anti-Ar antibody that lacks the CRI. These mice produce normal or moderately reduced concentrations of anti-Ar antibodies, despite their profound state of suppression with respect to CRI. Mice preinoculated with thymocytes

TABLE 1

SUPPRESSION OF SYNTHESIS OF IDIOTYPE BY INOCULATION
OF IDIOTYPE-CONJUGATED THYMOCYTES *

| | Antibody Response (Individual mice; day 38) | |
Preinoculations †	Anti-Ar Titer (μg/ml)	Anti-Ar Antibody Required for 50% Inhibition (ng)
None	400–1800	17, 36, 14, 28, 39, 7, 18
A/J thymocytes	200–5800	18, 7, 13, 12, 76
Conjugate, A/J thymocytes–anti-Ar	180–8100	>4600, >89 000, >4600, >46 000, >110 000, >150 000, >120 000, 190 000
Conjugate, A/J thymocytes–normal mouse IgG	200–15 000	25, 8, 10, 10
Anti-Ar antibody, 12 μg twice	470–2900	>29 000, 16, >72 000, >14 000, 35, 56, 90
Anti-Ar antibody, 100 μg twice	420–3200	8, >59 000, 52, 34, 51, 8
Mixture, A/J thymocytes + anti-Ar ‡	9–7500	25, 60, 70, 8, 300, 14, >190 000, 5300
KLH-Ar; conjugate, A/J thymo-cytes–anti-Ar §	1900–2900	28, 20, 60, 40, 55
Conjugate, C57BL/10 thymocytes–anti-Ar	10–6000	>500, >140 000, >39 000, 240, 11 000, >76 000, 40 000
Conjugate, Balb/c thymocytes–anti-Ar	240–7800	500, 80, 1100, 300, 650, 1500

* Data from Reference 12.

† Preinoculations were given on days −42 and −21 in complete or incomplete Freund's adjuvant, respectively. When thymocytes were injected, 25×10^6 were used. Conjugated thymocytes contained 12 ± 2 μg purified A/J anti-Ar antibody per 25×10^6 cells. All recipients received 0.25 mg KLH-Ar i.p. in CFA on days 0 and 28.

‡ 25×10^6 cells plus 12 μg Ab per injection.

§ Mice received 0.1 mg KLH-Ar i.p. in CFA on day −47. Inoculation of the conjugate and additional KLH-Ar were then given as specified above.

alone or with thymocytes conjugated with normal A/J IgG were not suppressed. When idiotype was injected alone or as a mixture with unconjugated thymocytes, only about one-third of the mice were suppressed. Thus, idiotype bound to a cell surface appears to be a potent means of inducing idiotype-specific regulation. The enhancement of suppression by conjugation to cells was found to be especially pronounced in F_1(A/J × Balb/c) and in C.AL-20 mice (see below). preinoculation of A/J CRI-conjugated thymocytes of Balb/c or C57BL/10 origin also induced a state of suppression in A/J mice with respect to the CRI, suggesting a lack of H-2 restriction in terms of the requirements of carrier cells.

Mice immunized with KLH-Ar five days before the inoculation of idiotype-coupled thymocytes produced normal amounts of CRI. The inability to suppress an ongoing idiotypic response had been previously observed when suppression was attempted with anti-CRI serum [3] or with anti-idiotypic T cells.[13] In subsequent experiments, T cells obtained from mice that had been given idiotype-conjugated thymocytes (without KLH-Ar immunization) were shown to transfer the suppressed state to untreated mice. As few as 1×10^7 T cells from an animal that had received two inoculations of idiotype-conjugated thymocytes were capable of causing suppression of the CRI in normal animals; the latter were immunized three days after adoptive transfer.

Studies of idiotype suppression induced by idiotype-conjugated thymocytes were also performed in C.AL-20 and $F_1(A/J \times Balb/c)$ mice.[12] C.AL-20 is a congenic strain that possesses the AL/N heavy chain allotype on a Balb/c background and normally produces CRI$^+$ anti-Ar antibody. In both strains, conjugation of idiotype to either Balb/c or A/J thymocytes was very effective in inducing a state of suppression. In C.AL-20 and $F_1(A/J \times Balb/c)$ mice, unconjugated mixtures of idiotype and thymocytes caused little, if any, suppression of the CRI.

Administration of idiotype presented in the context of a cell membrane therefore appears to induce the subsequent regulation of that same idiotype upon immunization with antigen. A probable mechanism is through the direct stimulation of anti-idiotypic suppressor T cells.

T Cell–Derived Suppressor Factors that Regulate the Idiotypic Component of the Humoral Anti-Ar Response

The existence of regulatory molecules derived from suppressor T cells has been reported in a variety of experimental systems. Such molecules have been shown to possess potent regulatory properties in both humoral and cell-mediated immune responses.[14-25] T cell–derived suppressor factors (TsF) reactive with a variety of haptens,[15-20] certain tumors,[21] and heterologous proteins[22] have been studied and TsF that control the production of a particular antibody class[23, 24] and allotype[25] have also been reported. In some cases, T cell–derived molecules have been shown to possess determinants that are serologically cross-reactive with the major idiotype of humoral antibodies reactive with the same antigen.[19, 26-29] In addition, products encoded by the major histocompatibility complex (MHC) are also present on many types of TsF.[14] It has been suggested that both idiotypic and MHC-encoded determinants present on TsF are crucial to their regulatory function *in vivo*.

It has been known for some time that administration of heterologous anti-idiotypic antiserum specific for A/J anti-Ar antibodies is capable of suppressing the major idiotypic component of the immune response.[2] In order to generate large numbers of anti-idiotypic suppressor T cells, animals must be subsequently immunized with a protein-Ar conjugate.[10] The T cells of such hyperimmunized suppressed (HIS) mice can transfer the suppressed state to untreated recipients.

To determine whether T cell–derived factor(s) can regulate the idiotypic component of the A/J anti-Ar humoral immune response, spleen cells from HIS mice were cultured *in vitro* for 24 h.[30] The cell-free culture supernatant thus obtained was incubated for four hours with normal spleen cells; the cells were then washed and transferred into irradiated syngeneic recipients that were subsequently immunized with KLH-Ar. The data in TABLE 2 show that normal A/J spleen cells incubated with cell-free supernatants from cultured cells of HIS mice can transfer a state of profound immunological suppression with respect to the CRI; this is indicated by the values for weight of anti-Ar antibody required for 50% inhibition in the standard radioimmune assay for CRI. The specificity of the suppression applies to the Ar hapten and not to the protein carrier. This is indicated by the results obtained with supernatants derived from suppressed mice immunized with KLH-Ar; when the recipients were sub-

TABLE 2

SUPPRESSION OF ID SYNTHESIS BY CELL-FREE CULTURE SUPERNATANTS
OF SPLEEN CELLS FROM IDIOTYPICALLY SUPPRESSED HYPERIMMUNIZED MICE *

Culture Supernatants (from A/J spleen cells)	Recipients Challenged with	Antibody Response (individual mice, day 35) †	
		Anti-Ar Titer (μg/ml)	Anti-Ar Ab Required for 50% Inhibition (ng)
Nonimmune	KLH-Ar	2600, 600, 3600, 2300, 1900	102, 8, 18, 13, 24
Nonimmune	Edestin-Ar	470, 210, 600, 540, 525	900, 105, 100, 21, 36
KLH-Ar-immunized	KLH-Ar	270, 560, 1190, 2000, 2400	560, 460, 30, 64, 25
Id-suppressed, KLH-Ar-immunized	KLH-Ar	310, 840, 560, 1050, 1700	7800, >21 000, >14 000 >26 000, 8400
Id-suppressed, KLH-Ar-immunized	Edestin-Ar	530, 360, 180, 530, 230	13 000, >9000, >4500 >13 000, >5800

* Each recipient was given 5×10^7 A/J spleen cells that had been incubated with culture supernatant from 5×10^7 spleen cells of the type specified in the first column. Idiotypically suppressed donor mice were allowed to rest for three weeks after hyper-immunization before culturing their cells. The recipients were inoculated i.p. with 0.1 mg KLH-Ar in CFA on days 3 and 17 after the adoptive transfer. Sera are from individual mice, taken 35 days after adoptive transfer.
† Data from Reference 30.

sequently immunized with edestin-Ar, they failed to produce the CRI. Culture supernatants obtained from spleen cells of nonimmune mice were nonsuppressive, while two out of five mice that received spleen cells treated with culture supernatants obtained from KLH-Ar immune spleen cells were mildly suppressed. The latter observation might relate to the presence of activated suppressor T cell populations in normally immunized mice.

Additional experiments showed that the factors involved are T cell–derived and that a minimum of 6–12 h is required for their optimal elaboration from HIS spleen cells *in vitro*.[30] Quantitative considerations indicated that the suppressor activity present in HIS spleen cell culture supernatants was not due to contaminating rabbit anti-CRI or A/J anti-Ar antibodies.

TsF obtained from HIS spleen cells was further characterized by affinity chromatography, using various proteins conjugated to Sepharose 4B. Although passage of TsF through columns containing insolubilized A/J anti-Ar antibody (idiotype) or rabbit anti-CRI antibodies failed to remove the suppressive activity, successive passage through the two types of immune adsorbents removed all the activity. This result indicates that TsF obtained from HIS spleen cells contains two types of molecules, one with idiotypic and one with anti-idiotypic receptors. In fact, molecules with suppressive activity could be eluted at low pH (2.8) from either idiotypic or anti-idiotypic immunoadsorbents. It was also shown that the factor with putative idiotypic receptors was bound by a column of BGG-Ar-Sepharose while the anti-idiotypic factor was not. Neither factor was retained by anti-Fab-Sepharose; this indicates the absence of conventional isotypic determinants.

The coexistence in solution of both idiotypic TsF and antiidiotypic TsF, rather than a complex of the two, is probably due to binding affinities that are inadequate to permit interaction at very low concentrations. Additional experiments showed that TsF is a protein with an approximate molecular weight of 50 000–100 000 daltons [30] and bears determinants encoded by the I-J subregion of the murine H-2 complex (Y. Hirai and A. Nisonoff, unpublished observations).

Thus, spleen cells obtained from mice treated with rabbit anti-CRI and subsequently immunized elaborate TsF with idiotypic and anti-idiotypic receptors. Lewis and Goodman have documented the presence of CRI[+] T suppressor cells (Ts) after challenging A/J mice with mouse IgG-Ar.[31] Suppressor T cells with anti-CRI receptors were discussed earlier. It seems likely that Ts cells with idiotypic receptors are generated first in HIS mice because the animals originally received rabbit anti-CRI antibodies. Once generated, the CRI[+] Ts may induce anti-CRI Ts. Although data obtained from studies of T cell responses (delayed-type hypersensitivity) to the Ar hapten indicate that a third order set of Ts actually mediates suppression in that system,[32] the class of Ts mediating suppression in the humoral system is not known.

Regulation of the Idiotype by Idiotopes Present on Monoclonal CRI[+] Anti-Ar Antibodies

Recent investigations with monoclonal CRI[+] anti-Ar antibodies have demonstrated that the major idiotype in the A/J strain constitutes a family of related molecules. A hybridoma product (HP) is designated CRI[+] if it causes more than 50% inhibition in the standard radioimmune assay for the idiotype using serum anti-Ar antibody as the labeled ligand. The heterogeneity of the family was demonstrated by serological [33, 34] and amino acid sequence analyses.[35–40] Heterogeneity was shown, first, by the marked variation among CRI[+] HP with respect to the weight required to cause 50% inhibition in the standard assay. Some CRI[+] HP are similar to serum anti-Ar in this respect, whereas others are weaker, with relatively large amounts required for inhibition. In addition, individual CRI[+] HP possess unique idiotypic determinants that are not found on most other CRI[+] HP and that are generally present only at low concentrations in pooled anti-Ar serum.[33]

It was found, however, that at least one idiotope is highly conserved within the family. This was shown by radioimmune assays in which anti-CRI directed against one CRI⁺ HP was allowed to interact with a different labeled CRI⁺ HP. This procedure was used to eliminate the role of antibodies directed to unique or "private" determinants on the labeled ligand. With this assay system it was found that 12 of 14 CRI⁺ anti-Ar HP were virtually identical as inhibitors in radioimmune assays. This provided strong evidence for the presence of at least one highly conserved idiotypic determinant.[34]

The available amino acid sequence data on monoclonal antibodies are, in general, consistent with these conclusions. First, microheterogeneity is seen within the family, with substitutions occurring both in the framework and in hypervariable regions.[35-40] On the other hand, there is a very close homology among the monoclonal antibodies. For example, among the five complete V_L sequences that have been determined by Siegelman and Capra, the number of differences between any pair of sequences up to residue 108 does not exceed seven and the average is three or four amino acid differences.[39] A high degree of homology (greater than 90%) is also observed when pairs of V_H sequences are compared, although the amount of data available so far is fairly limited.[35-38, 40]

Substantial differences are noted when comparisons are made with the previously published sequences of the V_L and V_H regions of serum anti-Ar antibodies.[41, 42] The reason for this discrepancy is not known; the fact that "unique" determinants of monoclonal antibodies are also found in serum antibody suggests that the monoclonal antibodies will prove to be representative of the serum pool.

The microheterogeneity of the CRI⁺ family raised the question of whether the idiotype response can be regulated by an individual member of the family or by anti-idiotypic antibodies directed against monoclonal CRI⁺ HP's. Our recent studies relating to these questions are described below. We will first summarize serological properties of the CRI⁺ HP, some of which were used in studies of regulation.

TABLE 3 presents data on the weight of serum anti-Ar or anti-Ar HP required for 50% inhibition in the standard radioimmune assay for idiotype, which uses purified labeled serum anti-Ar.[33] Experimental details are included in a footnote to the table. Hybridomas secreting monoclonal anti-Ar antibodies were produced by the technique of Köhler and Milstein[43] with spleen cells of A/J mice immunized with KLH-Ar. The tumor line used was Sp2/0-Ag14,[44] which does not secrete heavy or light chains before or after fusion. Affinity-purified HP, obtained from cloned cells, were determined to be monoclonal by isoelectric focusing and electrophoresis in polyacrylamide gels. Monoclonal CRI⁺ HP of each IgG subclass were obtained in pure form. An individual anti-Ar HP is considered CRI⁺ only if it can cause greater than 50% inhibition in the standard radioimmune assay.

The various anti-Ar HP possess a broad range of inhibitory capacities in the radioimmune assay. For example, R16.7 is comparable to serum anti-Ar as an inhibitor; R22.4 is more weakly inhibitory in the assay than purified serum anti-Ar, while R9.3 and R23.2 are intermediate in strength as inhibitors. Of particular interest is the fact that an individual HP, such as R16.7, can almost completely displace labeled serum anti-Ar antibody from rabbit anti-CRI. This indicates that a single monoclonal HP can possess virtually all the idiotopes recognized by the rabbit anti-CRI. In addition, individual HP also possess unique determinants not found on most other HP; most of these determinants are found at low concentrations in serum anti-Ar.[33] The capacity of individual anti-Ar HP to cause virtually complete displacement of labeled serum anti-Ar indicates that conventional rabbit anti-CRI reacts almost exclusively with "public" determinants possessed in common by members of the CRI⁺ family. A likely explanation for this is that the private determinants are so diverse, and are present at such low concentration in serum antibody, that they are poorly immunogenic.

TABLES 4, 5 and 7 show the results of three different types of experiments that were designed to ascertain whether the expression of the CRI⁺ family present in serum anti-Ar antibodies can be regulated by idiotypic determinants

TABLE 3

DISPLACEMENT OF LABELED A/J ANTI-AR FROM
ITS RABBIT ANTI-IDIOTPYIC ANTIBODIES BY UNLABELED A/J ANTI-AR ANTIBODIES
OR HYBRIDOMA PRODUCTS WITH ANTI-AR ACTIVITY *

Unlabeled Inhibitors	Amount Required for 50% Inhibition ‡ (ng)
A/J serum anti-Ar	11 (97) §
HP R16.7 (IgG1)	9 (94)
93G7 (IgG1)	12 (90)
R20.4 (IgG2b)	14 (86)
R26.5 (IgG3)	17 (85)
R13.4 (IgG3)	21 (87)
R10.8 (IgG2a)	180 (60)
R23.2 (IgG2b)	200 (66)
R9.3 (IgG2b)	300 (65)
121D7 (IgG1)	300 (71)
R17.5 (IgG2b)	460 (63)
R24.6 (IgG2a)	1800 (52)
123E6 (IgG1)	1900 (51)
124E1 (IgG1)	2900 (47)
R22.4 (IgG2a)	3200 (49)
R8.2 (IgG2b) †	>2000 (9)
R18.11 (IgG3) †	>2000 (20)
R19.9 (IgG2b) †	>2000 (15)
R21.10 (IgG1) †	>2000 (6)

* Each test used 10 ng ¹²⁵I-labeled, specifically purified A/J anti-Ar antibodies and slightly less than an equivalent amount of rabbit anti-idiotype. Complexes were precipitated by goat anti-rabbit Fc.
† HP R8.2, R18.11, R19.9, and R21.10 lack the major CRI.
‡ Data from Reference 33.
§ Values in parentheses are the percentages of inhibition by 2000 ng.

present on a single CRI⁺ HP. In one set of experiments, various CRI⁺ HP were conjugated to syngeneic thymocytes and administered to A/J mice before immunization with KLH-Ar. In the second, rabbit anti-Id antibodies were prepared against individual CRI⁺ HP and administered before antigen. The third set used monoclonal anti-idiotope antibodies.

The effect of the administration of CRI⁺ HP conjugated to thymocytes is shown by the data in TABLE 4. It is evident that four out of five CRI⁺ HP possess very potent regulatory capabilities when conjugated to thymocytes and

TABLE 4

SELECTIVE SUPPRESSION OF IDIOTYPE SYNTHESIS,
WITHOUT SUPPRESSION OF ANTI-AR SYNTHESIS,
BY INOCULATION OF CRI⁺ HYBRIDOMA PRODUCTS
CONJUGATED TO A/J THYMOCYTES *

	Antibody Response (individual mice; day 38) †	
Preinoculation	Anti-Ar Titer (mg ml⁻¹)	Anti-Ar Ab Required for 50% Inhibition ‡ (ng)
Conjugate, thymocytes– A/J anti-Ar Ab	0.7–22	700, 700, 5100, 27 000, 9700, >58 000, >61 000, >62 000, 310, 38 000, 9400, >190 000, >550 000
Conjugate, thymocytes– R16.7	0.03–9.4	>750, >38 000, >75 000, >120 000 >210 000, >240 000
Conjugate, thymocytes– R20.4	0.2–3.3	750, 6100, 9700, 280, 83 000
Conjugate, thymocytes– R23.2	0.02–2.9	>500, 7700, 4200, 7400, 59 000, 9100
Conjugate, thymocytes– R9.3	0.7–8.9	9200, 40, 760, 170 000, 2000, 4400, 220 000
Conjugate, thymocytes– R22.4	0.4–3.6	800, 13, 103, 260, 16, 1800
Conjugate, thymocytes- normal A/J IgG	0.8–10	16, 10, 29, 11, 11, 32, 9, 13, 21, 34, 14, 16, 39, 13
None	1.5–7.3	38, 39, 41, 32, 34

* A/J male mice received 25×10^6 thymocytes, conjugated with 11 ± 2 μg protein, i.p. on days -42 and -21. They were immunized i.p. with 0.2 mg KLH-Ar in CFA on days 0, 14, and 24, were bled on day 38, and their sera were tested for anti-Ar and CRI content.

† Data from Reference 45.

‡ In the standard radioimmune assay for the major idiotype.

administered before antigen. There was virtually complete suppression of CRI⁺ anti-Ar antibody in almost all of the animals studied, but little or no reduction in total anti-Ar titer. In addition, the degree of suppression was similar to that achieved with A/J serum anti-Ar conjugates. A fifth CRI⁺ HP, R22.4, induced suppression in approximately one-half the animals tested; the degree of suppression was considerably less than that achieved by the other CRI⁺ HP or serum CRI.

Subsequent experiments using R16.7 conjugates demonstrated that animals pretreated with conjugated thymocytes generate T cells capable of transferring the suppressed state to lightly irradiated recipients subsequently immunized with KLH-Ar.[45]

TABLE 5 shows the results of administering rabbit anti-CRI antibodies specific for three different CRI⁺ anti-Ar HP before immunization with KLH-Ar. Anti-CRI sera specific for R23.2, R16.7, and R22.4 were each capable of inducing virtually complete suppression with respect to the CRI⁺ component of an A/J anti-Ar antibody response. The degree of suppression was comparable to that achieved with anti-CRI specific for A/J serum anti-Ar; little or no reduction in total anti-Ar concentration was observed. It may be noted that anti-CRI specific for R22.4 was a strong inhibitor in this system, despite the poor inhibitory capacity of that HP in the standard radioimmune assay for CRI and the inability of that molecule to function as a strong regulatory force (in comparison to the other CRI⁺ HP) when conjugated to thymocytes.

These results are consistent with the view that at least one determinant in each CRI⁺ HP (even those CRI⁺ HP which are poor inhibitors in the serological assay for idiotype) is sufficiently conserved to be recognized by, and stimulate, the same suppressor T cells or set of cells. Further experiments, outlined below, lend support to the notion that the formation of any CRI⁺ antibody, or the suppression of its synthesis, may initiate a network of interactions that can affect most or all members of the CRI⁺ family.

Regulation of the Idiotype by Monoclonal Anti-Idiotope Antibodies

Formal proof of the existence of a conserved idiotope on CRI⁺ HP and CRI⁺ serum anti-Ar antibody has been obtained recently with monoclonal anti-idiotypic reagents.[46] Balb/c mice, which are CRI⁻, were hyperimmunized with purified A/J anti-Ar antibody that had been polymerized with glutaraldehyde. Spleen cells from a mouse making anti-CRI antibody were fused with the nonsecreting tumor line, SP2/0-Ag14. Three different fusion products elaborating anti-CRI antibody were cloned. All three anti-CRI HP are IgG₁, but exhibit distinct electrophoretic patterns in agarose electrophoresis. All three bind the CRI⁺ HP R16.7, which bears most of the "public" determinants present in anti-Ar antibodies obtained from a serum pool.[33] In addition, all

TABLE 5

SUPPRESSION OF CRI BY INOCULATION OF RABBIT ANTI-IDIOTYPIC ANTISERUM DIRECTED AGAINST CRI⁺ HYBRIDOMA PRODUCTS *

Preinoculation	Antibody Response (individual mice; day 28)		
	Anti-Ar Titer (μg ml⁻¹)	Anti-Ar Ab Required for 50% Inhibition † (ng)	Inhibition by 2 μg Anti-Ar Ab (%)
Anti-id *versus* serum anti-Ar	330–480	>3300, >3300, >3900, >3900, >4800	5, 39, 4, 7, 6
Anti-id *versus* HP R23.2	300–920	>3000, >3600, >4200 >5100, >5400, >9200	7, 4, 9, 8, 2, 7
Anti-id *versus* HP R16.7	290–550	>2900, >3200, >4400, >5000, >5500	24, 39, 17, 10, 18
Anti-id *versus* HP R22.4	310–590	>3100, >3300, >4200 >4700, >5900	35, 33, 20, 14, 14
None ‡	510–1200	12, 11, 10, 27, 10	95, 99, 100, 94, 100

* Mice were inoculated intravenously with anti-idiotypic antiserum (15 μg idiotype-binding capacity) on days −14 and −11. They were immunized with 0.2 mg KLH-Ar i.p. in CFA on days 0 and 14 and bled on day 28.

† Data from Reference 45.

‡ Inoculation with normal rabbit serum has been shown to have no effect on the expression of the CRI.

three monoclonal anti-CRI antibodies bind serum anti-Ar, although to varying degrees. One of the anti-CRI HP binds 60% of those CRI$^+$ serum anti-Ar molecules which are reactive with a rabbit anti-CRI serum specific for the CRI$^+$ anti-Ar HP, R16.7. Thus, as many as three out of five of the molecules bearing the major CRI are reactive with a single monoclonal reagent.

Data on the fine specificity of the three anti-CRI HP are presented in TABLE 6. Various unlabeled proteins were tested for their capacity to inhibit

TABLE 6

INHIBITION BY MONOCLONAL ANTI-AR ANTIBODIES
OF BINDING OF LABELED PURIFIED ANTI-AR ANTIBODY
TO IMMOBILIZED MONOCLONAL ANTI-CRI PREPARATIONS *

Unlabeled Inhibitor	Presence of CRI in Inhibitor	Immobilized Anti-CRI		
		7B7.10	2F6.4	1F2.1
		(ng required for 50% inhibition †)		
nMIgG	−	>5000(10)	>5000(0)	>5000(6)
HIS Serum ‡	−	>5000(50)	>5000(16)	>5000(49)
A/J Anti-Ar (serum)	+	47(100)	67(100)	25(100)
Purified serum A/J Anti-Ar	+	57(100)	82(97)	25(100)
HP R16.7	+	23(100)	22(100)	21(100)
HP R20.4	+	72(97)	61(96)	75(98)
HP R9.3	+	21(97)	25(93)	60(97)
HP R10.8	+	39(96)	76(93)	64(100)
HP R17.5	+	25(95)	58(93)	36(98)
HP R23.2	+	100(95)	64(93)	100(100)
HP R24.6	+	22(93)	78(92)	78(98)
HP R22.4	+	100(95)	56(93)	68(99)
HP 123E6	+	>5000(27)	85(91)	>5000(41)
HP 124E1	+	>5000(31)	>5000(7)	>5000(35)
HP R18.11 §	−	>5000(34)	>5000(1)	>2000(9)**
HP R19.9 §	−	>5000(22)	>5000(1)	>5000(10)
HP R21.10 §	−	>5000(15)	>5000(7)	>5000(15)

* Wells of polyvinylchloride microtiter trays were coated with anti-CRI HP 7B7.10, 2F6.4, or 1F2.1. Various amounts of unlabeled inhibitor proteins (anti-Ar) were added, followed by 10 ng ^{125}I-labeled purified A/J serum anti-Ar antibodies.

† Data from Reference 46. Values in parentheses show the percentages of inhibition by 5000 ng, or, where indicated (**), by 2000 ng unlabeled inhibitor.

‡ Hyperimmune suppressed mice were immunologically suppressed by preinoculation of rabbit anti-CRI serum, followed by hyperimmunization with KLH-Ar. The serum contains a high titer of anti-Ar antibody but lacks the CRI.

§ Representative of the "minor" A/J crossreactive idiotype.[33]

the interaction between purified radiolabeled serum CRI and each of the three monoclonal anti-CRI in a solid-phase radioimmune assay. Details of the experimental protocol are given in footnotes to the table. Normal mouse immunoglobulin, CRI$^-$ serum antibodies from mice that were immunologically suppressed and hyperimmunized, and three CRI$^-$ anti-Ar HP all failed to inhibit the interaction between each monoclonal anti-CRI and radiolabeled serum CRI. In contrast, A/J serum anti-Ar and eight out of ten CRI$^+$ anti-Ar HP were inhibitory in the assay. The degrees of inhibition by serum CRI and the eight CRI⁺ anti-Ar HP were roughly equivalent. Similar results were obtained when the same inhibitory proteins were tested as inhibitors of the interaction between each monoclonal anti-CRI and purified radiolabeled R16.7. Eight out of ten CRI⁺ anti-Ar HP were strongly inhibitory; CRI⁻ proteins failed to cause inhibition.

Subsequent experiments that tested the effects of free haptens on binding demonstrated that the idiotope recognized by each of the three different monoclonal anti-CRI was associated with, or close to, the hapten-binding site of the CRI⁺ anti-Ar HP, R16.7.[46]

The experiments shown in TABLE 7 were designed to determine whether a reagent specific for a highly conserved idiotope, present on CRI⁺ serum

TABLE 7

SUPPRESSION OF THE MAJOR CROSSREACTIVE IDIOTYPE
IN ADULT A/J MICE BY MONOCLONAL ANTIIDIOTYPIC HP *

Anti-CRI	Dose † (μg)	Anti-Ar Titer (mg ml⁻¹)	Anti-Ar Antibody Required for 50% Inhibition ‡ (ng)
None	—	0.44–1.8	13, 98, 22, 24, 54
7B7.10	300	2.0–4.4	1000, 710, 300, 1300
	100	1.0–3.1	160, 260, 130, 230
	10	0.7–3.4	>2000, 1800, >4000, 80, >4000
	1	1.0–5.2	840, 780, 490, >4000, 60
2F6.4	300	0.9–2.9	3200, 4000, 3000, 2100
	100	0.9–4.5	4000, 2000, 3800, 700
	10	2.2–7.9	4000, 150, 400, 58, 42, 75
	1	0.18–8.9	180, >4000, 70, 600, >4000, 50
1F2.1	100	1.0–2.2	400, 100, 100
	10	1.0–3.9	63, 29, 31, 23, 28
	1	1.9–4.6	89, 23, 92, 76, 39, 50

* Adult A/J mice were inoculated i.p. with various anti-CRI preparations on days —3 and 0, immunized on days 14 and 28 with 125 μg KLH-Ar emulsified in CFA, and bled on day 40. Each test used 10 ng labeled A/J anti-Ar antibody and slightly less than an equivalent amount of rabbit anti-CRI. Immune complexes were precipitated with goat anti-rabbit Fc.
† The values for the anti-CRI HP are weights of protein injected.
‡ Data from Reference 46.

anti-Ar and CRI⁺ anti-Ar HP, can suppress the appearance of the entire family of CRI⁺ molecules. Mice were treated with monoclonal anti-CRI antibodies before immunization with KLH-Ar. Sera from the immunized mice were then assayed quantitatively for the presence of CRI⁺ anti-Ar antibody by the standard radioimmune assay. Experimental details are included in a footnote to the table. It can be seen that two of the three monoclonal anti-CRI reagents are able to suppress the production of CRI⁺ antibody. In both cases, administration of as little as 1 μg protein was able to cause suppression in the majority of the animals tested. The third monoclonal anti-CRI (1F2.1) was unable to prevent the subsequent expression of the CRI in most of the animals when as much as

100 μg was inoculated. Thus, treatment of mice with a monoclonal anti-CRI reagent specific for a conserved idiotope found in CRI⁺ serum anti-Ar antibody and CRI⁺ anti-Ar HP can prevent the expression of the entire family of CRI⁺ anti-Ar antibodies. The suppression we obtained with monoclonal anti-idiotope antibody is similar to that reported for monoclonal antibodies specific for idiotopes associated with C57 anti-4-hydroxy-3-nitrophenylacetyl antibodies.[47]

ACKNOWLEDGMENT

Dr. Nelles is a recipient of a postdoctoral fellowship from the Arthritis Foundation.

REFERENCES

1. KUETTNER, M. G., A. WANG & A. NISONOFF. 1972. J. Exp. Med. **135**: 579–95.
2. HART, D. A., A. C. WANG, L. PAWLAK & A. NISONOFF. 1972. J. Exp. Med. **135**: 1293–1300.
3. PAWLAK, L. L., D. A. HART & A. NISONOFF. 1973. J. Exp. Med. **137**: 1442–58.
4. COSENZA, H. & H. KOHLER. 1972. Proc. Nat. Acad. Sci. USA **69**: 2701–5.
5. STRAYER, D. S., H. COSENZA, W. M. F. LEE, D. A. ROWLEY & H. KOHLER. 1974. Science **186**: 640–42.
6. EICHMANN, K. 1974. Eur. J. Immunol. **4**: 296–302.
7. EIG, B. M., S.-T. JU & A. NISONOFF. 1977. J. Exp. Med. **146**: 1574–84.
8. BROWN, A. R., C. L. DEWITT, M. J. BOSMA & A. NISONOFF. 1980. J. Immunol. **124**: 250–54.
9. OWEN, F. L., S.-T. JU & A. NISONOFF. 1977. Proc. Nat. Acad. Sci. USA **74**: 2084–88.
10. OWEN, F. L., S.-T. JU & A. NISONOFF. 1977. J. Exp. Med. **145**: 1559–66.
11. ROWLEY, D. A., H. KOHLER, H. SCHREIBER, S. T. KAYE & I. LORBACH. 1976. J. Exp. Med. **144**: 946–59.
12. DOHI, Y. & A. NISONOFF. 1979. J. Exp. Med. **150**: 909–18.
13. OWEN, F. L. & A. NISONOFF. 1978. J. Exp. Med. **148**: 182–94.
14. TADA, T. & K. OKUMURA. 1980. Adv. Immunol. **28**: 1–87.
15. TAKAOKI, M., M.-S. SY, J. NEPOM, R. FINBERG, B. WHITTAKER, A. NISONOFF, B. BENACERRAF & M. I. GREENE. 1981. J. Immunol. In press.
16. GREENE, M. I., A. PIERRES, M. E. DORF & B. BENACERRAF. 1977. J. Exp. Med. **146**: 293–96.
17. THEZE, J., J. A. KAPP & B. BENACERRAF. 1977. J. Exp. Med. **145**: 839–56.
18. THEZE, J., C. WALTENBAUGH, M. E. DORF & B. BENACERRAF. 1977. J. Exp. Med. **146**: 287–92.
19. OKUDA, K., M. MINAMI, S.-T. JU & M. E. DORF. 1981. Proc. Nat. Acad. Sci. USA **78**: 4557–61.
20. MOORHEAD, J. W. 1977. J. Immunol. **119**: 315–21.
21. GREENE, M. I., S. FUJIMOTO & A. H. SEHON. 1977. J. Immunol. **119**: 757–64.
22. TANIGUCHI, T. & J. F. A. P. MILLER. 1978. J. Immunol. **120**: 21–26.
23. KISHIMOTO, T., T. HIRAI, M. SUEMURA, N. NAKANISHI & Y. YAMAMURA. 1978. J. Immunol. **121**: 2106–12.
24. WATANABE, T., M. KIMOTO, S. MARUYAMA, T. KISHIMOTO & Y. YAMAMURA. 1978. J. Immunol. **121**: 2113–17.
25. HERZENBERG, L. A., K. OKUMURA, H. CANTOR, V. L. SATO, F.-W. SHEN, E. A. BOYSE & L. A. HERZENBERG. 1976. J. Exp. Med. **144**: 330–44.

26. BACH, B. A., M. I. GREENE, B. BENACERRAF & A. NISONOFF. 1979. J. Exp. Med. **149:** 1084–98.
27. BINZ, H. & H. WIGZELL. 1975. J. Exp. Med. **142:** 197–211.
28. PACIFICO, A. & J. D. CAPRA. 1980. J. Exp. Med. **152:** 1289–301.
29. GERMAIN, R. N., S.-T. JU, T. J. KIPPS, B. BENACERRAF & M. E. DORF. 1979. J. Exp. Med. **140:** 613–22.
30. HIRAI, Y. & A. NISONOFF. 1980. J. Exp. Med. **151:** 1213–31.
31. LEWIS, G. K. & J. W. GOODMAN. 1978. J. Exp. Med. **148:** 915–24.
32. SY, M.-S., A. NISONOFF, R. N. GERMAIN, B. BENACERRAF & M. I. GREENE. 1981. J. Exp. Med. **153:** 1415–25.
33. LAMOYI, E., P. ESTESS, J. D. CAPRA & A. NISONOFF. 1980. J. Immunol. **124:** 2834–40.
34. LAMOYI, E., P. ESTESS, J. D. CAPRA & A. NISONOFF. 1980. J. Exp. Med. **152:** 703–11.
35. ESTESS, P., A. NISONOFF & J. D. CAPRA. 1980. Mol. Immunol. **16:** 1111–18.
36. ESTESS, P., E. LAMOYI, A. NISONOFF & J. D. CAPRA. 1980. J. Exp. Med. **151:** 863–75.
37. MARSHAK-ROTHSTEIN, A., M. SIEKEVITZ, M. MARGOLIES, M. N. MUDGETT-HUNTER & M. L. GEFTER. 1980. Proc. Nat. Acad. Sci. USA **77:** 1120–24.
38. ALKAN, S. S., R. KNECHT & D. G. BRAUN. 1980. Hoppe-Seyler's Z. Physiol. Chem. **361:** 191–95.
39. SIEGELMAN, M. & J. D. CAPRA. 1981. Proc. Nat. Acad. Sci. USA. In press.
40. SIEGELMAN, M., C. SLAUGHTER, L. MCCUMBER, P. ESTESS & J. D. CAPRA. 1981. *In* Immunoglobulin Idiotypes and Their Expression, Proc. ICN-UCLA Symposium. C. Janeway, E. Sercarz, and H. Wigzell, Eds. Academic Press. New York. In press.
41. CAPRA, J. D., A. S. TUNG & A. NISONOFF. 1977. J. Immunol. **119:** 993–99.
42. CAPRA, J. D. & A. NISONOFF. 1979. J. Immunol. **123:** 279–84.
43. KOHLER, G. & C. MILSTEIN. 1976. Eur. J. Immunol. **6:** 511–19.
44. SHULMAN, M., C. D. WILDE & G. KOHLER. 1978. Nature (London) **276:** 269–70.
45. HIRAI, Y., E. LAMOYI, Y. DOHI & A. NISONOFF. 1981. J. Immunol. **126:** 71–74.
46. NELLES, M. J., L. GILL-PAZARIS & A. NISONOFF. 1981. J. Exp. Med. **154:** 1752–63.
47. RETH, M., G. KELSOE & K. RAJEWSKY. 1981. Nature (London) **290:** 257–59.

DISCUSSION OF THE PAPER

A. H. SEHON (*University of Manitoba, Winnipeg, Man.*): What cell do you use for fusion—SP-2/0?

NISONOFF: All the data I showed were obtained with the SP-2/0 nonsecreting line.

J. W. STREILEIN (*University of Texas Southwestern Medical School, Dallas, Tx.*): Is there a single species of responding cell types and molecules or is there a variety of anti-idiotypes responding to the idiotype in the A/J strain?

NISONOFF: The monoclonal anti-idiotypes are prepared by immunizing Balb/c mice with the A/J idiotype and then fusing the cells.

STREILEIN: Would you expect all the products of those fusions to be similar in type; that is, would they all share reactivity with the idiotype? Or would you expect them to be homogenous molecules from different cell types?

NISONOFF: They are homogeneous by physical criteria, such as electrophoresis and isoelectric focusing. They're monoclonal and, therefore, one would expect them to be homogeneous. They're not identical to one another.

STREILEIN: That's what I meant.

NISONOFF: There are three active anti-idiotypic antibodies that are not identical by these same criteria. Two of the three do suppress the idiotype.

Z. OVARY (*New York, N.Y.*): What classes of the monoclonal antibodies have you produced?

NISONOFF: In the case of anti-arsonate, we've seen virtually everything except IgE and IgD.

AUTOANTI-IDIOTYPE ANTIBODY PRODUCTION FOLLOWING ANTIGEN INJECTION AND IMMUNE REGULATION *

Gregory W. Siskind,[†] Takashi Hayama,[§] Gillian M. Shepherd,[†]
A. Faye Schrater[¶] Marc E. Weksler,[‡] G. Jeanette Thorbecke,[§]
and Edmond A. Goidl [†]

[†] Division of Allergy and Immunology
[‡] Division of Geriatrics and Gerontology
Department of Medicine
Cornell University Medical College
New York, New York 10021

[§] Department of Pathology
New York University School of Medicine
New York, New York 10016

[¶] Department of Medicine
Harvard Medical School
Boston, Massachusetts 02115

During the course of studies on antibody affinity at the plaque-forming cell (PFC) level, it was observed that, at times, more PFC were detected in the presence of low concentrations of hapten than in the absence of hapten.[1] This observation was clearly contrary to the usual view of this system, according to which adding hapten to the PFC assay medium should inhibit plaque formation or have no effect, depending upon the affinity of the antibody secreted and the concentration of hapten. We hypothesized that the increase in the number of PFC might be due to the "displacement" by hapten of autoanti-idiotype antibody (anti-id) from cell surface idiotype. According to this hypothesis, the binding of autoanti-id on the cell surface inhibits the secretion of antibody. This inhibition is reversible and, when the anti-id dissociates, secretion of antibody is reinitiated. Hapten and anti-id, in effect, compete for the same cell surface idiotype. Therefore, once dissociated in the presence of hapten, anti-id cannot cause further inhibition of secretion.

Under certain experimental conditions, the number of hapten-augmentable PFC is very great.[1] For example, when normal nonirradiated AKR mice received spleen cells from syngeneic mice that had received 10 μg 2,4,6-trinitrophenylated ficoll (TNP-F) seven days before their use as cell donors, the number of PFC observed in the presence of hapten was two or three times that seen in the absence of hapten. We took advantage of this situation to test the hypothesis that hapten-augmentable PFC are cells whose secretion of antibody had been inhibited by the binding of autoanti-id to cell surface antibody molecules. If the hypothesis were true, we would expect that incubation with hapten would elute material with properties of anti-id from immune cell populations

* This research was supported, in part, by grants from the National Institutes of Health of the United States Public Health Service, nos. AI–11694, AG–00541, AI–3076, AG–00239, AG–02347, and AG–01881.

that exhibited hapten-augmentable PFC. Such immune cells were incubated with 10^{-8} M TNP-ϵ-amino-n-caproic acid for 30 min, the cells were then removed by centrifugation, and the eluate was freed of hapten by extensive dialysis. This eluate caused hapten-reversible inhibition of anti-TNP plaque formation, but did not affect anti-sheep erythrocyte (SRBC) PFC.[2] Furthermore, the inhibitory activity was removed by passage over an anti-mouse gamma globulin (MGG) immunoadsorbent, but was not removed by passage over a TNP immunoadsorbent.[2] Finally, an immunoadsorbent prepared from anti-TNP antibody removed the PFC inhibitory activity.[2] In summary, the eluate is capable of causing a specific hapten-reversible inhibition of plaque formation and the inhibitory activity is present in a molecule having the following properties: (1) it bears antigenic determinants of MGG, (2) it is not anti-TNP antibody, and (3) it binds to anti-TNP antibody. The results are thus consistent with the view that PFC inhibitory activity is due to an anti-id and that hapten-augmentable PFC are cells whose secretion of antibody has been inhibited by the binding of autoanti-id to cell surface idiotype.

If autoanti-id is formed during the normal immune response to an injected antigen, we would expect to detect PFC inhibitory activity in the serum of immunized mice. In a series of studies using mice immunized with TNP-F, PFC inhibitory activity was detected and characterized.[2] The serum of mice seven days after antigen injection was found to contain a specific anti-TNP PFC inhibitory activity. The inhibition was reversed by hapten and the serum did not affect anti-SRBC PFC. The inhibitory activity was not removed on a TNP immunoadsorbent but was removed on both an anti-MGG immunoadsorbent and the anti-TNP antibody immunoadsorbent. The inhibitory activity was not removed by passage over an anti-dansyl antibody immunoadsorbent. Thus, immune serum, seven days after the injection of TNP-F, contained a PFC inhibitory factor that has the properties of an anti-id.

We have recently extended these observations to the anti-p-azophenylarsenate immune system, where there is a well-defined idiotype and specific anti-id reagents are available. Using materials kindly provided by Dr. Alfred Nisonoff, we have been able to demonstrate hapten-reversible inhibition of plaque formation in this well-characterized idiotypic system.[3]

Using the presence of hapten-augmentable PFC as an assay for autoanti-id-blocked antibody-secreting cells, we have obtained evidence for autoanti-id production after antigen injection in four mouse strains[1-6] and in chickens (unpublished observations). In addition, evidence has been obtained for the production of autoanti-id during the primary and secondary responses to both thymic-dependent and thymic-independent antigens.[4] The autoanti-id response after a second injection of the thymic-independent antigen, TNP-F, appears more rapidly and is of greater magnitude than that after the first injection of TNP-F, suggesting a secondary autoanti-id response. In contrast, the autoanti-id response after a second injection of TNP-bovine gamma globulin (BGG) is indistinguishable in timing and magnitude from the autoanti-id production after the first injection of antigen. This is probably because the response to TNP-BGG typically has greater heterogeneity and a larger shift in antibody affinity than the response to TNP-F. Thus, with TNP-BGG, different anti-TNP idiotypes are presumably elicited after boosting and a "primary" autoanti-id response is seen.

Using these assays, evidence was obtained that T cells are required for autoanti-id production.[5] Athymic nude mice and bone marrow–reconstituted irradiated thymectomized mice lack a hapten-augmentable PFC component in their anti-TNP-F response and do not develop detectable plaque-inhibiting activity in their sera. Comparing the kinetics of the decrease in antibody concentration in nude and euthymic mice, we are led to suggest that autoanti-id is one of the factors responsible for the normal *in vivo* down regulation of the immune response.[5]

Using hapten-reversible inhibition of plaque formation to detect anti-id and the corresponding idiotypes, we looked for changes in idiotype expression. It was found that there is a shift in idiotype expression with time after antigen injection (unpublished observations). In addition, the anti-TNP idiotypes expressed at the peak of the response to TNP-F change with age.[6] Thus, immune sera from three- to four-week-old mice will inhibit plaque formation by TNP-F immune spleen cells from most other three- to four-week-old mice but not by immune spleen cells from six- to eight-week-old or older mice. Immune serum from six- to eight-week-old mice will inhibit plaque formation by immune spleen cells from most six- to eight-week-old mice but will rarely inhibit plaque formation by immune spleen cells from three- to four-week-old or 21- to 22-month-old mice. Similarly, immune serum from 21- to 22-month-old mice inhibits plaque formation by anti-TNP-F immune spleen cells from 80% of 21- to 22-month-old, 50% of six- to eight-week-old, and only 20% of three- to four-week-old mice. Further studies on the effect of age on the autoanti-id response revealed that old mice have far more hapten-augmentable PFC than do young mice, suggesting an increase in down regulation of the immune response by autoanti-id in aged mice.[6]

Finally, we have recently observed that an autoanti-id preparation, obtained by incubation of TNP-F immune spleen cells with a low concentration of hapten for 10–30 min, will depress contact sensitization with trinitrobenzene sulfonic acid (TNBS). Treated mice showed an approximately 50% decrease in ear swelling in response to a subsequent local challenge with TNBS.[7]

Thus, evidence has been obtained that autoanti-id is produced in mice during the immune response following the injection of various TNP conjugates and that this autoanti-id functions in the regulation of the immune response.

The measurement of hapten-augmentable PFC can be used as an assay for cells whose secretion of antibody has been inhibited by the binding of autoanti-id.

Hapten-reversible inhibition of plaque formation can serve as an assay for anti-id antibody.

Autoanti-id antibody is produced during the primary and secondary responses to thymic-dependent and thymic-independent antigens. After the second injection of a thymic-independent antigen, a secondary autoanti-id response is observed.

Autoanti-id production is thymic dependent in young adult mice.

Old mice have an increased number of hapten-augmentable PFC, suggesting increased down regulation by autoanti-id.

There is an age-related change in id expression in response to the same epitope.

Autoanti-id can down regulate the PFC response and inhibit sensitization for contact reactivity.

REFERENCES

1. SCHRATER, A. F., E. A. GOIDL, G. J. THORBECKE & G. W. SISKIND. 1979. Production of auto-anti-idiotypic antibody during the normal immune response to TNP-ficoll. I. Occurrence in AKR/J and BALB/c mice of hapten-augmentable, anti-TNP plaque-forming cells and their accelerated appearance in recipients of immune spleen cells. J. Exp. Med. 150: 138–53.
2. GOIDL, E. A., A. F. SCHRATER, G. W. SISKIND & G. J. THORBECKE. 1979. Production of auto-anti-idiotypic antibody during the normal immune response to TNP-ficoll. II. Hapten-reversible inhibition of anti-TNP plaque forming cells by immune serum as an assay for auto-anti-idiotypic antibody. J. Exp. Med. 150: 154–65.
3. HAYAMA, T., E. A. GOIDL, G. M. SHEPHERD, G. W. SISKIND & G. J. THORBECKE. 1981. Hapten-reversible inhibition of PFC as an assay for anti-idiotypic antibodies. Fed. Proc. Fed. Am. Soc. Exp. Biol. 40: 994.
4. GOIDL, E. A., A. F. SCHRATER, G. J. THORBECKE & G. W. SISKIND. 1980. Production of auto-anti-idiotypic antibody during the normal immune response. IV. Studies of the primary and secondary responses to thymus-dependent and -independent antigens. Eur. J. Immunol. 10: 810–14.
5. SCHRATER, A. F., E. A. GOIDL, G. J. THORBECKE & G. W. SISKIND. 1979. Production of auto-anti-idiotypic antibody during the normal immune response to TNP-ficoll. III. Absence in nu/nu mice: evidence for T-cell dependence of the anti-idiotypic antibody response. J. Exp. Med. 150: 808–17.
6. GOIDL, E. A., G. J. THORBECKE, M. E. WEKSLER & G. W. SISKIND. 1980. Production of auto-anti-idiotypic antibody during the normal immune response: Changes in the auto-anti-idiotypic antibody response and the idiotype repertoire associated with aging. Proc. Nat. Acad. Sci. USA 77: 6788–92.
7. SHEPHERD, G. M., E. A. GOIDL, M. E. WEKSLER & G. SISKIND. 1981. Effect of auto-anti-idiotype antibody on delayed hypersensitivity. Clin. Res. 29: 530A.

DISCUSSION OF THE PAPER

F. L. ADLER (*St. Jude Children's Research Hospital, Memphis, Tenn.*): I have trouble visualizing the idiotype-secreting B cell sitting in the spleen and tolerating on its surface an accumulation of anti-idiotype. Intuitively, I would say that it should be pushing the anti-idiotype away all the time. Even if it were a nonsecreting cell that has the idiotype on the membrane, it should be busy cleansing itself by capping or endocytosis. Now, I could see these cells being in the state in which I think you visualize them if there were a huge excess of anti-idiotype in the serum. Do you find such anti-idiotype in a free state in fairly high concentration in the serum? Is it possible that your augmentable plaque formers are not B cells that would normally be secreting during your assay period, but are cells that you are activating into secretion by removing the anti-idiotype that may be sitting on them?

SISKIND: First, we are activating them into secretion by removing the anti-idiotype antibody that's on their surface. The hypothesis is that, indeed, these are cells that are, by virtue of the fact that they have anti-idiotype antibody bound-to-the-surface idiotype, inhibited in their secretion. They are certainly inhibited in the test tube and in the plate, and presumably that inhibition is reversible because, if you remove the anti-idiotype from their surface by incubation with hapten, you can see their production of a plaque, which means that they begin to secrete and produce anti-TNP antibody. Second, the question of a large excess—well, we have demonstrated anti-idiotype in the serum. Quantitatively, I don't know how much it is in terms of mg ml^{-1}, but my guess is that it's very low. What I would envision in terms of the cells sitting with anti-id on their surface is that they are in a steady-state situation in which they are constantly cleansing themselves, constantly internalizing the material, constantly shedding it, constantly having new material bound. In addition, the anti-idiotype antibody is bound only with a certain degree of affinity and is constantly dissociating and reassociating. So, I envision this as an extremely dynamic steady-state situation modulated very rapidly by changing conditions. And, of course, it can be modulated in a test tube by just a few minutes of incubation with hapten that displaces this autoanti-idiotype antibody. Perhaps the cells don't lyse because there are only a few molecules of the stuff on their surface. This is enough to send a signal to them, but is not enough to support binding of complement and lysing.

D. W. SCOTT (*Duke University Medical Center, Durham, N.C.*): This is a quick yes or no question. You presented some evidence for this autoanti-idiotypic response with both a thymus-dependent and a thymus-independent response. If you prepare the eluates from the two different kinds of responding populations, will they crossinhibit or is there a different repertoire?

SISKIND: With serum antibody they do crossinhibit to some extent, but there is also some degree of uniqueness.

H. BRALEY-MULLEN (*University of Missouri School of Medicine, Columbia, Mo.*): Do you see hapten-augmentable plaques after immunization with thymus-independent type-1 antigen?

SISKIND: Yes.

QUESTION: Have you attempted to present your spleen cell eluate (your autoanti-idiotype) in an immunogenic form, thereby raising an AB-3?

SISKIND: No, we have not.

NEGATIVE FEEDBACK REGULATION
OF CONTACT SENSITIVITY TO DNFB
BY AUTOANTI-IDIOTYPIC ANTIBODY *

John W. Moorhead

*Departments of Microbiology and Immunology
and of Medicine
University of Colorado Health Sciences Center
Denver, Colorado 80262*

INTRODUCTION

I would like to focus on one specific aspect of contact sensitivity (CS) to 2,4-dinitrofluorobenzene (DNFB), that being the effector phase of the primary response and its down regulation by autoanti-idiotypic (autoanti-Id) antibody. We have previously shown that the duration of the response is short lived, peaking on the sixth day after sensitization and then declining rapidly.[1] Further, we have shown that this rapid decline is due to the production, by the host, of autoanti-Id antibodies.[1] These anti-Id antibodies, which are detected in suppressive immune serum (SIS) 9–15 days after DNFB sensitization, specifically block the transfer of CS to DNFB. In addition to this naturally occurring autoanti-Id serum, I have prepared a syngeneic anti-Id serum in Balb/c mice by repeated immunization with purified DNFB-sensitized lymph node (LN) T cells (T_{DH}-DNP) from Balb/c mice.[2] Both anti-Id sera have similar properties and specificities. One important characteristic of both antisera is that they will block the transfer of CS to DNFB both with and without the use of complement (C). Reasoning that anti-Id inhibition of transfer of immunity without C might be relevant to *in vivo* regulation by anti-Id, I have examined the phenomenon in some detail. The results show that anti-Id without C has no discernible effect on the Id^+ T_{DH}-DNP effector cells. Rather, the inhibition is an active process, resulting from anti-Id activation of a subset of Ia^+ T cells in the immune LN population. The final suppression mediated by the anti-Id-activated T cells occurs locally and is antigen nonspecific.

MATERIALS AND METHODS

Mice

Male CBA/J mice were purchased from the Jackson Laboratory, Bar Harbor, Me.

Sensitization with DNFB or Oxazolone

Donors of immune LN cells were sensitized with DNFB by two daily paintings with 25 μl of 0.5% DNFB on the shaved abdomen and 5 μl on the

* This research was supported, in part, by a grant from the United States Public Health Service, no. AI–12993.

footpads and ears. Oxazolone (Ox) sensitivity was induced by two paintings of 50 μl of 3% Ox on the shaved abdomen and 5 μl on the footpads and ears. In some experiments, donor mice were doubly sensitized with DNFB and Ox. This was done by painting the left side of the clipped abdomen and the left forepaw and ear with DNFB and the right side of the abdomen and the right forepaw and ear with Ox.

Transfer of Contact Sensitivity

Three days after the last skin painting, single cell suspensions of draining LN cells were prepared and 5×10^7 cells were injected i.v. into normal syngeneic recipients. The recipients and negative controls were challenged within 1 h after cell transfer by applying 20 μl of 0.2% DNFB or 20 μl of 1% Ox on the dorsal side of each ear. Increased ear swelling was measured 24 h later with an engineer's micrometer and expressed in units of 10^{-4} in.

Antiserum

Anti-Ia^k serum was prepared by repeated injections of A.TH mice with spleen and LN cells from A.TL donors. Polyvalent rabbit anti-mouse immunoglobulin serum (anti-MIg) was prepared as previously described.[3] Before use, the antisera were heat inactivated at 56° C. The cytotoxicity and specificity of both antisera have been described.[3, 4]

Syngeneic anti-T$_{DH}$-DNP serum (anti-Id) was prepared by repeatedly immunizing Balb/c mice with purified LN T cells from DNFB-sensitized Balb/c mice.[2] SIS that contained autoanti-Id antibodies[1] was obtained by bleeding optimally DNFB-sensitized Balb/c mice 9, 12, and 15 days after sensitization and pooling the serum.

For treatment of immune LN cells, 10^8 cells per ml were suspended in 1:10 diluted anti-Ia^k or anti-MIg, 1:2 diluted SIS, or 1:20 diluted anti-Id and incubated for 1 h on ice. After washing, anti-Ia-, SIS- and anti-Id serum-treated cells were resuspended in 1:20 rabbit C (unless otherwise indicated) and anti-MIg-treated cells were resuspended in 1:6 guinea pig C. The cells were then incubated for 10 min on ice, followed by 30 min at 37° C.

Preparation and Use of Immunoadsorbant Columns

Affinity-purified normal mouse immunoglobulin (MIg) or Balb/c anti-DNP antibodies (MaDNP) were conjugated to Sepharose 4B beads (Pharmacia), according to the standard labeling protocol. 20 ml plastic syringes fitted with plastic discs were packed with 5–7 ml of the appropriate Sepharose conjugate. Before use, the columns were washed with 60 ml phosphate-buffered saline (PBS, pH 7.3), 30 ml of 0.1 M NH$_4$OH, and equilibrated with PBS. Then, 2.5 ml of 1:20 syngeneic anti-Id serum was added to the column and washed through slowly with 25 ml of PBS. 25 ml of effluent was collected and concentrated to 2 ml using an Amicon Ultrafiltration cell fitted with an XM50 Diaflo Ultramembrane (Amicon, Lexington, Me.). Column-bound material was eluted with 25 ml of 0.1 M NH$_4$OH. The eluate was neutralized immediately with 1 N HCl, dialyzed against PBS, and concentrated to 2 ml as described above.

RESULTS

Inhibition by Anti-Id Serum of Transfer of Immunity: Lack of Requirement for C

The basic phenomenon of C-independent inhibition of transfer of CS to DNFB by syngeneic anti-Id or autoanti-Id (SIS) is given in FIGURE 1. As shown, similar levels of inhibition occurred whether or not C was added.

All experiments have been done comparing autoanti-Id (SIS) and syngeneic anti-Id serum and similar results have been obtained. However, for ease of presentation, only those results obtained using the syngeneic anti-Id serum will be shown.

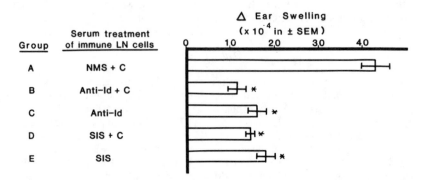

FIGURE 1. Complement-independent inhibition of transfer of contact sensitivity to DNFB by treatment with either syngeneic anti-Id or autoanti-Id (SIS) antibodies. * $p < 0.001$.

Inhibition of Transfer of Immunity by Anti-Id without C Requires Ia+ T Cells in the Immune LN Population

We considered three explanations that could account for the inhibition of transfer of immunity by anti-Id without C. These were (1) anti-Id antibodies blocking the antigen receptor on T_{DH}-DNP effector T cells, (2) C-mediated lysis of the effector T cells after transfer into the normal recipients, and (3) anti-Id activation of some T cell subset, resulting in suppression of the effector T_{DH}-DNP cells. The third explanation was considered because we have shown that DNFB-sensitized LN T cells are heterogeneous,[4] containing, among others, Ia+ auxiliary suppressor T cells (Ts-aux), which are required in order for suppressor T cells (Ts) to suppress effector functions of the T_{DH}-DNP cells.[5]

To examine the third possibility, DNFB-sensitized LN cells were depleted of Ia+ cells by treatment with anti-Ia^k serum plus C. These cells were then treated with anti-Id, both with and without C, and transferred to syngeneic recipients to assess their ability to transfer immunity. The results (FIGURE 2) show that pretreating the immune LN cells with anti-Ia serum plus C eliminated the inhibitory effect of the anti-Id serum alone. However, if the anti-Id serum

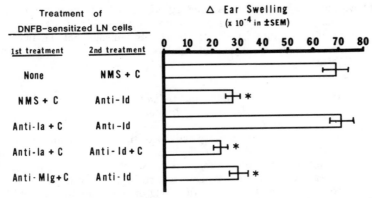

FIGURE 2. Complement-independent inhibition of transfer of contact sensitivity by anti-Id: Requirement of Ia$^+$ T cells. * p < 0.001.

was used with C, transfer of immunity was inhibited, presumably due to killing of the Id$^+$ T$_{DH}$-DNP effector cells. Depletion of B cells by treatment with anti-MIg plus C had no effect on the C-independent inhibition by anti-Id. Similar results have been obtained using nylon wool–purified DNFB-immune LN T cells (not shown). Thus, the results indicate that the C-independent inhibition by anti-Id of transfer of immunity requires the presence of Ia$^+$ T cells in the DNFB-sensitized LN population.

The Ia$^+$ T Cells Are Found in Sensitized but Not Normal LN Cell Populations

We next asked whether the Ia$^+$ T cell population was ubiquitous or whether it required antigen activation. 2×10^8 DNFB-immune LN cells depleted of Ia$^+$ cells were mixed with untreated LN cells from normal or sensitized mice. The cell mixtures were then treated with anti-Id serum without C and transferred to normal recipients, which were then ear challenged with DNFB. Ear swelling was measured 24 h later; the results are given in FIGURE 3. As previously described, immune LN cells depleted of Ia$^+$ cells were no longer inhibited by

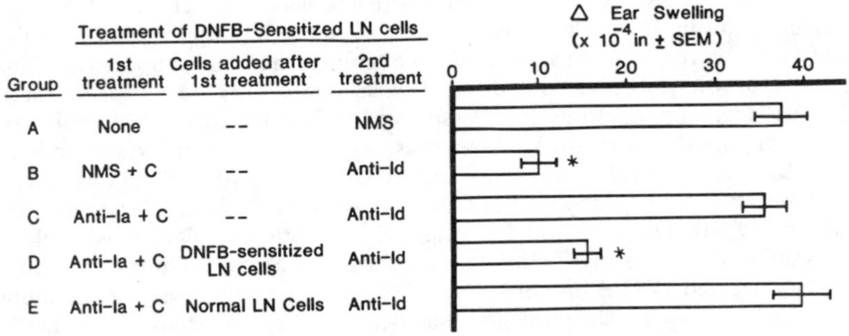

Group	1st treatment	Cells added after 1st treatment	2nd treatment	Δ Ear Swelling (x 10^{-4} in ± SEM)
A	None	--	NMS	
B	NMS + C	--	Anti–Id	*
C	Anti–Ia + C	--	Anti–Id	
D	Anti–Ia + C	DNFB-sensitized LN cells	Anti–Id	*
E	Anti–Ia + C	Normal LN Cells	Anti–Id	

FIGURE 3. Ia$^+$ T cells, which are required for complement-independent anti-Id antibody inhibition of transfer of contact sensitivity, are induced by antigen. * p < 0.001.

anti-Id without C (group C). Adding 10^8 untreated LN cells from DNFB-sensitized mice restored the inhibition (group D), while adding 10^8 normal LN cells had no effect (group E). Thus, the results indicate that the Ia^+ T cells necessary for C-independent anti-Id inhibition of transfer are induced by antigen (DNFB).

Anti-Id Antibodies Mediate the C-Independent Inhibition of Transfer of Immunity

We have shown that the inhibitory activity of the syngeneic antiserum when used with C is due to anti-Id antibodies.[2] Similar experiments were done to determine if anti-Id antibodies were also responsible for the C-independent inhibition of transfer of immunity. Diluted anti-Id serum was passed through Sepharose columns conjugated with either MIg or mouse anti-DNP antibodies. The column effluent and eluate were collected and tested without C on DNFB-sensitized LN cells for inhibition of transfer of immunity. The results are given in FIGURE 4. Passage of the antiserum through the MIg column had no effect, as all the inhibitory activity was present in the column effluent (group B). In contrast, when the anti-Id serum was passed through the MaDNP column, virtually all the inhibitory activity was found in the column eluate (group E). This indicates that anti-Id antibodies, which bind to the idiotype expressed by at least some anti-DNP antibodies, are responsible for the C-independent inhibition of transfer of immunity.

Suppression by Anti-Id-Activated Ia^+ T Cells is Antigen Nonspecific

To examine the specificity of suppression, LN cells from mice doubly sensitized with DNFB and Ox were treated with either normal mouse serum (NMS) or anti-Id. After washing, the cells were resuspended at 10^8 cells per ml and 0.5 ml was injected i.v. into normal recipients. DNFB ear challenges were made on half the recipients receiving NMS-treated cells and on half those receiving anti-Id-treated cells. The remaining recipients were challenged with Ox, and ear swelling in all recipients was measured 24 h later. As shown in FIGURE 5, transfer of CS to DNFB by LN cells from the doubly sensitized mice was inhibited by treating the cells with anti-Id (group B). In contrast, the ability of these same cells to transfer CS to Ox was unaffected by the anti-Id treatment (group D). These results indicate that the suppression is antigen specific. However, we considered the possibility that the suppressive signals delivered by the anti-Id-activated Ia^+ T cells might only occur locally at the skin test site. To explore this possibility, DNFB-sensitized LN cells were treated with NMS or anti-Id. After washing, the cells were resuspended at $3-4 \times 10^8$ cells per ml in medium and 10 μl ($3-4 \times 10^6$ cells) was injected intradermally into the dorsal side of the ears of normal mice. These mice then received 5×10^7 Ox-sensitized LN cells i.v. and were ear challenged with Ox. Ear swelling was measured 24 h later. As shown in FIGURE 6, intraear injection of anti-Id-treated DNFB-immune LN cells suppressed the transfer of immunity to Ox (group B). This suppression was dependent on Ia^+ cells in the DNFB-sensitized population. Depletion of Ia^+ cells before treatment with anti-Id reversed the suppression to an insignificant level (group C). Thus, it appears that suppression is antigen nonspecific and occurs locally at the skin test site.

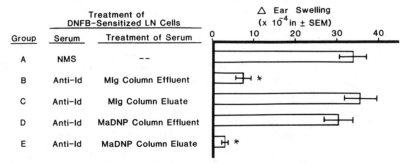

FIGURE 4. Anti-Id antibodies mediate the complement-independent inhibition of transfer of contact sensitivity. * p < 0.001.

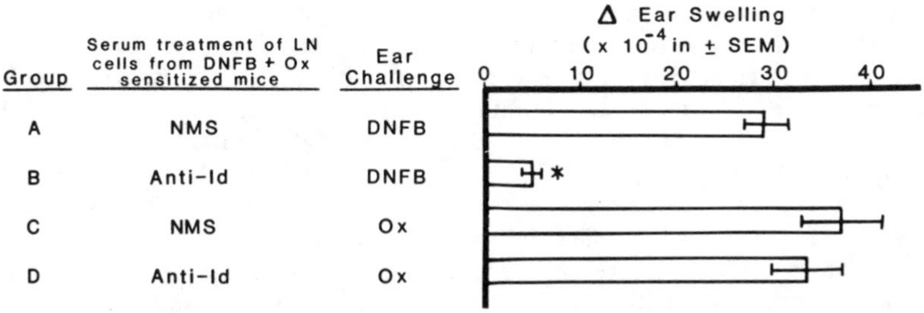

FIGURE 5. Passive transfer of systemic immunity: Complement independent inhibition by anti-Id antibody appears to be antigen specific. * p < 0.001.

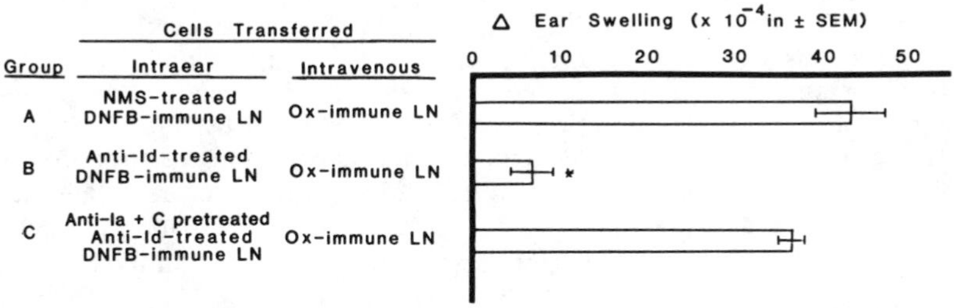

FIGURE 6. The final suppression induced by anti-Id antibody is antigen nonspecific, occurs locally, and requires Ia⁺ T cells. * p < 0.001.

DISCUSSION

Regulation of the immune response by interactions between Id and anti-Id has been established in several different experimental systems.[6-9] In some, production of autoanti-Id antibody has been shown to occur, correlating with down regulation of the immune response.[10-14] The mechanisms of the down regulation are poorly understood. We have previously shown that effector functions of DNFB-sensitized T cells (T_{DH}-DNP) are inhibited by autoanti-Id, which appears in the serum of Balb/c mice 9–15 d after optimal DNFB sensitization.[1] The experiments reported here were done to investigate the mechanisms involved in this regulation. Using either autoanti-Id or syngeneic anti-Id antibodies and transfer of CS to mimic the natural effector phase of the reaction, the results indicated that *in vivo* regulation by anti-Id is a complement-independent active process that requires anti-Id activation of a subset of Ia^+, Id^+ T cells. These T cells are present only in DNFB-sensitized LN populations and, once activated by anti-Id, they suppress effector mechanisms of the CS reaction antigen nonspecifically.

Although the effector T cells (T_{DH}-DNP) that mediate CS to DNFB are known to be Ia^-, functional subsets of DNFB-sensitized Ia^+ T cells have been identified.[4] Of relevance here is the subset we have termed auxiliary suppressor T cells (Ts-aux).[5] Ts-aux is a regulatory population. The cells are Ia^+ (I-J), and precursors are sensitive to cyclophosphamide.[5] In order for efferent-acting Ts to suppress T_{DH}-DNP effector cells, there is an absolute requirement for Ts-aux in the immune population. Thus, the target for the exogenous Ts is Ts-aux, rather than the effector T_{DH} population. We believe that Ts-aux and the Id^+, Ia^+ T cells we have identified here belong to the same T cell subset.

When Ts-aux was identified, we were somewhat surprised that this subset of regulatory cells was present in the immune population and apparently remained immunologically silent unless exogenous Ts were added. Since Ts are not present in immune populations, the role of Ts-aux cells in natural regulation was obscure. The results presented here clarify this issue and indicate that Ts-aux cells naturally regulate the CS response by interacting with anti-Id antibody. I believe that, after antigen (DNFB) stimulation, clones of Id^+ T_{DH} and Ts-aux cells are expanded. The CS response mediated by T_{DH} cells peaks six days after sensitization. By day 9, this response is no longer detectable; this down regulation is caused by autoanti-Id antibodies. These antibodies are produced against the Id receptors expressed on the expanded numbers of T_{DH} and Ts-aux cells. Regulation is affected by anti-Id binding to Id receptors on the Ts-aux population. This apparently activates the cells, which then suppress the effector T_{DH} cells. Suppression occurs locally at the skin test site and is antigen nonspecific. This scheme of regulation is shown in FIGURE 7. For reasons that are not clear at present, anti-Id antibodies do not sterically block the receptors on the T_{DH} cells, even though this binding occurs, as evidenced by adsorption [4] and by C-mediated lysis of the cells *in vitro*. It may be that, once anti-Id antibodies bind and crosslink these Id receptors, rapid shedding occurs with subsequent receptor re-expression.

This scheme—negative feedback regulation by anti-Id—is attractive because of its relative simplicity. In contrast to most other systems, it is not necessary to inject animals with excessive amounts of antigen, Id, or anti-Id antibodies.

Nor is it necessary to transfer lymphocytes from other animals treated with these reagents. All that is necessary is to sensitize the animals with an optimal dose of DNFB. The positive CS response, mediated by T_{DH}-DNP cells, is induced and peaks six days later. Simultaneously, cells that function to regulate this response are also induced (Ts-aux). The negative, or anti-, response, *i.e.*, anti-Id antibodies, is induced by receptors on these cells, as proposed by Jerne,[15] and feedback indirectly to down regulate the effector cells.

Ts-aux-like cells are present in other experimental systems and serve to regulate immune responses. These include antibody responses to hapten-protein conjugates [16] and delayed hypersensitivity to *p*-azobenzene arsonate [17, 18] and to phosphorylcholine.[19] We believe that further characterization of other experimental systems will reveal the presence of Ts-aux-like regulatory cells in immune lymphocyte populations.

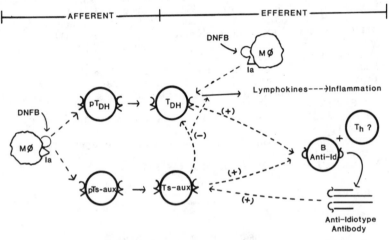

FIGURE 7. Negative feedback regulation of contact sensitivity to DNFB by auto-anti-Id antibody. (From Moorhead,[20] by permission.)

SUMMARY

Contact sensitivity to 2,4-dinitrofluorobenzene is maximal six days after sensitization but declines rapidly, due to autoanti-idiotypic antibodies produced by the host. The studies presented here indicate that this down regulation by anti-Id is a C-independent active process involving a subset of Ia^+ T cells in the immune lymph node cell population. Depleting immune LN cells of Ia^+ T cells renders them insensitive to inhibition by anti-Id alone, although the same population is inhibited by treatment with anti-Id plus C. This cell population is rendered sensitive to inhibition by anti-Id alone by adding untreated DNFB-sensitized LN cells but not by adding normal LN cells. Further studies showed that suppression by anti-Id-activated Ia^+ T cells occurs locally at the skin test site and is antigen nonspecific. These data indicate that the natural regulation of CS to DNFB by autoanti-Id antibodies involves a negative feedback regulatory loop.

REFERENCES

1. SY, M.-S., J. W. MOORHEAD & H. N. CLAMAN. 1979. J. Immunol. **123:** 2593–98.
2. MOORHEAD, J. W. 1982. J. Immunol. In press.
3. MOORHEAD, J. W., C. S. WALTERS & H. N. CLAMAN. 1973. J. Exp. Med. **137:** 411–23.
4. MOORHEAD, J. W. 1978. J. Immunol. **120:** 137–44.
5. SY, M.-S., S. D. MILLER, J. W. MOORHEAD & H. N. CLAMAN. 1979. J. Exp. Med. **149:** 1197–207.
6. BINZ, H. & H. WIGZELL. 1977. Prog. Allergy **23:** 154–98.
7. RAJEWSKY, K. & K. EICHMANN. 1977. Contemp. Top. Immunobiol. **7:** 69–112.
8. BONA, C. 1979. In Molecular Basis of Immune Cell Function. J. G. Kaplan, ed.: 161–80. Elsevier. Amsterdam.
9. BONA, C. & J. HIERNAUX. 1981. Crit. Rev. Immunol. **2:** 33–81.
10. KLUSKENS, L. & H. KOHLER. 1974. Proc. Nat. Acad. Sci. USA **71:** 5083–87.
11. BANKERT, R. B. & D. PRESSMAN. 1976. J. Immunol. **117:** 456–62.
12. COSENZA, H., A. AUGUSTIN & M. JULIUS. 1977. Eur. J. Immunol. **7:** 273–78.
13. KELSOE, G. & J. CERNY. 1979. Nature (London) **297:** 333–34.
14. SCHRATER, A. E., E. A. GOIDL, C. J. THORBECKE & G. W. SISKIND. 1979. J. Exp. Med. **150:** 138–53.
15. JERNE, N. K. 1974. Ann. Immunol. (Paris) **125C:** 373–89.
16. TADA, T. & K. OKUMURA. 1979. Adv. Immunol. **28:** 1–87.
17. SY, M.-S., A. NISONOFF, R. N. GERMAIN, B. BENACERRAF & M. I. GREENE. 1981. J. Exp. Med. **153:** 1415–25.
18. THOMAS, W. R., F. I. SMITH, I. D. WALKER & J. F. A. P. MILLER. J. Exp. Med. **153:** 1124–37.
19. SUGIMURA, K., T. KISHIMOTO, K. MAEDA & Y. YAMAMURA. 1981. Eur. J. Immunol. **11:** 455–461.
20. MOORHEAD, J. W. 1982. J. Exp. Med. **155:** 820.

DISCUSSION OF THE PAPER

B. BENACERRAF (*Harvard Medical School, Boston, Mass.*): When you speak of I-bearing cells in this system, do you use antisera that can also detect I-J, or do you think it's another type of I?

MOORHEAD: This antiserum does contain I-J.

BENACERRAF: So it could be I-J?

MOORHEAD: It could be.

BENACERRAF: Have you tried to determine whether or not the Fc part is necessary in your antibody? Will anti-F(ab′)2 carry the signal to the auxiliary cell?

MOORHEAD: We have not done that. An important question to be determined is, What is or are the signals that activate the auxiliary cell? Does the antibody do it by itself or are there other interactions that might be necessary with antigen or with other cells to activate this cell?

H. C. MAGUIRE, JR. (*Hahnemann Medical College, Philadelphia, Penn.*): Do you regard this as the only mechanism responsible for the rapid waning of contact sensitivity in the mouse? Have you looked for this anti-idiotypic antibody in other species, where you have a relative stability of contact sensitivity after sensitization, having in mind that the anti-idiotypic antibody might be epiphenomenal?

MOORHEAD: In answer to your first question: I'm not foolish enough to say that I think this is the only mechanism. I don't know how many other mechanisms there might be. We believe that this one operates in a relatively simple way. To answer your second question: We have not looked in other species for this antibody.

INDUCTION OF SPECIFIC TRANSPLANTATION TOLERANCE VIA IMMUNIZATION WITH DONOR-SPECIFIC IDIOTYPES *

Hans Binz,† Anu Soots,‡ Arto Nemlander,‡ Edward Wight,†
Martin Fenner,† Beat Meier,† Pekka Häyry,‡ and Hans Wigzell §

† Institute for Immunology and Virology
University of Zürich
POB, CH-8028 Zürich, Switzerland

‡ Transplantation Laboratory
IV Department of Surgery
University of Helsinki
Helsinki, Finland

§ Institute for Immunology
Uppsala University, Biomedicum
Uppsala, Sweden

INTRODUCTION

Induction of specific transplantation tolerance in adult immunocompetent individuals remains a primary focus of interest for those interested in transplantation immunology, whether at basic or at clinical levels. Various approaches to that goal have been used, involving such things as irradiation, more or less selective drugs, and antisera in conjunction with the grafting of foreign tissue.[1] Blood transfusions have been found to increase the survival of allogeneic kidney grafts, although the underlying mechanism is poorly understood.[2] Enhancement *via* the induction of anti-graft antibodies of particular specificities has been reported under some conditions.[1] Our approach, which we have been exploring for the last few years, has been to analyze the possibility of inducing autoanti-idiotypic immunity as a way to achieve a selective and long-lasting transplantation tolerance.[3, 4] The present article will try to summarize the findings obtained and inform the reader of our present state of knowledge.

METHODS

All material and methods used have been published in detail (see References 3, 6–8, 10, 13, 15, 18, 30, and 32).

RESULTS

The Idiotypic Systems of Anti-MHC Reactivity in Mice and Rats

A primary requisite for understanding of the autoanti-idiotypic approach is knowledge of the idiotypic systems involved, which are anti-MHC reactivity at the T cell and at the B cell levels, as analyzed by anti-idiotypic reactions.

* This research was supported by a grant from the Swiss National Science Foundation, no. 3.450–0.79, and by the Swedish Cancer Society.

0077–8923/82/0392–0360 $1.75/0 © 1982, NYAS

We have accumulated sizable amounts of data in this regard in two species, mice and rats.[3, 5, 6] TABLE 1 depicts, in a summary form, our basic knowledge of the build-up of T cell idiotopes in the anti-MHC systems. A primary finding was the discovery that T and B cells reactive against the same MHC antigens may share idiotypic determinants.[7] T cells could then be shown to be comparatively restricted with regard to idiotopes, *i.e.*, a virtually complete elimination of a specific anti-MHC reactivity could be achieved both at primary[8] and at secondary[9] set levels by suitable anti-idiotypic antisera. This is, of course, of prime importance if one wishes to eliminate a particular antigen-specific reactivity by the present approach. When we extracted soluble molecules in the body fluids from normal mice or rats using anti-idiotypic immunosorbant, we were struck by a second finding at the T cell level, that is, that seemingly all idiotype-positive molecules expressed the expected alloantigenic specificity, as measured by binding studies.[10] This is certainly in marked contrast to what is known to occur at the B cell level, where immunoglobulin molecules frequently may express idiotypes with perhaps only a statistically significant tendency to react with a particular antigenic determinant. We feel that this is, at least in

TABLE 1

SUMMARY OF BASIC RESULTS OBTAINED CONCERNING T CELL
IDIOTYPES IN ANTI-MHC SYSTEMS

Basic findings: B and T lymphocytes directed against the same antigens share idiotypes.[7, 26–28]

Biochemistry of T cell receptors: The dominating unit is a polypeptide chain of around 70 000 daltons.[3, 10, 11, 29] Such a single polypeptide chain can bind strongly to the antigen.[3, 5, 11]

Inheritance of T cell idiotypic determinants is linked to the heavy chain Ig loci.[12]

Lyt 1^+2^- anti-Ia proliferating and Lyt 1^-2^+ anti-K/D killer T cells express different idiotopes.[13]

part, due to the fact that our earlier studies on the anti-MHC-specific T cell receptors and factors had already led us to conclude that these molecules express highly specific and avid reactivity with the relevant antigen, despite the fact that they may exist as single polypeptide chains.[5, 9, 10, 11]

The genetics of the inheritance of anti-MHC reactive T cell receptors is also in agreement with this, though we have, so far, only been able to demonstrate that the heavy chain Ig genes are linked to T cell idiotypes—no linkage is demonstrable with light chain Ig genes.[12] No MHC linkage was found, disregarding the fact that the introduction of the "antigenic" MHC locus into the individual for reasons of immunological tolerance would result in a negative impact, that is, elimination of that particular group of antiallo-MHC-reactive idiotypic molecules and cells.[12]

As one might expect, it was also found that different T cell subsets with reactivity towards a foreign haplotype express different idiotopes, that is, Lyt 1^+2^-, anti-Ia, mixed leucocyte culture (MLC) proliferating T cells have idiotopes different from those of Lyt 1^-2^+, anti-K/D, killer effector T cells.[13] Likewise, in the rat, we could demonstrate by other means that T cells involved in graft *versus* host reactions (GVHR) may only in part have the same idiotopes as those which respond in a dominating manner in MLC.[1, 30] This represents the practical problem of determining what assays should be used to assure the investigator that functional *in vivo* transplantation tolerance has, indeed, been introduced *via* the autoanti-idiotypic protocol to be discussed below.

Autoanti-Idiotypic Immunity Represents a Possible Way to Achieve Long-Lasting Specific Transplantation Tolerance

After the initial discovery that it was, indeed, possible to induce autoanti-idiotypic immunity,[14] we applied the concept to the T cells involved in allo-MHC reactions.[3, 15] TABLE 2 describes our collected knowledge of the approach, using autoanti-idiotypic immunity to achieve specific suppression of transplantation immune reactions across the major histocompatibility complex (MHC) in animals over the last few years, summarizing the positive findings. It was thus found to be possible to use idiotypic receptors and molecules and, later, even idiotypic MLC-generated T blasts to induce autoanti-idiotypic immunity that could result in the select *in vivo* elimination of anti-MHC reactivity of the specificity corresponding to the immunogen used.[3, 15] Transplantation tolerance was induced in several species of animals, as measured either by *in vitro* immune assays or by actual tests for graft survival.[3, 4, 6, 15-17] The mechanism of auto-anti-idiotype-mediated suppression of this anti-MHC reactivity could be shown to reside at virtually all levels of the specific immune system, involving suppressor and killer T cells as well as helper T cells and B cells making anti-idiotypic antibodies.[18] Further positive elements in the system were the failures to find any damaging consequences of the autoanti-idiotypic immune reactions, *i.e.,* glomerulonephritis or the like, and the fact that, once induced, the specific suppression was long-lasting, perhaps life-long.[4] We believe this to be due to the fact that the idiotype-positive anti-MHC-reactive lymphocytes that would be constantly generated from the stem cells during life serve as a built-in self-boosting device to maintain the state of suppression.

Other workers have obtained evidence that similar autoanti-idiotypic immunity resulting in transplantation tolerance can be achieved in monkeys,[16, 17] and probably also in human beings, after conventional grafting protocols in a few patients.[19] Minor histocompatibility antigen differences, such as the male antigen[20] and tumor-associated antigens,[21-23] have also been studied, with results similar to those above.

In parallel with these highly positive results, we have also obtained results that should be grouped on the negative side; they are summarized in TABLE 3. Three major drawbacks have been encountered, out of which we have so far been able to fully solve only one. The first drawback is the frequency at which "positive," that is, autoanti-idiotype immune, individuals are reduced to unresponsiveness by the presently used immunization protocols. Here we have encountered drastic variations between experiments,[4] and, not too frequently, we have found that the specific immune reactivities of entire groups of experimental animals have been left largely untouched by the protocol used. The same protocols have, however, yielded highly significant and selective immune suppression in other experiments. This is due, at least in part, to matters of quantity, that is, the amounts of idiotypic material used as autoimmunogen,[4] where the law "the more the better" is seemingly correct. Some recent experiments to be presented below will reinforce this point. A second drawback

TABLE 2

SUMMARY OF AUTOANTI-IDIOTYPIC IMMUNITY IN ANTI-MHC SYSTEMS

Basic finding: Idiotypic anti-MHC receptors can evoke autoanti-idiotypic immunity.[3]

This can be shown to occur in mice, rats, guinea pigs, baboons,[4, 6, 15, 16] chimpanzees,[17] and, probably, man.[19]

Autoanti-idiotypic immunity can be induced by idiotypic soluble receptors and by idiotypic MLC T blasts.[3, 15]

Autoanti-idiotypic immunity can result in specific suppression of MLC, GVHR, Tc, and alloantibody production.[4]

Autoanti-idiotypic immunity can result in specific long-lasting transplantation tolerance.[4]

The mechanism for this specific immune suppression exists at the level of both T cells (suppressor, killer, and helper T cells with anti-idiotypic specificity) and B cells that produce anti-idiotypic antibodies.[18]

No negative side effects of autoanti-idiotypic immunity have been found in this system.[4, 24]

encountered has been the need for adjuvants, in particular Freund's complete type, to achieve the successful induction of autoanti-idiotypic immunity.[24] This adjuvant is not suitable for clinical use and most other adjuvants used have been found to be inefficient.[24] Recently, however, muramyl dipeptide adjuvants functioning *via* esther linkages have been found to be suitable in the successful induction of autoanti-idiotypic immunity in the present systems,[24] thereby largely solving the adjuvant problem. Finally, as already alluded to above, sizable variance in biological consequences was found in individual animals, *i.e.,* mixed leukocyte culture (MLC) was suppressed but not GVHR, etc.,[4] thereby making it difficult to use a single assay, such as the MLC system, to estimate the completeness of suppression achieved. A combination of serological determinations of idiotypic cells remaining in defined systems and MLC assays probably provides the best screening method for the *in vitro* evaluation of the degree of suppression achieved in animal experimental systems.

TABLE 3

PROBLEMS IN TRYING TO USE AUTOANTI-IDIOTYPIC IMMUNITY IN
ANTI-MHC SYSTEMS TO ACHIEVE TRANSPLANTATION TOLERANCE

Low frequency or high variability in successful induction of autoanti-idiotypic immunity.[4, 24]

A requirement for certain types of adjuvant to achieve efficient anti-idiotypic immunity.[4, 24]

The dichotomy between *in vitro* and *in vivo* results: Suppression in one assay not always paralleled in another system.[30]

New Biochemical and Serological Features of Anti-MHC Reactive
T Cell Receptors

In the present approach, we normally use T cells (or T cell–derived soluble molecules) with idiotypic antigen-binding properties as the auto-immunogen. In a situation where antigen-specific T cells were around in enriched form but there was a lack of anti-idiotypic antisera, it would be extremely useful to have antisera directed against the constant region(s) of IgT material available. We have recently been able to produce such anti-IgT sera by immunizing rabbits with purified Lewis anti-DA reactive T cell receptors.[11] These antisera react with mouse as well as rat antigen-specific T cell receptors. Using this antiserum, we found that it possible to obtain internally labeled molecules from Lewis anti-DA and C57BL/6-anti-CBA MLC supernatants (FIGURE 1). Molecules

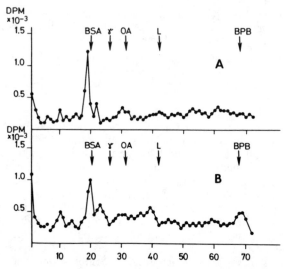

FIGURE 1. SDS gel analysis of rat and mouse T cell receptor material. The material was isolated from internally labeled supernatants from Lewis anti-DA (A) and C57BL/6 anti-CBA MLC (B) *via* rabbit anti-rat C_r immunosorbent.[11] After concentration, isolated material was analysed under reducing conditions on 10% SDS gel and radioactivity was determined in 1 mm slices, as described.[11]

with size distribution profiles identical to those of the molecules obtained using anti-idiotypic immunosorbents were obtained.[5, 10, 11] Thus, the dominating polypeptide chain was found around 70 000, with a minor, sometimes-observed chain around 60 000 daltons. Some experiments contained peaks of small magnitude at 50 000, 43 000, and 25 000 daltons; these are known to represent degradation products from the 70 000 chain. Plasmin degradation yielded two sharp fragments from the 70 000 chain, as shown in FIGURE 2. The antigen binding ability could be shown to reside in the 25 000-sized fragment, as demonstrated in FIGURE 3. Nearly identical fragmentation patterns using plasmin were found when we used T receptors from mouse T blasts isolated by this rabbit antiserum. The sizes of the molecules and their proteolytic susceptibility was the same, regardless of whether they were obtained from a mixture of

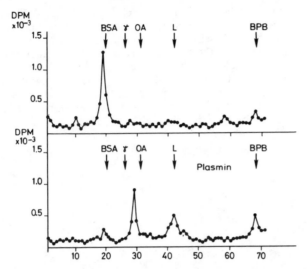

FIGURE 2. Splitting of rat T cell receptor material with plasmin. Lewis anti-DA T cell receptor material was purified from internally labeled supernatant *via* rabbit anti-rat C_r antiserum and digested with plasmin, as described.[11] Analysis of the products was made on 10% SDS gels under reducing conditions and radioactivity was determined in 1 mm slices, as described.[11]

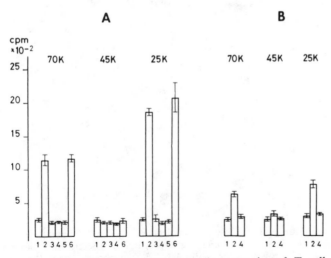

FIGURE 3. Demonstration of the antigen-binding capacity of T cell receptor material. Lewis anti-DA MLC supernatant was purified over rabbit anti-rat C_r immunosorbent, radiolabeled with ^{125}I, and digested with plasmin.[11] Peptides were fractionated over G-2000 Sephadex in 6 M urea and 0.1 M sodium acetate (pH 4.5). Fractions forming peaks of 45 000 and 25 000—as determined by counting the radioactivity—were pooled, dialysed, and concentrated; then 50.000 (A) or 100.000 (B) cpm were incubated with 1×10^6 cells, as indicated, for 1 h at 4° C. Columns represent the mean ± s.e. of quadruplicates. 1, Lewis; 2, DA; 3, August; 4, BN; 5, L.BN; and 6, AVN.

T blasts or from Lyt 1⁺2⁻3⁻ or Lyt 1⁻2⁺3⁺ blasts, as shown in FIGURE 4. This, in conjunction with the finding that rat T cell receptors isolated from both pooled MLC blasts and Lewis-anti-DA alloreactive, proliferating, noncytolytic clones behaved identically (FIGURE 5), leads us to conclude that we have, so far, been unable to separate anti-MHC reactive receptors into more than one class of molecule by size and proteolytic degradation patterns. Isotypic variability may certainly exist among the IgT molecules from different subsets of T lymphocytes, as indicated in the mouse in other systems,[25] but we have not yet discovered such variability in the allo-MHC systems.

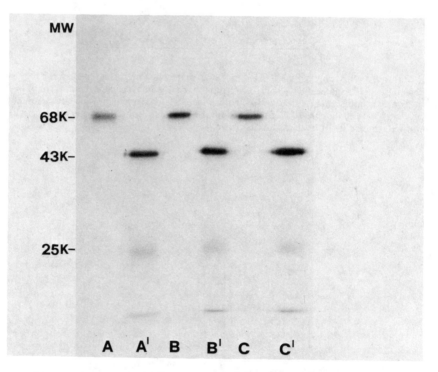

FIGURE 4. Similar T cell receptor molecules on T cell subpopulations. C57BL/6 anti-CBA MLC T subpopulations were prepared as described,[32] using anti-Lyt 1 and anti-Lyt 2,3 antisera. Internally labeled supernatants from these T cell subpopulations were absorbed on rabbit anti-rat C_r immunosorbent. Isolated material was exposed to plasmin, and the products, as well as undigested material, were analysed on 10% SDS gel. A, material from a mixture of Lyt 1⁺2⁻3⁻ and Lyt 1⁻2⁺3⁺ cells. B, material from Lyt 1⁻2⁺3⁺ cells. C, material from Lyt 1⁺2⁻3⁻ cells. A', B', C', the corresponding products after digestion with plasmin. Around 20.000 dpm were applied on A, B, and C and about double that amount on A', B', and C'. Gel was exposed to Ilford film for one month.

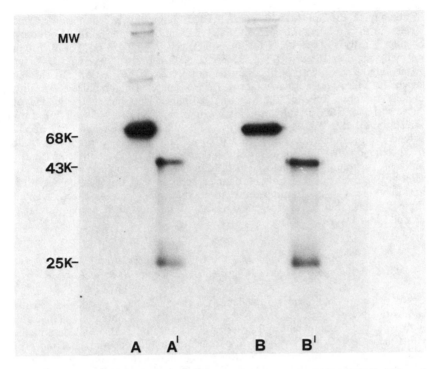

FIGURE 5. Internally labeled supernatants from Lewis anti-DA MLC (A) and from cloned Lewis anti-DA proliferative T cell clone (B) were absorbed and eluted from rabbit anti-rat C_r immunosorbent. Lewis anti-DA T clones were derived from Lewis anti-DA MLC after three *in vitro* restimulations. T cells were cloned on (Lewis × DA)F$_1$ macrophages in EHAA medium complemented with 10% FCS and 20% TCGF.[11] Purified material was analysed on 10% SDS slabgel as such or after digestion with plasmin (A'), (B').

Induction of Autoanti-Idiotypic Immunity in Tumor-Specific Systems

Reactions against weak histocompatibility antigens may, in time, play highly important roles in the rejection of allogeneic grafts. Successful induction of autoanti-idiotypic immunity, resulting in a reduction of the immune response against the Y antigen or tumor-associated antigens, has been reported.[21-23] Here we would just like to add yet another system, *i.e.*, chemically induced tumors in rats. Humoral and cellular immunity against the antigens associated with the tumor P_1 (7,12 dimethyl-benz(a)anthracen-induced sarcoma in DA rats) can be readily demonstrated *in vitro* after *in vivo* immunization by proliferation and selective killer T cell function. Purified anti-P_1 antibodies (absorbed and eluted from P_1 tumor cells) can be used in adjuvant to induce a state of autoanti-idiotypic immunity in a certain number of syngeneic rats, in analogy to the anti-MHC systems.[26] This immunity is manifested at two levels: in the production of autoanti-idiotypic antibodies and in the production of killer T cells with specificity for the anti-P_1-generated T blasts. The P_1 tumor normally requires 10^6 cells for a successful take in normal syngeneic DA rats. After immunization with purified anti-P_1 antibodies, 10^3 P_1 tumor cells showed successful takes and permanent growth in 3 out of 10 immunized DA rats, namely in those three of the rats that displayed the reported evidence of successful induction of autoanti-idiotypic immunity. The results of this study are summarized in TABLE 4. From this we deduced that we could confirm and extend the previous observation that it is, indeed, possible to produce a state of specific *in vivo* unresponsiveness against certain minor histocompatibility antigens, including tumor-associated histocompatibility structures, *via* autoanti-idiotypic immunization. It is, of course, possible that this can be used *via* anti-idiotypic T blast immunizations to produce the opposite effect, even in these systems, that is, an increased resistance against such weaker antigens as well.[22]

Induction of Specific Transplantation Tolerance towards Allogeneic Heart Allografts Using Donor-Specific Idiotypes

In order to obtain further evidence of the underlying mechanisms while trying to obtain specific tolerance *via* autoanti-idiotypic immunity, especially with regard to the adjuvants and doses of T blasts to be used, we made a major effort using 13 different protocols in parallel. The different immunization protocols used are summarized in TABLE 5, using various forms and doses of anti-DA or anti-BN idiotypic molecules in Lewis rats, assessing the success by grafting allogeneic hearts into the peritoneal cavity of the animals.

Effect of Anti-Idiotype Immunization of the Survival of L.BN and DA Heart Allografts in Lewis Rats

Without immunization, the survival of L.BN and DA heart allografts in Lewis recipients was 6.7 ± 0.3 and 6.0 ± 0.0 d, respectively. In groups I–VII, where the recipients were immunized with four injections of 2×10^7 2° MLC blasts, a significant prolongation of survival (to 26.8 ± 5.1 d) was observed only in group III, where complete and incomplete Freund's adjuvants were used. In the remaining groups, the prolongation of survival was either marginal or nonexistent. In group VIII, where Lewis anti-BN 4° MLC blasts expanded with T cell growth factors (TCGF) were used as immunogen and muramyl dipeptides (MDP) were used as adjuvant, a single injection of 3×10^8 blasts induced "indefinite" (more than 30 d) survival in six out of six occasions. The prolongation was specific, since the survival of DA heart allografts in similar recipients was only 6.0 ± 0.0 d. In groups IX–XIII, Lewis recipients had been immunized with Lewis anti-DA T cell receptor material derived from MLC-primed lymph node and spleen cell cultures and absorbed and eluted over anti-Id (pool 3)[8] or normal control serum (group XI) immunosorbent. One injection of receptor protein in complete Freund's adjuvant prolonged the survival of relevant DA heart allografts from 6.0 to 13.2 ± 0.8 or 9.0 ± 0.4 days, depending on the amount of antigen administered, while the procedure had no effect

TABLE 4

INDUCTION OF AUTOANTI-IDIOTYPIC IMMUNITY IN A TUMOR-SPECIFIC SYSTEM

Animal	Immunized with	Anti-ID (RIA) Antibodies	Anti-Id (restimulation) Antibodies	Tumor Growth
1		+	−	−
2		−	−	−
3		+	+	+
4		−	−	−
5	purified	+	+	+
6	DA anti-P_1	−	−	−
7		−	−	−
8		(+)	−	−
9		+	+	+
10		−	−	−
1		−	−	−
2		−	−	−
3		−	−	−
4		−	−	−
5	normal DA IgG	−	−	−
6		−	−	−
7		−	−	−
8		−	−	−
9		−	−	−
10		−	−	−

NOTES: DA anti-P_1 antibodies were obtained by repeated immunization of syngeneic DA rats with P_1 sarcoma cells (the P_1 tumor is a 7,12 dimethyl-benz(a)anthracen-induced sarcoma in DA rats). Anti-P_1 antibodies were absorbed and eluted from paraformaldehyde-fixed P_1 tumor cells, and specific antibodies were crosslinked with glutaraldehyde.[81] Ten rats were immunized either with 400 μg specific anti-P_1 antibodies (emulsified in Freund's adjuvant) or with normal DA Ig (ten control rats). Animals got one booster, using the same protocol, three weeks later and were bled three weeks after the first injection and one month after the second injection. Sera from individual rats were heat inactivated. Anti-idiotypic antibodies were tested in two independent assays. (1) In a solid-phase RIA using F(ab')$_2$ from DA anti-P_1 antibodies or from normal DA IgG as antigens. Immunoreactions were demonstrated by using a rabbit anti-rat Fc (IgG) and ^{125}I-labeled protein A. (2) By restimulation of *in vivo* primed DA anti-P_1 T lymphocytes *in vitro*. Putative anti-idiotypic antisera were used at concentrations of around 0.2%. Secondary proliferative responses were measured by ^{3}H-TdR incorporation.[82]

Animals that had been immunized with either purified DA anti-P_1 antibodies or DA normal Ig were injected with 1×10^3 P_1 tumor cells one month after the second immunization. Normal DA rats developed lethal tumors when 1×10^6 tumor cells were injected.

+, positive reaction (RIA, or restimulation and tumor growth with 1×10^3 tumor cells). Positive reactions were more than 200% over the control values.

−, negative reaction in RIA and restimulation or no tumor growth with 1×10^3 tumor cells.

TABLE 5

DIFFERENT SCHEDULES OF IMMUNIZATION AND THE IMPACT OF IMMUNIZATION ON THE SURVIVAL OF DA AND L.BN HEART ALLOGRAFTS IN LEWIS RECIPIENTS

Group	Immunogen	Adjuvant	Schedule of Immunizations	Transplant Donor	Transplant Survival		
					Number	Mean ± s.d. (d)	p ‖
Control a	—	—	—	Lewis	2	> 30.0	
Control b	—	—	—	L.BN	3	6.7 ± 0.3	
Control c	—	—	—	DA	3	6.0 ± 0.0	
I	Lewis anti-BN 2° MLC blasts	MPD-C *	4 injections of 2 × 10^7 blasts i.p.‡	L.BN	5	6.8 ± 0.3	N.S.
II		MDP-A		L.BN	5	6.0 ± 0.5	N.S.
III		CFA/IFA †		L.BN	4 (5)§	26.8 ± 5.1	0.004
IV		None		L.BN	5	6.4 ± 0.5	N.S.
V		MDP-B		L.BN	5	7.4 ± 0.5	N.S.
VI		MDP-E		L.BN	4 (5)§	8.8 ± 0.5	0.03
VII		MDP-D		L.BN	4 (5)§	7.3 ± 0.5	N.S.
VIIIa	Lewis anti-BN 4° MLC blasts expanded with TCGF	MDP-B	1 injection of 3 × 10^8 blasts i.p.	L.BN	6	> 30.0	0.000
VIIIb		MDP-B		DA	2	6.0 ± 0.0	N.S.

Group	Description	First immunization	Treatment	Strain	n	Survival (days)	p
IXa	Lewis anti-DA T cell receptor deriving from MLC-primed LNC and SC, adsorbed/eluted over an anti-ID pool 3 column	CFA	1 injection of 100 µg protein s.c.	DA	5	13.2 ± 0.8	0.000
IXb		CFA		L.BN	2	6.0 ± 0.0	N.S.
Xa	Control protein to Lewis anti-DA receptor deriving from MLC-primed LNC and SC, adsorbed/eluted over a normal F1 column	CFA	1 injection of 200 µg protein s.c.	DA	5	9.0 ± 0.4	0.000
Xb		CFA		L.BN	2	7.0 ± 1.4	N.S.
XI		CFA		DA	5	6.0 ± 0.0	N.S.
XII		MDP-B	1 injection of 100 µg protein s.c.	DA	6	10.0 ± 4.0	0.05
XIII	Lewis anti-DA T cell receptor deriving from MLC-primed LNC and SC, adsorbed/eluted over an anti-Id pool 3 column	MDP-B		DA	5	8.7 ± 2.6	0.05

* MDP-derivatives: MDP-B—*N*-acethylmuramyl-L-alanyl-D-isoglutaminyl-L-alanyl-2-(1',2'-dipalmitoyl-*SN*-glycero 3'-phosphoryl)-ethyl-amide; MDP-C, -D, and -E—these MDP derivatives contain biological inactive aminoacide stereoisomeres. All preparations were obtained through the courtesy of Dr. L. Tarcsay, Ciba-Geigy, Ltd., Basel, Switzerland.
† First immunization in complete Freund's adjuvant (CFA); subsequent immunizations in incomplete Freund's adjuvant (IFA).
‡ The immunizations were given approximately two, five, nine, and ten weeks before transplantation.
§ One graft in these groups was lost and excluded because of technical failure.
|| Student's *t* test to respective control.

on the survival of L.BN heart allograft in similar recipients. A similar prolongation of survival was observed when MDP was used as adjuvant (to 10.0 ± 4.0 or 8.7 ± 2.6 d, depending on the amount of antigen used), while immunization with control protein to the receptor protein had no effect (6.0 ± 0.0 d).

Effect of Immunization on the Alloantibody Response

In all groups demonstrating a prolonged graft survival, the alloantibody response to the relevant transplant donor strain was entirely abolished. Normal or, occasionally, slightly suppressed alloantibody responses were obtained in the remaining groups. The suppression was immunologically specific—rats in groups III and VIII responded with normal antibody production to DA heart allografts and rats in groups IX, X, XII, and XIII responded with normal responses to L.BN (data not shown). All animals responded with similar titers when immunized with BSA or uv-inactivated Sendai virus.

Proliferative and Cytotoxic Capacity of Lymphoid Cells Deriving from Idiotype-Immunized Recipients

At the time the animals were killed, spleen cells from randomly selected animals were used for stimulation and cytotoxicity assays in vitro. The spleen cells were tested for responses to concanavalin A (con A) and to relevant and irrelevant stimulator cells in MLC and (after stimulation) for cytotoxicity to relevant and irrelevant target cells in the cell-mediated lympholysis (CML) assays. All animals responded normally to con A, regardless of the antigen or type of adjuvant used for the immunization. Upon stimulation with 2500 rad–irradiated BN stimulator cells, the responses were significantly reduced or abolished in groups I–III and VIII, while normal responses to BN stimulator cells were obtained in groups IX–XIII. On the other hand, upon stimulation with irradiated DA spleen cells, normal responses were obtained in groups I–VIII and a significantly reduced response was obtained in groups IX, X, XII, and XIII. Animals in groups IV–VII and XI responded normally to both types of stimulator cells. In the Tc assay performed after stimulation in a relevant MLC, a significant suppression of cytotoxicity to BN targets was found in groups II, III, and VII and to DA target cells in groups IX, X, XII, and XIII. Thus, as in the MLC, suppression of Tc was immunologically specific. Tc responses using effector cells generated in irrelevant MLC were not suppressed.

Autoanti-Idiotypic Mechanisms Involved in Specific Suppression

In group VIII, where indefinite survival of a relevant heart allograft was observed, we tested the MLC-primed spleen cells for cytotoxicity against Lewis anti-BN and Lewis anti-DA T blasts in vitro. After priming with irradiated BN stimulator cells when no cytotoxicity to BN and DA target cells was demonstrable, a highly efficient killing on six out of six occasions was observed against Lewis anti-BN blasts. No cytotoxic effect was demonstrable against Lewis anti-DA T blasts. This would indicate the presence of anti-idiotypic killer T cells in these animals. The testing of possible anti-idiotypic antibodies in the immunized recipients is still under way. In group VIII, so far, three sera have been found positive with regard to reactivity to Lewis anti-BN blasts but none with regard to Lewis anti-DA.

In conclusion, the observed suppression using a new protocol (MDP-B with *in vitro* expanded Lewis-anti-BN blasts in very high numbers in a single dose) would appear to have autoanti-idiotypic immunity as its basis.

DISCUSSION

It has been known for some time that autoanti-idiotypic immunity can be induced, resulting in a selective loss *in vitro* and *in vivo* against the relevant transplantation antigens.[3] This has been found to be true in several species of animals,[3, 6, 15–17] including, possibly, man [19] and extends beyond allo-MHC antigens to include weaker histocompatibility antigens, such as the male antigen [20] and tumor-associated transplantation antigens.[21–23] The latter findings, as confirmed here, are important, for they show that the allo-MHC results are not unique, but perhaps representative of what may be achieved in several different transplantation systems. But, while theoretical progress has swiftly delineated possible methods of immune regulation in autoanti-idiotypic systems, possible clinical applications have been painfully slow in developing for several reasons. One of these reasons, the requirement for Freund's complete adjuvant,[24] has been solved (this study and Reference 24) by replacing the adjuvant with certain muramyl dipeptide reagents, allowing human applications.

The second major reason has been the comparatively low frequency of success using the hitherto applied immunization protocols,[4] which makes clinical applications questionable because of low efficiency. We have previously found that the quantity of idiotypic receptors would seem to be one important factor in obtaining a higher rate of success.[4] In the present study, use of a comparatively very high dose of syngeneic T blasts (3×10^8 specific MLC T blasts per rat) yielded complete tolerance *in vivo* and *in vitro,* as assessed by several parameters. This high dose of cells was obtained by using recently developed techniques with TCGF after primary MLC; corresponding numbers of cells could certainly be generated in human situations without too much difficulty. The underlying mechanism using this new protocol would still seem to be at the level of autoanti-idiotypic immunity, making it likely that tolerance is lifelong and without any noticeable complications. Further experiments using this revised protocol will be necessary before any general conclusions concerning its improved reproducibility can be made.

In parallel with the use of TCGF-expanded MLC T blasts for autoimmunization, the successful production of antisera reacting with constant regions of T cell receptor polypeptide chains also allows the molecules released into the supernatant to be isolated during the growth of the antigen-specific T cells in the absence of antigen. This should allow further significant improvement in the quantity of antigen-specific idiotypic material for analysis and immunization to be made.

We would thus conclude that, in addition to yielding new data on the basic composition of the antigen-binding receptors on T cells, improvements in the protocols used to induce autoanti-idiotypic immunity against allo-MHC structures indicate that this should still be considered a quite viable alternative approach in future clinical trials.

REFERENCES

1. 1981. Transplant. Proc. **13**.
2. OPELZ, G. & P. I. TERASAKI. 1980. Transplantation **29**: 153.
3. BINZ, H. & H. WIGZELL. 1976. J. Exp. Med. **144**: 1438.
4. BINZ, H. & H. WIGZELL. 1979. Transplant. Proc. **11**: 914.
5. BINZ, H. & H. WIGZELL. 1977. Prog. Allergy **23**: 154.
6. ANDERSSON, L. C., M. AGUET, E. WIGHT, R. ANDERSSON, H. BINZ & H. WIGZELL. 1977. J. Exp. Med. **146**: 1124.
7. BINZ, H. & H. WIGZELL. 1975. J. Exp. Med. **142**: 197.
8. BINZ, H. & H. WIGZELL. 1975. J. Exp. Med. **142**: 1231.
9. BINZ, H. & H. WIGZELL. 1977. Contemp. Top. Immunobiol. **7**: 113.
10. BINZ, H. & H. WIGZELL. 1977. Scand. J. Immunol. **5**: 559.
11. BINZ, H. & H. WIGZELL. 1981. J. Exp. Med. **154**: 1261.
12. BINZ, H., H. WIGZELL & H. BAZIN. 1976. Nature (London) **264**: 639.
13. BINZ, H., H. FRISCHKNECHT, F. W. SHEN & H. WIGZELL. 1979. J. Exp. Med. **149**: 910.
14. RODKEY, L. I. S. 1974. J. Exp. Med. **139**: 712.
15. ANDERSSON, L. C., H. BINZ & H. WIGZELL. Nature (London) **264**: 778.
16. MYBURGH, J. A. & J. A. SMIT. 1979. Transplant. Proc. **11**: 923.
17. STRONG, D. M. et al. 1979. Transplant. Proc. **11**: 928.
18. BINZ, H. & H. WIGZELL. 1978. J. Exp. Med. **147**: 63.
19. MIYJIMA, T., R. HIGUCHI, H. KASHIWABARA & T. YOKOYAMA. 1980. Nature (London) **283**: 306.
20. SUNDAY, M. E., J. Z. WEINBERGER, S. WOLFF & M. E. DORF. 1981. Eur. J. Immunol. **8**: 626.
21. FLOOD, P. M., M. L. KRIPKE, D. A. ROWLEY & H. SCHREIBER. 1980. Proc. Nat. Acad. Sci. USA **77**: 2209.
22. TILKIN, A. F., N. SCHAAF-LAFONTAINE, A. VAN ACKER, M. BOCCARDORO & J. URBAIN. 1981. Proc. Nat. Acad. Sci. USA **78**: 1809.
23. DUPREZ, V., S. BELUCCHI & J. P. LEVY. 1980. Eur. J. Immunol. **10**: 26.
24. BINZ, H., L. TARCSAY, H. WIGZELL & P. DUKOR. 1981. Transplant. Proc. **13**: 566.
25. OWEN, F. L., R. RIBLET & B. A. TAYLOR. 1981. J. Exp. Med. **154**: 801.
26. BINZ, H., J. LINDENMANN & H. WIGZELL. 1973. Nature (London) **246**: 146.
27. EICHMANN, K. & K. RAJEWSKY. 1975. Eur. J. Immunol. **5**: 661.
28. MCKEARN, T .J. 1974. Science **183**: 94.
29. RUBIN, B. et al. 1980. Bull. Inst. Pasteur Paris **78**: 305.
30. AGUET, M. et al. 1978. J. Exp. Med. **147**: 50.
31. DAUGHARTY, H., J. E. HOPPER, A. B. MCDONALD & A. NISONOFF. 1969. J. Exp. Med. **130**: 1047.
32. FRISCHKNECHT, H., H. BINZ & H. WIGZELL. 1978. J. Exp. Med. **147**: 500.

CONCLUDING REMARKS

David W. Scott

Division of Immunology
Department of Microbiology and Immunology
Duke University Medical Center
Durham, North Carolina 27710

Summarizing a meeting such as this one is, as Dr. Battisto noted in opening this conference, "an unenviable task." If I fail to mention some people's work, they will be upset because I have overlooked their contributions. However, those I may choose to cite will probably think that I have misquoted them. Therefore, I will not mention individual names, but will rather cite a few themes, which, I believe, have become apparent during this conference.

It is clear that self recognition (rather than the lack of same) is an intrinsic property of the immune system; unresponsiveness to self (or antigens associated with self markers) is, therefore, influenced by this property. However, not all self antigens are created equal (*sic*). Hence, the associative recognition emphasized throughout this meeting depends on which self markers a foreign antigen becomes associated with, the time during which this association occurs (*e.g.*, ontogenetically), and how such complexes are introduced to the immune system.

It is thus apparent that no single unifying theory can account for the multitude of observations presented in the last two and one half days. Surely, histocompatibility antigens, both class I and class II, are important guideposts in this regulatory process, as are the restrictions imposed by idiotypic markers. In addition, other kinds of carriers also provide different approaches and probes for manipulation of the immune system; these include synthetic carriers unrelated to self and isologous serum proteins, both of which may display intrinsic tolerogenic properties leading either to the induction of suppressor cells or to direct unresponsiveness.

An important set of observations emphasized how cells in the immune system may speak to one another *via* groups of soluble factors, including the interleukins and antigen- and idiotype-specific I-J$^+$ factors. Depending on the nature of the antigen presented and the presence or absence of interleukins, T cells decide whether to respond or become unresponsive. Suppressor factors also act to convey messages to activate or inactivate other members of the immune family circuit.

One is tempted to draw an analogy between T cell circuits and the famous dialogue between Abbott and Costello involving the names of players on a baseball team. When asked to identify players, Abbott replies, "Well, Who's on first, What's on second, and I Don't Know's on third," which leads to Costello's classic confusion. In reviewing the current state of our knowledge, as exemplified in the present meeting, I cannot but conclude that we have made significant progress. I believe that we now know Who's on first and What's on second and that we have a fairly good idea of the name of the character on third (although different names were used by different speakers at this meeting). With the advent of functional cloned cell lines representing different T cell subsets as well as B cell and antigen-presenting cells, and with the use of purified macromolecules from such cells, I believe that we will soon not only know Who's on first, etc., but also how they play the game!

PROLONGATION OF NEONATALLY INDUCED
B CELL TOLERANCE

A Role for the Thymus

R. B. Acres and A. J. Cunningham

Department of Medical Biophysics
University of Toronto

and

Ontario Cancer Institute
Toronto, Ontario, Canada M4X 1K9

Mice were rendered tolerant as neonates to fowl gamma globulin (FGG). Over the entire period that the mice were tolerant, B cell function and T cell–mediated immune regulation were studied. The objectives of the study were to determine the following.

(1) Whether tolerogen-specific B cell function is decreased for the entire period that mice are tolerant to an antigen that does not bind murine Fc receptors or murine complement (as does human gamma globulin (HGG), which has been used in previous studies [1, 2]).

(2) Whether FGG-specific cell-mediated immune regulatory mechanisms function in the spleens and thymuses of tolerant mice throughout the tolerant period or during the limited time intervals when mice are tolerant.

(3) Whether the thymus is required for the prolongation of neonatally induced tolerance to soluble antigens.

Neonatal CBA mice were injected with 6 mg FGG (hereafter referred to as Tol mice) or saline (control mice). FGG-specific B cell function in Tol mice of various ages was analyzed using the following protocol: Spleen cells were removed from Tol and age-matched control mice, treated with anti-Thy 1 and complement, supplemented with normal syngeneic thymocytes, and injected into irradiated syngeneic mice. Recipients were immunized with FGG and a control antigen, bovine serum albumin (BSA), in complete Freund's adjuvant and splenic plaque-forming cells (PFC) were enumerated one week later.

The results of these experiments suggest that Tol mice's FGG-specific B cells are hyporesponsive for the entire period that the mice remain hyporesponsive to FGG.

Cell mixtures in adoptive transfer experiments were used to analyze spleen and thymus cells from neonatally tolerized mice for FGG-specific suppressor capabilities. Spleen and thymus cells from Tol mice were able to specifically suppress the FGG PFC response of normal adult spleen cells only if the donor Tol mice were between the ages of six weeks and the age at which tolerance was lost.

The two series of experiments described above have been repeated using mice rendered tolerant as neonates to BSA, with similar findings, *i.e.*, BSA-specific B cell function was significantly decreased whenever mice were tolerant and BSA-specific regulatory cells could be found in spleens and thymuses of tolerant mice only if the tolerant donors were between six weeks of age and the age at which tolerance was lost. The finding that tolerogen-specific B cell function is decreased for the duration of neonatally induced tolerance agrees with work in other laboratories on tolerance to HGG induced neonatally [1] and *in utero*.[2] Our data, which suggest that tolerogen-specific immunosuppressive mechanisms function in the late stages of neonatally induced tolerance, agree with at least one previous study of tolerance to HGG induced *in utero*.[2]

To determine whether thymic-dependent regulation plays a role in the maintenance of B cell tolerance, neonatal nude mice and their euthymic litter-mates were injected with FGG. At various ages, their spleens were analyzed for B cell function, using the method described above. FGG-specific B cell tolerance in euthymic mice lasted two to three times longer than it did in nude mice. B cells from Tol euthymic mice were functionally depleted until 22 to 25 weeks of age, whereas those from Tol nudes were functionally depleted only until 8 to 11 weeks of age. Tolerance was specific in both nudes and euthymic littermates.

These results suggest that neonatally induced B cell tolerance to high doses of soluble antigens can be established and maintained, in the early stages, in the absence of T cell–mediated immune regulation. However, it is likely that thymic-dependent regulatory mechanisms are responsible for the prolongation of neonatally induced tolerance to soluble antigens.

REFERENCES

1. BENJAMIN, D. C. 1977. Neonatally induced tolerance to HGG: Duration in B cells and absence of specific suppressor cells. J. Immunol. **119:** 311.
2. WATERS, C. A., L. M. PILARSKI, T. G. WEGMAN & E. DIENER. 1979. Tolerance induction during ontogeny. I. Presence of active suppression in mice rendered tolerant *in utero* correlates with the breakdown of the tolerant state. J. Exp. Med. **149:** 1134.

SPECIFIC HUMAN PANCREATIC ISLET CELL PROTEINS RECOGNIZED BY ANTIBODIES IN DIABETIC CHILDREN

Steinunn Baekkeskov, Takahiro Kanatsuna, Jens H. Nielsen,
Birgitte Marner, and Åke Lernmark

Hagedorn Research Laboratory
2820 Gentofte, Denmark

Circulating antibodies that bind to the surface of viable pancreatic islet cells have been demonstrated in sera from many newly diagnosed insulin-dependent diabetic (IDD) patients. These antibodies can mediate a complement-dependent cytotoxic reaction and seem to bind mainly to the insulin-producing β-cells. These observations indicate that an autoimmune attack specific for β-cells may be involved in the pathogenesis of the disease. However, the target antigens for the circulating antibodies are unknown.

We have studied (1) whether autoantibodies in sera from newly diagnosed diabetic children can immunoprecipitate human islet cell proteins and (2) whether binding of the antibodies can affect the function of β-cells.

Human islets isolated from the pancreases of five cadaver kidney donors were labeled biosynthetically with ^{35}S methionine and lysed in 1% NP-40. After ultracentrifugation to remove cellular debris, the supernatant was incubated with normal human serum, followed by adsorption to formalin-fixed *Staphylococcus aureus*. Aliquots of the preabsorbed lysate were incubated with sera from ten newly diagnosed diabetic children or eight normal controls and the immune complexes were isolated by binding to Protein A Sepharose and analysed by SDS polyacrylamide gel electrophoresis, followed by autoradiography. To study the effect of the diabetic antibodies on β-cell function, the immunoglobulin fraction was isolated from the heat-inactivated sera of six newly diagnosed diabetic children and six normal controls by precipitation with 10% polyethylene glycol. After extensive dialysis against Swimms medium, the immunoglobulin fractions, at a final concentration of 10% (v/v), were used to perifuse dispersed rat islet cells supported in small Bio-Gel P-2 polyacrylamide columns. The dynamics of insulin release was determined by radioimmunoassay of fractions collected at various time intervals.

Sera from eight out of ten diabetic children precipitated a protein of M_r 64 000 from human pancreatic islet cell lysates. An additional protein at M_r 38 000 was precipitated by all four sera tested on islets isolated from a HLA-DR 3 positive pancreatic donor. Neither of these bands were precipitated by control sera, nor were they detected in immunoprecipitates of human lymphocyte lysates processed in parallel. While there was little effect at 5.5 mmol l^{-1} glucose, the immunoglobulin fractions of the sera from six diabetic children were found to inhibit insulin release from dispersed rat islet cells perifused with 30 mmol l^{-1} glucose. The results suggest that diabetic antibodies may be directed against 64 000 or 38 000 islet cell–specific proteins and that the binding of such antibodies to β-cells can block glucose-stimulated insulin release.

IMMUNOSUPPRESSIVE EFFECTS
OF POLYETHYLENE GLYCOL–MODIFIED ASPARAGINASES

Adrianne Bendich, David Kafkewitz, Abraham Abuchowski, and
Frank F. Davis

Rutgers University
Newark and New Brunswick, New Jersey 07102

Covalent attachment of methoxypolyethylene glycol (PEG) to the catalytically nonessential groups of enzymes can render the enzymes nonimmunogenic. Thus, an enzyme modified with PEG is not detected as a foreign protein, does not evoke an antibody response, does not react with any preformed antibody that might be present, and is not rapidly cleared from the bloodstream. Asparaginase is used to treat certain leukemias in children. The *Escherichia coli* asparaginase now in clinical use is recognized as a foreign protein by the immune system. The catalytic activities of this enzyme produce immunosuppressive side effects during therapy.

At present, it is not clear whether this immunosuppression is due to asparagine depletion or to glutamine depletion caused by the low level of glutaminase activity present in *E. coli* asparaginase. The anaerobic bacterium *Vibrio succinogenes* produces an asparaginase that is devoid of glutaminase activity. The elimination of immunogenicity by the covalent attachment of PEG permits one to compare the immunosuppressive effects of these two enzymes directly, without the complicating variable of the immune response.

The immunosuppressive effects of PEG-asparaginase from *V. succinogenes* (PEG-VS) and *E. coli* (PEG-EC) have been investigated in mice. Mitogen-induced blastogenesis of splenocytes harvested five days after *in vivo* administration of the PEG-enzymes show that PEG-VS is not immunosuppressive, whereas PEG-EC is immunosuppressive. Both enzymes cause some microsplenia. In mice with the L5178Y tumor and its associated LDH virus, which causes the circulating life of PEG-VS and native VS to be similar, tumor regression and its attendant immunological changes are identical in animals treated with PEG-VS and with native VS.

These data indicate that the glutaminase activity of the *E. coli* asparaginase is responsible for the enzyme's immunosuppressive side effects. The absolute substrate specificity of the *V. succinogenes* asparaginase eliminates its immunosuppressive effects; PEG modification of the *V. succinogenes* enzyme eliminates its immunogenicity. We suggest that the PEG asparaginase VS should prove to be the ideal asparaginase preparation for therapies requiring asparagine depletion.

MULTIPLE SIGNALS FOR THE INDUCTION
OF SPECIFIC SUPPRESSOR T CELLS

Jonathan S. Bromberg,* Terry L. Delovitch,† and
Mark I. Greene *

*Department of Pathology
Harvard Medical School
Boston, Massachusetts 02115

† C.H. Best Institute
University of Toronto
Toronto, Ontario, Canada

Work in the trinitophenyl (TNP) system of contact sensitivity revealed that intravenous injection of TNP-coupled syngeneic spleen cells tolerized recipient mice and generated a set of antigen-specific suppressor T cells (Ts). If high densities of antigen were coupled to the cell surface (10 mM trinitrobenzene sulfonic acid (TNBS)), then the Ts generated were genetically unrestricted by the MHC in their ability to transfer suppression. If low densities of antigen were coupled (0.01 mM TNBS), then specific suppression could be transferred to H-2 allogeneic but not syngeneic strains. This finding led to the hypothesis that suboptimal doses of antigen injected intravenously led to the priming of a set of precursor Ts (pre-Ts) that required a second signal, provided by an allogeneic effect, in order to express their suppressive potential. This hypothesis was confirmed by titrating putative pre-Ts and allogeneic cells into a strain syngeneic to the pre-Ts. Only pre-Ts plus allogeneic cells could suppress the recipient; neither was effective alone. A further analysis of the allogeneic effect showed that an I-J allogeneic effect was necessary and sufficient as a second signal. Allogeneic effects directed against K, D, I-A, Mls, or background allo-antigens were ineffective. Furthermore, parental and F_1 combinations revealed that the allogeneic effect was directed against the pre-Ts; whole haplotype bystander allogeneic effects were ineffective signals. If the allogeneic effect is taken to be a reflection of normal physiological processes, then high hapten epitope density may be equivalent to low density plus an I-J allogeneic effect, by virtue of the fact that high density could modify cell surface I-J determinants, generate "altered self," and hence create the equivalent of an I-J allogeneic effect.

These findings were duplicated in the suppression of the azobenzene arsonate (ABA) system of delayed hypersensitivity. The predominance of idiotypic and anti-idiotypic interactions in this system permitted a further analysis of pre-Ts and the signals that effect the induction of specific suppression. Cells that were induced by lightly haptenated cells and required an I-J allogeneic effect were found to be Thy 1.2+, Lyt 1+2-, I-J+, and idiotype-positive. Therefore, these resemble the fully active first order Ts (Ts_1) induced by heavily haptenated cells. Other protocols known to induce Ts_1 (e.g., anti-idiotype administered intravenously) were rendered ineffective when low or suboptimal doses of these reagents were given. However, the provision of an allogeneic effect resulted in very potent suppression, while neither signal alone (anti-idiotype, allogeneic effect) was suppressive. Idiotypic antibody given intravenously is not suppressive in this experimental system; however, it should be able to interact with anti-idiotypic second order Ts (Ts$_2$). Hence, idiotype plus an I-J allogeneic effect was able to induce suppression. Therefore, the second allogeneic signals can act on both Ts$_1$ and Ts$_2$ cells. A number of other idiotypic and anti-idiotypic reagents, which did not interfere with immunity when given by themselves, were found to be potent first signals for the induction of suppression when an I-J allogeneic effect was induced. Therefore, a two-signal model for the activation of Ts can be envisioned. The first signal interacts with a clonally distributed antigen-specific receptor, while the second interacts with a cell surface molecule that is presumably nonclonal (*e.g.*, I-J).

An I-J allogeneic effect was induced *in vitro* and the culture supernatant was analyzed for its ability to activate pre-Ts. Upon transfer with pre-Ts, the crude unfractionated supernatant was able to induce suppression, while neither pre-Ts nor factor alone were effective. Fractionation of the supernatant revealed that there were several distinct components that could independently activate pre-Ts. One of the components was 30 000–35 000 daltons, pI 4.0–5.0—presumably interleukin-2. A second was 80 000–100 000 daltons and genetically unrestricted in its activity. A third activity was 40 000–70 000 daltons, pI 5.5–6.0, and genetically restricted to the allogeneic effect stimulator, type H-2.

HAPTEN-SPECIFIC
CELL-MEDIATED LYMPHOLYSIS UNRESPONSIVENESS

Larry D. Butler, Stephen D. Miller, and Henry N. Claman

Departments of Medicine and of Microbiology and Immunology
University of Colorado Health Sciences Center
Denver, Colorado 80262

The induction of trinitrophenyl (TNP)-specific cell-mediated lympholysis (CML) unresponsiveness in mice has been difficult to achieve. Most protocols that are tolerogenic for TNP-specific delayed-type hypersensitivity and antibody responses have proven to be ineffective in preventing primary TNP-specific CML responses.[1-3] We have been studying the regulation of TNP-specific CML responses generated *in vitro* and have developed protocols that render mice specifically unresponsive to *in vitro* generation of CML activity. We have previously reported that the induction of TNP-specific CML unresponsiveness in adult mice following a single injection of water-soluble hapten (trinitrobenzene sulphonic acid, TNBS), is cyclophosphamide sensitive, adult thymectomy resistant, and associated with H-2 loci, in that H-2^d mice, but not H-2^k mice, can be rendered unresponsive.[4] Furthermore, TNP-specific CML activity could be partially restored in those mice tolerized as adults if concanavalin A–induced supernatants were added to the tolerant responder cells *in vitro*. Since tolerance to other antigens has been reported to be easier to induce during the neonatal period, in this study we have examined the capacity of several TNP-congeners to induce TNP-specific CML tolerance when the potential tolerogenic treatment is begun during the neonatal period and chronically maintained. Using this protocol, chronic treatment with heavily irradiated TNP-modified syngeneic lymphoid cells does not render mice tolerant but actually primes TNP-specific cytotoxic activity *in vitro*. In contrast, chronic treatment with TNP-modified syngeneic red blood cells induces TNP-specific CML tolerance in a strain-dependent manner, in that Balb/c, but not C3H/HeN, mice were rendered unresponsive. The most effective tolerogen was TNBS. Chronic treatment with TNBS induced TNP-specific CML tolerance in both Balb/c and C3H/HeN mice.

This observation is especially noteworthy, since we have previously shown that a single injection of TNBS does not induce tolerance in adult C3H/HeN mice.[4] The unresponsiveness induced following chronic TNBS treatment could be partially reversed if concanavalin A–induced supernatants were added to the tolerant responder cells *in vitro*. These latter results suggest that the TNP-specific CML tolerance induced with chronic exposure to tolerogen, TNBS, involves deficient amplifier T helper cell activity and, perhaps, altered precytotoxic T cell function. Furthermore, the effectiveness of the chronic TNBS treatment in the C3H/HeN strain, when compared to the inability to induce tolerance in adult C3H/HeN mice after a single injection of TNBS, suggests that different mechanisms may be responsible for the induction and maintenance of the TNP-specific CML unresponsiveness induced by chronic exposure to tolerogen, as opposed to that induced by a single exposure to tolerogen.

REFERENCES

1. FUJIWARA, H., R. B. LEVY, G. M. SHEARER & W. P. TERRY. 1979. Studies on *in vivo* priming of the TNP-reactive cytotoxic effector cell system. I. Comparison of effects of intravenous inoculation with TNP-conjugated cells on the development of contact sensitivity and cell-mediated lympholysis. J. Immunol. **123:** 423.
2. FINBERG, R., S. A. BURAKOFF, B. BENACERRAF & M. I. GREENE. 1979. The cytolytic T lymphocyte response to trinitrophenyl-modified syngeneic cells. II. Evidence for antigen-specific suppressor T cells. J. Immunol. **123:** 1210.
3. BULTER, L. D., H. L. WONG & J. R. BATTISTO. 1980. Use of immunotolerance to dissect the mechanisms regulating appearance of hapten-specific killer T cells *in vivo*. J. Immunol. **124:** 1245.
4. BUTLER, L. D., S. D. MILLER & H. N. CLAMAN. 1981. Unresponsiveness in hapten-specific cytotoxic T lymphocytes. I. Characteristics of tolerance induction in adult mice. J. Immunol. **127:** 1383.

INDUCTION OF SUPPRESSOR CELLS
FOR LYMPH NODE CELL PROLIFERATION
AFTER CONTACT SENSITIZATION OF MICE
WITH 3-HEPTADECYLCATECHOL

I. S. Dunn,* D. J. Liberato,† N. Castagnoli,† and V. S. Byers *

*Department of Dermatology
†Department of Pharmaceutical Chemistry
University of California, San Francisco
San Francisco, California 94143

Contact sensitivity with the general properties of delayed-type hypersensitivity (DTH) can be induced in mice by 3-heptadecylcatechol (HDC), a component of poison oak urushiol oil. Sensitization is routinely effected by painting on abdominal skin and is assessed by measuring ear swellings produced after ear challenge. Further studies of the nature of the sensitization process were made by monitoring the induction of lymph node cell (LNC) proliferation after cutaneous treatment with HDC. Proliferation was assessed by testing the ^{14}C-thymidine uptake of cell suspensions *in vitro*. After abdominal painting of mice with HDC, inguinal LNC proliferation was detectable, peaking after 5–6 d. Ear painting with the standard challenge dose of HDC alone resulted in cervical LNC proliferation, peaking after five days. However, if mice were sensitized on their abdomens before ear challenge, the cervical LNC proliferation was strongly suppressed. Investigations were then performed to determine whether HDC sensitization induced regulatory cells against the proliferative response. Transfer of pooled LNC from sensitized donors (at later times after sensitization) to normal recipients suppressed the induction of draining inguinal LNC proliferation subsequently arising after recipient sensitization. This suppression was more marked when the donor LNC were taken from mice at times after the normal peak of proliferation. As few as 10^7 LNC taken from mice 10 d after sensitization could transfer suppression. The HDC-induced suppressive effect appeared to have a nonspecific component, but such suppression was more effective against proliferation induced by HDC itself, implying that a specific component also existed. Cells mediating suppression were T lymphocytes, as evidenced by their sensitivity to treatment with anti-Thy-1.2 antibody and complement. However, LNC containing such suppressor cells could not suppress the *in vitro* activity of cells already proliferating at optimal levels, nor could such LNC block the induction of DTH in recipient mice. Hence, this afferent suppression may regulate the proliferation of specific lymphocyte subclasses involved in contact hypersensitivity to HDC without preventing the induction or expression of T cells mediating DTH.

SUPPRESSION OF CONTACT SENSITIVITY IN MICE BY CUTANEOUS APPLICATION OF A POISON IVY URUSHIOL ANALOGUE

I. S. Dunn,* D. J. Liberato,† N. Castagnoli,† and V. S. Byers*

*Department of Dermatology
†Department of Pharmaceutical Chemistry
University of California, San Francisco
San Francisco, California 94143

Abdominal painting of mice with 3-heptadecylcatechol (HDC) or 3-penta-decylcatechol (PDC) (components of poison oak and ivy urushiol oils, respectively) results in contact sensitization with characteristics of delayed-type hypersensitivity. Sensitivity is gauged by assessing ear swelling increases after ear challenge. It was found that HDC and PDC were completely crossreactive in this *in vivo* assay. Studies of the chemical reactivities of these catechols have been made to attempt to define the basis for their immunogenicity. It is known that attack by nucleophilic species (including those found on proteins) on the ring moiety of the *o*-quinone intermediate of PDC (derived from the oxidation of the catechol) operates regiospecifically, with amino-nucleophiles attacking only the 5-position, and thiol-nucleophiles attacking only the 6-position. An available series of PDC analogues monomethylated at the 4-, 5-, or 6-positions on the catechol ring were used to study molecular requirements for sensitization. These analogues are still capable of forming quinones and can be attacked by nucleophiles, except where sites on the ring are blocked by methyl groups. Under conditions where HDC or PDC produced strong sensitization, only 5-methyl-3-pentadecylcatechol (5-Me-PDC), and not the corresponding 4-methyl or 6-methyl analogues, was an ineffective sensitizer. However, 5-Me-PDC could still induce a proliferative response in inguinal lymph nodes after its abdominal application, as assessed by ^{14}C-thymidine uptake of cell suspensions *in vitro*. The possibility that 5-Me-PDC preferentially induced a suppressive response was then tested. A primary painting of mice with this analogue suppressed the subsequent development of sensitization after painting ten days later on a separate skin site with HDC. In contrast, similar pretreatment with HDC itself enhanced sensitization to the secondary painting, whereas the unrelated sensitizers picryl chloride and oxazolone had no effect. Neither the corresponding 4-methyl or 6-methyl PDC derivatives produced significant suppression; only the 4-methyl compound produced enhancement of sensitization to the second treatment with HDC. Lymph node cells taken from mice ten days after treatment with 5-Me-PDC, but not PDC, depressed the induction of PDC sensitization when transferred into normal recipients. These results suggest that cutaneous treatment of mice with 5-Me-PDC induces a cellular population with suppressive activity against the induction of HDC or PDC sensitization and that the suppression is related to the blocking of specific covalent binding sites on the catechol ring.

T CELLS DO NOT MEDIATE CLONAL DELETION IN TRANSPLANTATION TOLERANCE

Rebecca S. Gruchalla and J. Wayne Streilein

Department of Cell Biology
University of Texas Health Science Center
Dallas, Texas 75235

Both *in vitro* and *in vivo* assays were used to discover the nature of the processes underlying the unresponsive state in mice rendered tolerant of selected *H-2* antigens neonatally. By numerous criteria, tolerant mice appear to be clonally deleted of lymphocytes specific for the *H-2* antigens encountered at birth. Lymphocytes from tolerant animals do not respond to the tolerated alloantigens in mixed lymphocyte reactions (MLR), cell-mediated lympholysis (CML) assays, or graft *versus* host reactions (GVHR), nor do "tolerant" cells suppress these reactivities. In addition, precursors of antigen-reactive cells (ARC) cannot be unmasked by polyclonal lymphocyte activation with concanavalin A, nor can they be identified amongst thymocytes. These *in vitro* data support the hypothesis of a clonal deletion mechanism of tolerance maintenance.

In contrast to the *in vitro* studies, results from *in vivo* experiments indicate that the tolerance phenotype may not result from a passive process alone. The findings that tolerance is not easily abolished in class II tolerant mice after these animals are given normal lymphoid cells and that lymphocytes from Ia-tolerant animals are able to transfer the unresponsive state adoptively indicate that an active process does participate in the maintenance of unresponsiveness to certain *H-2* alloantigens. In light of these results, as well as those obtained from the *in vitro* studies, we conclude that transplantation tolerance of Ia alloantigens must be maintained by more than one mechanism. Since Ia-tolerant mice are devoid of ARC by all *in vitro* criteria, clonal deletion appears to be the mechanism by which tolerance is maintained in these animals. In addition, the ability of "tolerant" lymphoid cells to transfer unresponsiveness adoptively indicates that an active regulatory mechanism must also participate in the maintenance of tolerance.

Although deletion of ARC may be primarily responsible for tolerance maintenance in the intact animal, the failure of adoptive transfer recipients of unresponsiveness to reject Ia-disparate allografts cannot be explained by this mechanism. These animals, unlike intact tolerant mice, display an *in vitro* phenotype of reactivity, and, at the same time, bear impeccable Ia-disparate allografts. Thus, it appears that these two groups of animals may be maintaining *in vivo* unresponsiveness by different mechanisms. More specifically, the mechanism that is transferable and responsible for maintaining tolerance in the adoptive transfer recipient may not be the primary mechanism of tolerance maintenance in the intact animal. The finding that all neonatally tolerant animals, including Ia-tolerant mice, lack mature ARC and suppressor cells of MLR, CML, and GVHR suggests that maintenance of tolerance occurs at an early stage of lymphocyte development. Since adoptive transfer recipients of tolerance possess cells specific for the tolerated Ia alloantigens in their peripheral lymphoid tissues, the mechanism maintaining unresponsiveness in these animals must act on a mature lymphocyte population. In light of these observations, it would appear that the primary mechanism by which tolerance is maintained in intact Ia-tolerant mice is classical clonal deletion. The cell-mediated active mechanism that is detected by adoptive transfer may function only as a fail-safe mechanism should ARC escape deletion. Others, too, have suggested that tolerance may be maintained primarily by a deletion mechanism and that active regulatory processes play only an ancillary role.[1-3]

An attempt was made to identify the nature of the cells responsible for the active process detected in Ia-tolerant animals. The role that T cells play and the role played by semiallogeneic descendants of the original tolerance-inducing inoculum were examined. Using the adoptive transfer assay system, it was found that neither of these cell types are necessary to transfer unresponsiveness successfully to naive recipients. These results indicate that the unresponsive phenotype displayed by the adoptive transfer recipients is not mediated by suppressor T cells from the tolerant donor nor is it induced *de novo* by contaminating semiallogeneic cells present within the transfer inoculum. Thus, other cell types, possibly B cells or their products, must be responsible for the failure of adoptive transfer recipients to reject Ia-disparate allografts.

REFERENCES

1. ELKINS, W. L.   1972.   Cell. Immunol. **4:** 192.
2. WATERS, C. A., L. M. PILARSKI, T. G. WEGMANN & E. DIENER.   1979.   J. Exp. Med. **149:** 1134.
3. WEIGLE, W. O.   1980.   *In* Strategies of Immune Regulation. E. Sercarz and A. J. Cunningham, Eds.: 521. Academic Press. New York.

MECHANISMS OF SPECIFIC TOLERANCE INDUCED
BY CYCLOSPORIN A *

Allan D. Hess, Peter J. Tutschka, and George W. Santos

Bone Marrow Transplant Unit
Oncology Center
The Johns Hopkins University
Baltimore, Maryland 21205

Cyclosporin A (CyA) is a nonmyelotoxic immunosuppressive agent that facilitates the induction of transplantation tolerance across major histocompatibility barriers in several organ allograft animal models. The mode of action of CyA and its role in establishing specific immunological unresponsiveness remain unclear. The present studies were undertaken to determine the effect of CyA on T lymphocyte subpopulations responding in the human mixed lymphocyte response (MLR) and to determine if this agent can induce specific tolerance *in vitro*.

After adding CyA to MLR at doses (1.0 and 2.5 μg ml^{-1}) that resulted in minimal levels of proliferation, the formation of cytotoxic effector lymphocytes (Tc) was completely suppressed, while alloantigen-induced suppressor cells (Ts) were found at levels comparable to control cultures without CyA. The suppressor cells from CyA-treated and control MLR cultures were identified as Ia-positive T lymphocytes belonging to the OKT8 subclass, as defined in monoclonal antibody plus complement depletion experiments. Further studies revealed that CyA inhibited the production of T cell growth factor (TCGF) in primary MLR. More importantly, the precursor Tc did not acquire the ability to respond to TCGF in the presence of CyA, perhaps maintaining their immunological precursor status.

The disequilibrium between Ts and cytotoxic effector cells induced by CyA in primary MLR results in the establishment of specific immunological unresponsiveness. Primed lymphocytes from CyA-treated MLR harvested on day 12 of culture were unable to generate Tc upon rechallenge with the original sensitizing alloantigen, but were capable of generating normal levels of CML activity after stimulation with unrelated third party antigens when tested on day 7 of culture. Fractionation of the CyA-tolerized cells over nylon wool columns restored the capacity to generate Tc upon challenge (of the nonadherent cells) with the sensitizing alloantigen. Recombining adherent and nonadherent cell populations re-established the specific immunological unresponsiveness.

Efforts were undertaken to define the mode of action of the Ts activated in MLR in the presence of CyA. Suppressor cells added to fresh MLR suppressed the formation of TCGF. More importantly, the Ts inhibited the fresh responding cells from acquiring the ability to respond to this growth factor, perhaps explaining the ability of the Ts to maintain tolerance.

* This research was supported by grants from the National Institutes of Health. nos. AI–17256, AM–26502, and CA–15396.

From our data, it appears likely that CyA inhibits the maturation of the precursor cytotoxic T cell while allowing the activation of suppressor lymphocytes. Once this disequilibrium is achieved, the suppressor cells appear to maintain tolerance not only by controlling the production of TCGF, but also, more importantly, by controlling the development of responsiveness to this growth factor.

DEPRESSED SECONDARY RESPONSE
OF CYTOTOXIC T CELLS TO TNP-LABELED
SYNGENEIC CELLS IN ULTRAVIOLET-IRRADIATED MICE *

Pamela J. Jensen and Marcia A. Gray

NCI–Frederick Cancer Research Facility
Cancer Biology Program
Frederick, Maryland 21701

Ultraviolet (uv) irradiation of mice has previously been found to induce selective immunological unresponsiveness. Ultraviolet-irradiated mice show both a depressed delayed-type hypersensitivity response to contact sensitizers [1, 2] and an enhanced susceptibility to uv-induced tumor transplants.[3] Although the latter effect requires more radiation than the former, the unresponsiveness is associated, in each case, with the formation of antigen-specific T suppressor cells.[4, 5] A defect in the presentation of certain antigens, including contact sensitizers, is also found in uv-irradiated mice, and recent evidence suggests that this antigen-presenting cell defect may be responsible for the generation of suppressor cells in these animals.

To explore the immunological consequences of uv irradiation further, we compared the primary and secondary responses of cytotoxic T lymphocytes (Tc), both to 1,3,5-trinitrophenyl (TNP)-labeled syngeneic spleen cells and to allogeneic spleen cells in normal and uv-irradiated mice. Five to six days before the initiation of an experiment, Balb/c female mice were shaved of dorsal hair and exposed to 3 h of radiation from FS40 sunlamps. This source delivered an average dose rate of 4.5 J m^{-2} s^{-1}, with 80% of the total energy output in the wavelength range 280–340 nm.

To examine the primary Tc responses, spleen cells from control or uv-irradiated mice were stimulated in culture for 4–5 d either with TNP-labeled syngeneic spleen cells or with allogeneic (C57BL/6) spleen cells. In both cases, the spleen cells from uv-irradiated animals exhibited a primary *in vitro* cytotoxic response within the normal range.

To examine the secondary Tc responses, control and uv-irradiated mice were primed subcutaneously with either TNP-labeled syngeneic spleen cells or allogeneic (C57BL/6) spleen cells. Seven or eight days later, spleen cells from these immunized animals were restimulated *in vitro* with cells identical to those used for priming. The secondary *in vitro* cytotoxic response generated against TNP-syngeneic cells was dramatically depressed by uv radiation in comparison to a normal secondary response. In contrast, the secondary *in vitro* cytotoxic response to allogeneic stimulation was normal in spleen cultures from uv-irradiated mice.

These findings suggest that uv irradiation *in vivo* may be exploited not only for the induction of subtle and selective unresponsiveness, but also for the study of the differences in cellular interactions required for the production of various types of cytotoxic T cells.

* This research was supported by the National Cancer Institute of the Department of Health and Human Services under a contract with Litton Bionetics, Inc. no. NO 1–CO–75380.

REFERENCES

1. NOONAN, F. P., M. L. KRIPKE, G. M. PEDERSEN & M. I. GREENE. 1981. Immunology **43:** 527.
2. GREENE, M. I., M. S. SY, M. L. KRIPKE & B. BENACERRAF. 1979. Proc. Nat. Acad. Sci. USA **76:** 6591.
3. FISHER, M. S. & M. L. KRIPKE. 1977. Proc. Nat. Acad. Sci. USA **74:** 1688.
4. FISHER, M. S. & M. L. KRIPKE. 1978. J. Immunol. **121:** 1139.
5. NOONAN, F. P., E. C. DeFABO & M. L. KRIPKE. 1981. Photochem. Photobiol. **34:** 683.

NONSPECIFIC SUPPRESSOR CELLS
Modulation of Hyporesponsiveness in Tumor-Bearing Mice to Dinitrochlorobenzene

J. M. Jessup,* B. D. Kahan,† and N. R. Pellis †

*Department of Surgery
M. D. Anderson Hospital and Tumor Institute
Houston, Texas 77030

†Department of Surgery
University of Texas Medical School at Houston
Houston, Texas 77004

Modulation of the response to simple chemicals like dinitrochlorobenzene (DNCB) correlates with prognosis in both human patients [1] and animals [2] with neoplastic disease. C_3H/HeJ mice bearing a low passage syngeneic transplantable methycholanthrene–induced fibrosarcoma, MCA-F, do not respond to an otherwise sensitizing dose of 2 mg DNCB that is followed, 5 to 10 d later, by challenge with 50 μg DNCB in a hind footpad. Tumor-induced hyporesponsiveness is mediated by nonspecific suppressor cells (NSC), which reside in the spleen. The intraperitoneal adoptive transfer of as few as 10^6 spleen cells (SC) harvested from tumor-bearing (TB) mice 10 d after tumor initiation inhibits primary sensitization to DNCB of tumor-free syngeneic mice: $36 \pm 4\%$ footpad swelling (FPS) for NSC recipients *versus* $47 \pm 5\%$ FPS for DNCB sensitized mice or $29 \pm 3\%$ for controls, $p < 0.01$, $n = 9$–10 per group. The NSC is a macrophage, since it adheres to plastic, phagocytoses carbonyl iron, is radioresistant, and lacks Thy 1.2. Activation of NSC is independent of tumor immunity, since hyporesponsiveness to DNCB is demonstrable in mice bearing progressively growing tumors, but not in tumor immune mice.

NSC act upon the elicitation rather than the induction phase because adoptive transfer of lymph node cells (LNC) from hyporesponsive recipients of NSC confers delayed hypersensitivity (DH) upon normal mice when challenged in a footpad: $40 \pm 3\%$ FPS for recipients of LNC from donors made hyporesponsive to DNCB by NSC *versus* $41 \pm 3\%$ FPS for recipients of LNC from DNCB-sensitized mice *versus* $25 \pm 2\%$ FPS for control mice, $p < 0.001$, ten mice per group. Cotransfer of NSC and lymphoid cells from DNCB–sensitive donors indicates that NSC do not directly inhibit effector cells for DH to DNCB. Furthermore, NSC must be transferred within the first three days after sensitization with DNCB to inhibit elicitation of DH 10 d after sensitization. Transfer of NSC six or nine days after sensitization does not inhibit elicitation of DH. These results suggest that NSC suppress effector cell function by inhibiting an auxiliary cell or factor necessary for effector cell function rather than effector cells directly. Furthermore, the NSC induced by progressive neoplastic disease modulate *in vivo* delayed hypersensitivity to chemical sensitizers in TB hosts.

References

1. EILBER, F. R. & D. L. MORTON. 1970. Cancer **25**: 362.
2. JESSUP, J. M., M. H. COHEN, M. M. TOMASZEWSKI & E. L. FELIX. 1976. J. Nat. Cancer Inst. **57**: 1077.

CELL-CELL INTERACTIONS IN THE MOUSE THYMUS

B. Kyewski, R. V. Rouse,* and H. S. Kaplan

Cancer Biology Research Laboratory
Department of Radiology
* *Department of Pathology*
Stanford University School of Medicine
Stanford, California 94305

T cell differentiation can be divided into pre-, intra-, and postthymic stages. The induction of self-tolerance, T cell subset specification, and the selection of self H-2-restricted T cells have been ascribed to the intrathymic pathway of T cell maturation, the precise sites and mechanisms responsible for these events being unknown. It has been suggested that the thymic microenvironment consists of localized concentrations of soluble factors (*e.g.*, thymic hormones and interleukin 2) and/or direct receptor-mediated cell-cell interactions. We have isolated multicellular complexes from the mouse thymus by enzymatic dissociation and subsequent 1 g sedimentation in order to study intrathymic cell-cell recognition. Two distinct types of highly purified complexes were identified by their intra-thymic location and cellular composition.[1, 2]

Type I. Lympho-epithelial complexes comprising PNA+, Lyt 1,2,3+, medium-sized, cortisone-sensitive thymocytes within subcapsular and outer cortical I-A+ epithelial cells ("thymic nurse cells").

Type II. Rosette formations between PNA+, Lyt 1,2,3+ lymphoblasts and nonlymphoid cells (50% I-A+) located in the inner cortex (and medulla?). The nonlymphoid cells comprise a subpopulation of highly phagocytic cells. By electron microscopy it was possible to distinguish typical macrophages and dendritic (interdigitating?) cells in the nonlymphoid population.

The association between the thymocytes and the nonlymphoid cells in both types of complexes is not an *in vitro* secondary event, but pre-exists *in vivo*. Intact complexes cannot be recovered in the presence of metabolic inhibitors, EDTA, and cytochalasin B, which suggests that the binding between the lymphocytes and the nonlymphoid cells is an active receptor-mediated recognition event. Studies in semiallogeneic bone marrow chimeras revealed that: (1) the epithelial component of type I complexes was consistently of host origin, (2) some type II complexes were completely bone marrow–derived soon after reconstitution, and (3) in both complexes, association between semiallogeneic partner cells occurred. The first isolation of rosette-like structures (presumably type II) on day 14 of gestation coincides with the first detection of I-A antigen expression on nonlymphoid cells during ontogeny. Postirradiation kinetics suggest that the type II complexes represent a compartment that is the first site of repopulation by bone marrow immigrants.

The different types of cellular interactions in the thymus presumably represent locally and functionally separate microenvironments, which might be involved in the induction of self-tolerance and in the selection of T cell precursors *via* self-recognition. The isolation and purification of defined thymocyte subpopulations (less than 5% of the whole thymic population) that bind to autologous nonlymphoid cells *in vivo* offer a new approach to the analysis of recognition and selection events in the thymus.

393

REFERENCES

1. KYEWSKI, B. & H. S. KAPLAN. 1982. J. Immunol. **128:** 2287–94.
2. KYEWSKI, B., R. V. ROUSE & H. S. KAPLAN. 1982. Proc. Nat. Acad. Sci. USA. In press.

RESISTANCE TO EXPERIMENTAL AUTOIMMUNE ENCEPHALOMYELITIS IS ASSOCIATED WITH ANTIGEN-INDUCED INHIBITION OF LYMPHOCYTE RESPONSES *

W. D. Lyman, A. S. Kadish, C. F. Brosnan, and C. S. Raine

Department of Pathology
Albert Einstein College of Medicine
Bronx, New York 10461

Experimental autoimmune encephalomyelitis (EAE) has long served as a model for studies on delayed-type hypersensitivity [1,2] and the inflammatory demyelinating diseases.[3] EAE can be induced by sensitizing animals with whole white matter, myelin basic protein (MBP), which is the major EAE-associated antigen, or with fragments of MBP in complete Freund's adjuvant (CFA). The expression of disease depends upon T cells being sensitized to central nervous system antigens.[4]

It is known that variations in clinical susceptibility to EAE occur.[5] It has been suggested that resistance in animals that fail to develop clinical disease is the result of an immunological suppressor mechanism mediated by T cells.[6] Lymphocyte responses to EAE-associated antigens, both *in vivo* and *in vitro*, have been found to vary with clinical susceptibility or resistance to EAE.[7] These findings prompted us to examine the possibility that such variations may reflect different immunoregulatory mechanisms controlling disease and resistance. The present study investigated the responsiveness of guinea pig (GP) spleen cells (SC) to (1) MBP, (2) concanavalin A (con A), a T cell mitogen, and the effect of MBP on responses to con A. Similar studies also investigated SC responses to purified protein derivative (PPD) of tuberculin and the effect of PPD on SC responses to con A.

Random-bred Hartley, inbred Strain 2, and Strain 13 GP were inoculated with bovine whole white matter in CFA. 66% (69 out of 103) of the Hartley GP developed clinical signs of EAE, while the remaining 34% (34 out of 103) did not display any signs of disease. None of the Strain 2 and all of the Strain 13 GP developed clinical signs of EAE. Histological examination of sections taken from brain and spinal cord revealed that clinically ill Hartley and Strain 13 and all of the Strain 2 GP had pronounced lesions characteristic of EAE. In contrast, similar sections from clinically well Hartley GP showed fewer and less severe changes.

The lymphocyte transformation assay used to measure the blastogenic responses of SC to MBP and con A revealed four different sets of responses *in vitro:* (1) SC from all animals tested had blastogenic responses to con A, (2) only SC from clinically ill GP had a blastogenic response to MBP; (3) only SC from clinically resistant Hartley GP were inhibited from a blastogenic response to con A by MBP, and (4) in contrast, when SC from clinically resistant,

* This research was supported by grants from the United States Public Health Service, nos. NS–07098, NS–11920, and CA–22906.

clinically ill, and CFA control GP were exposed to con A in the presence of PPD, the blastogenic response was enhanced.

Although clinically resistant Hartley GP did not have a blastogenic response to MBP, the discovery of MBP-induced inhibition of the con A response suggested that the animals were indeed sensitized to MBP. To further confirm that clinically resistant Hartley GP were sensitized, other immunological parameters were examined. Plasmas collected from EAE-sensitized GP (both clinically ill and resistant) of all strains studied had equivalent titers of anti-MBP antibody, as demonstrated by immunodiffusion. Furthermore, skin testing also showed that all EAE-inoculated Hartley GP were sensitized to both MBP and PPD.

These experiments have shown that the clinical resistance and reduced histological changes characteristic of EAE correlated with an antigen-induced (MBP) inhibition of SC responses to a T cell mitogen. The data suggest that clinical resistance to EAE in Hartley GP is mediated by an immunological suppressor mechanism. Clinical resistance to EAE in Strain 2 GP appears to be controlled by a different mechanism.

REFERENCES

1. WAKSMAN, B. H.   1959.   Int. Arch. Allergy Suppl. 14: 1.
2. PATERSON, P. Y.   1976.   In Textbook of Immunopathology. P. A. Miescher and H. J. Muller-Eberhard, Eds.: 179–213. Grune & Stratton. New York.
3. RAINE, C. S.   1976.   In Progress in Neuropathology, Vol. 3. H. M. Zimmerman, Ed.: 225–51. Grune & Stratton. New York.
4. WEIGLE, W. O.   1980.   In Advances in Immunology, Vol. 30. F. J. Dixon and H. G. Kunkel, Eds.: 159–273. Academic Press. New York.
5. STONE, S. H.   1969.   Proc. Soc. Exp. Biol. Med. 132: 341.
6. LANDO, Z., D. TEITELBAUM & R. ARNON.   1980.   Nature (London) 287: 551.
7. LYMAN, W. D., A. S. KADISH & C. S. RAINE.   1981.   Cell. Immunol. 63: 409.

DONOR MARROW–DERIVED SUPPRESSOR CELLS IN SKIN ALLOGRAFT UNRESPONSIVENESS INDUCED IN ANTILYMPHOCYTE SERUM–TREATED MARROW-INJECTED MICE

Takashi Maki, Mary L. Wood, James J. Gozzo, and
Anthony P. Monaco

Department of Surgery
Harvard Medical School
Cancer Research Institute
New England Deaconess Hospital
Boston, Massachusetts 02115

Specific unresponsiveness to skin allografts can be induced in (C57BL/6 × A)F_1 (B6AF$_1$; H-2$^{b/k, d}$) mice treated with antilymphocyte serum (ALS) on days −1 and 2 relative to grafting with C3H (H-2^k) skin on day 0 by the injection on day 7 of 25 × 10^6 C3H whole marrow or 10^6 lymphoid cell–enriched fraction obtained by a unit gravity sedimentation of normal C3H marrow.[1, 2] Analysis of cell-mediated immune reactivity in marrow-injected B6AF$_1$ recipients shows prolonged suppression of the proliferative response to C3H alloantigens.[3] Therefore, the possible involvement of suppressor cells in this model was investigated.

When spleen cells of marrow-injected B6AF$_1$ recipients bearing intact C3H grafts were added to the mixed lymphocyte culture (MLC) of normal B6AF$_1$ responders and mitomycin-C-treated C3H spleen cells, marked suppression of the proliferative response occurred. Suppressor activity was C3H alloantigen specific, since the spleen cells failed to inhibit the B6AF$_1$ anti-B10.AKM (H-2^m) response, which is comparable in magnitude to the B6AF$_1$ anti-C3H response and the stronger B6AF$_1$ anti-B10.D2 response. Although spleen cells of control B6AF$_1$ mice given ALS and C3H skin grafts alone were also capable of suppressing the B6AF$_1$ anti-C3H response, the suppressor activity in these mice persisted for a much shorter time.

The origin of the suppressor cells present in the spleens of marrow-injected B6AF$_1$ recipients was investigated by pretreating the spleen cells with either anti-H-2, anti-Thy 1, or anti-I-J sera and complement (C) prior to MLC. Treatment with anti-H-2K^b or anti-Thy 1.2 serum plus C abrogated the anti-C3H as well as the anti-DBA/2 mixed lymphocyte reaction (MLR). When the antiserum-treated cells were added to the MLC of normal B6AF$_1$ and C3H spleen cells, cultures containing anti-H-2D^k or anti-Thy 1.2 serum–treated cells showed increased MLR, while those containing anti-H-2K^b serum-treated cells showed much greater suppression of the anti-C3H response. In contrast, anti DBA/2 MLR was significantly depressed in cultures containing anti-H-2K^b- and anti-Thy 1.2–treated cells. These results indicate that the suppressor cells present in marrow-injected B6AF$_1$ recipients are H-2D^k-bearing T cells of donor C3H marrow origin.

When these spleen cells were pretreated with either anti-I-J^b or anti-I-J^k serum plus C, abrogation of suppressor activity was obtained by anti-I-J^k serum, but not by anti-I-J^b serum. Since the suppressor activity of spleen cells obtained from control mice given ALS and grafts was abrogated by both anti-I-J^k and I-J^b sera, these results confirmed that the suppressor cells present late in the marrow-injected B6AF$_1$ mice are of donor (C3H) origin, whereas those present in the control mice are of host (B6AF$_1$) origin.

The suppressive activity of C3H marrow cells was further examined using fresh whole marrow cells and cells in various fractions obtained by a unit gravity sedimentation of normal C3H marrow cells. Addition of normal whole marrow cells or lymphoid cell–enriched fraction III cells to the MLC of normal B6AF$_1$ responders resulted in nonspecific suppression of the proliferative response, as well as the generation of cytotoxicity. Cells in other fractions had no inhibitory effects.

These results indicate that three sets of suppressor cells are involved in the unresponsiveness induced in B6AF$_1$ mice by ALS and C3H marrow cells: (1) host-derived suppressor cells induced by ALS, (2) early natural suppressor cells of donor marrow, and (3) late donor marrow-derived suppressor cells. Early natural suppressor cells might function as inhibitors of the graft *versus* host response by marrow cells in the ALS-treated host, while late marrow-derived suppressor cells inhibit the host response to donor antigens, thus maintaining the unresponsive state. Whether the natural suppressor cells present in normal C3H marrow are the precursors of late marrow-derived suppressor cells or these two suppressor cells belong to separate subsets is currently under investigation.

REFERENCES

1. Wood, M. L., A. P. Monaco, J. J. Gozzo & A. Liegeois. 1971. Transplant. Proc. **3:** 676.
2. Gozzo, J. J., D. Litvin, Y. M. Bhatnagar & A. P. Monaco. 1981. Transplant. Proc. **13:** 592.
3. Maki, T., R. Gottschalk, F. N. Homsy, H. Okazaki, M. L. Wood & A. P. Monaco. 1981. Transplant. Proc. **13:** 596.

ANTI-IDIOTYPIC IMMUNITY AND AUTOIMMUNITY
III. INVESTIGATIONS BY ELISA METHODS

J. P. McCoy, J. H. Michaelson, and P. E. Bigazzi

Department of Pathology
University of Connecticut Health Center
Farmington, Connecticut 06062

We have recently shown that autoantibodies to thyroglobulin (Tg) from rats with spontaneous autoimmune thyroiditis share idiotypic determinants and can be characterized using heterologous anti-idiotypic antibodies.[1] Similar studies, using sera from patients with autoimmune thyroiditis and rats with mercuric chloride–induced glomerulonephritis, are ongoing in our laboratory. Several types of enzyme-linked immunosorbent assays (ELISA) are being used in each of these studies, including those for the detection of circulating auto-antibodies and those for the evaluation of experimentally induced anti-idiotypic antibodies. Our experiments using thyroiditis sera indicate that ELISA detects titers of anti-Tg antibodies very similar to those detected by a more traditional coprecipitation radioimmunoassay (RIA). Simultaneous titration of a pool of human thyroiditis sera by the two methods produced similar titration curves, each detecting antibody activity in dilutions of the serum pool up to $1:10^5$. In experimental glomerulonephritis, ELISA has proven more sensitive, in our laboratory, than immunofluorescence for the detection of antiglomerular basement membrane (GBM) antibodies.[2] Indirect immunofluorescence titers of anti-GBM antibodies in this model rarely exceed 20 and are detectable in only 45% of the treated rats. By ELISA, 100% of the treated rats surveyed had detectable levels of anti-GBM, with titers as high as 10^3.

Heterologous anti-idiotypic antibodies have been developed for the disease models described above. ELISA techniques were used to monitor the reactivity of the anti-idiotypic antibodies against the idiotypes and normal immunoglobulins. In both the human and the rat systems, ELISA demonstrated residual activity specific for the idiotype after exhaustive absorption of the anti-idiotypes with normal immunoglobulins. In the human model, RIA were run with ^{125}I-labeled idiotype and labeled normal immunoglobulin, which confirmed the ELISA results. The ELISA techniques used in the assessment of these anti-idiotypic antibodies equalled or surpassed the sensitivities of RIA used for the same purpose, but proved to be quicker, easier, and safer to perform.

Current data have indicated the feasibility of using inhibition assays in ELISA methods. In the model systems described above for the detection of circulating autoantibodies, preincubation of the autoantiserum with homologous antigen has been shown to be capable of inhibiting the ELISA reaction. In addition, crossreactive heterologous antigens were capable of partially inhibiting the ELISA reactivity of autoantibodies. It may be possible to use similar inhibition-type assays to determine if anti-idiotypic antibodies are binding site specific; we are currently exploring this possibility in our laboratory.

REFERENCES

1. ZANETTI, M. & P. E. BIGAZZI. 1981. Eur. J. Immunol. **11:** 187–95.
2. MICHAELSON, J. H., J. P. McCOY & P. E. BIGAZZI. 1981. Kidney Int. **20:** 285–88.

ROLE OF UTEROGLOBIN AND TRANSGLUTAMINASE IN SELF AND NON-SELF RECOGNITION DURING REPRODUCTION IN THE RABBIT

Anil B. Mukherjee, Diane Cunningham, Arun K. Agrawal, and R. Manjunath

Molecular and Developmental Genetics Section
Pregnancy Research Branch
National Institutes of Health
Bethesda, Maryland 20205

Mammalian reproduction involves prolonged and intimate interactions between two genetically dissimilar individuals. The epididymal spermatozoa as well as the developing embryos have been demonstrated to be antigenic and the female reproductive tract is not an immunologically privileged organ. Nonetheless, the ejaculated spermatozoa or implanting embryos do not normally immunize the female. Many hypotheses have been proposed to elucidate the mechanism of this unique alloantigen tolerance during pregnancy, but none have, as yet, been conclusively proven.

Recently, we proposed a hypothesis explaining a possible mechanism by which the implanting mammalian embryo may be protected from maternal immunological assault. Using rabbit as a model, we proposed that uteroglobin (UG), a pregnancy-specific uterine protein, in conjunction with transglutaminase (TG), which is present in the uterus during implantation, may crosslink with antigens (*e.g.*, RLA, H-2, HL-A) on the embryonic cell surface. The crosslinked UG-antigen complex is not recognized by maternal lymphocytes. Similarly, the prostatic fluid contains UG as well as TG. During ejaculation, the epididymal sperm comes in contact with prostatic fluid, which masks the sperm antigens by a mechanism similar to that proposed for implanting embryo in the uterus.

Here, we present experimental evidence that suggests that, indeed, the two components of uterine and prostatic fluid (*e.g.*, UG and TG) can mask the antigenicity of developing embryos, as well as that of the epididymal spermatozoa, *in vitro*.

We used female splenocytes and lymphocytes as responder cells. Mitomycin-C inactivated blastomeres from implanting embryos and epididymal spermatozoa served as stimulator cells in a mixed culture with splenocytes/lymphocytes. The degree of incorporation of ^{3}H-thymidine into the lymphocytes was considered a criterion of recognition or nonrecognition of the embryonic or sperm antigens by these cells. The embryonic cells and spermatozoa were pretreated with various substances before their addition into the lymphocyte cultures, as shown in TABLE 1. Appropriate nontreated controls were also kept in each case. The results are shown in TABLE 1.

As shown in the table, both epididymal spermatozoa and blastomeres lost their antigenicity when they were pretreated with UG and TG, as determined by the low ^{3}H-thymidine incorporation into female lymphocytes. Inhibition of TG or pretreatment of TG with its antisera abolished this effect of UG and TG. Treatment of UG with anti-UG antisera yielded similar results. The effect of

401

UG was dose dependent and a nonspecific protein such as myoglobin did not have an antigen-masking effect as UG. These results, in addition to supporting our hypothesis, suggest that masking of antigens during mammalian reproduction may be one of the mechanisms by which the female of the species does not normally get immunized by alloantigens such as spermatozoa and the fetal cells during implantation.

TABLE 1

Incubation Conditions for Spermatozoa and Blastomeres	^{3}H-Thymidine Incorporation into Lymphocytes Spermatozoa as Antigen		^{3}H-Thymidine Incorporation into Lymphocytes Blastomeres as Antigen	
	(cpm ± s.e.)	Control (%)	(cpm ± s.e.)	Control (%)
Not pretreated	17 000 ± 500	(100%)	68 000 ± 800	(100%)
Pretreated with crude prostatic fluid	1800 ± 60	(10.5%)	—	— —
Pretreatment with crude pregnant uterine fluid	—	—	9000 ± 480	(16.0%)
Pretreated with crude nonpregnant uterine fluid			53 000 ± 1200	(89.0%)
Pretreated with UG	9100 ± 150	(53.5%)	43 013 ± 280	(63.0%)
Pretreated with UG + TG	600 ± 120	(3.5%)	950 ± 20	(2%)
Pretreated with UG + anti-TG-treated TG	11 000 ± 210	(64.7%)	65 000 ± 520	(95%)
Pretreated with anti-UG-treated UG + TG	18 500 ± 1150	(108.8%)	63 000 ± 680	(93%)
Pretreated with myoglobin + TG	17 200 ± 950	(101%)	64 000 ± 430	(94%)
Blastomeres pretreated with UG and NPCNU-treated TG	12 3000 ± 680	(72.3%)	66 000 ± 510	(97%)
Lymphocytes + Phytohemagglutinin	162 000 ± 1500 (238%)			

REFERENCE

1. MUKHERJEE, A. B. et al. 1980. Med. Hypoth. 6: 1043–55.

A NOVEL MECHANISM
FOR INACTIVATING CERTAIN SELF-REACTIVE CELLS

Shizuko Muraoka and Richard G. Miller

Department of Medical Biophysics
University of Toronto
and
Ontario Cancer Institute
Toronto, Ontario, Canada M4X 1K9

The immune system does not normally react against self components. Originally, it was postulated by Burnet that self-reactive cells were somehow deleted or blocked. More recent thinking is that such cells are suppressed by regulatory networks similar to those limiting the immune response against non-self determinants. Both mechanisms may exist. We are working on a type of suppression more closely related to the first type postulated.[1-3] When a subpopulation of some lymphoid organs is added to a one-way mixed lymphocyte reaction (MLR), only cytotoxic responses directing against H-2 antigens of the added cells are suppressed; cytotoxic responses against antigens unrelated to the added cells are not suppressed. This special subpopulation is found in normal or nude BM, nude spleen, and thymus, but not in normal spleen, lymph node, or peritoneal exudate cells. From the point of view of the added cells, anti-self reactions are being suppressed. The suppression of the anti-self H-2 response is induced much more effectively by the addition of lymphoid colony cells grown from normal or nude BMC than by intact BMC. Suppressor cells in BM are 900 rad irradiation sensitive but resistant to treatment with anti-Thy 1.2 plus complement, whereas suppressor cells in BM lymphoid colony are 1500 rad irradiation resistant but sensitive to anti-Thy 1.2 treatment. When the addition of BMC is delayed 40 h after MLR initiation, the suppression of anti-self reaction is not induced, but is rather enhanced. From the limiting dilution analysis, the addition of BMC results in the reduction of frequency of cytotoxic T lymphocyte precursor cells (CLP). Thus, the suppressor cell appears to act at the stage of CLP activation rather than at the stage of cytotoxic effector cell development.

The fact that the suppressor cells in nude spleen suppress an anti-TNP modified-self response only after they have been TNP-modified indicates that the initial event for suppression is the CLP recognizing the suppressor cell, not the suppressor cell recognizing the CLP via, *e.g.*, an anti-idiotype receptor.

The suppressive activity found in bone marrow may represent a precursor population that seeds to thymus in a normal mouse but seeds to spleen in an athymic nude mouse. In the thymus, the suppressor cell (probably a thymic epithelium cell) could inactivate cells recognizing the antigens on the suppressor cell before such cells are exported to the periphery.

REFERENCES

1. MILLER, R. G. & H. DERRY. 1979. A cell population in nu/nu spleen can prevent generation of cytotoxic lymphocytes by normal LN cells against self antigens of the nu/nu spleen. J. Immunol. **122:** 1502–9.

2. MURAOKA, S. & R. G. MILLER. 1980. Cells in bone marrow and in T cell colonies grown from bone marrow can suppress generation of cytotoxic T lymphocytes directed against their self antigens. J. Exp. Med. **152:** 54–71.
3. MILLER, R. G. 1980. An immunological suppressor cell which inactivates cytotoxic T lymphocyte precursor cells recognizing it. Nature (London) **287:** 544–46.

SYSTEMIC SUPPRESSION OF CONTACT HYPERSENSITIVITY BY *IN VIVO* UV IRRADIATION

Frances P. Noonan, Edward C. De Fabo, and Margaret L. Kripke

NCI-Frederick Cancer Research Facility
Cancer Biology Program
Frederick, Maryland 21701

Ultraviolet (uv) irradiation of Balb/c mice with FS40 sunlamps causes a systemic suppression of contact hypersensitivity (CHS) to trinitrochlorobenzene (TNCB) and dinitrofluorobenzene (DNFB).[1] We have investigated some of the photobiological and immunological characteristics of this effect and compared them to the previously reported characteristics of uv-induced suppression of tumor immunity.[2-5]

Mice were irradiated with a subcarcinogenic dose (2–20 J m^{-2}) of uv on the shaved dorsal skin and afterwards sensitized on the shaved abdomen. CHS was determined five days later by the measurement of ear swelling 24 h after challenge. Animals sensitized one day after uv responded normally, but sensitization 3–15 d after uv resulted in about 70% suppression of the response. CHS returned to normal levels about 21 d after irradiation. Irradiation of unshaved mice required 14 times more energy for 50% suppression than that required for shaved mice, suggesting that the exposed skin is the primary target for this effect. The suppression of CHS was proportional to $\log_{10}$ of the dose and was unaffected by dose fractionation over a five-day period or by changes in dose rate over a ten-fold range. Elimination of wavelengths below about 315 nm with a Mylar filter abrogated the suppressive effect of the sunlamps, even when the same dose was administered.

Contact sensitization of uv-irradiated, but not unirradiated, mice induced the appearance of antigen-specific suppressor cells in the spleen. These were shown to be suppressor T cells by nylon wool filtration and deletion by anti-Thy 1.2 serum.

Similar photobiological characteristics have been reported for the uv-induced suppression of immunity to uv-induced tumors.[4,5] Also, immunological characteristics, *i.e.*, a time delay in the expression of the effect after irradiation and the generation of specific suppressor T cells, in this case for uv-induced tumors, are similar. Because of these similarities, a common step is implied on the pathway for the uv-induced suppression of these two effects. There are, however, two differences: 13 times more energy is required to suppress tumor immunity and the addition of exogenous antigen is not necessary for the generation of tumor-specific suppressor cells.

Using these observations and the previously reported finding that there is an antigen-presenting defect in uv-irradiated mice,[6,7] a hypothesis for the mechanism of uv-induced suppression is suggested. A photoproduct (which may be soluble) is formed in the skin upon uv irradiation and causes a systemic alteration in antigen presentation such that, when a contact sensitizer is subsequently added, suppression, rather than active immunity, results. In the tumor system, it is suggested that the uv has two functions: firstly, to generate an antigen presentation defect and, secondly, to generate in the skin a tumor-related antigen that is responsible for triggering the formation of tumor-specific suppressor T lymphocytes.

REFERENCES

1. JESSUP, J. M., N. HANNA, E. PALASZYNSKI & M. L. KRIPKE. 1978. Cell. Immunol. **38:** 105–15.
2. FISHER, M. S. & M. L. KRIPKE. 1977. Proc. Nat. Acad. Sci. USA **74:** 1688–92.
3. FISHER, M. S. & M. L. KRIPKE. 1978. J. Immunol. **121:** 1139–44.
4. DE FABO, E. C. & M. L. KRIPKE. 1979. Photochem. Photobiol. **30:** 385–90.
5. DE FABO, E. C. & M. L. KRIPKE. 1980. Photochem. Photobiol. **32:** 183–88.
6. GREENE, M. I., M. S. SY, M. L. KRIPKE & B. BENACERRAF. 1979. Proc. Nat. Acad. Sci. USA **76:** 6592–95.
7. NOONAN, F. P., M. L. KRIPKE, G. M. PEDERSEN & M. I. GREENE. 1981. Immunology **43:** 527–33.

LYMPHOID CELL REGULATION
OF MHC ANTIGEN EXPRESSION
ON TERATOCARCINOMA CELLS *IN VIVO*

Suzanne Ostrand-Rosenberg and Allen Cohn

Department of Biological Sciences
University of Maryland–Baltimore County
Catonsville, Maryland 21228

Teratocarcinomas are malignant tumors of the testes or ovaries derived from sperm, ova, or early preimplantation embryos. They consist of metastatic undifferentiated stem cells (embryonal carcinoma) that do not express the major histocompatibility complex (MHC, H-2 in the mouse) antigens as well as benign differentiated cell types that express MHC antigens. The 402AX teratocarcinoma is a spontaneous tumor in 129 (H-2^b) mice that has lost the ability to differentiate either *in vitro* or *in vivo* (nullipotent). Recent studies in this laboratory have established that rejection of the 402AX tumor is under genetic control in the mouse [1] and that H-2 negative tumor cells modulate to become H-2^b antigen-positive when placed in genetically resistant host mice. Tumor cells grown in genetically susceptible mice remain H-2 antigen-negative.[2] These findings may reflect a direct *in vivo* requirement for H-2 antigen expression on target tumor cells for effective host cell–mediated cytotoxicity, and suggest a direct host induction for H-2 antigen expression on resident tumor cells. We have, therefore, further examined the *in vivo* mechanism of host-mediated regulation of H-2 antigen expression on 402AX cells. Reconstitution of lethally irradiated susceptible hosts (129/J) with resistant bone marrow (C57BL/6) extends the mean survival time of the reconstituted hosts, but does not confer complete resistance to the tumor. Teratocarcinoma cells placed in such reconstituted hosts do not express H-2 antigens. Two lines of evidence, however, suggest that tumor cell H-2 antigen expression and host resistance are mediated by lymphoid cells: (1) sublethal irradiation of genetically resistant hosts inhibits H-2 antigen modulation on teratocarcinoma cells placed *in vivo* and produces mice susceptible to the tumor and (2) immunological priming can overcome the loss of H-2 modulation and conversion to susceptibility that are normally associated with aging in genetically resistant hosts. Genetically susceptible mice can be fully reconstituted for tumor rejection and H-2 antigen expression on teratocarcinoma cells by reconstitution with both (1) genetically resistant bone marrow and (2) lymphoid cells from tumor-primed resistant hosts. These results (1) further indicate the necessity for H-2 antigens on tumor cells for an effective host cell–mediated immune response against the tumor and (2) indicate that host lymphoid cells regulate H-2 antigen expression on 402AX teratocarcinoma cells placed *in vivo*.

REFERENCES

1. OSTRAND-ROSENBERG, S., T. M. RIDER & A. TWAROWSKI. 1980. Immunogenetics **10:** 607.
2. OSTRAND-ROSENBERG, S. & V. COHAN. 1981. J. Immunol. **126:** 2190.

STUDIES ON THE ROLE OF THE SOLVENT IN THE INDUCTION OF TOLERANCE FOLLOWING HAPTEN FEEDING

Jerome R. Pomeranz

Department of Dermatology
Cleveland Metropolitan General Hospital
Case Western Reserve
University School of Medicine
Cleveland, Ohio 44109

The purpose of these studies was to investigate the role of the solvent in the immune response to hapten feeding.

In the past, all the methods used to induce immunological unresponsiveness to simple chemical sensitizers by oral feeding entailed the use of vegetable oil or organic solvents. In the present studies, the trinitrophenol ligand—in the form of picryl sulfonic acid (PSA) or picryl chloride (PC)—was fed in aqueous solvents. Feeding large doses of PSA, a readily water-soluble hapten, in an aqueous solvent (saline) to starved (24 h) guinea pigs did not result in significant unresponsiveness to contact sensitization with PCL in complete Freund's adjuvant (CFA).

In contrast, when PSA was fed in saline emulsified with varying amounts of vegtable oil or in Upjohn fat emulsion, from one-half to two-thirds of the animals fed PSA became unresponsive to subsequent sensitization with PC. Many guinea pigs fed PSA developed picryl-specific antibody, as demonstrated by passive cutaneous anaphylaxis (PCA), regardless of whether the hapten was given in saline or saline-lipid emulsions. The significance of the antibody is unclear.

Guinea pigs fed PC, a slightly water-soluble hapten, in saline-ethanol mixtures also showed a decreased capacity to become unresponsive to contact sensitization. Approximately 20% of the animals fed either 30 mg PC in 10% ethanol or 32 mg PC in 2% ethanol were unresponsive. PCA tests for antibody were negative. In contrast, previous experiments from this laboratory have shown that slightly over 70% of the animals fed 30 mg PC in olive oil alone become unresponsive to contact sensitization.

These experiments demonstrate that the solvent in which the hapten is fed influences the subsequent immunological response to sensitization with the haptenic ligand. The mechanisms of how the addition of vegetable oil alters the immune response to hapten feeding are unclear, but may be related to the way in which the hapten is absorbed and distributed as it comes into contact with gut-associated lymphoid tissue.

IDIOTYPE SHIFTS GENERATED BY NEONATAL EXPOSURE TO PHOSPHORYLCHOLINE TOLEROGEN IN BALB/C MICE *

J. Quintáns and Z. S. Quan

La Rabida–University of Chicago Research Institute
Chicago, Illinois 60649

We have followed the emergence of responsiveness to phosphorylcholine (PC) in Balb/c mice after neonatal exposure to PC conjugated to mouse gamma globulin (PC-MGG). Conventional Balb/c mice respond well to PC, with a preponderance of their anti-PC antibodies bearing the T15 idiotype. The injection of PC-MGG within 48 h of birth, however, eliminates all direct plaque-forming cell (PFC) responses to the thymus-dependent antigen PC–keyhole limpet hemocyanin (KLH) and the thymus-independent class II antigen PnCs in the neonatal period. Antigen reactivity appears after four weeks, but the magnitude of the PC-specific responses in tolerized animals does not approach that of normal Balb/c mice even seven months after birth. An idiotypic analysis of the anti-PC responses in mice breaking tolerance indicates that the earliest responses to emerge are T15+, but that these are supplanted by T15- clones, resulting in non–T15 dominance. At five months after birth, avidity profiles of these non–T15 clones, as determined by PFC inhibition with various concentrations of hapten, reveal that a heterogeneous anti-PC population arises, including clones with both higher and lower avidity than T15. As such heterogeneity can also be observed by two months after birth, there does not seem to be a distinct trend towards either a generally higher or lower avidity. The shift to T15- expression is not due to a loss of putative idiotype-specific help, since normal Balb/c splenic B cells transplanted into unirradiated neonatally tolerized animals will produce T15+ responses to the thymus-dependent antigen PC–KLH. In addition, carrier-primed lymph node cells from tolerized mice will help PC-primed normal Balb/c splenic B cells produce predominantly T15+ responses to PC–KLH. Adoptive transfer of tolerized splenic B cells to xid-bearing (CBA/N $\times$ Balb/c)F_1 male hosts, which do not produce anti-PC PFC but which have adequate T cell help for both T15 and non-T15 B cell clones, does not reverse the loss of T15 dominance; nor does the mixture of these tolerized B cells with those from normal Balb/c mice uncover any suppressor cells in *in vivo* experiments. Furthermore, the transfer of 10^7 tolerized spleen cells to normal Balb/c neonates does not reduce the recipients' anti-PC PFC responses from control levels by four weeks of age, implying that suppression of T15+ B cell precursors or progenitors does not occur. Thus, the idiotypic changes generated by neonatal exposure to PC tolerogen reflect changes in the emerging PC-specific B cell subpopulations. The transition to T15- expression has been observed under other experimental conditions as well, such as irradiation of normal Balb/c mice,[1] and the adoptive transfer of either Balb/c adult splenic B cells [2] or neonatal liver cells.[3] Since we have been unable to demonstrate either the loss

* This research was supported by a grant from the March of Dimes Birth Defects Foundation, no. I-736, and by grants from the National Institutes of Health, nos. RO1-AI-14530, AI-00268, and 5T32 GM07183.

409

of help or the acquisition of suppression, the idiotypic shifts seen in these studies suggest that clonal dominance in the PC system may be a function of processes other than active idiotype-anti-idiotype regulation; idiotype-specific T cells may play little or no role. The loss of T15 expression may be a consequence not so much of regulatory or network interactions at the level of idiotype expression as of a more nonspecific competition among PC-specific progenitors for the opportunity to develop into mature B cells.

REFERENCES

1. KAPLAN, D. & J. QUINTÁNS. 1978. J. Exp. Med. **148:** 987.
2. QUINTÁNS, J., M. R. LOKEN, Z. S. QUAN, R. F. DICK & B. REGUEIRO. 1981. Eur J. Immunol. **11:** 236.
3. QUAN, Z. S. & J. QUINTÁNS. 1981. J. Exp. Med. **154:** 1475.

IDIOTYPIC INTERACTIONS
OF T SUPPRESSOR CELL POPULATIONS INVOLVED
IN SUPPRESSION OF *IN VITRO* PFC RESPONSES

David H. Sherr and Martin E. Dorf

Department of Pathology
Harvard Medical School
Boston, Massachusetts 02115

It has been well documented that the manifestation of immune suppression is the result of interactions among several T lymphocyte subsets. These cellular interactions often depend upon the recognition of unique idiotypic determinants present on the various lymphoid elements.

We have previously characterized a system in which murine suppressor T cells (Ts), induced by the intravenous administration of syngeneic spleen cells covalently coupled with the 4-hydroxy-3-nitrophenyl acetyl (NP) hapten, specifically affected the responses of NP^b idiotype-bearing B lymphocytes both *in vivo* and *in vitro*.[1] The ability of these Lyt 1^-, 2^+, Igh-restricted suppressor T cells to bind idiotype and to function during the effector phase of an *in vitro* response suggested that they corresponded to the effector phase suppressor T cell (Ts^e or Ts_2) involved in the suppression of NP-specific delayed-type hypersensitivity and cutaneous sensitivity responses.[2] Effector phase suppressor T cells could also be induced by the injection of monoclonal Ts_1 factor *in vivo* or by the addition of this factor to normal spleen cells *in vitro*.[3] The purpose of the studies presented herein was to further investigate the specificity of the Ts_2 suppressor cell and to determine the nature of its target cell.

It is well established that many defined idiotypic systems are composed of a family of idiotypically related but nonidentical molecules. In the NP^b idiotypic system, for example, most monoclonal anti-NP antibodies exhibit only a fraction of the serum NP^b idiotypic specificities. In order to determine if T cell receptors recognize the same repertoire of NP^b idiotypic determinants as anti-idiotypic antiserum, the ability of effector phase suppressor cells to bind monoclonal anti-NP antibodies bearing different levels of NP^b idiotypic determinants was studied. The results suggest that anti-idiotypic effector phase suppressor T cells do not recognize the predominant serologically detected NP^b idiotypic determinants.

Although the Ts_2 population recognized molecules bearing NP^b idiotypic determinants and the overall effect of the suppression was idiotype specific, there was no direct evidence proving that this Ts_2 was, in fact, the final effector cell in the suppressor pathway. In order to determine if a third order suppressor T cell was required for the manifestation of immune suppression, Ts_2 suppressor cells were added to responder cultures pretreated with anti-I-J antiserum plus complement. The data indicate that treatment of responder populations with anti-I-J antiserum eliminates a population of T cells required for expression of immune suppression. This Ts_2 population was shown to be present in NP primed but not unprimed donors. Furthermore, the Ts_3 population specifically bound NP, was Lyt 1^-, 2^+, and $I-J^+$ and expressed NP^b idiotypic determinants.

Taken together, the data indicate that the interaction of at least three T cell

411

populations (Ts_1, Ts_2, Ts_3) is required for the suppression of NP^b idiotype-positive B cell responses *in vitro*. The ability of these populations to communicate with one another apparently involves the expression of complementary idiotypic or anti-idiotypic receptors.

REFERENCES

1. SHERR, D. H., S.-T. JU, J. Z. WEINBERGER, B. BENACERRAF & M. E. DORF. 1981. Hapten-specific T cell responses to 4-hydroxy-3-nitrophenyl acetyl. VII. Idiotype specific suppression of plaque forming cell responses. J. Exp. Med. **153:** 640.
2. SHERR, D. H. & M. E. DORF. 1981. Hapten specific T cell responses to 4-hydroxy-3-nitrophenyl acetyl. IX. Characterization of idiotype specific effector phase suppressor cells on plaque forming cell responses in vitro. J. Exp. Med. **153:** 1445.
3. OKUDA, K., M. MINAMI, D. H. SHERR & M. E. DORF. 1981. Hapten-specific T cell responses to 4-hydroxy-3-nitrophenyl acetyl. XI. Pseudogenetic restrictions of hybridoma suppressor factors. J. Exp. Med. **154:** 468.

NEITHER SELF-EYE NOR SELF-PITUITARY IMPLANTS ARE REJECTED BY FROGS DEPRIVED OF THEIR EYE OR PITUITARY ANLAGEN AS EMBRYOS *

Louise A. Rollins-Smith and Nicholas Cohen

Department of Microbiology
Division of Immunology
School of Medicine and Dentistry
University of Rochester
Rochester, New York 14642

Self tolerance to organ-specific antigens is thought to result from the contact of cells of the maturing lymphoid system with these antigens early in development. If this idea is valid, then failure of the animal to encounter self-antigens during this critical developmental period could result in tissue destruction when the antigens are presented to an immunocompetent individual for the first time. We have adopted the amphibian model of Triplett [1] to test this hypothesis with tissue-specific antigens of the eye and pituitary. Eye anlagen or pituitary anlagen were extirpated from tail bud frog embryos (*Xenopus laevis* and *Xenopus laevis-gilli* hybrid clones, stages 26–32 of Nieuwkoop and Faber; [2] *Rama pipiens*, stages 17–18 of Shumway [3]). In some experiments, the anlagen were grafted on sibling embryos, allowed to differentiate, and then returned to their now immunocompetent original owners. In other experiments, immunocompetent larval or post-metamorphic *Xenopus* that had been enucleated as embryos were given eye grafts from isogenic donors. None of the self-eyes implanted on larval *R. pipiens* ($N = 7$) or larval *Xenopus* ($N = 10$) were rejected by their enucleated hosts for as long as they were observed (some, more than one year), whereas allogeneic eyes were rejected by about half the intact larvae of both species. Similarly, all the self-eyes implanted on postmetamorphic *Xenopus* (enucleated as embryos) survived for as long as they were observed (some, more than one year; $N = 5$), whereas allogenic eyes were invariably rejected by adult hosts ($N = 9$).

These results are in marked contrast to those that would be predicted by the observations of Triplett on the survival of self-pituitary implants in embryonically hypophysectomized tree frogs (*Hyla regilla*).[1] Triplett observed that 10 out of 13 self-implants were rejected, with a mean survival time of about 40 d, when they were implanted on 45-day-old larval hosts. To try to resolve the apparent conflict, we repeated Triplett's protocol with *R. pipiens* embryos. Consistent with our results with eye implants, all self-pituitary implants returned to embryonically hypophysectomized larval hosts survived and continued to function (as assayed by the recipients' pigmentation and growth) for at least 50 d ($N = 5$; observations are continuing). In contrast, only 28% of the allogeneic pituitaries survived in hypophysectomized hosts for 50 d ($N = 7$). Most were rejected within 20 d.

The reasons for the differences between our observations and those of

* This research was supported by grants from the United States Public Health Service, nos. HD 07901, CA 06375, and AI 18319.

Triplett are not clear. In our experiments, the hypophyseal anlagen were implanted orthotopically on previously hypophysectomized sibling embryos. At later larval stages, the "parked" pituitaries could be recovered by dissection of the brain of the "parking" host and returned as a discrete organ. In contrast, Triplett implanted the anlagen intradermally. At this site it would be difficult to remove the organ discretely. Thus, the rejections that Triplett observed may have been a response to contaminating allogeneic cells rather than to pituitary-specific antigens.

Our results suggest that the period in which tolerance to organ-specific antigens can be induced is not confined to the early embryonic period. Rather, it may extend throughout larval and adult life in amphibians. The nature of this unresponsive state and the mechanism(s) for its maintenance will be intensively studied employing this unique amphibian model.

REFERENCES

1. TRIPLETT, E. L. 1962. On the mechanism of immunologic self recognition. J. Immunol. **89:** 505–10.
2. NIEUWKOOP, P. D. & J. FABER. 1967. Normal table of *Xenopus laevis* (Daudin): 1–252. North Holland Publishing Co. Amsterdam.
3. SHUMWAY, W. 1940. Stages in the normal development of *Rana pipiens*. I. External form. Anat. Rec. **78:** 139–47.

CONTROL OF MACROPHAGE Ia EXPRESSION IN NEONATAL MICE
POSSIBLE RELEVANCE TO INDUCTION OF SELF-TOLERANCE

D. S. Snyder, C. Y. Lu, and E. R. Unanue

Department of Pathology
Harvard Medical School
Boston, Massachusetts 02115

We have reported that neonatal mouse peritoneal and splenic macrophages are deficient in the basal expression of surface I region–associated antigens (Ia) and in antigen presentation to T lymphocytes. Since Ia⁺ antigen-presenting cells are required to initiate specific immune responses and their absence leads to the induction of tolerance, we postulated that this deficiency in neonatal mice may contribute to the induction of self-tolerance during the first weeks of life.

In our current studies, we have shown that neonatal mice not only have a defect in their basal number of Ia⁺ macrophages but also fail to respond to immune stimuli that generate exudates enriched for these cells. Adult mice produce peritoneal exudates rich in Ia-bearing macrophages in response to intra-peritoneal injection of either *Listeria*-immune T cells and heat-killed *Listeria* or a soluble T cell product called macrophage Ia-recruiting factor (MIRF). Neonates fail to generate such exudates. In contrast, neonates respond normally to nonimmune inflammatory stimulation by thioglycollate with an influx of Ia⁻ macrophages.

We have identified a suppressor system operating in neonates that significantly reduces the recruitment of Ia⁺ macrophages. Initial studies *in vitro*, which indicate that neonatal phagocytes can express Ia when stimulated by T cell mediators, underscore the significance of this suppressor mechanism. Suppressor activity is found in neonatal spleen, adult bone marrow, and adult peritoneal exudate cells, but neither in adult spleen nor neonatal thymus cells. When freshly harvested from neonatal spleens, the suppressor cell lacks T cell markers, is radiosensitive, and is poorly adherent to plastic dishes and nylon wool columns, unlike mature B cells and macrophages. However, after four days in culture, suppressor activity is enriched in a population of radioresistant cells characterized as classical phagocytes. Suppression is reversed by indomethacin and aspirin. Thus, our data suggest that phagocytes autoregulate their expression of Ia *via* prostaglandins. Indeed, preliminary experiments with purified prostaglandins have shown that these compounds markedly suppress macrophage Ia expression both *in vitro* and *in vivo*.

Neonatal liver and spleen, as hematopoietic organs, contain large numbers of phagocyte precursors. These cells may give rise to prostaglandin-producing monocyte-macrophages, which suppress Ia expression by local macrophages. The resulting absence of Ia⁺ antigen-presenting cells may promote the induction of self-tolerance during ontogeny.

THE SELECTIVE ROLE OF MEMBRANE IgG
IN THE ANTIGEN-INDUCED INHIBITION
OF HUMAN *IN VITRO* ANTIBODY PRODUCTION

Ronald H. Stevens, Etty Benveniste, and David Dichek

Departments of Microbiology and Immunology
University of California–Los Angeles School of Medicine
Los Angeles, California 90024

IgG-anti-tetanus toxoid-producing B cell precursors from recently immunized individuals can be stimulated by pokeweed mitogen (PWM) and T cells to produce IgG-anti-tetanus toxoid antibodies (IgG-Tet) *in vitro*.[1, 2] Several lines of evidence suggest that these PWM-reactive antibody-producing cells represent a population of short term memory cells. First, these cells appear in the circulation after the *in vivo* production of IgG-Tet has already occurred, and they are only detectable for 10–12 weeks after immunization.[2] These cells are also somewhat larger than the majority of circulating B cells and appear committed *in vivo* to the production of a single antibody isotype when stimulated by PWM *in vitro*.[3, 4]

Other studies in which B cell subpopulations were separated on the basis of surface Ig isotype expression indicated that the cells responsible for the *in vitro* IgG-Tet production may or may not express μ or δ on the cell surface but uniformly express γ.[4-6]

More recently, we have discovered an additional property of these IgG-Tet-producing B cells, that is, the ability to be functionally inactivated by brief treatment with antigen.[6-9] Treatment of the B cell fraction with as little as 10 μg ml^{-1} TT for as little as 1 h can inhibit the majority of the *in vitro* IgG-Tet production. The *in vitro* production of IgM-Tet and of IgG-Dip were not affected by this treatment, indicating that the inhibition is antigen specific and restricted to antibodies of the IgG isotype. As the B cell precursors of IgG-Tet synthesis can express multiple Ig isotypes, we wished to determine if all isotypes participated equally in the inhibition or if one isotype was selectively involved. Positive selection of μ^+ and δ^+ B cell subsets followed by antigen treatment indicated that the susceptible cells were in all four resulting B cell subsets (μ^+, μ^-, δ^+, δ^-). Further studies examining the effects of anti-isotype antisera on the IgG-Tet B cells revealed that the inhibitory effect of antigen could be mimicked by anti-γ antibodies but not by anti-μ or anti-δ, suggesting a role of the γ receptor in the antigen-induced inhibition of IgG-Tet production. This was substantiated by experiments showing that the removal of membrane IgG receptors by antibody modulation followed by antigen treatment did not show inhibition of antibody synthesis. A similar removal of IgM or IgD followed by treatment of the cells with TT did not prevent the inhibited state. Lastly, similar studies with IgG subclass-specific reagents have demonstrated that it is IgG$_1$ that is responsible for conveying the inhibitory signal.

These studies indicate that short term memory B cells in humans can be functionally inactivated by treatment with native antigen and that this inhibition is mediated by membrane IgG molecules.

REFERENCES

1. STEVENS, R. H. & A. SAXON. 1978. Immunoregulation in humans. Control of antitetanus toxoid antibody production after booster immunization. J. Clin. Invest. **62:** 1154–60.
2. STEVENS, R. H. & A. SAXON. 1979. Reduced in vitro production of anti-tetanus toxoid antibody after repeated in vivo immunization with tetanus toxoid. J. Immunol. **122:** 592–98.
3. THIELE, C. J., C. D. MORROW & R. H. STEVENS. 1981. Multiple subsets of anti-tetanus toxoid antibody-producing cells in human peripheral blood differ by size, expression of membrane receptors and mitogen reactivity. J. Immunol. **126:** 1146–53.
4. THIELE, C. J. & R. H. STEVENS. 1980. Antibody potential of human peripheral blood lymphocytes differentially expressing surface membrane IgM. J. Immunol. **124:** 1898–904.
5. THIELE, C. J. & R. H. STEVENS. 1981. Expression of surface membrane IgG on pokeweed mitogen-reactive anti-tetanus toxoid antibody-producing cells. J. Clin. Immunol. **1:** 174–80.
6. STEVENS, R. H. & A. SAXON. 1980. Antigen-induced suppression of human in vitro pokeweed mitogen-stimulated antibody production. Cell. Immunol. **55:** 85–93.
7. STEVENS, R. H. 1981. Immunoglobulin bearing cells are a target for the antigen induced inhibition of pokeweed mitogen stimulated antibody production. J. Immunol. **127:** 968.
8. STEVENS, R. H., E. BENVENISTE & E. PINEDA. 1982. The selective role of membrane IgG in the antigen induced inhibition of human in vitro antibody synthesis. J. Immunol. **128:** 398–401.

GENERATION OF GENETIC RESTRICTIONS IN THE SUPPRESSION OF DELAYED-TYPE HYPERSENSITIVITY

Muneo Takaoki, Man-Sun Sy, Baruj Benacerraf,
and Mark I. Greene

Department of Pathology
Harvard Medical School
Boston, Massachusetts 02115

A soluble suppressor factor (TsF_1) produced by first-order suppressor T cells in the azobenzene arsonate (ABA)-specific delayed-type hypersensitivity (DTH) reaction bears crossreactive idiotypic (CRI) determinants of anti-ABA antibodies and determinants encoded in the I–J subregion of the H–2 gene complex. TsF_1, when injected i.v. into naive mice, induces second-order suppressor T cells that produce a soluble suppressor factor, TsF_2. TsF_2 suppresses the effector phase of DTH and can bind to CRI. TsF_2 can also be induced in a CRI⁻ strain by injecting CRI-coupled spleen cells, but such TsF_2 works only in CRI⁺ (V_H restriction) and H-2 matched (H-2 restriction) strains.[1]

To investigate how these restrictions are generated, either TsF_1 extracted from spleen cells of A/J(H-2ᵃ, CRI⁺) mice or monoclonal TsF_1 produced by F12, a suppressor T cell hybridoma line of A/J origin,[2] was injected i.v. into various strains of mice daily for five days. TsF_2 were extracted from the spleen cells of these mice by freezing and thawing on day 7 after the first injection. Mice were injected i.v. with TsF_2 on days 4 and 5 after s.c. immunization with ABA-coupled syngeneic spleen cells and challenged into the hind footpad with ABA solution on day 5. The footpad response was measured 24 h later.

TsF_2 of A/J mice suppressed only A/J DTH. TsF_2 induced by A.By (H-2ᵇ, CRI⁺) mice suppressed A.By DTH, but not A/J DTH, despite the fact that A/J TsF_1 was used for its induction. Similarly, TsF_2 induced in C57BL/6 (H-2ᵇ, CRI⁻) mice suppressed A.By DTH, but not A/J DTH. To do intra H-2 mapping of the restriction, TsF_2 were raised in B10.A(3R) (bbbbkdd) and B10.A(5R) (bbbkkdd), and tested in A/J and A.By. TsF_2 of B10.A(3R) suppressed A.By DTH but not A/J DTH, while TsF_2 of B10.A(5R) suppressed A/J DTH but not A.By DTH. It was concluded that the H-2 restriction was determined by the I-J subregion of the H-2 complex of the mice that produce TsF_2. It may relate to recognition of I-J determinants by a subset of suppressor cells. I-J determinants expressed on TsF_1, however, did not seem to play a role in the determination of the restriction. On the other hand, V_H restriction may be generated by the recognition of the CRI determinants of the TsF_1 molecule.

REFERENCES

1. Sy, M. S., M. H. Dietz, R. N. Germain, B. Benacerraf & M. I. Greene. 1980. J. Exp. Med. **151:** 1181–95.
2. Takaoki, M., M. S. Sy, B. Whitaker, J. Nepon, R. Finberg, R. N. Germain, A. Nisonoff, B. Benacerraf & M. I. Greene. 1982. J. Immunol. In press.

ANTIGEN-PRESENTING CELLS
IN IMMUNITY AND SUPPRESSION

Akira Tominaga, Sophie Lefort, Muneo Takaoki,
Baruj Benacerraf, and Mark I. Greene

Department of Pathology
Harvard Medical School
Boston, Massachusetts 02115

It is well documented that the route of administration of antigen influences whether immunity or suppression is induced. It was observed that the intravenous route of administration of ligand-coupled cells activates the suppressor pathway, while the subcutaneous administration of ligand-coupled cells activates the helper pathway. This suggests different modes of antigen presentation for the two routes.

We have evaluated the role of specialized antigen-presenting cells (APC) in the induction of T cell immunity *in vitro*. By using the bovine serum albumin flotation method, we have been able to isolate a potent APC source for the generation of primary and secondary cytolytic responses to azobenzene arsonate (ABA)-coupled cells *in vitro*. This APC population, which can turn on the helper circuit, has the following characteristics: low density, 1500 rad x-ray resistance, uv sensitivity, and I-A$^+$.

In *in vivo* studies, we observed that uv-treated mice inoculated with uv-treated hapten-coupled APC developed a population of hapten-specific suppressor T cells capable, upon adoptive transfer, of inhibiting the generation of T cell immunity in normal mice.

This suggests the possibility that, in the absence of I-A$^+$ APC, special uv-resistant presenting cells capable of activating certain suppressor cells remain or certain subsets of suppressor cells are activated in the absence of any APC. In order to clarify this, we developed a suppressor factor–sensitive killer cell generation system. We observed that the so-called first-order suppressor factor secreted by hybrid cells can suppress the secondary ABA killer generation.

CHANGES IN SURFACE MARKERS
AND FUNCTIONAL PROPERTIES
OF H-2 SENSITIZED T CELL SUBPOPULATIONS
IN MOUSE SPLEEN AFTER AN ALLOGRAFT *

Vincent K. Tuohy and Helen G. Durkin

Department of Pathology
State University of New York Downstate Medical Center
Brooklyn, New York 11203

Male Balb/c *H-2*^{k} (Balb.K) skin was transplanted to male Balb/c *H-2*^{d} congenic partners; all grafts were rejected by day 13. On days 6–28 after transplantation, recipient spleen cells were separated on discontinuous bovine serum albumin (BSA) density gradients into subpopulations AB (least dense), C, D, E, and pellet. The relative numbers of Thy 1, Lyt 1, or Lyt 2 or Ig-bearing cells (immunofluorescence, cell suspensions), and phagocytic cells were determined, as was the capacity of these subpopulations to respond (^{3}H-thymidine uptake) to allogeneic (x-irradiated Balb.K or Balb/c *H-2*^{b} (Balb.B) spleen cells (mixed lymphocyte reaction; MLR) and to mitogens.

Cells specifically responsive to *H-2*^{k} alloantigens were consistently found in AB (FIGURE 1). Reactivity appeared on day 6 and increased 10- and 15-fold in magnitude by days 12 and 21, respectively. AB never responded to Balb.B spleen cells. Although total spleen cell numbers did not change with time after transplantation, there was a progressive increase in the numbers of low density cells, predominantly in AB, but also in C and a concomitant decrease in the numbers of cells in E and pellet. In unsensitized mice, AB accounted for 2% of all spleen cells (FIGURE 1). Yields obtained on days 6, 12, and 21 after transplantation were, respectively, 2-, 4-, and 8-fold greater than normal AB. The number of T cells in AB also progressively increased with time after transplantation (FIGURE 1). AB cells from unsensitized mice did not express Thy 1, Lyt 1, or Lyt 2 surface markers. On day 6, 15% of all AB cells were Thy 1+; 50% were Thy 1+ on days 12–28. Lyt 1+ cells represented 15% of AB on day 6, reached peak values on day 12 (65%), and dropped to <3% on day 21. Lyt 2+ cells were not detected until day 12 (10%), and reached peak values on days 21–28 (~50%). Thus, on day 21, when the magnitude of specific MLR was highest, there were virtually no Lyt 1+ cells in AB. This was accompanied by the appearance of specific suppressor activity in spleen. AB contained virtually no sIg+ cells at any time, and on days 12–28, <2% phagocytic cells. Lyt 2+ cells purified (99%) (anti-Lyt 1 plus complement, fluorescence-activated cell sorter, FACS) from AB on day 21 gave high-magnitude specific MLR. They did not respond to a third party challenge.

AB cells did not respond to concanavalin A or PHA on days 12–28, but gave high-magnitude responses to lipopolysaccharide (LPS). Thy 1+ cells purified (99%) (FACS) from AB on day 12 gave high magnitude responses both to donor-specific H-2 alloantigens and to LPS.

* This research was supported by grants from the American Cancer Society, no. IM-145, and from the United States Public Health Service, no. AI-1560303.

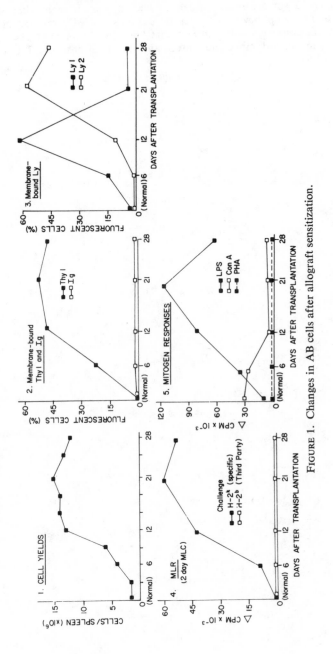

FIGURE 1. Changes in AB cells after allograft sensitization.

Therefore, distinct subsets of H-2-sensitized T lymphocytes, bearing either Lyt 1 or Lyt 2 surface markers, can be separated from each other and from other T and B lymphocytes in spleen on days 12 and 21 after transplantation. Our data are consistent with the idea that both Lyt 1+ and Lyt 2+ T cells can proliferate in mixed lymphocyte culture and that H-2-sensitized T cells can respond to LPS.

T LYMPHOCYTE REGULATION
OF THE ANTIBODY RESPONSE TO ALTERED SELF

Susanne E. Urban and John J. Jandinski

Department of Immunology
Merck Institute for Therapeutic Research
Rahway, New Jersey 07065

Spleen cells from mice rendered unresponsive by the injection of TNP-modified (trinitrophenylated) syngeneic lymphoid cells contain hapten-specific suppressor cells capable of regulating the B cell response to TNP. Analysis of the suppressor T cells induced *in vivo* suggested that these cells were either Lyt $1^+2^+3^+$ or a mixture of Lyt 1^+ and Lyt 2^+3^+ cells.

To further dissect the cellular events in both the induction and effector phases, we developed an *in vitro* "double stage" culture system. The "double stage" system consisted of culturing 5×10^6 CBA/J spleen T cells together with 1.5×10^6 irradiated TNP-modified syngeneic spleen cells (2100 rad) in Mishell-Dutton macrocultures for 40–48 h. Cultures were then harvested and washed and 5×10^5 cells were added to 5×10^5 fresh B cells with trinitrophenylated brucella (TNP-BA) as antigen. The cells were further cultured for 72 h in microcultures. The anti-TNP plaque-forming response was measured by the Cunningham assay.

To identify the Ly phenotypes of the subpopulation functionally responsible for regulating hapten-specific suppression, selection procedures for Lyt subsets using monoclonal anti-Lyt 1 and anti-Lyt 2 antibodies plus complement were used to examine cells at the precursor and effector stages. Selected nylon wool column–passed T cell subsets were analyzed both by function (suppression of TNP-specific antibody production) and by fluorescence-activated cell sorter (FACS) analysis.

When T cells were preselected on the basis of their Ly phenotype before the primary incubation, Lyt 1^+ cells exhibited profound suppression on B cells in the secondary cultures. Lyt 2^+ cells did not show any suppressor activity. A mixture of precultured Lyt 1^+ and Lyt 2^+ cells was also suppressive when added to B cells.

Analysis performed at the effector stage after unselected T cells were incubated with inactivated TNP spleen cells for 48 h demonstrated that suppressor activities were sensitive to both anti-Lyt 1 and anti-Lyt 2 treatment. Mixtures of anti-Lyt 1 and anti-Lyt 2 treated cells failed to generate any suppressor activity, indicating that the effector cell was a Lyt $1^+2^+3^+$ cell. These findings contradicted the observations obtained at the precursor stage, which was found to be Lyt 1^+2^-.

To further explore these results, the following experiments were conducted to determine if the effector cell was distinct from the precursor cell or if it represented the expression of new Ly phenotypes by the precursor cell.

The purity of the Lyt 1^+ subpopulation was supported by FACS analysis, demonstrating that fluorescein conjugated anti-Lyt 2 antibody stained less than 5% of the total cells after the primary incubation period. To further support the concept of two cell types, precultured Lyt 1^+ cells were treated with either anti-Lyt 1 or anti-Lyt 2 antibodies plus complement. Anti-Lyt 1 was cytotoxic for the majority of cells and abrogated the suppressor activity, while anti-Lyt 2 had no significant effect on either cell death or the suppressor function.

In addition, functional studies and FACS analysis demonstrated that these T cells did not passively take up any Lyt antigens that might have been shed from the irradiated TNP spleen cell population. By using irradiated T cell–depleted TNP spleen cells instead of TNP whole spleen cells, no differences were observed either in suppressor function or in phenotype expression. Thus, Lyt 1+ cells, in the absence of Lyt 1+2+3+ cells during the induction period, could develop into effector suppressor cells. However, when both Lyt 1+ and Lyt 1+2+3+ cells are present, it appears that the Lyt 1+2+3+ cells preferentially develop into suppressor cells. We therefore postulate that either Lyt 1+ cells induce Lyt 1+2+3+ to become suppressors or Lyt 1+2+3+ cells become suppressors without an inducing signal from another subset.

PRESENCE OF HOST-REACTIVE T CELLS IN LYMPHOHEMATOPOIETIC CHIMERAS

J. Douglas Waterfield and Ian D. King

ICRF Tumour Immunology Unit
Department of Zoology
University College London
London, England WC1 6BT

Richard W. Dutton

Department of Biology
University of California, San Diego
La Jolla, California 92093

The generation of the immunological repertoire is a crucial problem in immunology. It is our intention to investigate whether T cell tolerance (deletion from the repertoire) is a natural consequence of the generation of H-2-restricted responses *in vivo* by thymic influence. In this report, we have investigated lymphohematopoietic chimeras for the presence of self-reactive T lymphocytes. B6→BDF$_1$ chimeras were produced by conventional methods: BDF$_1$ mice were irradiated with 950 rad and reconstituted with 20×10^6 fetal liver cells. The chimeras were tested three to six months after reconstitution. Lymphocytes from individual B6→BDF$_1$ mice were tested for their ability to respond to DBA/2 host determinants in mixed lymphocyte reactions (MLR) or MLR-generated cell-mediated lympholysis (CML). It was found that they failed to respond in both assays, although they were immunologically competent as judged by their ability to respond to third party stimulators. However, after activation with concanavalin A (con A), the B6→BDF$_1$ lymphocytes displayed a significant lectin-independent cytotoxic effector activity against P815 (H-2^d) targets, demonstrating that precursors of host-reactive cytotoxic effector lymphocyctes were present in the chimeric mice. It should also be noted that the B6→BDF$_1$ lymphocytes failed to kill EL4 targets, indicating that killing was only directed towards surface antigens displayed by the nonshared parent in the radiation-induced chimeras.

We then tested these lymphocytes for their ability to recognize DBA/2 host determinants in other experimental systems of alloreactivity: the ability to exert helper function (positive allogeneic effect) in the induction of a humoral response to sheep red blood cells and the ability to suppress the secondary antibody-forming cell response of antigen-primed lymphocytes (negative allogeneic effect). It was found that B6→BDF$_1$ T lymphocytes failed to recognize host determinants in the allohelper and allosuppressor assay systems. It was then of interest to determine whether precursors of host-reactive lymphocytes exist *in situ* together with precursors of T cells capable of mediating H-2-restricted responses to both parental haplotypes. B6→BDF$_1$ chimeras were primed *in vivo* with 10^7 mitomycin-C-treated Balb/c × Balb.B (H-2^d × H-2^b) splenic lymphocytes. It was again found that con A–activated lymphocytes from individual mice could kill the P815 targets. Furthermore, these cells could

425

be induced to respond to Balb minor histocompatibility antigens in the context of H-2^b and H-2^d. Cold target competition experiments comparing P815, DBA/2, and B10.D2 blocking populations suggest that class I major histocompatability complex antigens are the target structures for this anti-host reactivity. We then investigated the mechanism by which these mice are nonresponsive *in vivo* and *in vitro*. Two possibilities were considered. Suppressor cells and/or suppressor factor(s) may be active as a "fail-safe" mechanism to suppress any anti-self immune response. It was also possible that unresponsiveness reflects a lesion of an amplifier or helper cell necessary for the induction of cytotoxic T lymphocytes. *In vitro* transfer experiments were carried out in which "putative" suppressor cells from the chimeric mice were added to normal B6 T cells to suppress their MLR response to DBA/2 stimulator cells. No suppression could be demonstrated. This suggests that suppressor cells may not be involved. However, addition of x-irradiated B6 T cells (helpers) from normal animals to B6→BDF$_1$ chimera T cells reconstituted the *in vitro* anti-DBA/2 cytotoxic lymphocyte response, suggesting that the defect may be the absence of a required amplifier cell in the chimeras. We conclude that, in radiation-induced chimeras, T cell tolerance may not be a natural consequence of the generation of the T cell repertoire.

TOLERANCE SENSITIVITY OF IMMATURE B CELLS IS A CARRIER-RELATED FUNCTION

A POTENTIAL VIOLATION OF THE CLONAL ABORTION THEORY FOR SELF TOLERANCE

C. A. Waters, R. C. von Borstel, U. E. Diner, and E. Diener

Department of Immunology
MRC Group on Immunoregulation
University of Alberta
Edmonton, Alberta, Canada T6G 2H7

To circumvent the development of autoimmune reactivities during the maturation of immunocompetent cells, a number of investigators have proposed a clonal abortion mechanism to provide for the deletion of autoreactive lymphocytes as they arise during ontogeny. According to this theory, immature B lymphocytes pass through a tolerance-sensitive phase, during which contact with antigen constitutes an obligatory negative signal, the result of which is irreversible inactivation of the clone. No proviso is made for any differences among the abilities of various antigens to deliver the negative signal, nor for the signaling to be of a highly dose-dependent nature.

We have examined both the universality and irreversibility of the clonal abortion theory in experiments in which antigen is introduced at birth and administered repeatedly until the functional maturation of the immune system is complete. Both T cell–dependent carriers selected for these initial studies, bovine serum albumin (TNP-BSA) and human γ-globulin (TNP-HGG), induced complete and specific IgG unresponsiveness for the trinitrophenyl (TNP) epitope when immunogenic challenge was with the original hapten-carrier conjugate used to induce the unresponsiveness. Nevertheless, a carrier-associated discriminator function was observed: Only with HGG as carrier for the TNP epitope was tolerance irreversible. Challenge of TNP-BSA-treated animals with the epitope presented on two different and, furthermore, "T cell–independent" carriers, lipopolysaccharide (TNP-LPS) and *Brucella abortus* (TNP-BruA), with which IgG responses can be generated, indicated that either complete tolerance was not induced in all B cell subsets with TNP receptor specificity or that the unresponsiveness was not irreversible. Neither of these explanations is permissible within the restrictions of the clonal abortion theory. Furthermore, rosette inhibition studies demonstrated that the reversibility of TNP-BSA-induced tolerance *vis-à-vis* TNP-HGG tolerance could not be attributed to any significant differences in the ability of the TNP-BSA to bind to B cells of appropriate receptor specificity.

In order to directly assess the ability of a TNP-carrier conjugate to interact with immature B cells in the absence of potential T cell regulation, we used a nonimmunogenic carrier to present the TNP epitope to both neonatal B cells and B cells in stem cell–reconstituted mice. TNP-methyl cellulose (TNP-MC) and TNP-carboxymethyl cellulose (TNP-CMC) have been shown to be potent tolerogens for both T cell–dependent and T cell–independent B cells in adult

427

animals challenged with TNP presented on the immunogenic carrier ficoll (TNP-F).[1]

Oxidation followed by subsequent reduction of the vicinal hydroxyl groups of CMC and MC results in carriers that are nontolerogens in adults, but have the same molecular weight as, and no loss of avidity for, TNP-specific B cells.[2] Clonal abortion, nonetheless, would predict that such changes in the intrinsic tolerogenicity of carriers for mature B cells should be irrelevant in the context of the immature immune system. Studies in irradiated fetal liver–reconstituted mice and neonatal mice demonstrated, however, that tolerance induction in the immature immune system is as carrier-dependent as that in adult mice. These results are consistent with our earlier experiments using the *in utero* model, in which only mammalian γ-globulin carriers were able to induce tolerance.[3]

REFERENCES

1. DINER, U., D. KUNIMOTO & E. DIENER. 1979. J. Immunol. **122:** 1886.
2. DIENER, E., U. DINER, C. A. WATERS & R. C. VON BORSTEL. 1982. In preparation.
3. WATERS, C. A., E. DIENER & B. SINGH. 1981. *In* Cellular and Molecular Mechanisms of Immunological Tolerance. T. Hraba and M. Hašek, Eds.: 483–91. Marcel Dekker. New York.

SUPPRESSOR CELLS INDUCED BY SELF ANTIGENS
PREVENT GENERATION OF Tc
TO ALTERED SELF ANTIGENS

Henry L. Wong and Jack R. Battisto

Department of Biology
Case Western Reserve University

and

Department of Immunology
Cleveland Clinic Foundation
Cleveland, Ohio 44106

In the past, attempts that have been made to generate cytotoxic T lymphocytes (Tc) to hapten-modified self antigens *in vivo* have failed due to the presence of a naturally occurring cyclophosphamide (Cy)-sensitive T suppressor cell [1,2] that maintains an interleukin-2 (IL-2) inhibitor in serum.[3] Recently, a method whereby Tc can be generated without the use of Cy has been described.[4] This protocol necessitates a simultaneous injection into footpads of C3H/HeN mice of two stimulating antigens: trinitrophenyl (TNP)-modified syngeneic spleen cells and H-2 compatible, minor histocompatibility locus (Mls)–disparate auxiliary CBA/J spleen cells. The auxiliary cell's Mls-disparate antigens are thought to stimulate the host's T helper cells to produce various helper lymphokines needed as a second signal by precytotoxic cells that are triggered by hapten–altered self antigen(s). In this way, the naturally occurring suppressor cell, or the inhibitor of serum IL-2, is circumvented. Five days after the footpad injections, draining popliteal lymph nodes are removed and used as effectors in a standard 3 h ^{51}Cr release assay with TNP-modified concanavalin A (con A) C3H blast spleen cells as targets.

In previous reports, we have shown that Tc can be regulated *in vivo* at the level of the hapten and at the level of the Mls antigen.[4,5] In this report, we provide evidence for still another regulatory level: suppression generated through exposure to self antigens. During experiments in which we attempted to augment the Tc response by priming mice with certain antigens, we observed that injecting unmodified normal syngeneic spleen cells (20×10^6) into footpads one week before sensitization caused complete suppression of the Tc response. Injecting TNP-modified syngeneic spleen cells into footpads, on the other hand, did not. In addition, preinjecting TNP-modified spleen cells along with normal spleen cells resulted in only a 50% decrease in the Tc response. Thus, some normal spleen cell characteristic (antigen?) eliminated by haptenation elicits the suppressive effect.

To determine the length of time required for suppression to become detectable, normal syngeneic spleen cells were injected into footpads of C3H mice and sensitization was attempted at various times thereafter. Mice sensitized on day 0 and day 1 after receiving syngeneic spleen cells in the footpad showed full Tc responses. When sensitization was initiated at day 2, the Tc response decreased to 50% of control values and, by day 3, the response was absent.

In order to understand the mechanism by which this down regulation occurs, suppressor cells were sought in popliteal lymph nodes of mice injected in the footpads with syngeneic spleen cells seven days earlier. Host mice given 100×10^6 lymph node cells i.v. were sensitized within one hour and assayed for Tc five days later. The recipients developed suppressed Tc responses. On the other hand, recipients of normal syngeneic cells from non-injected donors showed normal responses. These results clearly indicate that the suppression is mediated by an inducible transferrable cell.

A further experiment was carried out to determine if the suppression was due to any influence contributed by the spleen. Mice that were splenectomized (SPLx) or sham SPLx were injected in the footpads with syngeneic spleen cells, rested for one week, and then subjected to sensitization.

The results showed that splenectomy did not alter the degree of suppression from that observed in sham SPLx control animals. Thus, the spleen is, apparently, not essential to the suppressive mechanism.

Earlier, Howe et al. described a phenomenon where proliferation, as measured by ^{3}H-thymidine uptake, occurred in in vitro cultures of syngeneic spleen and neonatal thymic cells.[6] This reaction, as well as the response between T and B cells from autologous spleens and lymph node cells or peripheral blood, has been termed the autologous mixed lymphocyte reaction (AMLR). Several investigators have detected the presence of nonspecific T suppressor cells arising from such in vitro cultures.[7-9] Whether the phenomenon described in this report can be explained on the basis of an in vivo AMLR occurring between the injected spleen cells and those of the draining popliteal lymph node is an attractive possibility currently under investigation.

REFERENCES

1. ROLLINGHOFF, M., A. STARZINSKI-POWITZ, K. PFIZENMAIER & H. WAGNER. 1977. J. Exp. Med. 145: 455.
2. TAGART, V. 1977. Transplantation 23: 287.
3. HARDT, C., M. ROLLINGHOFF, K. PFIZENMAIER, H. MOSMANN & H. WAGNER. 1981. J. Exp. Med. 154: 262.
4. BUTLER, L. D. & J. R. BATTISTO. 1979. J. Immunol. 122: 1578.
5. BUTLER, L. D., H. L. WONG & J. R. BATTISTO. 1980. J. Immunol. 124: 1245.
6. HOWE, M. L., A. L. GOLDSTEIN & J. R. BATTISTO. 1970. Proc. Nat. Acad. Sci. USA 67: 619.
7. BURNS, F. D., P. C. MARRACK, J. W. KAPPLER & C. A. JANEWAY. 1975. J. Immunol. 114: 1345.
8. HODES, R. J. & K. S. HATHCOCK. 1976. J. Immunol. 116: 167.
9. SMITH, J. B. & R. P. KNOWLTON. 1979. J. Immunol. 123: 419.

TRUNCATED MATURATION OF ALLOREACTIVE T CELLS IN NEONATALLY H-2 TOLERANT MICE

Peter J. Wood and J. Wayne Streilein

Department of Cell Biology
University of Texas Health Science Center
Dallas, Texas 75235

Experiments performed almost exclusively in adult mice have provided support for the roles of both clonal deletion and peripheral suppression in the maintenance of neonatal tolerance to transplantation antigens (see Reference 1). Two questions crucial to a full understanding of neonatal tolerance, however, concern how soon after injection tolerance is induced and at what stage of T cell differentiation it occurs. To gain an insight into the answer to the first of these questions, the ontogeny of neonatal tolerance was studied.

Neonatal (less than 24 h) mice were injected i.v. with 15×10^6 semiallogeneic bone marrow and spleen cells that contained a whole *H-2* disparity. At various times after birth, their thymuses and spleens were removed and the cells tested for their ability to proliferate in response to the foreign alloantigens present on the injected cells (mixed lymphocyte reaction, MLR) and to generate specific cytotoxic cells against these antigens (cell-mediated lympholysis, CML). Similar studies were performed on control, uninjected, and saline-injected mice. Positive MLR (SI > 2) and CML ($>10\%$ cytotoxicity at an E:T of 20:1) were first detectable in the spleens of 3–4-day-old mice and gradually rose to adult levels by 2–3 weeks of age. By contrast, neither CML nor MLR against the injected antigens could be detected with spleen cells from neonatally injected mice, although reactivity against third parties developed normally.

CML responses were less reliably obtained with thymus cells than with spleen, although cells from younger mice did seem to give better responses. However, the lesion in the CML responsiveness of neonatally injected mice was apparent at the level of the thymus, as judged by the fact that 46% of the thymuses from 22 normal mice gave a positive CML compared to 0% of the thymuses from 19 neonatally injected mice, this lack of response again being specific. In light of previous reports that thymus cells taken at, or just before, birth respond in an MLR,[2] it was of particular interest to see what would happen to this responsiveness after neonatal injection of F_1 cells. It was confirmed that thymus cells taken on the day of birth (*i.e.,* before injection of cells) did respond in an MLR; in neonatally injected mice, this response declined rapidly during the second to fourth days of life so that, by day 7, these mice were unresponsive, in a specific manner, to the foreign alloantigens present on the injected cells. Thus, it can be concluded that tolerance is rapidly induced and that, within a week of neonatal injection, the mice have acquired the *in vitro* phenotype characteristic of adult mice rendered tolerant by our protocol.[3] Studies on the level of chimerism in these mice have excluded the possibility that the rapid loss of reactivity is due to repopulation of the host's tissue with F_1 cells and indicate a deficit in the ability of the hosts own cells to respond.

The rapid loss of MLR from the thymuses of neonatally injected mice could be due to events within the thymus or could be a consequence of prethymic events, resulting in the loss of supply of antigen-specific precursors of the thymus. As a first step in analyzing these two possibilities, immature and mature thymocytes from neonatally injected mice were separated on the basis of their binding to peanut agglutinin and tested in an MLR against the putative tolerogen and against third party alloantigens. Since the procedure of agglutination with PNA requires large numbers of cells, it was not possible to test very young mice; however, both 21-day-old and adult (8 week) mice bearing perfect skin grafts of the injected phenotype were available and both gave the same results. Neither PNA⁻ (mature) nor PNA⁺ (immature) thymocytes, the latter in the presence of concanavalin A culture supernatant as a source of interleukin-2 (IL-2), from neonatally injected mice responded to the foreign alloantigens present on the neonatal inoculum, whilst responses against third party alloantigens were normal. These results suggest either that tolerance is being induced in cells at a very early early stage during thymocyte maturation, possibly in a population of cells that is too small for responses to be detected using current techniques or too immature to respond even with the addition of IL-2, or that tolerance is being induced prethymically. The fact that the level of chimerism in the thymus is extremely low ($\leq 0.1\%$), whilst that in the bone marrow is some 5–10-fold higher, would tend to favor the latter interpretation.

REFERENCES

1. STUART, F. P. & F. W. FITCH. 1979. Immunological Tolerance and Enhancement. University Press. Baltimore.
2. WIDMER, M. B. & E. L. COOPER. 1978. J. Immunol. **122:** 291.
3. STREILEIN, J. W. & R. S. GRUCHALLA. 1981. Immunogenetics **12:** 161.

DEXTRAN INTERFERES WITH TOLERANCE INDUCTION TOWARD A CONTACT SENSITIZER

B. Yen-Lieberman, K. Beckman, and J. R. Battisto

Department of Immunology
Cleveland Clinic Foundation
Cleveland, Ohio 44106

In the past, we have reported that intravenously administering clinical grade dextran to mice before applying a sensitizing dose of hapten to the skin caused induction of heightened delayed-type hypersensitivity (DTH) to the hapten.[1] Three plausible ways in which dextran could cause greater DTH are: (1) release of helper factor(s), (2) interruption of DTH down regulation, and (3) activation of macrophages. The latter explanation was excluded by adoptive transfer of the heightened DTH from dextran-treated mice using lymphoid cells from which macrophages had been removed.[1] To determine whether subpopulations of lymphoid cells concerned with down regulation of DTH were being affected, we examined dextran's effect on tolerance induction to picryl chloride.

Accordingly, dextran or its saline vehicle was administered intravenously to mice (10 mg per 25 g) two hours before injecting the tolerogen (trinitrophenylated-(TNP) spleen cells, 50×10^6, syngeneic with the host).[2] Seven days thereafter, 0.1 ml picryl chloride in ethanol (7%) was applied to the shaved abdomen in an attempt to induce cutaneous hypersensitivity. The development of DTH was detected six days later by applying picryl chloride in olive oil (1%) to the dorsum of the right ear immediately after the ear thickness was determined with a micrometer. A second reading on the next day determined whether any change in thickness had occurred.

We have observed that dextran given to mice shortly before tolerogen abrogated hapten-specific tolerance. Thus, whereas tolerant animals developed only 5% of the sensitivity seen in positive control mice, dextran-treated animals exposed to tolerogen developed 60% of the control hypersensitivity.

A time study to determine the optimal point at which to administer dextran relative to the tolerogen indicated that it was 2 h before tolerogen injection. The optimal dose of dextran found to be effective to prevent tolerance induction was 1–10 mg per 25 g mouse.

Experiments designed to elucidate the mechanism by which dextran abrogates tolerance have shown that dextran is capable of preventing efferent suppressor T cells from acting upon DTH effector cells. Precisely how dextran is able to interrupt the function of suppressor T cells is our present focus of interest.

REFERENCES

1. ALEVY, Y. G. & J. R. BATTISTO. 1979. J. Immunol. **121:** 255.
2. BATTISTO, J. R. & B. BLOOM. 1966. Nature (London) **212:** 158.

433

Index of Contributors

(Italic page numbers refer to comments made in discussions.)